Maternal Medicine
Medical Problems in Pregnancy

For Elsevier

Commissioning Editor: Ellen Green
Development Editor: Janice Urquhart
Project Manager: Anne Dickie
Designer: Erik Bigland
Illustrator: Richard Morris

Maternal Medicine
Medical Problems
in Pregnancy

Edited by

Ian A. Greer MD FRCP(Glas) FRCPE FRCP FRCPI FRCOG FMedSci

Dean and Professor of Obstetric Medicine, Hull York Medical School, UK

Catherine Nelson–Piercy MA FRCP FRCOG

Consultant Obstetric Physician, Guy's and St Thomas' Foundation Trust, Queen Charlotte's & Chelsea Hospital, London, UK

Barry N. J. Walters FRACP FRANZCOG

Clinical Associate Professor, Obstetric Medicine, Department of Women's and Infant's Health, University of Western Australia, Perth, Australia

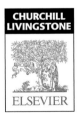

CHURCHILL LIVINGSTONE

ELSEVIER

EDINBURGH   LONDON   NEW YORK   OXFORD   PHILADELPHIA   ST LOUIS   SYDNEY   TORONTO   2007

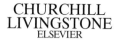

CHURCHILL
LIVINGSTONE
ELSEVIER

An imprint of Elsevier Limited

First published 2007

ISBN: 978 0 443 10129 8

British Library Cataloguing in Publication Data
A catalogue record for this book is available from the British Library

Library of Congress Cataloging in Publication Data
A catalog record for this book is available from the Library of Congress

Notice
Knowledge and best practice in this field are constantly changing. As new research and experience broaden our knowledge, changes in practice, treatment and drug therapy may become necessary or appropriate. Readers are advised to check the most current information provided (i) on procedures featured or (ii) by the manufacturer of each product to be administered, to verify the recommended dose or formula, the method and duration of administration, and contraindications. It is the responsibility of the practitioner, relying on their own experience and knowledge of the patient, to make diagnoses, to determine dosages and the best treatment for each individual patient, and to take all appropriate safety precautions. To the fullest extent of the law, neither the Publisher nor the Editors assume any liability for any injury and/or damage to persons or property arising out or related to any use of the material contained in this book.

The Publisher

Preface

Over the last few years, obstetric medicine has evolved from a niche area practiced in a few highly specialized centers to a branch of medicine that deserves representation wherever pregnant women require care. Increasing numbers of physicians are seeking training in the specialty so that they will feel confident in dealing with the medical problems of pregnant women. In addition, many obstetricians have developed an interest in the medical problems of their patients, and seek expertise in collaborative management of such disorders, together with an understanding of the 'medical' elements underlying many of the 'obstetric' disorders they have dealt with over the years. This growth in knowledge and interest in obstetric medicine is global, as exemplified by the formation of the International Society of Obstetric Medicine, the development of specific training programs in several countries, and the inclusion of obstetric medical content in curricula for certain medical specialties.

The clinical importance of this area is highlighted by reports such as those of the Confidential Enquiries into Maternal Death in the United Kingdom. As in other developed countries, these show that the leading causes of maternal death are 'medical conditions'. Thromboembolism and hypertension are the leading direct causes in the UK, and most of the indirect causes are also medical, particularly including cardiac disease, infectious, neurological, hematological, respiratory and gastroenterological problems. Moreover, cancer and psychiatric disturbance are also major causes of death. Furthermore, medical complications clearly contribute to many of the direct deaths, namely those attributed to 'obstetric' calamities. Massive obstetric hemorrhage and pre-eclampsia are often complicated by disseminated intravascular coagulation, renal failure, adult respiratory distress syndrome,

sepsis and multi-organ failure. Management of the seriously ill obstetric patient, therefore, requires a substantial and sophisticated knowledge of medicine in general and obstetric medicine in particular.

There is a shortage of reliable information from detailed research into severe maternal morbidity, as distinct from mortality. The cases reported in documents such as the UK Confidential Enquiries into Maternal Deaths represent the tip of a large iceberg of severe maternal morbidity. Pre-existing medical disorders are common in pregnant women and those planning pregnancy. For example, depending on the population studied, up to 8% of women have asthma, 2-5% suffer from chronic hypertension, 1% from epilepsy and 1% from thyroid disease while many other women have renal, cardiac, neurological and other problems. Thus, substantial numbers of women enter pregnancy with a pre-existing medical condition and would benefit from specialist advice and care both before and during pregnancy. Societal changes and advances in assisted reproductive therapy are also resulting in increases in the number of older, obese women becoming pregnant. Increased age and body mass index independently increase the risk of superimposed medical complications in pregnancy. The combination of a multiple IVF pregnancy in a woman with a pre-existing medical problem is now commonplace.

This book does not confine its attention to the customary nine-month duration of pregnancy itself. Care of women with medical problems is required long before pregnancy. Pre-pregnancy care and advice allow the woman to make an informed choice not only about whether she wishes to conceive, but how to minimize any risks by optimizing the management of her medical condition before embarking on pregnancy. No less deserving of attention from those who practice obstetric medicine are the medical problems after pregnancy, in the first days of the puerperium, and in the weeks that follow, a vulnerable time when many complications may arise. In this book, we have taken a systematic approach, seeking to address, specifically and practically, the key issues for each condition with regard to pre-pregnancy care, antenatal care, management in labor and postpartum care, while including the implications for the fetus and neonate.

We have presented an international approach to the practice of obstetric medicine such that its content and recommendations should be applicable wherever these problems are seen. It is not our intention to give a full and detailed review of the literature. Indeed within obstetric medicine there is often insufficient evidence to support a single approach, and management therefore depends heavily on experience and a sound interdisciplinary knowledge of internal medicine, obstetrics and perinatal medicine. For these reasons, management advice may need to be drawn from internationally recognized experts to provide practical clinical information based not only on evidence but also on experience gathered over years of practice that has been agreed by consensus after debate. The editors share the hope that the book will stimulate thought in young practitioners dealing with medical problems in pregnancy and provoke them to be involved in research to provide answers where formal evidence is not yet available.

We believe the book will contribute to the training of both obstetricians and physicians, as the conditions dealt with herein must be understood thoroughly by all those who seek to manage the medical complications of pregnancy.

Ian A. Greer
Catherine Nelson-Piercy
Barry N. J. Walters

Contributors

Dawn L. Adamson BSc MBBS MRCP PhD
Interventional Fellow and Obstetric Cardiologist, Hammersmith Hospital, London; Cardiology Specialist Registrar in Obstetric Cardiology, Queen Charlotte And Chelsea Hospitals, London, UK

Philip N. Baker DM FRCOG
Professor of Maternal and Fetal Health, Maternal and Fetal Health Research Centre, St Mary's Hospital, Manchester, UK

Simon E. Barton BSc MD FRCOG FRCPEd FRCP
Consultant Physician and Honary Senior Lecturer, Directorate of Sexual Health and HIV Medicine, Chelsea and Westminster Hospital, London, UK

N. Wah Cheung MBBS FRACP PhD
Senior Staff Specialist, Department of Diabetes and Endocrinology, Westmead Hospital; Clinical Senior Lecturer, Discipline of Medicine, University of Sydney, Sydney, Australia

Rachel Collis MBBS FRCA
Consultant Obstetric Anaesthetist, University Hospital of Wales, Cardiff, UK

David P. D'Cruz MD FRCP
Honorary Senior Lecturer and Consultant Rheumatologist, The Lupus Research Unit, The Rayne Institute, St Thomas' Hospital, London, UK

Michael de Swiet MD FRCP
Emeritus Professor of Obstetric Medicine, Imperial College, London; Consultant Obstetric Physician, Queen Charlotte's Hospital, University College Hospital, Whittington Hospital, London, UK

Mandish K. Dhanjal BSc MBBS DFFP MRCP MRCOG
Consultant Obstetrician and Gynaecologist, Queen Charlotte's and Chelsea Hospital, London; Honorary Senior Lecturer, Imperial College, London, UK

Rosalind Foster MRCP MBChB MSc
Immunology Specialist Registrar, Department of Immunology, St Thomas' Hospital, London, UK

Peter W. Fowlie MBChB MSc DRCOG MRCGP MRCP FRCPCH
Consultant Paediatrician, Neonatal Intensive Care Unit, Ninewells Hospital and Medical School, Dundee, UK

Caroline Gordon MA MD FRCP (UK)
Reader in Rheumatology, University of Birmingham; Consultant Rheumatologist, Sandwell and West Birmingham Hospitals and University Hospital Birmingham NHS Trusts, Birmingham, UK

Ian A. Greer MD FRCP(Glas) FRCPE FRCP FRCPI FRCOG FMedSci
Dean and Professor of Obstetric Medicine, Hull York Medical School, UK

John Griffiths MBBS MA MRCP FRCA DICM
Specialist Registrar and Hononary Research Fellow, Nuffield Department of Anaesthetics, John Radcliffe Hospital, Oxford, UK

William M. Hague MD(cantab) FRCP FRCOG
Senior Consultant in Obstetric Medicine, Clinical Senior Lecturer in Obstetrics, University of Adelaide Women's and Children's Hospital, Adelaide, South Australia, Australia

David Arnold Hawkins BSc MBBS FRCP
Consultant Physician, Directorate of Sexual Health and HIV Medicine, St Stephen's Centre, Chelsea and Westminster Hospital NHS Foundation Trust; Honorary Senior Lecturer, Division of Medicine, Imperial College, London, UK

Alexander P. Heazell MBChB
Clinical Research Fellow, Maternal and Fetal Health Research Centre, St Mary's Hospital, Manchester, UK

Mary Hepburn BSc MD MRCGP FRCOG
Consultant Obstetrician and Gynaecologist, Princess Royal Maternity Hospital, Glasgow , UK

Saadiya Aziz Karim MBBS FCPS FRCOG
Professor and Chairperson, Obstetrics and Gynaecology, Karachi Medical and Dental College, Karachi, Pakistan; Dean, Faculty of Medicine, University of Karachi, Pakistan

Máiréad M. Kennelly MB BCH BAO MRCOG MRCPI MD
Subspecialty Training Fellow, Department of Fetal Medicine, Royal Victoria Infirmary, Newcastle-upon-Tyne, UK

Munther Khamashta MD PhD FRCP (UK)
Senior Lecturer and Consultant Rheumatologist, Lupus Research Unit, St Thomas' Hospital, London, UK

Manjiri M. Khare MD MRCOG
Consultant in Maternal-Fetal Medicine, Women's and Perinatal Services, University Hospitals of Leicester NHS Trust, Leicester Royal Infirmary, Leicester, UK

Milind D. Khare MD MRCPath MRCP(UK) MRCPCH
Consultant Microbiologist, Derby Hospitals NHS Foundation Trust, Derby, UK

Terence T. Lao MBBS MD FRCOG FHKAM(O & G) FHKCOG
Professor, Department of Obstetrics and Gynaecology, The University of Hong Kong; Honorary Consultant to the Hong Kong Hospital Authority, Queen Mary Hospital, Hong Kong

Gwyneth Lewis MSc FFPH FRCOG
National Director for Maternity Care, Department of Health, London, UK; Director of the United Kingdom Confidential Enquiries into Maternal Deaths; Member of the Make Pregnancy Safer Team, World Health Organization, Geneva, Switzerland

Liz Lightstone MA MBBS PhD FRCP
Senior Lecturer in Renal Medicine, Renal Section, Division of Medicine, Faculty of Medicine, Imperial College, Hammersmith Hospital, London, UK

Sandra A. Lowe MBBS FRCP MD
Visiting Obstetric Physician, Royal Hospital for Women, Sydney, Australia; Conjoint Senior Lecturer, School of Women's and Children's Health, University of New South Wales, Sydney, Australia

William McGuire MD MRCPCH
Associate Professor of Neonatology, Australian National University Medical School, Canberra, Australia

Catherine Nelson-Piercy MA FRCP FRCOG
Consultant Obstetric Physician, Guy's and St Thomas' Foundation Trust, Queen Charlotte's and Chelsea Hospital, London, UK

Margaret R. Oates MBChB MRCPsych FRCPsych
Senior Lecturer in Psychiatry, Department of Psychiatry, University Hospital, Queen's Medical Centre, Nottingham, UK

Raymond O. Powrie MD FRCP(C) FACP
Associate Professor of Medicine and Obstetrics and Gynaecology, Brown University School of Medicine; Inpatient Director, Division of Obstetric and Consultative Medicine, Women and Infants' Hospital, Providence, Rhode Island, USA

Margaret Ramsay MB Bchir MA MD MRCP FRCOG
Consultant Senior Lecturer in Fetomaternal Medicine, Queen's Medical Centre, Nottingham, UK

Steven C. Robson FRCOG MD
Professor of Fetal Medicine, Department of Fetal Medicine, Royal Victoria Infirmary, Newcastle-upon-Tyne, UK

Robin Russell MBBS MD FRCA
Consultant Anaesthetist and Honorary Senior Clinical Lecturer, Nuffield Department of Anaesthetics, University of Oxford, Radcliffe Infirmary, Oxford, UK

Rebekah A. Samangaya MRCOG
Clinical Research Fellow, Maternal and Fetal Health Research Centre, St Mary's Hospital, Manchester, UK

Mahmood I. Shafi MB BCh MD DA FRCOG
Consultant Gynaecological Surgeon and Oncologist, Addenbrooke's Hospital, Cambridge University Hospitals NHS Foundation Trust, Cambridge, UK

Samantha Vaughan Jones MD FRCP
Consultant Dermatologist, Ashford and St Peter's Hospital Trust, Chertsey, Surrey, UK

Isobel D. Walker MPHIL MD FRCP(Ed) FRCP(Glas) FRCPath
Consultant Haematologist and Honorary Professor of Perinatal Haematology, Department of Haematology, Glasgow Royal Infirmary, Glasgow, UK

Barry N. J. Walters FRACP FRANZCOG
Clinical Associate Professor, Obstetric Medicine,
Department of Women's and Infant's Health,
University of Western Australia, Perth, Australia

David Williams PHD MRCP
Consultant Obstetric Physician and Honorary Senior
Lecturer, Elizabeth Garrett Anderson and Obstetric
Hospital, University College Hospital London,
London, UK

Catherine Williamson BSc MB CHB MRCP MD
Senior Lecturer and Honorary Consultant in
Obstetric Medicine, Institute of Reproductive
and Developmental Biology, Imperial College, London,
UK

Chee-Seng Yee MBBS MRCP
Clinical Research Fellow, Department of Rheumatology,
Medical School, University of Birmingham,
Birmingham, UK

Contents

Chapter 1

Maternal mortality: the global picture

G. Lewis, M. de Swiet

SYNOPSIS

Maternal mortality in the developing world
    Introduction
    Where, in the world, are women dying?
    What, in the world, are pregnant women
      dying of?
    Why, in the world, are these women dying?
    What, in the world, is being done about this?

Medical factors in maternal death: the developed world
    Introduction
    Venous thromboembolism
    Hypertension and pre-eclampsia
    Heart disease
    Other indirect deaths
    Conclusion

Maternal mortality in the developing world
G. Lewis

INTRODUCTION

Every minute of every day, every day of every year, year in year out, somewhere in the world a woman dies of complications arising from pregnancy or childbirth. The majority die without skilled care, perhaps lying on a dirt-ridden floor, probably in a simple dwelling and attended only by the women of her family or an untrained birth attendant. They die in pain, fear and in vain. More than 80% of these women's deaths could be prevented or avoided through actions that are proven to be effective and affordable, even in the poorer countries of the world. Their deaths represent the largest public health discrepancy in the world today, and, in some parts of the world, it is getting worse.

Globally, more than half a million women die every year of pregnancy-related causes, including 69 000 deaths from unsafe abortion (World Health Organization [WHO] 2003, 2004a). Less than 1% of these women die in high-income countries. In developing countries as many as one woman in 16 may die of a pregnancy-related complication compared to one in 5000-9000 in developed countries. In developing countries, a woman's lifetime risk of dying from a pregnancy-related complication can be up to 200 times higher than in many developed countries (WHO 2005).

In parts of Sub-Saharan Africa a young girl may face a lifetime risk of dying from maternal causes as high as one in eight. Fifteen million adolescent girls give birth at an age when the risks are particularly high. Girls under the age of 15 are five times more likely to die of a pregnancy-related cause than women in their 20s (United Nations [UN] 1991).

Death is not the only problem. The WHO estimates, globally, over 300 million women currently suffer from short- or long-term complications arising from pregnancy or childbirth (WHO 2005) with around 20 million new cases arising every year (Pittrof et al 2002). Problems include infertility, severe anemia, uterine prolapse and vaginal fistula. It is estimated that, mainly in Sub-Saharan Africa but also Asia, more than 2 million young women live, usually in isolation and shame, with untreated obstetric fistulas (UN Populations Fund [UNFPA]/International Federation of Gynecology & Obstetrics [FIGO] 2002).

Each death or long-term complication arising from pregnancy or childbirth not only represents an individual tragedy for the woman, her partner and her surviving children but also an economic loss to her family, community and society. Apart from housework and raising children, women are often the backbone of the economy. It has been estimated that, in Nigeria, for example, each year about US$102 million productivity losses are incurred due to maternal and newborn death and disability (Islam & Gurdtham 2005). And, as the latest World Health report states 'Children are the future of society, and their mothers are the guardians of that future. Mothers are much more than caregivers and homemakers, undervalued as these roles often are' (WHO 2005).

If these figures were not harsh enough, every year, 3.3 million babies are stillborn and more than another 4 million will die in the first month of life (WHO 2005). Millions of other children are left motherless following a maternal death, and the risk of death for children under five is doubled if their mother dies in childbirth. Babies who survive the death of their mother seldom reach their first birthday. The loss of the mother is especially risky for female infants (UNICEF 2001). Surviving children are more at risk of long-term health and social problems.

WHERE, IN THE WORLD, ARE WOMEN DYING?

Over 99% of maternal deaths occur in developing countries. While the largest numbers of maternal deaths, and consequently also pregnancies that result in severe morbidity, are to be found in countries with very high population and fertility rates, such as India, the highest mortality rates are in Africa, followed by Asia and Latin America. However, intraregional differences are also high, especially in Asia.

To help better understand the true level of maternal death and disability in each country, given that vital statistic reporting systems in many countries are underdeveloped, WHO, UNICEF and UNFPA have developed an approach to estimate more accurately the true number of maternal deaths and the maternal mortality ratios (MMR). Given the uncertainty of the available data, the estimates made are subject to wide margins of error and cross-country comparisons should also be treated with caution. Nonetheless, the approach, with some variations, was used to develop estimates for maternal mortality in 1990, 1995 and most recently in 2000 (WHO 2004a). It is on these estimates that the Millennium Development Goals are based.

Actual numbers

In 2000, an estimated 529 000 women died from maternal causes worldwide. These deaths were almost equally divided between Africa (251 000) and Asia (253 000), with about 4% (22 000) occurring in Latin America and the Caribbean. Less than 1% occur in the more developed regions of the world

Due to the size and fertility rates of its population, the country with the highest estimated number of maternal deaths is India although the *rate* of maternal deaths is now falling quite considerably in many states of the country as the results of safe motherhood initiatives are beginning to be seen. Other countries with high overall actual numbers include Nigeria, Pakistan, Democratic Republic of Congo, Ethiopia, the United Republic of Tanzania, Afghanistan, Bangladesh, Angola, China, Kenya, Indonesia and Uganda. These 13 countries account for 70% of all maternal deaths.

Rates

However, the number of maternal deaths does not give a reliable indicator of the state of the healthcare services provided to women in each country. The most useful indicator of the problems countries continue to face in overcoming maternal mortality and morbidity is the MMR. The International Classification of Diseases (ICD-10) defines the MMR as the number of direct and indirect maternal deaths per 100 000 live births per annum. This describes the obstetric risk a pregnant woman in that country faces per total number of births.

In terms of the MMR, the global figure is estimated to be 400 per 100 000 live births. By region, Africa has the highest MMR, followed by Asia, Oceania, Latin America and the Caribbean. In the worst affected countries the MMR exceeds 1000 deaths per 100 000 live births. In the UK the figure is 12 maternal deaths per 100 000 live births (Islam & Gurdtham 2005).

When comparing on a risk per birth basis, the list of countries facing the severest difficulties looks rather different from that with the highest actual number of deaths. With the exception of Afghanistan, the countries with the highest MMRs are in Sub-Saharan Africa. Countries with MMRs of 1000 or greater, are, in rank order, Sierra Leone, Afghanistan, Malawi, Angola, Niger, the United Republic of Tanzania, Rwanda, Mali, Somalia, Zimbabwe, Chad, Central African Republic, Guinea Bissau, Kenya, Mozambique, Burkina Faso, Burundi and Mauritania (WHO 2004a).

As Table 1.1 shows, the MMR is highest in Africa followed by Asia, Oceania, Latin America and the Caribbean. These figures hide wide, inter-country variations and even within countries, major discrepancies exist between the rich and poor and urban and remote areas. Discrepancies also exist between ethnic or tribal groups and the educated or most disadvantaged groups in society. Even in the UK the latest report of the Confidential Enquiries into Maternal Deaths (2004) 'Why Mothers Die 2000-02' shows excluded and vulnerable women face a risk of maternal death 23 times greater than professional women living in comfortable surroundings.

WHAT, IN THE WORLD, ARE PREGNANT WOMEN DYING OF?

A breakdown of the major causes of global maternal deaths is shown in Figure 1.1. A maternal death is defined as the death of a woman while pregnant or within 42 days of termination of pregnancy, from any cause related to or aggravated by the pregnancy or its management, but not from accidental or incidental causes. Around 80% of maternal deaths in developing countries are due to *direct* obstetric causes and 20% due to *indirect* causes. ICD-10 defines direct deaths as those deaths resulting from obstetric complications of the pregnant state (pregnancy, labor and puerperium), from interventions, omissions, incorrect treatment or from a chain of events resulting from any of the above. ICD-10 defines indirect deaths as those resulting from previous existing disease, or disease that developed during pregnancy and that was not due to direct obstetric causes, but which was aggravated by the physiologic effects of pregnancy.

Direct deaths are due to complications that can only arise because of pregnancy, such as hemorrhage, obstructed labor, eclampsia or sepsis. Long-term permanent/chronic and disabling conditions associated with these conditions include chronic anemia, obstetric fistula with urinary and or fecal incontinence, foot drop or palsy, scarred uterus or pelvic inflammatory disease. Indirect conditions leading to death or long-term complications include, for example, HIV/AIDS, malaria, hepatitis, tuberculosis and cardiovascular disease.

Table 1.1 Maternal mortality estimates by WHO/UN regions, 2000

Region	Maternal mortality ratio (maternal deaths per 100 000 live births)	Number of maternal deaths	Lifetime risk of maternal death (1 in)
World total	400	529 000	74
Developed regions[a]	20	2 500	2800
Europe	24	1 700	2400
Developing regions	440	527 000	61
Africa	830	251 000	20
Northern Africa	130	4 600	210
Sub-Saharan Africa	920	247 000	16
Asia	330	253 000	94
Eastern Asia	55	11 000	840
South-Central Asia	520	207 000	46
South-Eastern Asia	210	25 000	140
Western Asia	190	9 800	120
Latin America and the Caribbean	190	22 000	160
Oceania	240	530	83

[a]Includes Canada, United States of America, Japan, Australia and New Zealand which are excluded from the regional totals.

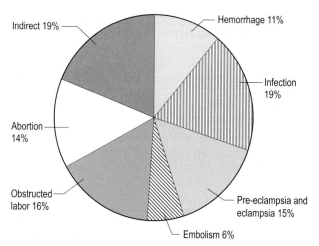

Figure 1.1 Leading causes of maternal deaths worldwide.

Table 1.2 Estimated incidence of major global causes of *direct* maternal deaths: 2000[a]

Cause	Incidence of complication (% of live births)	Number of cases	Case fatality rate (% of cases)	Maternal deaths	Percentage of all direct deaths
Hemorrhage	10.5	13795000	1	132000	28
Sepsis	4.4	5768000	1.3	79000	16
Pre-eclampsia, Eclampsia	3.2	4152000	1.7	63000	13
Obstructed labor	4.6	6038000	0.7	42000	9
Abortion	14.8	19340000	0.3	69000	15

[a]These estimates have been developed for WHO's calculations of the global burden of disease and are based upon both literature review and expert consensus.

WHO has developed estimates of mortality and morbidity related to the five leading direct causes of maternal death: postpartum hemorrhage, puerperal sepsis, pre-eclampsia and eclampsia, obstructed labor and abortion. These are shown in Table 1.2. Overall deaths from direct causes comprise around 80% of the global deaths due to direct complications of pregnancy. The other 20% comprise deaths from conditions such as ectopic pregnancies, anesthetic complications and thrombosis. These are very different from the leading causes of maternal death in the UK where, for 2000-2002 (Lewis 2004), the five global leading causes of death only comprised 39% of all such cases combined. In the UK the leading cause of *direct* death is thromboembolism which accounts for 28% of these deaths.

Abortion

Some 46 million women face an unwanted pregnancy every year (UN Department of Economic and Social

Affairs [DESA] 2002) and 20 million women may risk an unsafe abortion as a result (UNFPA 1997, WHO 2004a). Of these, more than 69000 women a year will die and many more are left with psychological and physical scars including infertility, chronic pelvic pain or infections, and genital tract trauma. Unsafe abortion is an issue particularly affecting younger women, as two-thirds of unsafe abortions occur among women between 25-30 years of age. Around 2.5 million abortions in developing countries are among adolescent girls or young women of less than 20 years of age (WHO 2004a).

Women who have unwanted pregnancies but continue with their pregnancies face the same risk of maternal death and disability as all other pregnant women. It has been estimated that up to 100000 maternal deaths a year could be prevented each year if women who do not wish to become pregnant had access to, and used, effective contraception (Marston & Cleland 2003). Further, the UK Department for International Development (DfID 2004) estimates that delaying the age of marriage and first birth, preventing unwanted pregnancy and eliminating unsafe abortion will avert one-third of maternal deaths, and that birth spacing and prevention of pregnancy in very young women may reduce neonatal mortality by one-quarter.

Indirect causes of death

Indirect causes account for some 20% of maternal deaths worldwide. Infectious or vector-borne diseases aside, the leading causes of *indirect* deaths are similar to those in the UK. Countries such as Sri Lanka, who have made major gains in reducing maternal mortality through the introduction of national safe motherhood programs report that, as with the UK, cardiac disease is the leading cause of death. However, infectious diseases are a rising cause of maternal death in certain parts of the world, reversing the gains made in the last few decades.

HIV/AIDS is now the leading cause of maternal death in most African countries. An estimated 2 million women living with HIV become pregnant each year and evidence from some African countries indicates that the HIV epidemic is reversing past gains in reducing maternal morbidity and mortality (Bicego et al 2002). In addition more than 30 million women in Africa who become pregnant in malaria-endemic areas are at risk of malaria infection (WHO 2002). This increases the risk of dying directly from severe malaria or indirectly from malaria-related severe anemia, the presence of which also contributes to death from hemorrhage. Although worldwide *indirect* deaths comprise a small proportion of maternal deaths overall, in the UK the picture is different and *indirect* deaths are now the leading cause of death, comprising around 60% of maternal deaths.

WHY, IN THE WORLD, ARE THESE WOMEN DYING?

Poor women

Women are not dying during pregnancy and childbirth of complicated conditions that are hard to manage. Women are dying because they do not receive the healthcare that they need, such as access to basic maternity care and a skilled attendant during childbirth. On a more fundamental level they are dying because they are poor, malnourished, lack education, have lower social status than the decision-makers in their families and communities, have no voice and many live in societies that, to date, have not invested in maternal health.

Birth spacing, preventing and managing unwanted pregnancies

Addressing women's reproductive rights and providing access to free or affordable effective contraception could avert up to 35% of maternal deaths (Bicego et al 2002). However, addressing issues such as the age at first pregnancy, optimal family size and the need for birth spacing is beyond the ability of the many health services. Deeply embedded cultural and social values, and systems of beliefs continue to form barriers that prevent young women from being able to manage their own lives and bodies. Where safe alternatives are not available, unsafe abortion can kill up to 15% of women undergoing abortion (Bicego et al 2002). In countries where abortion is legal, safe affordable abortion services should be available and in all settings post-abortion care should be routinely provided.

Skilled care for pregnancy and childbirth

Skilled care before and after birth, but particularly during labor, can make the difference between life and death for women and their babies yet only a half of women in developing countries receive assistance from a skilled attendant during delivery (WHO 2003). The recent WHO (2004b) publication 'Global action for skilled attendants for pregnant women' sets out the evidence and responsibilities for increasing access to skilled professionals at delivery as well as identifying steps to maximize the effectiveness of current staff in countries where trained professionals are scarce.

Obtaining access to suitably equipped facilities for antenatal care and safe childbirth is usually difficult, especially in rural settings where health centers able to provide basic emergency obstetric care may be 70 km away, with no easy or affordable form of transport. Basic essential obstetric care (BEOC) includes the availability of parenteral antibiotics, oxytocics, treatments for eclampsia, assisted vaginal delivery (vacuum extraction), manual removal of placenta and removal of retained products (MVA). Even where such centers exist there is often a lack of accessible referral facilities, even further away, that can provide comprehensive emergency obstetric care such as Cesarean section. Comprehensive essential obstetric care (CEOC) should include all elements of BEOC plus 24-hour facilities for Cesarean section and blood transfusion. Even if women manage to travel to these facilities they are often required to provide their own gloves, dressings, etc. for a clean delivery and may be required to pay official, and often unofficial, costs. For a poor family living in extreme poverty the costs of an emergency Cesarean section can be crippling and some families cannot afford them, or are left in debt for many years as a result (Women's Dignity Project 2003). A recent study in rural Tanzania estimated the average cost of an emergency Cesarean section to be US$135 compared to the average family annual income of US$115 (Kowalewski et al 2002).

Assessing the barriers to effective services

Many of those who work in the field of international women's health use the model of the 'Three Delays' to try to explain the barriers pregnant women face in receiving the care they need (Thaddeus & Maine 1994). These barriers may be erected by the family, the community or the healthcare system and are often interlinked. For example, are women dying because of:

> *A delay associated with the decision to seek care.* Were these women or their families unaware of the need for care, unaware of the warning signs of problems in pregnancy, or did financial, family or socio-cultural barriers prevent them seeking help?

> *or*

> *A delay in arriving at a place of care.* Did the services exist in the first place? If so how far away were they? Was there a lack of transport? Were they too expensive? Or were the facilities inaccessible for other reasons such as poor reputation or socio-cultural barriers?

> *or*

> *A delay in the provision of appropriate care.* Was the facility equipped and staffed appropriately and was the care they received inadequate or actually harmful?

Answering these questions is vital for program planners, managers and service providers. In order to help address this, the WHO's Making Pregnancy Safer initiative has recently published 'Beyond the Numbers' (WHO 2004c) a practical guide that describes a number of strategies and approaches to review cases of maternal death or disability to help understand why mothers really die, thus enabling healthcare planners to take the necessary actions based on the results. The methodologies described in BTN range from community (verbal autopsy) and facility based reviews, confidential enquiries into maternal deaths, near miss reviews and clinical audit. These approaches will enable, and empower, health professionals and authorities to act to answer these and other important questions about why women die during pregnancy and childbirth.

WHAT, IN THE WORLD, IS BEING DONE ABOUT THIS?

In 2000, 194 Governments, as member states of the UN, endorsed the Millennium Development Goals (UN 2000). A 75% reduction in the MMR between 1990 and 2015 is the fifth of these key goals. However, the recent World Health Report, published on World Health Day 2005, which focused on maternal and newborn health, describes the position today as 'a patchwork of progress, stagnation and reversal' (WHO 2005).

The reasons for this are complex. This lack of progress is not due to a lack of international or, for some countries, national effort. UN agencies such as UNICEF and UNFPA, in addition to WHO, all have major programs offering in-country support, assisted by donors such as the World Bank, the United States Agency for International Development (USAID), the UK's DfID and many other organizations. However, to date, the best efforts by all the agencies and countries working towards safe motherhood have been hampered by maternal, newborn and reproductive health not being seen as a top priority by many resource poor countries. The emergence of HIV/AIDS has had a particularly harsh effect on the funding for safe motherhood initiatives, as has the change in policy directions of some major donors in relation to reproductive health. The continuing exodus of skilled doctors and midwives from the countries that need them the most compounds the situation.

With the renewed focus on maternal health, given impetus in the World Heath Report for 2005, and other initiatives, it is hoped that finally a concerted effort can be made to address the problem of why so many women continue to die in a world where the knowledge and resources to prevent such deaths are already available or attainable.

Acknowledgement

The views in this chapter are those of the author and should not be taken to represent those of the organizations for which they work.

Medical factors in maternal death: the developed world

M. de Swiet

INTRODUCTION

A review of maternal mortality in the developed world might be expected to elicit a completely different response from that arising from knowledge of maternal mortality in the developing world. The message that comes from the first section of this chapter relating to the developing world is brutally clear: all people should care more for women and their place in society. But even in the developed world where far fewer women die in pregnancy the message is the same. If there were more respect for women and consideration of their health in general, then the outcome of pregnancy would be better.

As shown in the previous section the maternal mortality ratio in the developed world is about 20 per 100 000 pregnancies compared to 400 in the developing world. The most recent UK data for the triennium 2000-2002 give a maternal mortality ratio of 13 but such differences between countries in the developed world are trivial by comparison with the huge discrepancy between the developing and developed worlds.

The remainder of this section will concentrate on the UK data and draw particular conclusions relating to medical problems in pregnancy. The reason why UK data are so important for consideration of maternal mortality in the developed world is that the Confidential Enquiries into Maternal Mortality and Child Health (CEMACH) have been published in a consistent format since 1952. No other country has such a record. Substandard care has been noted and commented on and any comments on individual cases, which are in all cases anonymized, are at present unacceptable in British courts of law.

The series was originally confined to England and Wales but in 1985 it was extended to Scotland and Northern Ireland in order to include the whole of the UK.

Maternal mortality in the UK was already declining during the 1940s (Fig. 1.2) and this decrease has continued during the period of the Confidential Enquiries (Fig. 1.3). The marked decline seen in the 1940s is thought to have been due in part to the introduction of sulfonamides, the first effective treatment for puerperal sepsis, part to the start of universal antenatal care, part to blood transfusion and part to the general increase in standards of living. But along with the overall reduction in maternal mortality has come a marked change in the pattern of causes of maternal death.

In the triennium 1952-1954 in England and Wales there were 1086 direct and 316 indirect maternal deaths; the maternal mortality (direct and indirect deaths) was 68 per 100 000 pregnancies. In the triennium 2000-2002 there were 106 direct and 155 indirect deaths in the whole of the UK; the maternal mortality had been reduced to 13.1 per 100 000 pregnancies.

The principal causes of maternal death in 1952-1954 and 2000-2002 are shown in Table 1.3 and their relative importance in Figure 1.4, i.e. the percentage of maternal mortality accounted for by each principal cause. Table 1.3 and Figure 1.4 show that not only are fewer women dying from hemorrhage, early pregnancy problems (including septic abortion), hypertension, prolonged labor and trauma but also that these direct causes of maternal death are relatively less important when compared with indirect deaths. This is a remarkable tribute to advances in obstetrics, although the increase in deaths from post-partum hemorrhage from one in 1997-1999 to 10 in 2000-2002 leaves no room for complacency. With the exception of hypertension these are all 'surgical' type deaths amenable to prevention by the attendance of a well trained obstetrician. By contrast deaths from venous thromboembolism, heart disease and other indirect causes have all become more significant (Table 1.3). These, including nearly all indirect deaths are of a more 'medical' nature. Hypertension, heart disease, venous thromboembolism (VTE), and other indirect causes have been grouped together as 'medical' causes of maternal mortality in Figure 1.4. 'Medical' causes now account for 81% of maternal mortality. It is likely that any significant further reduction in maternal mortality will only be made by improving medical care in pregnancy.

The CEMACH are an audit tool giving unique information relating to the outcome of medical

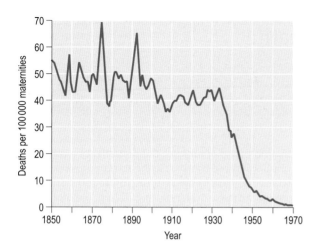

Figure 1.2 Maternal mortality by year. Engalnd and Wales, 1850-1970. *Source:* Registrar General for England and Wales.

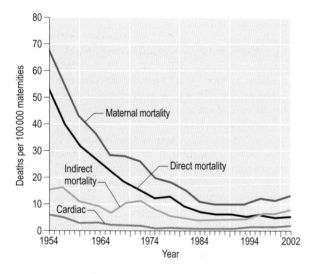

Figure 1.3 More recent UK maternal mortality by year: 1952-2004, deaths per 100 000 maternities.

Table 1.3 Maternal deaths in England and Wales (1952-1954) and the UK (2000-2004) by cause

Year	Hemorrhage	Early	Toxemia	VTE[a]	Prolonged labor and trauma	Sepsis	Other direct	Cardiac	All other indirect	Total
1952	234	212	200	138	119	42	141	121	195	1402
2000	17	15	14	30	1	11	18	44	111	261

[a]Venous thromboembolism.

problems in pregnancy. Conclusions relating to some of these conditions and arising from the enquiries will now be considered in more detail. The medical conditions themselves are of course considered elsewhere in this book

VENOUS THROMBOEMBOLISM
(see also Ch. 8)

In 1952-1954 there were 138 deaths from VTE. In the most recent 2000-2002 report there were 30 deaths from

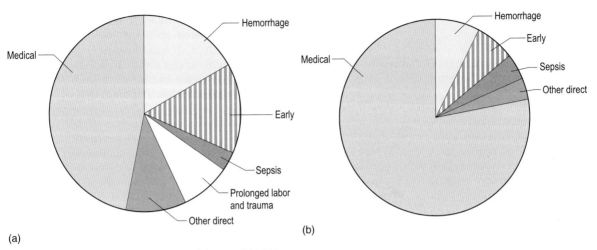

Medical

Hemorrhage

Early

Sepsis

Prolonged labor
and trauma

Other direct

(a)

Medical

Hemorrhage

Early

Sepsis

Other direct

(b)

Figure 1.4 Maternity mortality by cause: (a) 1952; (b) 2004.

pulmonary embolus. This enormous reduction was probably the result of less traumatic management of delivery and of patients being mobilized more vigorously afterwards. No longer do puerperal women 'lie-in' for over a week following childbirth. The CEMACH have also highlighted the relation between VTE mortality, increasing age and increasing parity. The association between estrogen suppression of lactation and VTE mortality was a major reason for discontinuing the use of estrogens to suppress lactation.

More recently there has been a marked reduction in deaths from pulmonary embolism following Cesarean section, which were reduced from 15 in 1994-96 to 4 in 1997-99; it is likely that this reduction was due at least in part to the publication in 1995 of the Royal College of Obstetricians and Gynaecologists (RCOG) guidelines recommending thromboprophylaxis for all but the most low risk Cesarean sections. These guidelines have been accepted and acted upon by most delivery suites in the UK.

In the 1997-99 report, there were 14 antenatal deaths, none during labour and 14 after delivery. So the antenatal period may be just as dangerous as the puerperium. Furthermore of the 14 antenatal deaths, 9 occurred in the first trimester. This has important implications for pre-pregnancy counselling regarding thromboprophylaxis. In patients who are at high risk because of previous VTE, decisions should be made before pregnancy about thromboprophylaxis. Since patients currently book after the first trimester, it is too late to leave such decisions until after booking. Typical risk factors for thromboembolism are previous VTE, known thrombophilia, family history of VTE, obesity and increasing age. These should be identified by those such as physicians and general

practitioners caring for women before pregnancy. Not only should obstetricians think more about obstetric medicine but so too should those not directly involved in obstetrics. This will be hard. Physicians of all specialties are usually very insecure if asked how patients even with problems in their own specialty should be managed in pregnancy.

Traditionally puerperal thromboprophylaxis has been reserved for those being delivered by Cesarean section. However, in 1997-1999 there were 10 deaths following vaginal delivery compared to four following Cesarean section, and therefore thromboprophylaxis should be considered for high-risk women who have vaginal deliveries. Risk factors were present in a high proportion of those who died following vaginal delivery (prolonged bed rest in one, obesity in seven, increasing age in three and previous VTE in two). Guidelines are available for thromboprophylaxis antenatally, in labor and following vaginal delivery.

Clinicians in all disciplines should also be more aware of the possibility of VTE, particularly pulmonary embolus in those complaining of chest pain, breathlessness and cough in pregnancy, notwithstanding the difficulty of evaluating breathlessness in pregnancy. They should be prepared to treat before the diagnosis is established. Among the 14 antenatal deaths from VTE in 1997-1999 the assessors considered that there was a failure to diagnose in 9 and in the 14 postnatal deaths a failure to diagnose in 6. Typical mistakes are to consider only infection as a cause of chest symptoms and to think that chest X-rays are contraindicated in pregnancy. By contrast there were only 4 failures of treatment in the 28 deaths. Once women are treated with heparin they tend to survive.

HYPERTENSION AND PRE-ECLAMPSIA
(see also Ch. 3)

There has also been a reduction in deaths resulting from hypertensive disease from 246 in England and Wales (1952-1954) to 14 in the whole UK (2000-2002). Table 1.4 shows the relative contributions of cerebral, pulmonary, hepatic and other causes of maternal mortality from hypertension between 1988 and 2002. Note that there is no separate section for kidney disease. Indeed there have been no deaths from renal failure due to hypertension between the years 1994 and 2002. Therefore strenuous attempts to maintain urine output in the erroneous belief that this will prevent renal failure and reduce maternal mortality are unjustified. Indeed aggressive fluid therapy will exacerbate the risk of pulmonary edema. Table 1.4 shows how this has decreased over the last six years. This has probably occurred because clinicians have been more sparing in their use of fluids after delivery realizing that oliguria is common after delivery and that it does not need to be 'treated' with overzealous intravenous fluid therapy. Also several triennial reports have emphasized the importance of fluid balance and recommended that there should be a single obstetrician coordinating fluid therapy.

The principal cause of death in hypertensive disease is now cerebral; usually cerebral hemorrhage. Better blood pressure control when patients are acutely ill is therefore needed. This can only be achieved by frequently reviewing the patient and being prepared to use the currently available drugs aggressively. Systolic hypertension should be treated as well as diastolic. The threshold for treatment of systolic blood pressure is likely to be 160-170 mmHg. If the patient is undelivered, delivery may be the only way to control blood pressure whatever the gestation.

Most automated sphygmomanometers have not been validated in pregnancy, let alone in severe pre-eclampsia. When they are tested they frequently underestimate blood pressure, sometimes by up to 30 mmHg diastolic. The most recent CEMACH report therefore recommends caution in the use of electronic machines to monitor the blood pressure of women with severe pre-eclampsia. At the very least, an initial recording should be made with a mercury sphygmomanometer to check the accuracy of the automatic machine in each patient where it is used.

General practitioners and hospital staff are often unaware of the importance of new onset epigastric pain and headache as symptoms of severe pre-eclampsia. The last two CEMACH reports recommend that women who have such symptoms severe enough to take them to their doctors, should at the very least have their blood pressure measured and urine tested. In addition severe pre-eclampsia can present very quickly sometimes within one week, the very shortest time interval at which women are routinely reviewed in pregnancy. Therefore pregnant women should be warned of the symptoms of severe pre-eclampsia and told to seek medical advice should they arise. This may be unpopular with some healthcare attendants as an example of the 'medicalization' of pregnancy; but those women who have suffered as a consequence of not being aware of the importance of headache and epigastric pain, are usually very angry because they have been left in ignorance.

HEART DISEASE (see also Ch. 2)

In 2000-2002 there were 44 deaths in the UK from heart disease, 14 more than the 30 deaths from the most frequent direct cause, thromboembolism. This underlines the importance of indirect causes of maternal mortality and of medical conditions in general. Not surprisingly, the pattern of mortality from heart

Table 1.4 UK deaths from pre-eclampsia, 1988-2002 (CEMACH 2004)

Cause of death	1988–1990	1991–1993	1994–1996	1997–1999	2000–2002
Intracerebral hemorrhage	10	5	3	7	9
Cerebral other	4	0	4	0	0
Cerebral total	14	5	7	7	9
Pulmonary	10	11	8	2	1
Hepatic	1	0	3	2	0
Other	2	4	2	5	4
Total	27	20	20	16	14

disease has also changed since the 1950s chiefly because of the decline in incidence of rheumatic fever. Between 1952 and 1960 there were 239 maternal deaths from rheumatic heart disease in the UK and the majority of these were due to mitral stenosis. Between 1991 and 2002 there was a total of 150 cardiac deaths of which no more than six were due to rheumatic heart disease and only three were due to mitral valve disease.

In the UK in 2000-2002 the pattern of death from heart disease in pregnancy has changed completely from that in evidence in 1952. The principle causes are now cardiomyopathy, dissection of the thoracic aorta or its branches, myocardial infarction and pulmonary vascular disease in approximately equal numbers. All other causes of cardiac mortality account for the remaining fifth.

Pulmonary vascular disease is quite rare but it has an extraordinarily high mortality in pregnancy, for example, 30-50% in Eisenmenger's syndrome. There is no other condition where the risk of dying in pregnancy is so great. Yet many obstetricians, some physicians and a few cardiologists are unaware of the risk of pulmonary vascular disease. Unfortunately there is no specific treatment and even the reason why the patients die is uncertain. Typically they die after delivery with slowly developing hypotension and increasing cyanosis. Probably blood is shunted away from the lungs due to a relative increase in pulmonary vascular resistance compared to systemic resistance. These patients need sensitive counseling in adult congenital heart disease (ACHD) clinics so that they come to realize that they should not become pregnant. But the desire for pregnancy is so strong in some women, that this counseling may alienate them from antenatal care should they decide to become pregnant despite receiving advice to the contrary. Eisenmenger's syndrome is only one cause of pulmonary vascular disease. There are many other causes, in particular primary pulmonary hypertension and connective tissue diseases such as scleroderma.

Pregnant women with significant heart disease should be managed at least in part in a specialist tertiary care center. They are probably the most demanding of all women with medical problems in pregnancy in their requirements. They need input from obstetricians who are genuinely interested and experienced in high-risk pregnancy, cardiologists and physicians with specific knowledge of pregnancy, hematologists because of the specific problems of anticoagulation in pregnancy and obstetric anesthetists who understand high-risk pregnancy.

OTHER INDIRECT DEATHS

These are also dominated by medical causes and the principal classification is shown in Table 1.5. Heart disease has already been considered. The next most frequent category is diseases of the central nervous system (CNS) (see also Ch. 14) followed by suicide. Suicide is outside the scope of this discussion but its importance as a cause of maternal mortality, certainly underlines the need for psychiatric services specifically orientated to the needs of pregnancy. Such services are not available in most maternity units in the UK.

In 2000-2002 the majority of the 40 CNS deaths were from 'stroke': subarachnoid (17) or intracerebral (3) hemorrhage and cerebral thrombosis (4). None of these events occurred in relation to labor nor were there any cases of stroke in relation to labor in the previous two reports, i.e. over a total period of 12 years in the UK. Therefore there is probably much misplaced anxiety about the method of delivery in women who are known to have berry aneurysms or a-v malformations. It is often thought that the 'strain' of labor will cause these lesions to bleed so that women are advised to be delivered by Cesarean section if they are 'allowed' to get pregnant at all. But there will have been many women with undiagnosed vascular brain lesions who have labored; and none of them seem to have died in the UK in the last 12 years because of cerebral bleeding occurring at the time of labor. So women with known vascular lesions may be reassured that it is relatively safe for them to become pregnant.

The other major cause of CNS death is epilepsy. In the 2000-2002 report there were 13 such deaths. It is insufficiently recognized that epilepsy is an inherently dangerous condition. Patients can die because of seizures, either because they become unconscious

Table 1.5 UK indirect deaths, 2000-2002

Cardiac	44
Psychiatric	16
Malignancy	5
Other indirect	
Diseases of the central nervous system	40
Infectious diseases	14
Diseases of the respiratory system	10
Endocrine metabolic & immunity diseases	7
Diseases of the gastrointestinal system	7
Other	16
Total	155

during a hazardous activity such as bathing, or because they choke, or because of sudden unexplained death in epilepsy (SUDEP).

SUDEP is recognized to be a cause of death in epilepsy. Patients die suddenly and no cause of death is identified. Poor epileptic control is a major risk factor and women are at risk of this in pregnancy; either because they reduce or stop anticonvulsant therapy due to fear of the effect of the drugs on the fetus; or because the increased metabolism of pregnancy decreases free drug levels. In the interval between 1994 and 2002 there were 20 maternal deaths in epileptic women that could have been due to SUDEP, emphasizing the need for good control of epilepsy in pregnancy. This is best given by either neurology specialists working in antenatal clinics or by obstetric physicians.

CONCLUSION

In the UK, a developed society, about 80% of maternal mortality is due to medical causes, such as thromboembolism, hypertension, heart disease and other indirect causes. It is likely that serious morbidity follows a similar pattern. Now that traditional surgical causes of maternal mortality such as postpartum hemorrhage, puerperal sepsis and ruptured uterus are being successfully addressed, more attention must be paid to the medical aspects of pregnancy. Input will come from obstetric physicians but obstetricians must also think more about medical matters. As in the developing world obstetricians, midwives and others caring for women in pregnancy must have respect and take responsibility for the general health of women; and not just pay lip service to the dogma of traditional obstetric practice. In addition, all healthcare practitioners who care for pregnant women or those who may become pregnant need more knowledge of the interaction between medical conditions and pregnancy.

Further reading

Bicego G, Boerma J T, Ronsman C 2002 The effects of AIDS on maternal mortality in Malawi and Zimbabwe. AIDS 16:1078-1081

DfID 2004 Reducing maternal deaths: evidence and action. A strategy for DFID. DfID, London

DHSS 1979 Report on confidential enquiries into maternal deaths in England and Wales, 1973-1975. HMSO, London

DoH 1957 Reports on public health and medical subjects No. 97. Report of confidential enquiries into maternal deaths in England and Wales, 1952-1954. HMSO, London

Islam K, Gurdtham U G 2005 A systematic review of the estimates of costs-illness associated with maternal and newborn ill-health. WHO, Geneva

Kowalewski M, Mujinja P, Janh A 2002 Can mothers afford maternal health care costs? User costs of maternity services in rural Tanzania. African Journal of Reproductive Health 6(1):65-73

Lewis G 1998 Why mothers die. Report on confidential enquiries into maternal deaths in the United Kingdom 1994-1996. HMSO, London

Lewis G 2001 Why mothers die 1997-1999. The confidential enquiries into maternal deaths in the United Kingdom. RCOG, London

Lewis G 2004 Why mothers die 2000-2002. The Confidential Enquires into Maternal Deaths in the United Kingdom (CEMACH). RCOG, London

Marston C, Cleland J C 2003 Do unintended pregnancies carried to term lead to adverse outcomes for mother and child? An assessment in five developing countries. Population Studies 57:77-93

Nilsson L, Farnhmand B Y, Persson P G, et al. 1999 Risk factors for sudden unexpected death in epilepsy: a case control study. Lancet 353:888-893

Penny J A, Shennan A H, Halligan A W, et al. 1997 Blood pressure measurement in severe pre-eclampsia (research letter). Lancet 349:1518

Pittrof R, Cambell O, Filippi V G A 2002 What is quality maternity care? An international perspective. Acta obstetricia et gynecologica Scandinavica 81:277-283

Royal College of Obstetricians and Gynaecologists 1995 Report of the RCOG working party on prophylaxis against thromboembolism in gynaecology and obstetrics. RCOG, London

Royal College of Obstetricians and Gynaecologists 2004 Thromboprophylaxis during pregnancy, labour and after normal vaginal delivery. Guideline No. 37. RCOG, London

Thaddeus S, Maine D 1994 Too far to walk: maternal mortality in context. Social Science and Medicine 38:1091-1110

UN DESA 2002 World contraceptive use 2001. New York, UN DESA

UNFPA 1997 State of the World's Population 1997. UNFPA, New York

UNFPA/FIGO 2002 Second Meeting of the Working Group for the Prevention and Treatment of Obstetric Fistula, Addis Ababa

UNICEF 2001 The Progress of the Nations 2001. UNICEF, New York

UN 1991 The world's women. Trend and statistics 1970-90. United Nations, New York

UN 2000 United Nations Millennium Declaration. UN, New York

Womens Dignity Project 2003 Faces of dignity. Online. Available: http://www.womensdignity.org/ Publications.asp

WHO 2003 Maternal mortality in 2000: estimates developed by WHO, UNICEF and UNFPA. WHO, Geneva

WHO 2004a Unsafe abortion. Global and regional estimates of the incidence of unsafe abortion and associated mortality in 2000. WHO, Geneva

WHO 2004b Global action for skilled attendant for pregnant women. Report RHR/02.17. 2004

WHO 2004c Beyond the numbers – reviewing maternal deaths and complications to make pregnancy safer. WHO, Geneva. Online. Availabe: http://www.who.int/reproductive-health

WHO 2005 The World Health Report 2005. WHO, Geneva

Chapter 2

Cardiac disease in pregnancy

D. L. Adamson, M. K. Dhanjal, C. Nelson-Piercy, R. Collis

Heart disease and its management in obstetrics
D. L. Adamson, M. K. Dhanjal, C. Nelson-Piercy

INTRODUCTION

Pregnancies complicated by significant heart disease are uncommon in the UK, Europe and the developed world. However cardiac disease is now the leading cause of maternal death in the UK. There were 44 indirect deaths attributed to cardiac disease in 2000-2002, giving a death rate of 2.2 per 100 000 maternities. The maternal mortality rate from cardiac disease has continued to rise in the UK since the early 1980s. The major causes of cardiac deaths over the last 10 years are cardiomyopathy (predominantly peripartum), myocardial infarction (most commonly due to coronary artery dissection), dissection of the thoracic aorta and pulmonary hypertension. In the UK, rheumatic heart disease is now rare in women of childbearing age and mostly confined to immigrants.

Women with congenital heart disease are surviving longer thanks to corrective or palliative surgery in childhood. They are therefore not uncommonly encountered in pregnancy. These women may have complicated pregnancies. Women with mechanical prosthetic valves face difficult decisions regarding anticoagulation in pregnancy.

Because of significant physiological changes in pregnancy, symptoms, such as palpitations, and signs such as an ejection systolic murmur are very common innocent findings. Not all women with significant heart disease are able to meet these increased physiological demands. The care of the pregnant and parturient woman with heart disease requires a multidisciplinary approach, involving obstetricians, cardiologists and anesthetists, preferably in a dedicated antenatal cardiac clinic. This allows formulation of an agreed and documented management plan encompassing management of both planned and emergency delivery.

PHYSIOLOGICAL CHANGES IN PREGNANCY

Blood volume starts to increase by the fifth week after conception secondary to estrogen- and prostaglandin-induced relaxation of smooth muscle that increases the capacitance of the venous bed. Plasma volume increases and red cell mass rises but to a lesser degree, thus explaining the physiological anemia of pregnancy. Relaxation of smooth muscle on the arterial side results in a profound fall in systemic vascular resistance and together with the increase in blood volume, determines the early increase in cardiac output. Blood pressure falls slightly but by term has usually returned to the pre-pregnancy value. The increased cardiac output is achieved by an increase in stroke volume and a lesser increase in resting heart rate of 10-20 beats/min. By the end of the second trimester the blood volume and stroke volume have risen by between 30 and 50%. This increase correlates with the size and weight of the products of conception and is therefore considerably greater in multiple pregnancies as is the risk of heart failure in heart disease.

Although there is no increase in pulmonary capillary wedge pressure (PCWP), plasma colloid oncotic pressure is reduced. The colloid oncotic pressure-pulmonary capillary wedge pressure gradient is reduced by 28%, making pregnant women particularly susceptible to pulmonary edema. Pulmonary edema may be precipitated if there is either an increase in cardiac pre-load (such as infusion of fluids), increase in left atrial and pulmonary venous pressure (such as in mitral stenosis) or increased pulmonary capillary permeability (such as in pre-eclampsia), or a combination of these factors.

In late pregnancy in the supine position, pressure of the gravid uterus on the inferior vena cava causes a reduction in venous return to the heart and a consequent fall in stroke volume and cardiac output. Turning from the lateral to the supine position may result in a 25% reduction in cardiac output. Pregnant women should therefore be nursed in the left or right lateral position wherever possible. If the mother has to be kept on her back, the pelvis should be rotated so that the uterus drops to the side and cardiac output as well as uteroplacental blood flow are optimized. Reduced cardiac output is associated with a reduction in uterine blood flow and therefore in placental perfusion; this can compromise the fetus.

Labor is associated with further increases in cardiac output (15% in the first stage and 50% in the second stage). Uterine contractions lead to autotransfusion of 300-500 mL of blood back into the circulation and the sympathetic response to pain and anxiety further elevate heart rate and blood pressure. Cardiac output is increased more during contractions but also between contractions. The rise in stroke volume with each contraction is attenuated by good pain relief and further reduced by epidural analgesia and the supine position. Epidural analgesia or anesthesia cause arterial vasodilation and a fall in blood pressure. General anesthesia is associated with a rise in blood pressure and heart rate during induction, but cardiovascular stability thereafter. Prostaglandins given to induce labor have little effect on hemodynamics but ergometrine causes vasoconstriction and syntocinon can cause vasodilation and fluid retention.

Following delivery of the baby up to 1 L of blood may be returned to the circulation due to the relief of inferior vena cava obstruction and contraction of the uterus. The intrathoracic and cardiac blood volumes rise, cardiac output increases by 60-80% followed by a rapid decline to pre-labor values within about 1 h of delivery. Transfer of fluid from the extravascular space increases venous return and stroke volume further. Those women with cardiovascular compromise are therefore most at risk of pulmonary edema during the second stage of labor and the immediate postpartum period. All the changes revert quite rapidly during the first week and more slowly over the following six weeks but even at a year significant changes still persist and are enhanced by a subsequent pregnancy.

NORMAL FINDINGS ON EXAMINATION OF THE CARDIOVASCULAR SYSTEM IN PREGNANCY

Normal findings on cardiovascular examination may include a loud first heart sound with exaggerated splitting of the second heart sound and a physiological third heart sound at the apex. A systolic ejection murmur at the left sternal edge is heard in nearly all women and may be remarkably loud and be audible all over the precordium. It varies with posture and if unaccompanied by any other abnormality it reflects the increased stroke output. Venous hums and mammary souffles may be heard. Because of the peripheral vasodilation the pulse may be bounding and in addition ectopic beats are very common in pregnancy.

CARDIAC INVESTIGATIONS IN PREGNANCY

The electrocardiographic (ECG) axis shifts superiorly in late pregnancy due to a more horizontal position of the heart. Small Q-waves and T-wave inversion in the right precordial leads are not uncommon. Atrial and ventricular ectopics are both common.

The amount of radiation received by the fetus during a maternal chest X-ray (CXR) is negligible and a CXR should never be withheld if clinically indicated in pregnancy. Transthoracic echocardiogram is the investigation of choice to exclude, confirm or monitor structural heart disease in pregnancy. Transesophageal echocardiograms (TEE) are also safe with the usual precautions to avoid aspiration. Magnetic resonance imaging (MRI) and CT pulmonary angiography are considered safe in pregnancy (see Ch. 21). Routine investigation with electrophysiological studies and angiography are normally postponed until after pregnancy but angiography should not be withheld if required, for example in acute coronary syndromes.

CONGENITAL HEART DISEASE

Congenital heart disease (CHD) in adults is increasing in frequency as a result of the success of congenital cardiology and cardiac surgery. It is the commonest birth defect with just under 1% of newborns having CHD. Half the CHD population are women, and are usually well enough to contemplate and undergo pregnancy. The majority of women with CHD who reach childbearing age do so because they either have a lesion which is associated with long-term survival or because they have had successful surgery. Whilst some may not be able to tolerate the hemodynamic changes of pregnancy, the majority will have enough cardiac reserve to carry a pregnancy to term. CHD is infrequently associated with maternal mortality, however, there may be a significant deterioration in the maternal condition. These complex patients should be jointly cared for by obstetricians, obstetric physicians and cardiologists with expertise in pregnancy and adult congenital heart disease and provide a challenge for such a team.

Pre-pregnancy counseling and assessment

Most women with congenital heart disease are known to a cardiologist prior to pregnancy. It is extremely important that such women are appropriately counseled about their individual health risks with pregnancy. If pregnancy carries an unacceptable risk, this should be explained and appropriate contraceptive advice given. Advising an individual may be difficult, particularly those with corrected complex disease, as data remain sparse for pregnancy outcomes following some forms of corrective and palliative surgery.

Maternal risk of pregnancy is assessed by obtaining an accurate history, which will define the functional status, examination and undertaking relevant investigations. This also provides a baseline of the cardiovascular status, allowing any change occurring in pregnancy to be objectively assessed. It may be necessary to treat the woman prior to pregnancy in order to minimize risk.

Poor maternal functional class (see Table 2.1), cyanosis, history of transient ischemic attack (TIA), heart failure, left arrhythmia, left heart outflow obstruction and impaired ventricular function have all prospectively been found to be associated with poor maternal outcome. Maternal cyanosis is also a risk factor for fetal and neonatal complications. There is only a 12% likelihood of a live birth if the resting arterial saturation is $\leq 85\%$ whilst $\geq 85\%$ is associated with a 63% likelihood of a live birth.

Most CHD is inherited in a multifactorial manner, however single gene disorders, chromosome abnormalities and maternal disease can be the cause. The risk of recurrent CHD is summarized in Table 2.2. The risk of cardiac malformation secondary to maternal diabetes mellitus is approximately 2-3%, while in single gene or chromosomal abnormalities such as Marfan, Noonan and Holt-Oram syndromes the risk of inherited heart disease is 50%.

Table 2.1 New York Heart Association (NYHA) functional classification

Class	Description
I	No breathlessness/uncompromised
II	Breathlessness on severe exertion/slightly compromised
III	Breathlessness on mild exertion/moderately compromised
IV	Breathlessness at rest/severely compromised

Table 2.2 Risk of congenital heart disease in a future pregnancy

Risk factor	Risk of CHD in future pregnancy (%)
One previous child with CHD	2
Two previous children with CHD	10
Mother with CHD	6
Father with CHD	2

The mode of delivery may also require some consideration prior to conception, although events in pregnancy may influence this. Cardiologists in the past have traditionally favored a Cesarean section (CS). In the majority of cases, however, vaginal delivery is safest for the mother. In comparison to CS, vaginal delivery is associated with a reduction in both blood loss and thromboembolic risk. There are also less abrupt hemodynamic changes, particularly when assisted by effective analgesia and a short second stage of labor. Vaginal delivery has to be balanced against the lack of predictable delivery time where a team can be prepared for all eventualities. Absolute indications for CS are Marfan syndrome with an aortic root dilated beyond 4.5 cm, aortic aneurysm and an acutely unwell mother.

Acyanotic heart disease

Septal defects

Atrial septal defects (ASD) are the most common congenital lesions found in adults, making up between 10-17%, while ventricular septal defects (VSD) are the commonest form in children (1.5-3.5 per 1000 live births). ASDs are often left uncorrected unless there is either a large hole or significant left to right shunt causing right ventricular overload and dilatation. If small or corrected, they cause no specific or significant problems during pregnancy and do not require antibiotic prophylaxis (Table 2.3). In an uncorrected defect, the effect of an increase in cardiac output on a volume-loaded right side is counterbalanced by the decrease in peripheral vascular resistance. The two main areas of concern are paradoxical embolus or arrhythmia. The former is rare but if the pregnant woman is immobilized or has other risk factors for thrombosis, thromboembolic prophylaxis is advised. The risk of atrial arrhythmias is well established with ASDs and remains even with correction. These should be treated dependent upon the rhythm (see arrhythmia section).

VSDs are less common and often corrected in childhood, unless they are small and hemodynamically insignificant. The only risk is that of endocarditis and prophylaxis is advised for delivery (see Table 2.3).

Valve disease

While all valves can be congenitally affected, the commonest lesion is that of a bicuspid aortic valve leading to aortic stenosis. This results in a fixed cardiac output. The majority of young women are asymptomatic and pregnancy is likely to be tolerated well. It is important to assess these women prior to pregnancy to determine whether it would be safer undergoing a pregnancy with the native valve or whether surgery should be contemplated prior to conception. Pregnancy is likely to be well tolerated if:

1. Resting ECG has no ST segment depression.
2. On exercise testing, there is an appropriate increase in BP and HR and no ST change.
3. The pressure across the aortic valve measures less than 80 mmHg at peak and mean pressure gradient is less than 50 mmHg.
4. There is good LV function

Women should be monitored throughout pregnancy to identify symptoms and signs suggestive of decompensation, such as an exaggerated tachycardia or dyspnea, angina, pulmonary edema or new ECG changes. A fall in pressure gradient across the aortic valve is suggestive of a reduction in LV function. Women with symptomatic aortic stenosis should be managed with bed rest to prevent the requirement of an increased cardiac output, and beta blockade which reduces cardiac output as well as lengthening diastole to aid coronary filling. In extreme cases of decompensation, emergency balloon aortic valvotomy or aortic valve replacement can be considered

Table 2.3 Risk of infective endocarditis with different cardiac conditions

Degree of risk of infective endocarditis	Prophylaxis required	Cardiac condition
High	Yes	Previous bacterial endocarditis
		Prosthetic heart valves or other foreign material
		Surgically created systemic or pulmonary conduits
		Complex cyanotic congenital heart diseases
Moderate	Yes	Acquired valvular heart disease
		MVP with MR or severe valve thickening
		Non-cyanotic congenital heart diseases (except secundum type ASD) including bicuspid aortic valves
		Hypertrophic cardiomyopathy
Negligible	No	Isolated secundum/sinus venosus ASD
		Surgically repaired ASD, VSD, PDA (provided no left valve abnormalities)
		MVP without regurgitation
		Physiological heart murmurs
		Cardiac pacemakers
		Pulmonary valve stenosis and post-operative valvotomy
		Total anomalous pulmonary drainage
		Well repaired tetralogy of Fallot with no shunts, aortic regurgitation, or valve grafts

but are associated with significant maternal and fetal morbidity and mortality. Where the woman has progressed well through pregnancy, a vaginal delivery can be considered but hypovolemia and vasodilators should be avoided. Some women with bicuspid aortic valves have post stenotic dilatation of the aorta and as such are at risk of aortic dissection. A history of chest pain should thus be taken extremely seriously.

Aortic pathology

The commonest problems encountered are aortic dissection (see later) and coarctation of the aorta. Although women with aortic coarctation have usually undergone corrective surgery prior to pregnancy, re-coarctation or aneurysm formation at the site of surgery can occur. The aorta should therefore be assessed prior to conception or as early in pregnancy as possible, preferably with MRI. If there is no significant defect, then a woman should be able to undergo a vaginal delivery with a short second stage. Patients with coarctation or aneurysm should have aggressive blood pressure management to minimize the risk of dissection (see aortic dissection). Pregnancy is usually well tolerated by all groups and mortality is low.

Congenitally corrected transposition of the great arteries

In this condition the ventricles are switched round, i.e. the right atrium drains into the left ventricle which is positioned where the right ventricle should be and then it drains back out into the pulmonary artery. De-oxygenated blood is still directed to the lungs, and oxygenated blood to the body. However, the morphological right ventricle now has to support a systemic circulation and pressure, which it is not designed to do. Additionally, the tricuspid valve between the left sided atrium and ventricle is prone to regurgitation in this higher-pressure system. If patients are well and have no deterioration in right (systemic) heart function, they will probably tolerate pregnancy well. However, right heart function as well as systemic tricuspid atrioventricular valve regurgitation may deteriorate in pregnancy. Finally, the atrioventricular node is absent and thus patients often have heart block requiring pacing.

Hypertrophic cardiomyopathy

This condition, previously thought to be rare, may affect up to 2 in 1000 people. Up to 70% of cases are familial with autosomal dominant inheritance. The diagnostic criteria for hypertrophic cardiomyopathy (HCM) are unexplained asymmetrical myocardial hypertrophy on echocardiography. Diagnosis is usually made as the result of echocardiography to investigate symptoms, a heart murmur or as part of familial screening.

Many women encountered in pregnancy are asymptomatic. Clinical features do not relate to the degree of left ventricular outflow tract obstruction and include chest pain, breathlessness, pre-syncope, syncope, atrial or ventricular arrhythmias, heart failure and sudden death. The overall risk of disease-related complications such as sudden death, endstage heart failure, and fatal stroke is roughly 1-2% per year. Risk factors for sudden death include a positive family history with 2 or more sudden cardiac deaths at < 40 years (as the risk of sudden cardiac death may be increased in certain genotypes), abnormal blood pressure response to exercise (failure of systolic blood pressure to rise by > 25 mmHg from baseline values) and ventricular tachycardia. Most sudden deaths occur in patients with left ventricular wall thickness less than 30 mm, so the presence of mild hypertrophy cannot be used to reassure patients that they are at low risk.

There are case reports of sudden death in pregnancy in patients with HCM however large series report few problems with pregnancy in patients with HCM. It is thought that deaths recorded may reflect the background expected rate and pregnancy seems not to be associated with an increased risk.

In pregnancy, beta-blockers should be commenced in women with symptoms. Caution is needed with regional anesthesia/analgesia since vasodilation may be poorly tolerated. Any hypovolemia or blood loss should be aggressively corrected and the patient kept 'well filled' during labor and delivery. Asymptomatic HCM is not an indication for Cesarean section and most of these women may deliver in their local units.

Cyanotic heart disease

Cyanotic heart disease with pulmonary hypertension

Eisenmenger's syndrome is a broad term applied to any cardiac anomaly in which the pathological process of increased pulmonary flow leads to obliterative pulmonary vascular disease. The result is pulmonary hypertension (PH), which is severe enough to reverse the left-to-right shunt to right-to-left. The PH is usually irreversible even after corrective surgery. Pulmonary hypertension of any cause carries a 40-50% risk of maternal death even if pulmonary pressures are only half of systemic.

Women with PH should be strongly advised against pregnancy and adequate contraception is imperative. The subdermal progestogen implant Implanon® is the most suitable contraceptive in view of its effectiveness and lack of cardiovascular risk. It is more effective than sterilization, which requires a general anesthetic. It can be inserted even with those on warfarin. If the patient is on the enzyme inducer Bosentan which renders Implanon® less effective, oral progestagen-only oral contraception should be added. IUCDs are usually best avoided due to the risk of a vagal response with cervical dilatation.

Women with PH who do become pregnant should be advised of the high risk of mortality and termination of pregnancy advised. Termination of pregnancy can be performed medically or surgically depending on facilities available. A medical termination can be performed at any gestation using mifepristone and then misoprostol or gemprost. The disadvantages are that it may take several days to complete during which there may be significant pain and bleeding. This can result in a tachycardia that may not be tolerated well. Adequate analgesia is essential. The procedure should be performed in a high dependency area with full monitoring. Expulsion of the products of conception or delivery of the fetus can be unpredictable. Products of conception may be retained requiring surgical evacuation.

Surgical termination can be performed by suction, or at gestations over 13 weeks, by dilatation and evacuation. Both procedures can be planned with appropriate medical staff available. The risks of a vagal response, uterine perforation and bleeding are reduced with skilled operators.

If women decline termination of pregnancy, they require careful management with a multidisciplinary team with expertise in PH. Bosentan has been shown to be teratogenic in the first trimester in animal studies, but it continued use may be necessary for maternal health. Prophylactic heparin throughout the pregnancy and elective admission for bed rest and oxygen therapy (which acts as a vasodilator) from 20-24 weeks' gestation onwards are usually recommended. Most women with Eisenmenger's syndrome who die as a result of pregnancy, do so soon after delivery. There is no evidence that Cesarean versus vaginal delivery, nor regional versus general analgesia/anesthesia reduces this risk. The dangers relate to increasing the right-to-left shunt and escalating pulmonary hypertension often despite intensive and appropriate care. The principles of management include multidisciplinary discussion and planning of elective delivery. Postpartum management should be in an intensive care environment by intensivists, anesthetists, cardiologists and obstetricians. Supplemental oxygen reduces pulmonary vascular resistance. It is important to avoid hypovolemia and acidosis, maintain pre-load, continue thromboprophylaxis and avoid pulmonary artery catheters, which carry a risk of potentially devastating in situ thrombosis. Systemic vasodilators (nitrates, epidural anesthesia and syntocinon) should be avoided but selective pulmonary vasodilators, e.g. inhaled nitric oxide, i.v. prostacyclin, sildenafil and the endothelin antagonist bosentan may be helpful although many women die despite optimal use of these measures.

Cyanotic heart disease in the absence of pulmonary hypertension

In complex cyanotic heart disease without PH maternal risk is dependent upon:

1. Ventricular function (see Table 2.1).
2. Hemorrhage due to impaired clotting factors and platelet function.
3. Paradoxical embolus as all cyanotic patients shunt from right to left.
4. Heart failure.
5. Increasing cyanosis secondary to the vasodilatation of pregnancy.

Cyanosis is associated with adverse effects on the fetus with an increased incidence of low birth weight, prematurity and fetal loss (see Table 2.4).

These patients need careful monitoring in a unit that understands the complex physiology of the maternal circulation. Women often require bed rest and oxygen which may reduce cyanosis and, as such, improve fetal well-being.

While spontaneous vaginal delivery is best for the mother, fetal growth restriction or fetal distress often precipitates a Cesarean section. It is important in these situations to maintain the circulatory volume and avoid significant vasodilation. The use of aspirin in these women is controversial because of the increased bleeding risk associated with poor platelet function.

Table 2.4 Livebirth rates with varying degrees of maternal cyanosis

Maternal oxygen saturation (%)	Livebirth rate (%)
>90	92
≥85–90	63
<85	12

Post surgical correction

The majority of women who have had definitive correction of simple lesions such as ASD, VSD, patent ductus arteiosus (PDA) can be treated as normal provided there is no significant residual lesion. The increased risk of arrhythmias, particularly atrial arrhythmias remains. In normal pregnancy, right ventricular volumes increase and this may lead to problems in women with right ventricular dysfunction. The more complex procedures, particularly those with shunts are prone to specific complications and are discussed below.

Repaired tetralogy of Fallot

Despite the complexity of the original lesion, a successful correction is likely to lead to an uncomplicated successful pregnancy. One report of 40 pregnancies in 27 women demonstrated no serious complications in any of the pregnancies and an incidence of miscarriage comparable to that of the general population. A second report of 63 pregnancies in 29 women reported that 13 ended in termination and 6 pregnancies were complicated by arrhythmias and/or right sided heart failure.

These women require assessment to confirm that there is no significant right ventricular outflow obstruction, pulmonary regurgitation (PR) or reduction in right ventricular function. The PR may get worse as the pregnancy progresses causing increasing tiredness and breathlessness which is best treated with bed rest and diuretics.

Repaired transposition of the great arteries

The Mustard operation uses a baffle (conduit) to direct pulmonary venous return into the right ventricle and transposed aorta, and the systemic venous blood via the mitral valve and left ventricle. Essentially, this allows blood to go in the right direction but through the wrong ventricle. Therefore the right ventricle and tricuspid valve support the systemic circulation with the same problems as in congenitally corrected transposition (see above).

The Senning operation is physiologically the same as the Mustard. The difference is that with the Senning, the baffle is created from right atrial wall and atrial septal tissue whilst the Mustard creates the baffle using pericardium or synthetic material.

The Rastelli repair operation uses a valved conduit for certain complex congenital lesions including transposition with pulmonary stenosis. Women with either subaortic stenosis or residual conduit obstruction can develop greater obstruction in pregnancy.

The main complication from repaired transposition of the great arteries is narrowing of the pulmonary venous pathway because of the baffle structure. This fixed obstruction acts as a physiological equivalent of mitral stenosis. These women require complete assessment before or early in pregnancy. However, providing the right ventricular function is good, pregnancy is usually well tolerated.

Post-Fontan procedure

The Fontan circulation was developed for patients with a functional single ventricle. The single ventricle supports the systemic circulation while the systemic venous return is directed to the pulmonary artery directly through a baffle. This means there is no pump directing the blood through this shunt. While this repairs any shunts and thus abolishes cyanosis, the circulation is prothrombotic, has a limited ability to increase cardiac output and poorly tolerates atrial arrythmias and hypovolemia. However, in those women with good ventricular function and few symptoms, pregnancy may be well tolerated.

ACQUIRED HEART DISEASE

Peripartum cardiomyopathy

Peripartum cardiomyopathy (PPCM) is a rare illness where there is an onset of heart failure with no identifiable cause in the last month of pregnancy or within the first 5 months postpartum, in the absence of heart disease before the last month of pregnancy. It is associated with increased maternal age, Afro-Caribbean race, multiparity, multiple pregnancy and hypertension. It is similar in its clinical presentation to dilated cardiomyopathy, but the latter is not related to pregnancy.

Clinical features

Presentation varies from an incidental finding during echocardiography through to severe heart failure and death. Cardiac decompensation in an otherwise stable patient may occur with iatrogenic fluid or syntocinon infusions, beta-agonists for tocolysis and steroids for fetal lung maturity, which may all cause fluid overload.

Clinically the patient may be tachycardic and tachypneic with congestive cardiac failure and may have an arrhythmia. A CXR will show an enlarged heart and pulmonary edema. The ECG confirms a tachycardia with possible atrial or ventricular arrhythmias, the signs of either left heart strain (ST depression and T-wave inversion in the chest leads) or left bundle branch block (LBBB). Complications include renal and hepatic dysfunction from low cardiac output, life threatening pulmonary edema, systemic or pulmonary emboli from mural thrombus, fatal arrhythmias and death.

The diagnosis is made with the temporal relationship with pregnancy and echocardiography which shows increased cardiac dimensions, left ventricular systolic dysfunction often with global/biventricular involvement (left ventricular ejection fraction < 45%; fractional shortening < 30% in M-mode; left ventricular end-diastolic dimension > 2.7 cm/m^2; and dilatation, often of all four chambers).

Management

Treatment is supportive as the underlying condition can only be treated with delivery. Pulmonary edema should be treated by sitting the patient up, giving oxygen, diamorphine and loop diuretics. Vasodilators such as nitrates, isosorbide or hydralazine will help reduce afterload. These can be replaced with ACE inhibitors postpartum, which may also help with cardiac remodeling. Thromboprophylaxis is essential and low molecular weight heparin (LMWH) such as enoxaparin is valuable. A higher dose may be required particularly in those with associated arrhythmias. In such cases warfarin should be used postnatally and breast feeding can continue. Digoxin can be safely used for atrial fibrillation or flutter and beta-blockers may be used with caution for rate control in those with preserved cardiac output.

In many cases preterm delivery will be iatrogenic due to maternal cardiac deterioration. Caution should be used with the administration of steroids for fetal lung maturation in such cases as further fluid overload can occur. A pre-emptive increase in diuretics may prevent sudden deterioration.

In the patient who remains hypoxic and hypotensive, intubation, ventilation and inotropic support is necessary. Delivery by Cesarean section will assist in reducing the cardiac requirement. Occasionally an intra-aortic balloon pump or a left ventricular assist device may be needed in the interim until myocardial recovery occurs or until cardiac transplantation is performed.

Delivery

Vaginal delivery is appropriate in those who have relatively mild disease or in those who are adequately treated. Invasive monitoring in labor is recommended with arterial and central venous lines. Pulmonary wedge pressure readings are not usually necessary. Elevations in central venous pressure (CVP) should be treated with diuretics. Intravenous beta-blockers such as metoprolol may be required for tachycardia. However extreme caution must be used because of their negative inotropic effect. They should be avoided in women in frank pulmonary edema. Analgesia in the form of an epidural needs to be administered with due care and consultant anesthetic involvement is imperative.

Induction of labor is often considered in such patients to allow for insertion of lines, and to plan for all relevant senior staff to be available for labor and delivery. Often patients are on twice daily LMWH preparations, and induction of labor allows the heparin dose to be omitted prior to the onset of labor, thereby allowing the use of regional anesthesia which is very useful for pain control and hence prevention of maternal tachycardia.

In the event of an obstetric indication, or if there is significant maternal compromise or severe disease, a Cesarean section should be performed. Delivery should be planned and is often carried out in operating theatres with access to cardiothoracic facilities.

A dilute infusion of 5 units of syntocinon is used for the third stage. In the event of a postpartum hemorrhage, ergometrine can be used. Misoprostol is useful as an efficient uterine contractor. Thromboprophylaxis should be continued postpartum when there are no bleeding concerns.

Prognosis

There is a highly variable outcome that may not always be predicted by the initial severity of the left ventricular systolic dysfunction or dilatation. Patients may improve with treatment and return to normal (50%), improve slowly and be left with a degree of LV impairment which may over years improve, or may deteriorate despite full medical intervention and require heart transplant. Cardiomyopathy is the cause of almost a quarter of cardiac maternal deaths. In one study, the five-year survival was 94% but data from this study are likely to be over-reassuring as half of the patients with a diagnosis of PPCM had myocarditis on endomyocardial biopsy.

Subsequent pregnancy

Such women should have pre-pregnancy counseling where the risk of cardiac decompensation and maternal death should be discussed frankly.

In those with persistent LV dysfunction or dilatation 6 months after the initial diagnosis of PPCM, pregnancy should be actively discouraged as the risk of worsening heart failure is 50% and maternal death 25%. Adequate contraception should be used such as the intra-uterine progestogen-only system or the subdermal progestogen-only implant.

It is difficult to predict the outcome of a subsequent pregnancy in those whose LV function returns to normal. The contractile reserve may be diminished and this may only become apparent with the hemodynamic stress of a future pregnancy. A study using modified dobutamine stress echocardiography has shown that women who have 'recovered' with normal LVEF on standard echocardiography have impaired contractile reserve suggesting an increased risk of deterioration in a future pregnancy. There will be a few women who will tolerate another pregnancy, but it is currently not possible to identify this group. Approximately 20% will develop cardiac failure.

If the cardiac function has returned to normal and the woman wishes to embark on another pregnancy, she should have full hospital combined obstetric and cardiology care. A baseline echocardiogram should be performed. At booking it is essential to ensure that teratogenic medications are discontinued and replaced as necessary. If the pregnancy is unplanned consideration should be given to termination. Echocardiography should be arranged at regular intervals. If clinical or echocardiographic deterioration occurs, serious consideration should be given to discontinuation of the pregnancy either as a termination of pregnancy or as a preterm delivery.

Other dilated cardiomyopathies

These may be idiopathic or related to other conditions such as SLE (see Table 2.5). Women with known impaired LV function from any cause have high-risk pregnancies because they may be unable to meet the demands for an increased cardiac output and deterioration in LV function may occur in pregnancy. In patients with idiopathic dilated cardiomyopathy (DCM) outside pregnancy, their three-year survival falls from 92% in patients with an ejection fraction of greater than 40% to 71% in patients with an ejection fraction of less than 30%. These risks are higher than the mortality risk from peripartum cardiomyopathy. Pregnancy is contraindicated if the patient is New

Table 2.5 Causes of dilated cardiomyopathy

Group	Examples
Infections	Viral, e.g. coxsackie B, HIV, Ebstein–Barr virus, varicella, echovirus, measles, mumps, polio Other: bacterial, e.g. TB; rickettsia; parasites; fungi
Neuromuscular	Muscular dystrophies
Nutritional deficiencies	Niacin, thiamine, selenium deficiencies, Kwashiorkor
Connective tissue diseases	Rheumatoid arthritis, systemic lupus erythematosus, dermatomyositis
Vascular	Kawasaki disease
Hematological	Thalassemia, sickle cell disease, iron deficiency anemia
Drugs	Alcohol, chloroquine, iron overload, cyclophosphamide
Endocrine	Hypo- and hyperthyroidism, hypoparathyroidism, phaeochromocytoma
Metabolic	Hemochromatosis, glycogen storage diseases

York Heart Association (NYHA) grade 3-4 (see Table 2.1) or if Left Ventricular Ejection Fraction (LVEF) is less than 30%.

Acquired valvular heart disease

Mitral valve prolapse

This is predominantly a benign condition that should not cause concern in pregnancy. An echocardiogram should be performed to exclude mitral regurgitation. If present, antibiotic prophylaxis against bacterial endocarditis is required (see Table 2.8).

Rheumatic heart disease

In young women most cases of acquired valvular heart disease are due to rheumatic heart disease, or previous endocarditis. Of these, mitral stenosis is the most common and potentially the most likely to cause maternal and fetal compromise.

Stenotic heart lesions

In mitral stenosis, the restriction in outflow from the left atrium results in higher left atrial pressures, left atrial enlargement and eventually right sided heart failure. The reduced blood to the left ventricle causes stroke volume to be reduced. A compensatory tachycardia occurs to maintain cardiac output. This however

will reduce the time for filling of the left ventricle in diastole, and results in further increases in left atrial pressure. Thus a vicious circle is begun, ultimately causing pulmonary edema and PH. Left atrial dilatation predisposes to atrial arrythmias.

Deterioration in pregnancy may occur due to a number of factors including the physiological increase in vascular volume that is maximal at around 20-24 weeks gestation, autotransfusion after delivery of the placenta, iatrogenic fluid infusions, or related to further tachycardia which may be due to pain at delivery, exercise, anxiety, intercurrent infection or arrythmias.

Pre-pregnancy advice This is essential for women with valvular heart disease. It allows for a full cardiological clinical and echocardiographic assessment prior to embarking on pregnancy. The following points should be considered

1. Is surgical or interventional treatment of valve lesions required pre-pregnancy to optimize maternal and fetal well-being in pregnancy?
2. Is adaptation of potentially teratogenic medication required prior to pregnancy?
3. Is pregnancy contraindicated?

Pregnancy is absolutely contraindicated in women with associated PH, and those with two or more risk factors (see below), due to maternal death rates of 30-60%. Fetal and neonatal risks are also higher. Such women should be given adequate contraception such as a subcutaneous progesterone implant.

Assessment of the degree of cardiac compromise should be made in the remainder. Those women exhibiting any of the risk factors below should be advised of the higher rates of adverse maternal events including pulmonary edema, sustained brady- or tachyarrhythmias requiring treatment, stroke, cardiac arrest or death:

- Reduced left ventricular systolic function with ejection fractions of < 40%.
- Left heart obstruction – aortic or mitral stenosis with valve areas of < 1.5 cm^2 or < 2.0 cm^2, respectively.
- Previous cardiovascular events including heart failure, transient ischemic attacks or stroke.
- Reduced functional capacity: disease of NYHA class II or higher (see Table 2.1).

The absolute risks of these adverse events are 4% in women with no risk factors, 27% with one and 62% with two or more risk factors. The fetal and neonatal risks (preterm delivery, intrauterine growth restriction, respiratory distress syndrome, intraventricular hemorrhage and death) are increased in those with left heart obstruction and NYHA class II or higher disease.

Surgical intervention with either balloon valvuloplasty or valve replacement pre-conception (especially if NYHA class III or IV, or mitral valve area < 1 cm²), will change the risk factor profile, allowing many of these women to undergo a relatively less complicated future pregnancy and labor than those treated medically.

Women should be advised to give up smoking and to start folic acid preconceptionally.

Booking visit Arrangements should be made for full hospital care with combined obstetric and cardiological input. A baseline echocardiogram, ECG and U+E should be performed. The ECG may show right axis deviation and P mitrale.

If the pregnancy is unplanned, detailed assessment of functional capacity, left ventricular function, degree of valvular obstruction and history of heart failure or embolic events should be made to see whether the pregnancy can continue or termination should be advised.

Antenatal care A combined assessment with a cardiologist or obstetric physician should be made each trimester at least, and more frequently if clinical deterioration occurs. Although routine echocardiography is unnecessary, it should be performed if there is any change in function.

With mitral stenosis, the heart rate should be controlled with beta-blockers which will allow more filling of the left ventricle in diastole and hence reduces the already elevated pressure in the left atrium. The benefits of this far outweigh the small risk of fetal growth restriction with beta-blockers.

The onset of palpitations warrants a 24-h ECG and echocardiography to establish the degree of heart chamber enlargement and to exclude mural thrombus. If an arrhythmia is detected it should be treated medically or by DC cardioversion (see later). Such a patient should be fully anticoagulated with treatment doses of LMWH.

Pulmonary edema should be treated with oxygen and loop diuretics. Diamorphine will assist in reducing anxiety. A CXR usually shows a small heart with an enlarged left atrium, and pulmonary congestion.

Further deterioration despite optimal drug treatment may require surgical intervention in pregnancy. Percutanous balloon valvuloplasty of mitral and aortic valves has been performed in the second trimester with good outcome. Mitral valvotomy is best done using transesophageal echocardiography which

eliminates the need for radiation. There is a 1% risk of major complications with this procedure which include dislodging of thrombi, cracking of a stenotic valve resulting in regurgitation which may be severe enough to require immediate valve replacement, and death. Comparatively, closed mitral valvotomy has a 3% maternal complication rate, which rises to 5% with open valvotomy. Fetal mortality is 5-15% with closed valvotomy increasing threefold if the procedure is open. The success of open valve replacements in pregnancy for severe mitral stenosis is similar to the non pregnant state, but the stillbirth rate is 10-30%.

Delivery Antibiotic prophylaxis should be administered to prevent bacterial endocarditis (see Table 2.8).

Vaginal delivery should be the aim unless there is an obstetric indication for Cesarean section. The 'cardiac position' is best adopted with the legs lower than the abdomen. Lithotomy and supine positions should be avoided. An epidural will provide adequate analgesia and will allow an instrumental delivery to be performed in the second stage. Those with moderate or severe mitral stenosis should ideally have invasive monitoring with an arterial line and CVP. Critical mitral stenosis may require pulmonary arterial (PA) catheterization though this has to be balanced with the risks of leaving a catheter in the PA in a pro-thrombotic patient. Pushing causes rises in the heart rate that may not be tolerated and hence assisted vaginal delivery is often performed.

A dilute infusion of syntocinon should be administered for the third stage (see peripartum cardiomyopathy). A degree of blood loss is tolerated well as it is the autotransfusion just after delivery which often precipitates pulmonary edema in those with critical mitral stenosis.

Regurgitant valve disease The systemic vasodilation and tachycardia that occurs in pregnancy reduces the regurgitant flow of blood allowing pregnancy to be tolerated far better than in those with stenotic valvular lesions. Arrythmias can however result in pulmonary oedema, and severe regurgitation with ventricular decompensation may cause problems.

Artificial heart valves

Bioprostheses are superior to mechanical (metal) prostheses in all aspects except durability. They are less thrombogenic with reduced thromboembolism rates and hence do not require anticoagulation. The 10-year mortality in women with bioprosthetic valves is lower than with mechanical valves despite the re-operations required when bioprostheses require replacement. It is the mandatory anticoagulation requirement of mechanical valves that complicates pregnancy. Pregnancy in a woman with a metal valve is associated with a maternal mortality rate of 1-4% with death usually as a result of thrombus formation on the valve. The thrombotic risk varies and is out-lined in Table 2.6.

There are four regimes for anticoagulation in preg-nant women with mechanical heart valves:

1. Warfarin throughout pregnancy and unfraction-ated heparin (UFH) or LMWH close to term.
2. Warfarin throughout pregnancy except weeks 6-12 and near term when UFH or LMWH is used.
3. UFH throughout pregnancy.
4. Dose adjusted LMWH throughout pregnancy maintaining anti-Xa level at 0.5-1.2 U/mL

Table 2.6 Thrombotic risk with mechanical heart valves

	Risk of thrombosis
Type of mechanical valve	Single tilting disc valves (e.g. Bjork Shiley) > Ball and cage valves (e.g. Starr–Edwards) > Bileaflet valves (e.g. carbomedics)
Position of mechanical valve	Mitral > aortic
Number of mechanical valve	2 > 1
Past history of embolic events	Yes > no

Table 2.7 shows the fetal and maternal effects of these regimes, which are all associated with signifi-cant risks. In general, warfarin is safer for the mother but more harmful for the fetus, whereas heparin is the converse. Warfarin and UFH have similar fetal wastage of one-third of all pregnancies. Warfarin is more protective against thrombosis and subsequent maternal death than UFH, but is associated with sig-nificant embryopathy in surviving babies. The risks of congenital malformations and fetal loss are dose dependent, being significantly higher if doses of greater than 5 mg are required to maintain an inter-national normalized ratio of greater than 2.0. Although heparins do not cross the placenta, UFH is associated with a 2% incidence of maternal osteoporosis and thrombocytopenia.

LMWH is an attractive option as it has consider-ably less maternal side effects of osteoporosis (0.04%) and thrombocytopenia than UFH, less fetal wastage and is easier to use. LMWHs have been used in preg-nancy in women with mechanical heart valves, but are not licensed for use and are specifically not rec-ommended by the manufacturers as anticoagulants in patients with prosthetic heart valves. This was fol-lowing a series of maternal deaths resulting from valve thromboses in women who had fixed dosing of LMWH in pregnancy without monitoring anti-Xa levels. More recent reports where dose adjusted regimes have been used are much more encouraging. Before using LMWHs, careful consideration should be given to the individual's thrombotic risk taking the factors in Table 2.6 into consideration as well as the presence of atrial fibrillation and impaired left ventricular function. If used, an initial therapeutic dose is advisable which is adjusted to maintain the anti-Xa level between 0.5-1.2 U/mL.

Table 2.7 Fetal and maternal risk with different anticoagulation regimes in women with metal heart valves

Anticoagulant regime	Fetal risks			Maternal risks	
	Spontaneous miscarriage (%)	Embryopathy (%)	Overall fetal loss[b] (%)	Thrombosis (%)	Maternal death (%)
Warfarin[a]	24.7	6.4	33.6	3.9	1.8
UFH (dose-adjusted)	25	0	43.8	25	6.7
UFH (<6-12 weeks) + warfarin[a]	14.7	0	16.3	9.2	4.2
LMWH[c]	7.4	0	12.35	12.35	1.23

[a]Warfarin replaced by unfractionated heparin (UFH) at term.
[b]Spontaneous miscarriages, stillbirths and neonatal deaths.
[c]Only 10% of patients were dose-adjusted according to anti-Xa levels.

Every case should ideally be evaluated pre pregnancy and the woman fully counseled concerning the risks of each treatment regimen. If she has a small Bjork Shiley valve in the mitral position with a previous history of embolic events or arrhythmia and requiring <5 mg warfarin daily then counseling should be directive towards warfarin throughout pregnancy. For a woman with a carbomedics valve in the aortic position and no history of previous embolic or arrhythmic events requiring >5 mg of warfarin then LMWH throughout pregnancy with careful monitoring would seem a reasonable option. Often the decision is not so straightforward and the woman may be unwilling to contemplate any risk of warfarin embryopathy especially if she has had a previously affected fetus.

Delivery
If warfarin is used, it should be stopped about 10 days pre-delivery to allow for clearance of the drug from the fetal circulation. Unfractionated heparin or LMWH treatment dose can be used until delivery. In labor or during induction, heparin should be stopped, but recommenced after delivery. Conversion back to warfarin should be delayed for at least 3 days postpartum to minimize the risk of obstetric hemorrhage.

The effects of unfractionated heparin can be reversed with protamine sulfate. This also partially reverses the effects of the longer acting LMWHs. Warfarin is reversed with fresh frozen plasma and vitamin K. Such agents may be required if bleeding occurs or if urgent delivery is necessary in the fully anticoagulated patient. It is best to avoid vitamin K if possible as anticoagulation with warfarin postpartum then becomes very difficult.

In the event of a valve thrombus occurring in pregnancy, thrombolytic treatment should be used. The risks of this treatment causing embolism, bleeding or placental abruption are lower than the risks associated with cardiothoracic surgery.

Antibiotic prophylaxis is mandatory to cover delivery in all women with artificial heart valves.

ENDOCARDITIS PROPHYLAXIS

Infective endocarditis is not common in pregnancy, but can have fatal consequences for both mother and fetus. The risk lies with any procedure causing bacteremia and hence can occur antenatally as well as in labor. Indeed most maternal deaths from bacterial endocarditis in the Confidential Enquiries have not occurred in association with delivery. A propagation of bacteria occurs on a heart valve, mural endocar-dium or on implanted prosthetic material in the heart and can embolize to the pulmonary vasculature or systemically. Alternatively abscesses or fistulae can occur in the heart or valve prostheses can dehisce.

The indications for antibiotic prophylaxis are given in Table 2.3 and the recommended antibiotics in Table 2.8. Antibiotics should be given before a bacteremia is expected. If antibiotic prophylaxis is not given before this event, antibiotics may help a late clearance if given intravenously within 2-3 h.

When to give endocarditis prophylaxis

Prophylaxis against bacterial endocarditis should be given when any obstetric procedure is performed in the presence of infection. The vagina contains commensals some of which can cause systemic infection and endocarditis in the presence of ruptured membranes. Screening for vaginal infection is not routinely performed, hence prophylaxis should be given to women who have ruptured their membranes, at the onset of labor, or before Cesarean section. Insertion of cervical cerclage and urinary catheterization should also be covered. Procedures not requiring prophylaxis include choriovillous sampling, amniocentesis, vaginal examination, transvaginal ultrasound scanning and insertion of regional analgesia.

AORTIC DISSECTION

Rupture of the thoracic aorta and its branches has resulted in 19% of cardiac deaths in the UK 1991–2002.

Risk factors are Marfan syndrome with known aortic root dilatation (see above) and hypertension. More recently bicuspid aortic valves have been implicated.

Table 2.8 Bacterial endocarditis prophylaxis regimens

Group	Penicillin allergy	½–1 h before procedure	6 h later
High risk	No	Amoxycillin 2 g i.v. + Gentamicin 1.5 mg/kg i.v.	Amoxycillin 1 g p.o.
	Yes	Vancomycin 1 g i.v. over 1-2 hr + Gentamicin 1.5 mg/kg i.v.	–
Moderate risk	No	Amoxycillin 2 g i.v.	Amoxycillin 1 g p.o.
	Yes	Vancomycin 1 g i.v. over 1-2 h	–

In pregnancy half of all reported aortic dissections are in women with Marfan syndrome. Most dissections will be Type A, which involve the ascending aorta with 88% of these occurring antenatally and 22% being fatal. Only 20% are Type B involving only the descending aorta which is not associated with previous aortic root enlargement or aneurysm.

The risk of Type A aortic dissection occurring in pregnant patients with Marfan syndrome increases with:

- Aortic root dilatation >4 cm.
- Progressive aortic root dilatation in pregnancy.
- Gestational age (most common in the third trimester).
- Maternal age.
- Family history of dissection.

However women with Marfan have a 1% risk of dissection during pregnancy, even in the presence of a normal sized aorta. Even women with no pre-existing cardiac disease can dissect, thought to be due to the increased cardiovascular stress in the aortic wall and the hormonal changes, which affect collagen tissue.

Pathology

Pregnancy causes alterations in the arterial wall with fragmentation in the reticulin fibers, and reduction in acid mucopolysaccharides and elastic fibers. When occurring in a woman with an inherited or acquired defect in the arterial wall, dissection may result. In Marfan syndrome there is a mutation within the fibrillin gene on chromosome 15q21 which often affects the cardiovascular system and predisposes to aortic root dilatation.

Preconception counseling

Women with Marfan syndrome or BAVD where the aortic root diameter is >4.5 cm should be offered pre-pregnancy aortic root replacement. The use of a composite graft (i.e. an aortic root replacement with an aortic valve replacement) will require anticoagulation with warfarin which can be changed to heparin in pregnancy (see artificial valves). Advice is less clear-cut for those with aortic roots of 4-4.5 cm.

Antenatal management

Where there is aortic root dilatation > 4 cm or a progression of aortic root enlargement, beta-blockers should be commenced. There is a small risk of intra-uterine growth restriction which is far outweighed by the benefits. Hypertension must be aggressively controlled as otherwise this can lead to intimal tears.

Echocardiography should be performed monthly, and delivery considered if the aortic root progressively dilates.

A patient having an aortic dissection will have sudden onset tearing chest pain radiating to the back associated with dyspnoea. Signs include new onset aortic regurgitation murmur and as the dissection advances, MI, CVA and hypotension. A dissection of the descending aorta may have few symptoms. Diagnosis is made with echocardiography, the transoesophageal route being far more sensitive, or CT.

Delivery and treatment of aortic dissection

In those with aortic root dilatation or aneurysm, it is imperative to prevent peaks of hypertension which may result in aortic dissection. The safest mode of delivery in such patients is by elective Cesarean section under regional blockade. Aortic repair should be performed postnatally as the risk of dissection remains.

If there is a Type A dissection, immediate surgery should ensue. In general after 28-30 weeks gestation a Cesarean section under GA should be followed by cardiac surgery which will usually involve replacement of the aortic root, aortic valve and reimplantation of the coronary arteries. Where the gestation is earlier than 28 weeks, aortic repair with the fetus in utero is recommended if there is no distal aortic involvement. Cardiopulmonary bypass will be required. A high-flow, high-pressure normothermic perfusion and a perfusion index of 3.0 is considered to be the safest for the fetus. Hypothermia can cause a fetal bradycardia resulting in hypoxic ischemic encephalopathy or even fetal death.

If there is associated distal involvement of the aorta in a Type A dissection, the fetus will need to be delivered as hypothermia is necessary for the open distal repair. It has been suggested that selective antegrade cerebral perfusion for maternal brain protection and moderate hypothermia (28 °C) can be used in this circumstance at gestations less than 28 weeks with the fetus left in utero. However, as this technique requires stopping cardiopulmonary bypass whilst the distal aorta is repaired, the fetus will not be perfused and hence this method is not recommended.

In those with a Type B dissection, conservative medical treatment should be used in the absence of rupture or hypotension. Delivery of the fetus should be considered as the fetal mortality is high. If there are any complications with a Type B dissection, immediate surgical intervention should proceed with delivery of the fetus and aortic repair.

ISCHEMIC HEART DISEASE

While acute coronary syndrome (ACS) is rare in pregnancy, as women delay childbirth until their late 30s and 40s, coronary artery problems and myocardial infarction (MI) are becoming more common pregnancy. Recent data from a retrospective study in the USA identified a threefold increase in the incidence of MI during pregnancy from 1 in 73 400 pregnancies in 1990 to 1 in 24 600 in 2000.

Atherosclerosis is the predominant pathogenesis outside pregnancy, whereas in pregnancy coronary artery dissection and embolus in the absence of atheroma are more frequent. In the last Confidential Enquiry into maternal mortality, 18% of cardiac deaths were from MI with 63% of these secondary to spontaneous coronary dissection rather than plaque rupture. There is still on-going debate about the role of pregnancy-associated plasma protein A (PAPP-A) in ACS, which is a potential proatherosclerotic metalloproteinase.

Diagnosis outside pregnancy relies on a combination of history, ECG changes and elevation of cardiac enzymes. ECG changes may require careful review as there is an incidence of up to 50% of abnormalities of unknown significance in women undergoing Cesarean section. Troponin I (TnT) and Troponin T (TnT) are thought not to be increased above the upper limit of normal both peri- and postpartum in healthy pregnant women and TnI is not affected by anesthesia or Cesarean section. It does however increase in pre-eclampsia, pulmonary embolism, atrial fibrillation and myocarditis.

While some drugs used in ACS are known to be safe in pregnancy (low dose aspirin, nitrates, heparin, beta-blockers and opiates) there are few data for the use of clopidogrel. Animal data appear promising, however experience is limited to isolated case reports. Statins and ACE inhibitors are contraindicated because of teratogenic side effects. There are no published data on either the safety or efficacy of GIIb/IIIa inhibitors, such as abciximab (antiplatelet agents used in the management of ACS).

Cases of MI during pregnancy have been described in a variety of patients however, all appear to be associated with a high maternal and fetal mortality. Coronary angiography should not be withheld in pregnant patients. Percutaneous coronary intervention may provide a better alternative to thrombolysis in these situations as it is associated with less bleeding risk and also allows management of spontaneous dissections with stent implantation. However, stent implantation may be associated with an increased risk of coronary dissection in a vulnerable vessel.

While evidence is scarce, it appears that women who have had ACS prior to conception should ideally delay pregnancy for a year after their event. These women should preferably be revascularized prior to conception or managed very aggressively if they present in pregnancy. Whether revascularized or medically managed, all women should ideally undergo stress testing prior to pregnancy to assess their residual ischemic burden so they may be best advised about the safety of pregnancy. Coronary artery bypass surgery (CABG) in pregnancy, has no increase in maternal risk compared to non-pregnant women, however is associated with a high fetal mortality.

Delivery is often influenced both by the maternal state as well as coexisting conditions such as diabetes and pre-eclampsia. If there is no subsequent angina, vaginal delivery is recommended. Agents that increase blood pressure such as beta-agonists, and ergot derivatives are best avoided or used in small doses.

ARRHYTHMIAS

The management of arrhythmias in pregnancy provides a complex dilemma for the physician. Many cardiologists do not have extensive experience in treating these women and the knowledge that therapy may have an adverse effect on the fetus is intimidating. Diagnosing arrhythmias with Holter monitoring can often be fruitless but treating arrhythmias blind means exposing the fetus to potentially unnecessary drugs. Once diagnosed, arrhythmia treatment requires a balance between maternal symptom control while avoiding or reducing any fetal complications from anti-arrhythmic medication. While there have been no documented maternal deaths from primary arrhythmias in the last UK Confidential Enquiry into maternal mortality, 9% of deaths were defined as sudden adult death syndrome, which raises the possibility of death from a primary arrhythmia. In women with heart disease arrhythmia is one of the five independent predictors of having a cardiac event during the pregnancy and should therefore be treated seriously.

Incidence of arrhythmia during pregnancy

The incidence of new onset and pre-existing arrhythmias are increased in pregnancy. As cardiac arrhythmias can be identified on Holter recordings in up to 60% of normal people under 40, it is not surprising that the antenatal clinic sees its fair share of palpitations. The increase in circulating hormones and cardiac physiological changes, may explain why some women will present for the first time in pregnancy. The incidence of serious arrhythmias remains low in pregnancy despite the 25% increase in heart rate (HR).

There is no significant increase in arrhythmias in laboring women apart from isolated atrial premature beats (APBs) which can occur in up to 90% of women.

Cause of arrhythmias

The main causes of arrhythmias are similar in pregnant and non-pregnant women. Theories explaining the increase in arrhythmia frequency in pregnancy include: heightened awareness; increased plasma catecholamine concentrations and adrenergic receptor sensitivity; atrial stretch and increased end-diastolic volumes due to intravascular volume expansion; and hormonal and emotional changes. Patients with known underlying structural heart disease have a higher incidence of arrhythmias and many patients may already have a diagnosis prior to conception. Increased ectopy is benign and generally well tolerated but may trigger a more significant arrhythmia in a susceptible individual.

Symptoms

Palpitations, breathlessness, chest pain or pre-syncope may occur with arrhythmias. In the third trimester, patients may become more symptomatic with activity and thus even minor arrhythmias may present with these symptoms. An accurate history of the onset and offset of arrhythmias as well as the frequency, duration and character of the attacks aids the diagnosis of an arrhythmia and helps distinguish it from the physiological symptoms of advancing pregnancy.

Diagnosis

- ECG
- 24- or 48-h Holter monitor
- patient activated event recorder
- implantable loop recorders

In a symptomatic patient with palpitations, an arrhythmia must be distinguished from physiological awareness of the heart beat. An ECG is essential, although the paroxysmal, short-lived nature of most palpitations means they may have subsided by the time the patient reaches an ECG machine. If an ECG is obtained, the normal changes due to pregnancy should be remembered (see earlier). If not a 24-h or 48-h Holter ECG may be necessary, although capture

may still be difficult. An accurate symptom diary is necessary which can be related to any abnormality on the Holter.

Asymptomatic arrhythmias should not be treated unless felt to be life threatening.

Less frequent episodes or those which have evaded detection are best documented using a patient activated event recorder. These come in a number of models: a continuous Holter recording; a solid state recorder placed on the chest when the patient is having an attack; or a wristwatch with a recording electrode. These devices record approximately 30 s of ECG which can either be stored or transmitted down a household telephone line to a central recording analyzer. They have the advantage of recording a sequential number of events as well as the ability to make remote diagnosis away from the hospital.

Finally, implantable loop recorders are increasingly being used to make diagnoses particularly in patients with unexplained syncope. There is no experience of these devices in pregnancy, however there is no theoretical reason why they would not be able to be used.

Types of tachyarrhythmia

Once an arrhythmia has been captured then it is important to correctly interpret the ECG.

Broad complex tachycardias

A broad complex tachycardia is likely to be either ventricular tachycardia (VT) or a supraventricular tachycardia (SVT) (Fig. 2.1) with aberrant conduction.

VT in the structurally abnormal heart

Cardiomyopathy
Those with cardiomyopathy, arrhythmias are the commonest cause of death outside pregnancy. Those with an ejection fraction under 35% post myocardial infarction are candidates for automatic implantable cardio-defibrillator (AICD) implantation. The data in the non-ischemic cardiomyopathies are less robust.

Hypertrophic cardiomyopathy (HCM) Non-sustained ventricular tachycardia (NSVT) is found in approximately 25% of adult patients with HCM although sustained monomorphic VT occurs in less than 1% of patients Studies suggest that VT is the single best indicator of risk of sudden death in patients with hypertrophic obstructive cardiomyopathy.

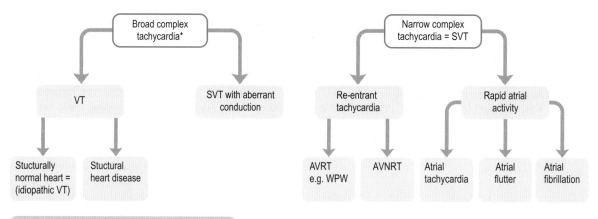

Figure 2.1 Pathological arrhythmias.

Arrhythmogenic right ventricular cardiomyopathy
Arrhythmogenic right ventricular cardiomyopathy (ARVD) is a disease characterized by progressive fibrofatty replacement of right ventricular myocardium, initially with regional and later global involvement of the right ventricle. It presents in adolescents or young adults with a mean age of presentation in their mid-30s with a male predominance of up to 80%. The disease can be familial with an autosomal dominant inheritance and incomplete penetrance. Presentation is usually with arrhythmias, mainly ventricular and sudden death is common, particularly in the young. It can be diagnosed in its earlier stages using MRI and later by echocardiography. Those women diagnosed because of presentation with ventricular arrhythmias often have implantable defibrillators already inserted at the time of pregnancy

Long QT syndromes   In one study of 111 pregnancies, women with long QT had no increase in risk of cardiac events in pregnancy, but they did have a significant risk in the postpartum period. There is concern that the increase in heart rate after delivery coupled with the stress of caring for an infant may increase the risk of torsade. It is therefore imperative that women should continue their treatment (usually beta-blockers) throughout the pregnancy and puerperium.

Idiopathic VT

The incidence of VT in women of childbearing age is low unless they have significant underlying heart disease. VT in a young woman with a structurally normal heart, is more likely to be an idiopathic VT, which is associated with a good prognosis and low likelihood of degradation to ventricular fibrillation (VF). Right ventricular outflow tract (RVOT) tachycardia, as identified by left bundle branch block (LBBB), inferior axis and palpitations, is more common in women and states of hormone flux are the most common trigger. It is important to take a careful family history of collapse or sudden cardiac death and to review the 12 lead ECG when in sinus rhythm to confirm the patient does not have a condition associated with prolonged QT interval.

Supraventricular tachycardia

Premature atrial beats can be found in 50% of pregnant women but are generally well tolerated. In patients with documented SVT, sustained arrhythmias are infrequent (2 to 3 per 1000 pregnancies), but patients with paroxysmal SVT have exacerbation in 20% of pregnancies. New onset supraventricular tachycardias are also increased during pregnancy. Whilst SVTs are narrow complex because ventricular activation is via the Hiss–Purkinje system, it is important to identify the differences between them and not treat them all as 'SVTs'. They can be broadly divided into two types, those that use an additional connection between the atria and ventricles that set up a re-entrant circuit, and those that result from rapid, abnormal atrial activity (Fig. 2.1).

There are two re-entrant tachycardias: those that have an accessory pathway outside the node atrioventricular re-entrant tachycardia (AVRT), and those that have the additional pathway within the AV node, atrioventricular nodal re-entrant tachycardia (AVNRT). Both these arrhythmias are common with AVNRT being more common in women. The duration and frequency of attacks differs between patients and, in some, attacks are precipitated by exercise. The rate is usually between 130 and 250 beats per minute and is influenced by the sympathetic nervous system. As the circulating impulse re-enters the atria after ventricular activation, there will be no normal p waves, though each QRS complex may be followed by an inverted p wave (retrograde p). If the tachycardia is fast, this may not be detectable on the surface ECG.

The atrial arrhythmias are divided into atrial tachycardia, flutter and fibrillation. The mechanism is confined to the atria and the AV node merely transmits the impulses. Atrial fibrillation is the most easily diagnosed arrhythmia because of its irregular features, however this irregularity may be difficult to see with rapid rates. The typical 'sawtooth' flutter waves are not always seen in flutter especially at rates over 100 however a regular ECG at a rate of 150 should alert the clinician to think about atrial flutter with 2:1 conduction. The difference between atrial flutter and tachycardia is that in the latter, the atrial rate is slower therefore the 'sawtooth' pattern is not seen. It maybe therefore be difficult to distinguish atrial tachycardia from the re-entrant tachycardias.

The diagnosis of an SVT is often helped by adenosine, which can be safely given in pregnancy. One of the problems of using this drug is that, blocking the AV node, may encourage conduction down an accessory pathway and thus accelerate an arrhythmia. As such, experienced personnel should give it in a monitored area with equipment available for resuscitation.

Electrophysiological studies in pregnancy

While electrophysiological studies (EPS) are important in making accurate diagnoses of arrhythmias as well as providing the mapping for the curative radiofrequency ablation, they are often not required as an emergency. The vast majority of arrhythmias can be managed with anti-arrhythmic drugs alone and certainly for the duration of the pregnancy. They are often long procedures and involve a significant amount of radiation exposure. As such, both from the logistics of a pregnant women lying flat for many hours and the X-ray dose to the fetus even if screened, the experience of EPS studies in pregnancy is limited.

There are however case reports of women who were refractory to medical therapy and were experiencing recurrent hemodynamically significant arrhythmias, who underwent successful pathway ablation with limited fluoroscopy.

Acute management of cardiac arrhythmias

Cardiac arrest

Cardiac arrests are rare but if they occur it is important to be aware of the differences in management of pregnant women compared to other patients. In order to optimize maternal outcome, resuscitation should proceed following established guidelines from the resuscitation council. An obstetrician and pediatrician should be involved from an early stage. In addition to the standard causes of cardiac arrest, amniotic fluid embolism, pulmonary embolism, peripartum cardiomyopathy and acute coronary or aortic dissection are important causes in pregnant or recently delivered women. Cardiac resuscitation is more difficult in a pregnant woman because of:

- aortocaval compression;
- enlarged breasts;
- splinting of the diaphragm.

In the supine position the enlarged uterus can reduce venous return by aortocaval compression. It is imperative to relieve this using sand-bags or a 'Cardiff wedge' under the right side of the patient, manual displacement of the uterus to the left or raising of the woman's right hip. Chest compression may be more difficult because of the enlarged breasts and splinting of the diaphragm. As gastric emptying is delayed in pregnancy, early intubation is recommended to prevent aspiration. After five minutes of resuscitation, the uterus should be emptied by Cesarean section. There are a number of reports where this has been associated with successful resuscitation of the mother.

DC Cardioversion

DC cardioversion is safe in all stages of pregnancy. The amniotic fluid buffers and protects the fetus, hence the amount of current reaching the fetus is small, and is associated with only a small risk of inducing fetal arrhythmias. There have been reports of the need for emergency CS because of fetal arrhythmia particularly in women who are compromised; hence the fetus should be carefully monitored before, and throughout the procedure. One case report concluded that DC cardioversion had led to sustained uterine contraction and fetal distress necessitating urgent CS, but this is rare. In the latter stages of pregnancy, some anesthetists prefer to carry out the procedure using full general anesthetic and intubation in view of the more difficult airway and increased risk of gastric aspiration. Women should be nursed in the wedged position as for a cardiac arrest, otherwise the procedure is the same as for non-pregnant women.

Sustained ventricular tachycardia

Women with sustained VT who are compromised with hypotension and circulatory collapse should be treated immediately with cardioversion. An obstetrician should be involved and the fetus should be monitored. VT with hemodynamic stability can be safely treated with anti-arrhythmics. The most appropriate area to nurse the woman is often in the coronary care unit (CCU) or intensive care unit (ITU), which are familiar with the use of the drugs, and where appropriate monitoring and surveillance systems are in place. Lignocaine is the drug of choice because it is both effective and has been extensively used in pregnancy because of its local anesthetic properties. It is known to cross the placenta and result in fetal concentrations around half that of the mother but no fetal adverse effects have been reported. Oral beta-blockers have been successfully used in many pregnancies particularly in women with mitral stenosis or aortic dilatation. Sotalol and procainamide have also been reported to be safe in pregnancy. Disopyramide should be avoided as it has been reported to stimulate uterine contractions. As the efficacy of intravenous drugs in terminating arrhythmias is 50% or less, alternative methods have been explored. Reports are available of successful arrhythmia termination with anti-tachycardia pacing following the use of a floatation wire thus avoiding the radiation.

Re-entrant supraventricular tachycardias

Vagal maneuvers are easily and quickly administered and should be attempted first while drugs or anesthetists are being sought. Their success ranges widely from 20 to 90% and some studies report a greater success with carotid sinus massage, whilst others favour the Valsalva maneuver. The re-entrant tachycardias using the node (AVNRT) are more likely to be successfully terminated than those that involve an accessory pathway. An ECG should be used to monitor the effect of therapies as even when unsuccessful, valuable diagnostic information can be gained for the electrophysiologist.

If unsuccessful, termination with IV adenosine should be attempted. Adenosine is a naturally occurring purine nucleotide that transiently depresses sinus node activity and slows atrioventricular (AV) conduction. It has an efficacy of nearly 100% for terminating SVTs when given as a rapid bolus injection through a large bore cannula or central line. As the half-life of this drug is less than 10 seconds, it is rapidly metabolized by the maternal metabolism and has no appreciable effect on the fetus. Adenosine has been shown to be safe and effective in pregnancy. Most women respond to doses between 6 and 12 mg.

Verapamil is an effective second line treatment for the treatment of SVTs and can be used in doses up to 10 mg without effecting fetal heart rate. It should be given in 5 mg doses and repeated after 5 min if the first bolus is unsuccessful. Fetal distress has been associated with verapamil induced maternal hypotension.

Beta-blockers are the drugs of choice in women with Wolff–Parkinson-White syndrome (WPW), as AV nodal blocking drugs may accelerate conduction through the accessory pathway and cause a deterioration in maternal condition.

As with all arrhythmias, those associated with hemodynamic compromise should be treated with DC cardioversion.

Atrial fibrillation and flutter

These arrhythmias are uncommon in young women. If seen in pregnancy they are usually associated with congenital or valvular heart disease as well as metabolic disturbances such as thyrotoxicosis or electrolyte disturbance. Though they may be well tolerated in conditions other than severe mitral stenosis, it is advantageous to terminate the arrhythmia to avoid the need for anticoagulation, particularly as pregnancy is a pro-thrombotic state. Quinidine was thought to be safe in pregnancy, but now it is rarely used outside pregnancy due to the risk of torsade de pointes. Procainamide is a safe alternative. Beta-blockers, verapamil and digoxin can all be used to control ventricular rate. Mexiletine, sotalol and amiodarone (in the acute management) have also been used in small numbers of cases with success.

Chronic management

Drug treatment in pregnancy

The decision to treat a woman for chronic arrhythmias depends upon the frequency, duration and tolerability of the arrhythmia. It is a balance between the benefit of arrhythmia reduction or termination and the maternal and fetal side effects of any drug therapy. The smallest recommended dose should be used initially and be accompanied by regular monitoring of maternal and fetal clinical condition. Various drugs have been used to terminate fetal arrhythmias which provide useful data, although reports are predominantly case reports or small case series. Drugs used include digoxin, adenosine, amiodarone, flecainide, procainamide, propranolol, propafenone,

quinidine, sotalol and verapamil (Table 2.9). The majority of drugs available only have class C evidence for use in pregnancy. For most women beta-blockers are first-line treatment for prophylaxis of SVT and VT in pregnancy unless they enter pregnancy already on alternative effective therapy such as flecainide. Amiodarone has the potential to cause thyroid dysfunction in the fetus and is usually therefore avoided.

Pregnancy and automatic implantable cardio-defibrillators

While the world experience is still low, with the increasing use of these devices, more reports of pregnancies in women with automatic implantable cardio-defibrillators (AICDs) are to be expected. Successful pregnancies are reported, but women with frequent

Table 2.9 Anti-arrythmic drugs

Drugs	Safety profile	Listed complications	Breastfeeding
Adenosine	Safe to use in pregnancy with no detectable effect on fetal cardiac rhythm	Pregnant women may respond to lower doses due to a reduction in adenosine deaminase	Safe as short halflife
Atropine	Unknown but has been used for resuscitation	Insufficient data	Unknown
Amiodarone	Only for short-term use in emergencies	If prolonged use; fetal hypo- and hyperthyroidism, goitre, IUGR, prematurity	Avoid
Beta-blockers	Avoid atenolol in first trimester because of concern over IUGR	IUGR, bradycardia, apnoea, hypoglycemia hyperbilirubinemia	Safe
Digoxin	Good safety profile	Miscarriage and fetal death in toxicity	Safe
Diltiazem	Too little experience to comment	Skeletal abnormalities, IUGR, fetal death	Unknown
Disopyramide	Too little data to recommend regular use	Premature uterine contractions	Unknown
Flecainide	Limited literature for treatment of maternal arrhythmias however maternal ingestion used to treat fetal SVT	Insufficient data but no reported significant complications. Concerns over its pro-arrhythmic potential in fetus have limited its use in past.	Unknown
Lignocaine	Good	Fetal distress may occur in fetal toxicity	Safe
Quinidine	Good safety profile in pregnancy however not used because of concern over safety profile in non-pregnant women	Rarely; mild uterine contractions, prem labor, neonatal TP, fetal VIIIn damage	Safe
Procainamide	Possibly as safe as quinidine short term in pregnancy	Chronic use may be associated with lupus like syndrome, GI disturbance, hypotension, agranulocytosis	Safe
Propafenone	Unknown	Insufficinet data	Unknown
Sotalol	Safe	Transient fetal bradycardia	Safe
Verapamil	Safe (first choice class IV drug)	Rapid injection may cause reduced maternal BP and fetal distress	Safe

arrhythmias require intensive management by a multidisciplinary team and often prolonged admission. One study reported a series of 44 women who underwent a pregnancy with an AICD implant in situ. They reported no increases in either device or therapy complications and no increases in the number of shocks the women received compared to pre-conception. In addition to standard AICD management, after each administered shock, monitoring of the baby with a cardiotocograph to ensure satisfactory fetal well-being may be considered.

Some groups have also reported the insertion of the AICD in women already pregnant using echocardiography to guide the positioning of the leads and avoiding radiation exposure to the fetus. AICD implantation may represent a safe alternative to medical therapy for ventricular tachycardia.

Bradyarrhythmias

Pathological bradycardia in pregnant women is rare. Some women who have physiological brady-cardia may, in the second trimester feel dizzy and their blood pressure falls, however treatment is rarely required. Congenital heart block (CHB) is rare (prevalence 1: 20 000) and the majority of these present before childbearing age. It does not usually pose a problem during the pregnancy. Temporary pacing is recommended during the delivery as the Valsalva associated with vaginal delivery increases the chance of worsening bradycardia and syncope as well as allowing for an adequate heart rate response for the increased cardiovascular stress.

Spinal anesthesia for CS can be associated with a high incidence of all grades of bradycardia (up to 13%). Rarely, symptomatic bradycardia has been attributed to aortocaval compression by the gravid uterus which responds to changing the maternal position.

In the rare case of a pregnant woman requiring a pacemaker transesophageal guided lead placement should be considered which avoids the standard X-ray screening techniques used.

Obstetric anesthetic management of the mother with cardiac disease
R. Collis

ANESTHETIC ANTENATAL ASSESSMENT AND CLASSIFICATION OF MOTHERS WITH CARDIAC DISEASE

Allocating risk associated with pregnancy and delivery for mothers with cardiac disease is based on the combination of the functional class of the New York Heart Association (NYHA) see Table 2.1 and the accurate assessment of the underlying lesion.

The NYHA classification is based purely on patient function. A careful evaluation should include recording activities such as walking up stairs and ability to carry out day-to-day activities such as shopping and housework. Formal assessment by exercise testing may occasionally be helpful in some women (e.g. ischemic heart disease).

Mothers with cardiac disease can be divided into three groups. The assessment and allocation of mothers into these groups is very important because it will determine where the mother should be looked after both during her pregnancy and delivery, and how often key members of a multidisciplinary team should see her.

Group one

These mothers (Box 2.1) should have a normal pregnancy. Operative delivery (elective or emergency Cesarean or instrumental vaginal delivery) should be based purely on obstetric indications.

These mothers should still have an early assessment and many should have one echocardiogram

---

Box 2.1 Group 1

Mothers with well-controlled and stable ischemic
   heart disease
      Good biventricular function
      No history of heart failure or pulmonary oedema
      No history of major dysrhythmias
Congenital heart disease which has been surgically
   completely corrected
      Complete closure of patent ductus arteriosis
      Complete closure of atrial or ventricular septal
         defect without residual pulmonary
         hypertension
Repaired coarctation of aorta
Small atrial or ventricular defects without a major
   shunt
Minor and asymptomatic pulmonary, aortic and
   mitral stenosis
Minor and asymptomatic mitral or aortic
   incompetence

Box 2.2 Group 2

Deteriorating NYHA: Any cardiac lesion
Continuing episodes of symptomatic ischemia
      Moderately impaired left ventricular function
         EF <40%
      Treated heart failure or pulmonary edema
      Episodes of symptomatic dysrhythmias
Palliative or partial correction of congenital heart
   disease
      Partial correction of tetralogy of Fallot
         without cyanosis
      Mustard's or Senning's procedure for
         transposition of the great vessels
Cardiomyopathy with mild to moderate ventricular
   impairment
      Congenital; e.g. hypertrophic cardiomyopathy
      Acquired; e.g. peripartum cardiomyopathy or
         secondary to viral infection or multisystem
         disease
Moderate pulmonary, aortic and mitral stenosis

---

during their pregnancy to confirm the patient's history, unless otherwise well documented. Early and rapid availability of cardiology services is therefore required.

The obstetric anesthetist should have the opportunity to see the mother at least once during her pregnancy at the beginning of the third trimester and careful plans should be documented in the notes. The basis for seeing all mothers with cardiac disease antenatally however asymptomatic is so that analgesia and anesthesia can be given without delay once in labor, especially in an emergency. Ideally there should be 24-h anesthetic and obstetric cover on the delivery suite, but anesthetic intervention either anesthesia or analgesia can usually be considered routine with the normal provisos of pregnancy.

Group two

There is an intermediate group of mothers with cardiac disease (Box 2.2) that can present with deteriorating parameters during pregnancy or delivery, but usually tolerate the physiological demands of pregnancy without major problems. These mothers can usually tolerate labor without difficulty (with the possible exceptions of asymptomatic Marfan syndrome and aortic stenosis associated with a dilated aorta > 4 cm or any dilatation in pregnancy), but the anesthetic care may need to be modified.

These mothers should be seen from the early second trimester by a multidisciplinary team, including an obstetric anesthetist, and they are best looked after in a hospital that can offer 24-hour specialist care in case of sudden cardiac problems and obstetric emergencies. Detailed anesthetic plans should be made from the early part of the third trimester with desirable analgesia, levels of monitoring and the appropriate grade of the attending anesthetist recorded.

In many situations a routine low dose epidural for labour analgesia is a safe and appropriate choice, with pulse oximetry and non-invasive blood pressure for monitoring. If a mother needs an emergency caesarean section, the different physiological demands resulting from an extensive and dense regional block, a general anesthetic or blood loss more commonly associated with emergency Cesarean delivery, often require a greater level of experience and monitoring than can routinely be provided in many smaller hospitals. The major demands on this level of service provision are problems that arise outside office hours, even if an elective Cesarean section / delivery is planned.

Group three

These mothers have a high risk of deterioration during pregnancy (Box 2.3). The mother may present in the first or the early part of the second trimester with heart failure, where a termination of pregnancy may be necessary or may need delivery, usually by Cesar-

---

Box 2.3 Group 3

Pulmonary hypertension
    Primary
    Eisenmenger's syndrome (reverse shunt with
        cyanosis and pulmonary hypertension
        associated with congenital heart disease)
    Chronic veno-occlusive disease associated
        with anti-phospholipid syndrome and other
        connective tissue diseases.
Cyanotic congenital heart disease not associated
    with pulmonary hypertension
Palliative shunts from vena cava to pulmonary
    artery
Severely impaired ventricular function EF < 30%
Severe mitral or aortic stenosis especially if
    associated with pulmonary edema, angina,
    dysrrythmias and collapse

---

ean section, early in the third trimester when the baby is viable.

A multidisciplinary team of an obstetrician, obstetric anesthetist and a physician with training in pregnancy, must assess these mothers early in pregnancy at around 20-24 weeks gestation. A pulmonary physician may need to be included if the mother has pulmonary hypertension. Flexible and ongoing assessment will be required throughout pregnancy as plans may rapidly change. The woman will need to be seen every two to four weeks in the mid-trimester of pregnancy and weekly from 30 weeks gestation. She will require monitoring (which may include invasive monitoring) in a high dependency area or intensive care setting at the time of delivery and all plans must be possible on any day and at any time.

ANESTHETIC INTERVENTIONS

Cardiac output increases during pregnancy and again during labor. Part of the increase in cardiac output in labor is caused by autotransfusion during uterine contractions and part by the physiological stress response to pain. Regional analgesia (epidural or combined spinal epidural) is the only form of pain-relief that can reliably obtund the pain response and is frequently offered to mothers with cardiac disease.

Mothers who fall into group one and many from group two will have tolerated pregnancy without difficulty and from the cardiovascular point of view will tolerate delivery well. These mothers can be offered regional analgesia safely, but those that feel they would prefer not to have an epidural need not have one.

Blood pressure and cardiac output control during anesthesia

To maintain blood pressure during anesthesia and prevent detrimental maternal problems (such as reduced coronary filling) and fetal distress, the anesthetist must control preload, afterload and heart rate.

Blood pressure (BP) is a function of cardiac output (CO) and systemic vascular resistance (SVR) and cardiac output is a function of heart rate (HR) and stroke volume (SV). This is summarized in the equation: $BP = (HR \times SV) \times SVR$.

Regional and general anesthesia can affect all of these parameters and it is the attention to the details of parameter control, rather than the absolute method of anesthesia, that will provide safe analgesia and anesthesia for the mother with cardiac disease.

Preload

Aortocaval compression
The majority of mothers will have a degree of aortocaval compression at term. For many mothers it will be asymptomatic, until they are given an anesthetic, where it can be a major contributing factor to significant hypotension in up to 80% of elective Cesarean sections under spinal anesthesia.

For the mother with cardiac disease with either poor ventricular function or a poorly compliant ventricle (especially in association with stenotic valvular lesions), the ability to maintain an adequate stroke volume will be heavily dependent on good venous return (preload) to the right side of the heart. Minor degrees of aortocaval compression causing even a small fall in venous return can cause serious cardiac decompensation either in relation to a fall in systemic vascular resistance associated with regional anesthesia or a further decline in ventricular contractility associated with the commonly used general anesthetic drugs. Mothers with cardiac disease should be nursed in the full lateral position to minimize aortocaval compression, especially in relation to establishing all regional anesthetic blocks. She should be placed on her back with visible left uterine displacement for the shortest possible time, should it be necessary, e.g. for delivery by Cesarean section, and hypotensive episodes treated with an increase in table tilt.

Hemorrhage
Hemorrhage will severely effect preload and may lead to early, rapid decompensation. This can be a problem

when there is no anesthesia and early aggressive fluid management needs to be instituted. If hemorrhage is associated with anesthesia, a fall in blood pressure and coronary filling can be even more alarming.

Monitoring preload

Early use of central venous pressure (CVP) monitoring can be very helpful to assess preload and should be considered in all mothers who have poor ventricular function and stenotic valvular lesions. An absolute filling pressure is very much less important than gradual changes or sudden falls in CVP readings. A sudden drop in CVP reading, which is usually rapidly followed by a drop in blood pressure, is often associated with aortocaval compression and re-positioning the mother is urgently required.

Fluid therapy

Gradual changes in CVP readings over the course of labor can indicate under filling due to dehydration or over filling associated with over enthusiastic intravenous fluid therapy. Both are detrimental, especially for the mother with poor ventricular function. An under filled mother will decompensate rapidly at delivery, should there be any hemorrhage. A mother who has been given too much fluid may suddenly develop pulmonary oedema at delivery, because of the additional burden of uterine autotransfusion.

In normovolemia, a CVP reading is unnecessary but intravenous fluids should be given to judiciously maintain a good urine output with a mother who is clinically warm and well perfused. In the face of hemorrhage, aggressive and early maintenance of hemoglobin concentration and intravascular volume must be instituted.

Cardiac factors

Heart rate

A normal HR is essential for maintaining cardiac output and blood pressure. In normal pregnancy, the mother's increase in cardiac output is largely achieved by an increase in HR. For the mother with cardiac disease it is important to maintain the HR she tolerates best.

Tachycardia is especially poorly tolerated if the mother has ischemic heart disease, stenotic valvular disease or hypertrophic cardiomyopathy. Bradycardia is poorly tolerated in heart failure, a poorly compliant ventricle or regurgitant valvular disease.

Vasopressors

If anesthesia is associated with a drop in blood pressure, then having excluded aortocaval compression, the vasopressor of choice will be the drug that maintains or changes maternal heart rate to within the range tolerated best by that mother.

Ephedrine has traditionally been the vasopressor of choice in the obstetric population, with a mild inotopic and chronotropic effect. It is a useful drug in 3-6 mg boluses if the mother's heart rate is below 80 beat/min or a mild tachycardia is desirable.

Phenylephrine has traditionally been avoided in obstetrics because it was feared that blood flow to the fetus may be affected by its pure alpha agonist, vasoconstrictor action. Recent studies have demonstrated that in the normal fetus, pH at birth may be improved by phenylephrine compared to ephedrine. This has led to a reassurance that phenylephrine can be used safely for the mother with cardiac disease. It can be given either as an infusion at 10-20 µg/min or boluses of 12-25 µg as required. It usually causes a reflex slowing of the maternal heart rate to 60-70 beat/min and blood pressure is well maintained.

Cardiac contractility

Regional anesthesia does not have an effect on cardiac contractility and cardiac output is well maintained as long as HR and preload are maintained. Regional anesthesia is particularly appropriate where cardiac function is poor and is the anesthetic of choice in cardiomyopathy and ischemic heart disease.

General anesthesia may be poorly tolerated in the mother with poor ventricular function as all general anesthetic drugs have a negatively inotropic action. If general anesthesia is required, then extreme care must be taken to maintain an appropriate heart rate using vasopressors and vagolytic drugs as required. Inotropic drugs may also be needed.

Afterload

Both regional and general anesthetic techniques are associated with a fall in afterload. This facilitates the forward flow of blood from the heart and blood pressure tends to fall.

As cardiac contractility is not affected by regional techniques, the fall in afterload can be beneficial in some conditions. For ischemic problems, cardiac work is reduced and the risk of cardiac failure improved. Regional techniques are also ideal for mothers with regurgitant valvular lesions, with improved forward flow and a reduction in ventricular dilatation and ventricular work.

A fall in afterload is particularly detrimental for the mother with aortic stenosis and a right to left cyanotic shunt. In aortic stenosis a fall in afterload can be associated with a dramatic fall in blood pressure leading to poor coronary filling, acute ischemia and dysrhythmias.

In cyanotic shunts a fall in afterload is associated with an increase in right to left shunt resulting in an increase in cyanosis. Phenylephrine is the agent of choice, as its pure alpha affect will minimize these changes.

The argument in these conditions is that general anesthesia is preferable to regional anesthesia, as it may be associated with a smaller fall in afterload. There are however many good descriptions in the literature of regional anesthesia being safely used in these conditions. It is the understanding of the pathophysiology of the condition and its management with tight, early control of cardiovascular parameters that is very much more important than the actual technique used.

ANESTHETIC TECHNIQUES

General anesthesia

For the mother with severe cardiac disease, a modified general anesthetic technique with a small intravenous induction dose of thiopentone or etomidate and intravenous opioids; fentanyl, alfentanil or remifentanil is appropriate. The mother is vulnerable to gastric regurgitation and aspiration and suxamethonium should still be given. The baby may have significant opioid induced respiratory depression due to this technique and the attending pediatrician must be made aware.

Regional techniques

Labor

For mothers with significant disease all regional techniques should be titrated slowly against analgesic requirements. A 0.1% bupivacaine solution with fentanyl or sufentanil given in 5 ml boluses is well tolerated. If analgesia is madequate combined spinal epidural technique can be considered but intrathecal local anesthetics should be avoided and intrathecal fentanyl 25 µg or sufentanil 10 µg used as a sole agent. The epidural component can then be used to supplement the analgesia.

Cesarean section

Epidural anesthesia is tolerated if given in small incremental doses. To establish a block for Cesarean section, 3-5 ml boluses of 0.5% bupivacaine given every 10-15 min can be given. When establishing a regional block in this way it may take 45-60 min with a total of 25-30 mL of solution. Very careful assessment of the block is required to avoid problems of inadequate anesthesia during the surgery.

A combined spinal epidural technique can also be useful. A 5 mg intrathecal dose of bupivacaine can usefully provide sacral anesthesia with little in the way of hemodynamic instability and the epidural component can then be used in small incremental top-ups, until the desired block is achieved. Sacral anesthesia is more assured with this technique and a smaller dose of epidural bupivacaine will be required.

Uterotonics

Oxytocin

Oxytocin is the drug most commonly used to enhance uterine contractility after delivery and reduce the risk of postpartum hemorrhage. As stated above, the risks of hemorrhage are significant to the mother with cardiac disease. It is therefore important she is given oxytocin but the usual method of giving a bolus of 5-10 units at delivery should be avoided.

Women with right heart problems and pulmonary hypertension may tolerate the autotransfusion from natural uterine contraction poorly. Additional uterine contraction associated with oxytocic drug use may make the situation worse. Gentle manual rubbing of the uterus followed by a slow infusion (40 u over 4-6 h) to maintain uterine contractility is preferable.

Oxytocin also causes a profound fall in afterload and a reflex tachycardia with a significant increase in cardiac output. These physiological parameters are frequently detrimental to the mother with significant cardiac disease and bolus doses should be avoided if possible. A slow infusion will avoid these problems and should be given as above.

Ergometrine

Ergometrine, usually given with oxytocin, can counter the vasodilation effect of oxytocin alone, but the effects are unpredictable and resulting hypertension can in itself be detrimental. In all but the most straightforward cases this combination should be avoided.

Carboprost

Carboprost is a prostaglandin used to treat post partum hemorrhage due to uterine atony in patients unresponsive to ergometrine and oxytocin. This drug can cause bronchospasm and hypertension, but when faced with severe hemorrhage its use should be considered, although myocardial ischemia is a known side-effect.

Physical methods

The mother with significant cardiac disease will not tolerate major and ongoing hemorrhage. If hemorrhage occurs after vaginal delivery then early transfer to theatre for examination under anesthesia is important. Early initiation of invasive monitoring (blood pressure and CVP) should be considered.

The early use of a uterine compression or brace suture such as a B-Lynch suture can lead to early control of hemorrhage due to placenta previa and uterine atony. Its use at laparotomy can avoid the consequences of major ongoing hemorrhage and avoids the continued use of the above drugs, in mothers who are intolerant of them.

Further reading

Bachet J, Guilmet D 2002 Brain protection during surgery of the aortic arch. Journal of Cardiac Surgery 17:115-124

Boyle R K 2003 Anaesthesia in parturients with heart disease: a five year review in an Australian tertiary hospital. International Journal of Obstetric Anesthesia 12:173-177

Chan W S, Anand S, Ginsberg J S 2000 Anticoagulation of pregnant women with mechanical heart valves. Archives of Internal Medicine 160:191-196

Clapp J F III, Capeless E 1997 Cardiovascular function before, during, and after the first and subsequent pregnancies. American Journal of Cardiology 80:1469-1473

Cotrufo M, De Feo M, De Santo L, et al 2002 Risk of warfarin during pregnancy with mechanical valve prostheses. Obstetrics and Gynecology 99:35-40

de Swiet M, Nelson-Piercy C 2004 Cardiac disease. In: Confidential enquiries into maternal and child health. Why mothers die, 2000-2002. 6th Report of Confidential Enquiries into Maternal Deaths in UK. RCOG, London

Elkayam U, Ostrzega E, Shotan A, et al 1995 Cardiovascular problems in pregnant women with the Marfan syndrome. Annals of Internal Medicine 123:117-122

Elkayam U, Tummala P P, Rao K, et al 2001 Maternal and fetal outcomes of subsequent pregnancies in women with peripartum cardiomyopathy. New England Journal of Medicine 344:1567-1571

Felker G M, Thompson R E, Hare J M, et al 2000 Underlying causes and long-term survival in patients with initially unexplained cardiomyopathy. New England Journal of Medicine 342:1077-1084

Immer F F, Bansi A G, Immer-Bansi A S, et al 2003 Aortic dissection in pregnancy: analysis of risk factors and outcome. Annals of Thoracic Surgery 76:309-314

Khairy P, Quyang DW, Fernandes S et al 2006 Pregnancy outcomes in women with congenital heart disease. Circulation 113:1564-1571

Ladner HE, Danielsen B, Gilbert WM 2005 Acute MI in pregnancy and the puerperium: a population based study. Obstet Gynecol 105:480-484

Lovell A T 2004 Anaesthetic implications of grown-up congenital heart disease. British Journal of Anaesthesia 93:129-139

Ngan Kee W D, Lee A 2003 Analysis of factors associated with umbilical arterial pH and standard base excess after Caesarean section under spinal anaesthesia. Anaesthesia 58:125-130

Oran B, Lee-Parritz A, Ansell J 2004 Low molecular weight heparin for the prophylaxis of thromboembolism in women with prosthetic mechanical heart valves during pregnancy. Thrombosis and Haemostasis 92:747-751

Pearson G D, Veille J C, Rahimtoola S, et al 2000 Peripartum cardiomyopathy. National Heart, Lung and Blood Institute and Office of Rare Diseases (NIH). Workshop Recommendations and Review. Journal of the American Medical Association 283:1183-1188

Reimold S C, Rutherford J D 2003 Valvular heart disease in pregnancy. New England Journal of Medicine 349:52-59

Robson S C, Hunter S, Boys R J, et al 1989 Serial study of factors influencing changes in cardiac output during human pregnancy. American Journal of Physiology 256: H1060–1065

Robson S K, Hunter S, Boys R, et al 1986 Changes in cardiac output during epidural anaesthesia for caesarian section. Anaesthesia 44:465-479

Sadler L, McCowan L, White H, et al North R 2000 Pregnancy outcomes and cardiac complications in women with mechanical, bioprosthetic and homograft valves. BJOG 107:245-253

Siu S C, Sermer M, Colman J, et al 2001 Prospective multicenter study of pregnancy outcomes in women with heart disease. Circulation 104:515-521

Task Force on Infective Endocarditis of the European Society of Cardiology 2004 Guidelines on prevention, diagnosis and treatment of infective endocarditis. European Heart Journal 25:267-276

Thorne S A 2004 Pregnancy in heart disease. Heart 90:450-456

Thorne S, Nelson-Piercy C, McGregor A et al 2006 Pregnancy and contraception in heart disease and pulmonary arterial hypertension. Journal of Family Planning and Reproductive Health Care 32:75-81.

Weiss B M, Zemp L, Seifert B, Hess O M 1998 Outcome of pulmonary vascular disease in pregnancy: a systematic overview from 1978 through 1996. Journal of the American College of Cardiology 31(7):1650-1657

Chapter 3

Hypertension in pregnancy

R. A. Samangaya, A. P. Heazell, P. N. Baker

INTRODUCTION

Hypertensive disorders are the most common medical problems encountered in obstetric practice, affecting between 10-15% of all pregnancies. In the last Confidential Enquiry into Maternal and Child Health (CEMACH 2004) for the period 2000-2002, 14 deaths were directly attributed to hypertensive disorders, with 46% of cases classified as receiving substandard care. However, in the developing world, it is estimated that hypertensive disorders of pregnancy lead to 160 000 maternal deaths per annum. The detection and appropriate management of hypertensive disorders in pregnancy is essential in the delivery of effective obstetric care.

Although they are grouped under a single title, hypertensive disorders in pregnancy encompass a variety of clinical situations, namely: chronic hypertension (usually originating in essential hypertension), pregnancy induced hypertension (PIH), pre-eclampsia and eclampsia. The enormous clinical spectrum of these disorders reflects underlying differences in their pathophysiology and natural history that have important consequences for intervention and treatment.

CARDIOVASCULAR CHANGES IN NORMAL PREGNANCY

The maternal cardiovascular system undergoes important physiological changes during pregnancy. Plasma volume increases from approximately 2600 to 3800 mL, by 32 weeks gestation. There is an increase in red cell mass from 1400 to 1650-1800 mL. Cardiac output increases by 40% from 4.5 L/min to 6 L/min by 30 weeks gestation, mainly due to an increase in stroke volume. The majority of this extra output is directed to the uterus and kidneys. Despite the increase in cardiac output, blood pressure falls reaching its nadir at around 20 weeks gestation and then slowly increases towards term. This fall in blood pressure reflects a substantial reduction in total peripheral resistance (see also Ch. 2.1).

ETIOLOGY

The exact etiology of pre-eclampsia remains unclear, although recently significant advances have been made in our understanding of the pathophysiology. The placenta is central to the development of pre-eclampsia. There is a failure of conversion of the maternal spiral arteries supplying the placenta, an increase in apoptosis (programmed cell death) within the placenta and an increased loss of placental syncytial fragments. Although systemic changes may not be overt until the late second or third trimester, the initial pathological events begin early in pregnancy at the time of placentation. One hypothesis proposes that circulating factors are released from the placenta in response to hypoxia as a result of underperfusion. These circulating factors are responsible for initiating the widespread endothelial cell dysfunction and multisystem disorder that is evident in pre-eclampsia (Fig. 3.1(a)). An alternative hypothesis suggests that there is an increased maternal immune response to syncytial trophoblast debris. This may be increased in response to noxious stimuli (e.g. hypoxia or reperfusion injury) or from a larger placental mass (e.g. multiple pregnancy).

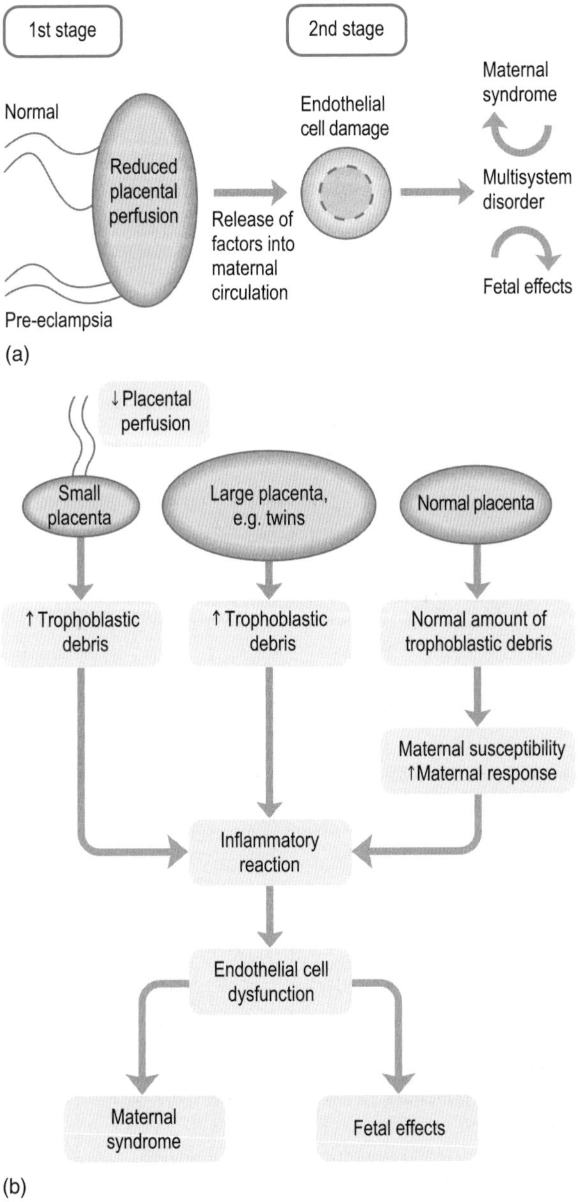

Pathophysiological process in pre-eclampsia
- genetic predisposition;
- inadequate trophoblast invasion of spiral arteries;
- reduced uteroplacental perfusion;
- placental damage (leading to apoptosis);
- release of circulating factors or placental syncytial fragments;
- exaggerated maternal immune response; and
- endothelial cell dysfunction.

RISK FACTORS

There are many risk factors for the development of pre-eclampsia (Table 3.1).

- Socio-demographic factors
  - Extremes of reproductive age
  - Socio-economic status
  - Ethnic group
- Genetic factors
- Pregnancy factors
  - Multiple pregnancies
  - Primigravidae
  - Assisted reproduction techniques
  - Previous pre-eclampsia
- Personal medical history
  - Obesity
  - Chronic renal disease
  - Chronic hypertension
  - Diabetes mellitus
  - Thrombophilia

Figure 3.1 (a) Two-stage model of pre-eclampsia; (b) continuum theory of inflammatory response to trophoblastic debris.

Table 3.1 Relative risks of developing pre-eclampsia for individual pre-pregnancy risk factors

Risk factor	Relative risk of developing pre-eclampsia
Chronic renal disease	20
Chronic hypertension	10
First-degree relative with hypertension in pregnancy	5
Twin pregnancy	4
Nulliparity	3
Maternal age over 40 years	3
Obesity (BMI > 25)	2.7
Diabetes mellitus	2

PRE-CONCEPTION CARE

In an ideal situation, a patient at high risk of developing pre-eclampsia should be seen prior to conception. This provides an opportunity to optimize management of pre-existing medical conditions, establish baseline observations and to consider prophylaxis for pre-eclampsia (Boxes 3.1 and 3.2). Patients who are likely to benefit from pre-conception care include those with a history of:

- Previous pre-eclampsia
- First-degree relative with pre-eclampsia
- Chronic hypertension
- Cardiac disease
- Renal disease
- Systemic lupus erythematosus (SLE), anti-phospholipid syndrome
- Thrombophilia

ANTENATAL CARE

The booking appointment is an opportunity to assess a woman's risk of developing hypertensive disorders of pregnancy, to measure blood pressure and to assess

---

Box 3.1 Pre-conceptional care

Investigations
- Blood pressure – 24-h blood pressure monitoring in selected patients.
- Urinalysis plus album creatinine ratio (ACR)/protein creatinine ration (PCR) if dipstick proteiuria.
- Urea and electrolytes.
- 24-h urine collection for proteinuria and creatinine clearance if significant renal dysfunction.
- Further specific investigations will be required if additional disorders such as SLE or thrombophilia are suspected.

Counselling
- Risk of pre-eclampsia and its effects.
- Risk of IUGR.
- Drugs – no known teratogenicity with any anti-hypertensives, but some fetotoxicity with ACE inhibitors and angiotensin receptor blockers. These should be stopped before pregnancy
- Early referral for obstetric care, ideally to a specialist high-risk obstetric clinic.
- Consider prophylaxis against pre-eclampsia.

Box 3.2 Evidence for prophylaxis against pre-eclampsia

Aspirin
- Imbalance of prostacyclin and thromboxane in pre-eclampsia, favoring vasoconstriction and platelet aggregation. Aspirin inhibits cyclo-oxygenase activity in platelets, altering the prostatcyclin : thromboxane ratio.
- Cochrane meta-analysis: overall 19% reduction in pre-eclampsia with aspirin in moderate- and high-risk women, irrespective of dose or gestation at drug commencement.
- No increase in maternal or neonatal complications associated with low dose aspirin.

Antioxidants
- Oxidative stress is a pathological state with an excess of damaging reactive oxygen species in comparison to buffering antioxidants. Oxidative stress is increased in pre-eclampsia.
- A small randomized placebo-controlled trial of the antioxidants, vitamin C and E demonstrated a lower incidence of pre-eclampsia (8%); compared to placebo group (26%).
- However, a recent large multi-center trial using vitamins C and E showed no difference in the incidence of pre-eclampsia between the treatment and placebo groups.

Calcium supplementation
- Ethnic groups with high dietary calcium intake have a low incidence of pre-eclampsia.
- A Cochrane meta-analysis has demonstrated a reduction in pre-eclampsia with calcium supplementation. This effect is greater in high-risk women, and those with a low dietary intake of calcium.

Fish oil supplementation
- Populations with a high consumption of fish oils have a low incidence of cardiovascular disease.
- Multi-center trials have shown no difference in incidence of pre-eclampsia.

Anti-hypertensives
- In women with chronic hypertension, anti-hypertensives reduce the risk of severe hypertension.
- Anti-hypertensives do not affect the incidence of pre-eclampsia.

Box 3.3 Manual measurement of blood pressure

- Woman should be seated and relaxed.
- The arm must be supported with *no* tight clothing constricting the upper arm.
- The air bladder must cover *at least* three quarters of the circumference of the upper arm and preferably the whole upper arm. If the arm has a circumference of > 33 cm, or the air bladder does not cover three-quarters of the circumference of the arm then a large cuff should be used.
- The cuff should be inflated to above systolic pressure, and the pressure slowly released listening for the first Korotkoff sound (when the pulse is first heard) for the systolic measurement, and the fifth Korotkoff sound (when the pulse disappears) for the diastolic measurement.

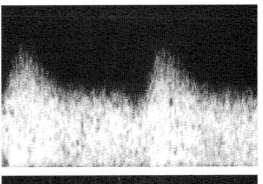

(a)

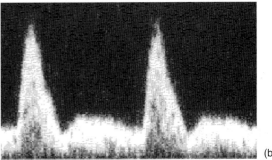

(b)

Figure 3.2 (a) Normal Doppler flow velocity waveform from the uterine artery at 24 weeks gestation; (b) abnormal Doppler flow velocity waveform from the uterine artery at 24 weeks with a uterine notch in early diastole.

the urine for proteinuria. It is important to note that the booking appointment often occurs around 12 weeks of gestation, when blood pressure may be lower than in the non-pregnant situation and therefore will not represent a true baseline by which to assess a chronic hypertensive problem. The patient should be classified as high or low risk for pre-eclampsia and should be managed accordingly.

As pre-eclampsia is asymptomatic in its early stage, much of antenatal care is directed towards screening of blood pressure and urine, to enable early detection. Accuracy in the measurement of blood pressure is essential and it is important that this is done in a consistent manner (Box 3.3).

Recently, the use of automated sphygmomanometers has become more common in obstetric practice. However, they may be inaccurate and it is essential to confirm their accuracy in the clinical situation by comparison with manual sphygmomanometry.

Patients at low risk of pre-eclampsia should have blood pressure measurement and urinalysis at 3-4 week intervals between 12 and 34 weeks, and 2 week intervals from 34 weeks until delivery. All patients should be educated regarding the symptoms of pre-eclampsia including headache, visual disturbance and epigastric pain.

Patients at high risk of pre-eclampsia can be identified by their risk factors and by Doppler ultrasound scanning. There is evidence that Doppler ultrasound of the uterine arteries performed between 22 and 24 weeks may be useful in the prediction of women who will later develop pre-eclampsia (Fig. 3.2).

CLASSIFICATION OF HYPERTENSIVE DISORDERS OF PREGNANCY

Due to the wide clinical spectrum of hypertensive disorders of pregnancy it is important to utilize an accurate classification of the nature of the condition, as this may have implications for the management of each condition (Box 3.4). Hypertension itself is defined as a blood pressure ≥ 140/90 mmHg on two separate occasions, at least four hours apart.

MANAGEMENT OF HYPERTENSION IN PREGNANCY

Chronic hypertension

These women are at increased risk of developing superimposed pre-eclampsia and require regular blood pressure measurements and urinalysis. However, even in chronic hypertension alone, there is an increased risk of intrauterine growth restriction and placental abruption (Box 3.5).

Box 3.4 Hypertension

- Chronic/essential hypertension – hypertension prior to pregnancy or occurring before 20 weeks gestation.
- Pregnancy induced hypertension/gestational hypertension – hypertension occurring after 20 weeks gestation without proteinuria.
- Pre-eclampsia – hypertension occurring after 20 weeks gestation with proteinuria (> 300 mg/24 h or ++ using urine dipstick on two consecutive urine samples in the absence of urinary tract infection. Urine protein/creatinine ratios and urine microalbumin/creatinine ratios may also be used, although the normal reference ranges and changes in pre-eclampsia have yet to be fully established).
- Superimposed pre-eclampsia – pre-eclampsia occurring in a patient with pre-existing chronic hypertension.

Box 3.5 Management of women with chronic hypertension

- Regular antenatal checks – blood pressure, urinalysis and bloods to assess renal function at baseline and then regular assessment of blood pressure and urianlysis.
- Education – on the symptoms of pre-eclampsia.
- Anti-hypertensives – change ACE inhibitors and angiotensin receptor blockers prior to pregnancy; dose reduction or cessation of anti-hypertensive therapy may be possible during the second trimester due to the physiological fall in blood pressure; increased dosage as necessary as pregnancy progresses; and use drug combinations e.g. labetalol or methyldopa and long-acting nifedipine.
- Monitor fetal growth with ultrasound scans every four weeks from ~26 weeks.
- Consider induction of labor approaching term.

Pregnancy induced hypertension (PIH)

Pregnancy outcomes in women with mild PIH are similar to those of normotensive women. However, such women are at risk of developing pre-eclampsia, and this risk is increased in those women who develop PIH at early gestation (Box 3.6).

Box 3.6 Management of women with pregnancy induced hypertension

- Regular antenatal checks – blood pressure, urinalysis and antenatal day unit management.
- Education – on the symptoms of pre-eclampsia.
- Anti-hypertensives may be required if the blood pressure is persistently ≥ 150/90 mmHg. Women with severe hypertension (≥ 160/110 mmHg) will require urgent treatment with oral or intravenous anti-hypertensives as necessary (see Tables 3.2 and 3.3).

Box 3.7 Pre-eclampsia subdivisions

Mild/moderate pre-eclampsia
BP ≥ 140/90 mmHg, proteinuria ≤ ++, no renal/hepatic/coagulation dysfunction, plasma urate concentration usually raised.

Severe pre-eclampsia
BP ≥ 160/110 mmHg, proteinuria ≥ +++, biochemical evidence of renal/hepatic dysfunction/coagulation dysfunction, plasma urate concentration elevated.

Pre-eclampsia

Pre-eclampsia can be subdivided into disease severity (Box 3.7). Several models and scoring systems have been used in patients with pre-eclampsia to try to determine those at most risk of adverse outcomes. However, due to the multi-systemic and sometimes rapidly progressive nature of this disorder, these boundaries are often artificial and do not always equate to outcomes. It is important however, to determine the level of severity. It is essential to take account of any changes in clinical symptoms such as the incidence of headaches, visual disturbances, epigastric pain or vomiting, and to monitor trends in blood pressure, proteinuria and biochemical tests as well as fetal condition.

Pre-eclampsia is a multi-systemic disorder affecting both the mother and fetus, and there can be significant complications (Box 3.8).

Presentation of pre-eclampsia

In the majority of mild to moderate cases of pre-eclampsia, the patient is asymptomatic. However,

Box 3.8 Complications of pre-eclampsia

Maternal
- Eclampsia
- Cerebral hemorrhage
- Placental abruption
- Renal failure
- Pulmonary edema, ARDS
- Disseminated intravascular coagulopathy
- HELLP syndrome, liver hemorrhage and rupture
- Thromboembolism
- Cortical blindness
- Laryngeal oedema

Fetal
- Intrauterine growth restriction
- Intrauterine death
- Iatrogenic preterm delivery

presenting complaints may include: headache; visual disturbance; nausea; vomiting; epigastric/right upper quadrant pain; edema – particularly rapid onset or oedema of the hands or face; and general malaise.

Examinations of women with hypertension in pregnancy should concentrate on:

- General appearance – facial oedema and jaundice.
- Cardiovascular system – blood pressure, pulse, peripheral and sacral edema.
- Respiratory system – fine-inspiratory crepitations, which may indicate pulmonary edema.
- Abdominal examination – right upper quadrant or epigastric tenderness, symphysio-fundal height, fetal presentation, liquor volume and fetal heart auscultation.
- Neurological system – hyperreflexia or clonus (thought to result from 'cerebral irritability') and papilledema.

Investigations of women with hypertension in pregnancy should encompass:

- Urinalysis and PCR.
- Twenty-four hour urine collection.
- In early onset severe PIH or pre-eclampsia: urine for catecholamines to exclude phaeochromocytoma. Also exclude other potential problems such as undiagnosed coarctation of the aorta or renal or connective tissue disease.
- Full blood count, urea and electrolytes, liver function tests, urate.

- Cardiotocograph (CTG) (gestation > 26 weeks).
- Ultrasound scan – fetal growth, liquor volume, umbilical artery Doppler flow velocity waveform.

The management of women with pre-eclampsia should include:

- Inpatient management if BP > 140/90 with significant proteinuria.
- Regular blood pressure monitoring (at least 4 hourly).
- Anti-hypertensives as necessary.
- Urinalysis and 24-h urine collection.
- Fluid input–output charts.
- Bloods – full blood count, urea and electrolytes, liver function tests, urate.
- Daily CTG.
- Fetal growth and liquor volume should be assessed via ultrasound to exclude intrauterine growth restriction.

Pharmacological agents commonly used in the management of hypertension in pregnancy include labetalol, nifedipine and methyldopa. There is no evidence that a single agent is more effective than another, and therefore, clinicians should use the drug with which they are most familiar. The aim of treatment is to prevent maternal complications of severe hypertension such as cerebral hemorrhage while not causing underperfusion of the placenta. There is no consensus as to the optimal level of blood pressure control for this group of patients, but most agree it should be at least < 150/100 mmHg to reduce the risk of cerebral hemorrhage and lessen the chance of delivery because of uncontrolled hypertension . The mode of action, dose ranges, and common side effects of these agents are shown in Table 3.2. Since each of these drugs is in a different class with different modes of action, they may be used in combination with synergistic effects. However, the following are not recommended for use in pregnancy: diuretics as they decrease intravascular volume, which is already reduced in pre-eclampsia; atenolol as it has been associated with intrauterine growth restriction; angiotensin converting enzyme (ACE) inhibitors and angiotensin II receptor antagonists as they have been associated with fetal toxicity.

Controlling maternal blood pressure with anti-hypertensives is essentially a holding mechanism for expectant management, and will not alter the underlying endothelial cell dysfunction. The only truly effective treatment for pre-eclampsia is delivery, since this removes the pathological placenta, which triggers the maternal response. However, at early gestations, delivery is associated with significant perinatal mor-

Table 3.2 Oral pharmacological agents used to treat hypertension in pregnancy

Agent	Receptor	Dose range	Side effects	Contraindications
Labetalol	α- and β-adrenoreceptor	200–1600 mg tds	Bradycardia, bronchospasm, gastrointestinal disturbances, fatigue, scalp tingling	Asthma Phaeochromocytoma
Nifedipine	Calcium channel antagonist	20–90 mg od Long acting form	Headache, flushing, dizziness, lethargy, tachycardia, palpitations, edema, rash nausea, visual disturbances	Aortic stenosis Liver disease
Methyldopa	Central action	250 mg–3 g tds	Gastrointestinal disturbances, dry mouth, stomatitis, bradycardia, postural hypotension, edema, sedation, headache, dizziness	Phaeochromocytoma Liver disease Depression

bidity and mortality. There is therefore, a fine balance at early gestations between employing expectant management to delay delivery in order to obtain the maximum possible maturity for the baby, and the risk of the maternal condition worsening.

Indications for delivery in women with PIH or pre-eclampsia, may be divided into maternal and fetal groups:

Maternal
- Severe hypertension > 160/110 mmHg unresponsive to pharmacological therapy.
- Deteriorating renal function as measured by oliguria, or increased urea and creatinine.
- Rapidly falling platelet count below 100×10^{12}/L and/or rising or profoundly elevated alanine aminotransferase (ALT) or aspartate aminotransferase (AST) levels (suggestive of HELLP syndrome).
- Evidence of coagulopathy.
- Persistent symptoms.

Fetal
- Intrauterine growth restriction with abnormal umbilical artery Doppler velocimetry – absent or reversed end diastolic flow.
- Suspected fetal distress identified on CTG.

If delivery before 34 weeks gestation is likely, corticosteroids should be administered to promote fetal lung maturity. It is vital to liaise with the neonatal services before delivery to ensure there is a cot available and to determine an appropriate time for delivery for all personnel. It is also important that a neonatologist discusses issues regarding prematurity with the mother. Ideally, patients with pre-eclampsia should not be transferred. However, if there are no cots available, and the patient is stable, they may be transferred to another unit where appropriate neonatal services are available. If the patient is unsuitable for transfer, she will have to be delivered, and the baby stabilized and then transferred exutero to another neonatal unit.

Management of acute severe hypertension or Pre-eclampsia

Acute severe hypertension is defined as a patient with a blood pressure greater than 160/110 mmHg. However, severe isolated systolic hypertension > 160 mmHg is also associated with an increased risk of maternal complications, most notably cerebral hemorrhage. The failure to identify and treat acute severe hypertension was identified as a cause of maternal death in the most recent UK report on maternal mortality (see Ch. 1). All maternity units should be equipped with a protocol for the management of acute severe hypertension that is easily available to all obstetric and midwifery staff. Treatment aims to control maternal hypertension and reduce the risk of eclamptic seizures. This requires a multidisciplinary approach involving senior obstetric, medical and anesthetic clinicians:

- Where possible the patient should be moved to a clinical area where they can receive 1:1 care.
- Blood pressure should be checked using a manual sphygmomanometer as automated readings tend to underestimate diastolic blood pressure.
- Oral anti-hypertensives for acute lowering include:
  - 200 mg oral labetalol, repeated as necessary;

Table 3.3 Intravenous agents for the treatment of severe acute hypertension

Agent	Receptor	Dosage	Side effects	Contraindications
Labetalol	α- and β-adrenoreceptor	50 mg (in 0.9% sodium chloride) over 1 min followed by infusion of 20 mg/h increased to maximum of 160 mg/h	Bradycardia, bronchospasm, gastrointestinal disturbances, fatigue	Asthma Phaeochromocytoma Known cardiac disease
Hydralazine	Vasodilator	5 mg (in 0.9% sodium chloride) over 5 min followed by infusion of 5 mg/h	Tachycardia, palpitations, flushing, fluid retention, gastrointestinal disturbances; headache, dizziness.	Severe tachycardia

- Intravenous anti-hypertensive agents can be employed if blood pressure is not controlled by oral agents, or if the patient is unable to tolerate oral agents for any reason.
- Commonly used agents include labetalol and hydralazine, which appear equally effective. The clinician should use the agent they are more familiar with. Doses and side effects are shown in Table 3.3.
- Sub-lingual nifedipine is to be avoided as the resultant fall in blood pressure may be too profound and has been associated with fetal distress.
- If blood pressure is very high and difficult to control, invasive monitoring such as peripheral arterial cannulation should be considered.
- Monitor urinary output.
- Blood should be taken for renal and liver function, urate, full blood count, clotting studies and blood for cross matching if delivery is anticipated.
- Fluid balance should be recorded. Strict fluid balance is necessary due to the risk of pulmonary edema. This requires a fluid restriction of 2 L/24 h (83 mL/h). Most cases require a urinary catheterization to determine hourly urine output
- If there is uncertainty regarding fluid status, central venous monitoring may rarely be considered.
- If there is no coagulopathy, and immediate surgery is not planned, consideration should be given to thromboprophylaxis (compression stockings and low molecular weight heparin), due to the increased risk of venous thromboembolism. Even if surgery is planned, compression stockings can still be employed.

- When the mother's clinical condition is stabilized, fetal well-being should be confirmed using CTG (if greater than 26/40).

Delivery is indicated in the following cases of:

- hypertension remaining uncontrolled despite maximal anti-hypertensive therapy;
- renal (including poor urine output), hepatic or coagulation impairment;
- pulmonary edema;
- eclampsia; and
- fetal distress.

Prior to delivery the clinical condition of the mother should be optimized, including the use of invasive monitoring of arterial and occasionally central venous pressure. Any coagulopathy should be corrected using blood products (e.g fresh frozen plasma and cryoprecipitate) as required.

Management of delivery

The choice of mode of delivery is dependent on the severity of pre-eclampsia, the gestation of the pregnancy and the patient's obstetric history. Induction of labor can be an option, although the time that this takes may be too long if the patient has rapidly progressing disease. If the patient is suitable for labor, good analgesia is important and epidural anesthesia is usually preferred (with a platelet count $>80 \times 10^{12}/L$). A patient in labor should have:

- continuous electronic fetal monitoring throughout labor;

- regular blood pressure monitoring;
- fluid balance chart (especially if receiving intravenous fluid);
- intravenous access (increased risk of postpartum hemorrhage);
- high concentration syntocinon infusion if required to allow use of reduced fluid volume; and
- active management of the third stage using 5iu i.m. syntocinon. Ergometrine should be avoided as this produces widespread vasoconstriction and may exacerbate hypertension.

If a patient requires delivery by Cesarean section, regional anesthesia is preferable to a general anesthesia, because of the association of endotracheal intubation with an increase in maternal blood pressure and all the other factors that favor regional analgesia in pregnancy (see Ch. 18). Most anesthetists will employ spinal anesthesia if the platelet count is greater than $80 \times 10^{12}/L$ provided there is no other evidence of coagulation disturbance. Patients should have cross-matched blood available, due to the increased incidence of postpartum hemorrhage and intra-operative blood loss in patients with pre-eclampsia who have thrombocytopenia or other abnormal coagulation profile.

Magnesium sulfate reduces the incidence of eclampsia, and women with severe pre-eclampsia should receive intravenous magnesium sulfate, usually around the time of delivery (Box 3.9).

Immediate postpartum care

Women with severe pre-eclampsia require careful postpartum monitoring, since they still remain at high risk of complications. This monitoring should preferably be in a high dependency environment, where 1:1 care can be provided. In this period, patients should have:

- Regular blood pressure monitoring (every 15 min).
- Strict input–output fluid chart:
- hourly urine via urinary catheter; and
- input should be ~83 mL/h including all infusions and oral intake to reduce the risk of pulmonary edema.
- Magnesium sulfate infusion (1 g/h) to reduce incidence of eclamptic seizures is generally continued for 24 h after delivery.
- Anti-hypertensives should be continued, or reduced slowly. Intravenous medication can usually be changed to oral preparations within 12 h of delivery. ACE inhibitors are safe to use and indeed are very effective, postpartum. Enalapril has reassuring breast milk data.

Box 3.9 Magnesium sulfate for severe pre-eclampsia

10% magnesium sulfate is used for the prevention of eclamptic seizures
Magnesium sulphate is given intravenously through a peripheral line. A bolus loading dose of 4 g should be given over 10 min. Following this an infusion of 1 g/h should be administered. Magnesium is excreted via the kidneys, hence particular caution is required in cases of renal impairment.

During magnesium sulfate administration, signs of toxicity must be assessed:

- pulse oximetry and ECG;
- hourly urine output;
- hourly respiratory rate; and
- deep tendon reflexes (every 4 h).

If deep tendon reflexes are absent, the respiratory rate is <12/min or there is oliguria, the infusion should be stopped or reduced to 0.5 g/h.

Serum magnesium levels are not routinely checked (therapeutic range 2–4 mmol/L, toxicity >5 mmol/L, respiratory depression >7 mmol/L).

In the case of cardiorespiratory arrest (levels normally >10 mmol/L) attending staff should:

- stop infusion of magnesium sulfate;
- get help, maintain airway – intubate if possible, commence CPR; and
- give 10 mL 10% calcium gluconate intravenously.

- Check full blood count, clotting function, renal function, liver enzymes and urate every 24 h until the patient's clinical condition has improved. The frequency will depend on the patient's clinical condition and previous evidence of renal, hepatic or hematological dysfunction.
- In the absence of coagulopathy or any obstetric bleeding such as wound or vulval hematoma the patient should receive low molecular weight heparin, in a prophylactic dose and compression stockings to reduce the risk of developing venous thromboembolism.
- Diuretics, such as frusemide should only be given if there is evidence of pulmonary edema. This may occur if fluid therapy, such as crystalloid infusions in large volume, have been administered, particularly if hypertension has been severe, and in older women. If it is impossible to arrive at a confident clinical conclusion about the state of

fluid balance, central venous pressure monitoring or Swann–Ganz catheter should be considered. These are very rarely necessary.

The majority of patients with severe pre-eclampsia will have a natural diuresis in the first 24 h after delivery. A patient may be transferred from the high dependency area when her blood pressure is controlled, urine output is satisfactory and any serious laboratory disturbance is resolving. While on the postnatal ward, blood pressure should be checked regularly, and hematological and biochemical blood tests should be repeated to ensure that they are returning to normal levels. Anti-hypertensive medication should be reduced gradually, but often patients will require oral anti-hypertensives at discharge (see Postnatal care, below).

Medication should be gradually reduced, rather than being stopped abruptly to avoid rebound hypertension; this process may take up to 6 weeks. Patients should be discharged when their blood pressure is well controlled, and when any impairment of liver, kidney or clotting function is resolving.

Eclampsia

Eclampsia is defined as one or more seizures occurring in the presence of pre-eclampsia. Eclampsia can occur antenatally (38%), intrapartum (18%) or postnatally (44%). The incidence of eclampsia in developed countries is 1 in 2000 deliveries, but is much higher in developing countries where eclampsia is estimated to complicate between 1 in 100 and 1 in 1700 deliveries.

The main priority for those caring for with a patient presenting with a seizure is to maintain oxygenation and stop the convulsion. Eclampsia is an obstetric emergency that all staff should be familiar with and should take part of regular obstetric drills.

The maternal condition is the priority at all times in the management of eclampsia, and it is vital that the woman is stabilized before any attempt is made to deliver the baby.

Following a seizure, further history and examination are required. It is important to determine if the seizure was related to eclampsia, or one of the differential diagnoses (Box 3.11). However, all seizures occurring in the third trimester should be considered as eclampsia until proven otherwise. Pulse, blood pressure and oxygen saturations should be monitored, and blood pressure controlled as necessary using intravenous agents. Bloods should be sent for full blood count, urea and electrolytes, urate, liver function tests and group and save serum. A urinary catheter should be inserted to monitor urine output and fluid balance.

Box 3.10 Treatment of eclampsia

Primary
- Get help – obstetric emergency phone number.
- Personnel required:
  - obstetric consultant, registrar and SHO;
  - anesthetic consultant, registrar and SHO; and
  - midwife in charge
- ABC:
  - airway – protect airway and give oxygen;
  - breathing – assess; and
  - circulation – left lateral tilt, IV access.
- Stop fit – IV diazepan then administer magnesium sulfate (IV bolus 4 g over 10-15 min [can be given i.m.], then IV infusion 1 g/h).

Secondary
- Second bolus of magnesium sulfate (2 g over 10 min [if < 70 kg], or 4 g over 10 min [if > 70 kg]).
- Diazepam 10 mg IV if still fitting.
- Thiopentone 50 mg IV
- Intubation, muscle relaxant and ventilation.

Box 3.11 Differential diagnoses of convulsions in pregnancy

- Eclampsia
- Epilepsy
- Intracerebral or subarachnoid hemorrhage
- Meningitis
- Drug or alcohol related
- Head trauma
- Pseudoseizures
- Thrombotic thrombocytopenic purpura and hemolytic uraemic syndrome
- Metabolic disorders, e.g. hypoglycemia

When the maternal condition has been stabilized, if the seizure occurred antenatally, it is important to assess the fetal condition by CTG. The subsequent management will depend on the gestation of the pregnancy, the previous obstetric history and the maternal and fetal condition. If the CTG recording is normal, a cervical assessment may be performed, and induction of labor considered. In cases with suspected fetal compromise, an unfavorable cervix or previous obstetric history (e.g. previous Cesarean section), a Cesarean section will be indicated.

Box 3.12 Management following eclamptic seizure

- High dependency care
- Stabilization of mother
- Anti-hypertensives as necessary
- Assess fetus with CTG
- Deliver
- Induction of labor
  - Cesarean section
- Magnesium sulfate for 24 h
- Fluid balance

Box 3.13 Diagnosis of HELLP syndrome

- Hemolysis:
  - peripheral blood film;
  - raised unconjugated bilirubin levels; and
  - raised lactate dehydrogenase (LDH) levels.
- Elevated liver enzymes:
  - raised ALT;
  - raised AST; and
  - raised LDH.
- Low platelets (< 100×10^9/L).
- Ultrasound scan:
  - liver (exclude cholecystitis, gallstones, hepatic hematoma); and
  - fetal growth, umbilical artery Doppler, liquor volume.

Eclampsia is estimated to be fatal in 1.8% of cases, and up to 35% can have at least one major complication such as coma, focal motor deficit, cortical blindness and CVA. It is therefore important that a CT scan is performed on any patient that has persistent neurological symptoms following a seizure. Concerted post-seizure management is crucial (Box 3.12).

HELLP syndrome

HELLP syndrome is a further part of the spectrum of pre-eclampsia and consists of Hemolysis, (infrequent) Elevated Liver enzymes and Low Platelets. It can occur antenatally (70%) or postnatally (30%), and complicates 20% of severe pre-eclampsia cases.

Symptoms are often non-specific with malaise, epigastric or right upper quadrant pain, nausea and vomiting. Women may also present with jaundice, or hematuria. While most women will also have hypertension, blood pressure is not usually as high as in severe pre-eclampsia alone. A proportion of women with HELLP syndrome do not have hypertension or proteinuria.

HELLP syndrome has a maternal mortality of 1 to 24% and is also associated with a high perinatal mortality rate (7 to 60%). Once a diagnosis of HELLP syndrome is made, the care of such women follows the same principles as the treatment of severe pre-eclampsia (Box 3.13).

Patients with HELLP syndrome require careful platelet count monitoring, liver function tests and clotting. They may need anti-hypertensives, and antenatal steroids for fetal lung maturity for women at less than 34 weeks gestation. The ultimate treatment for these women is delivery, and in those women at early gestations, the balance of risks of expectant management to delay delivery has to be assessed.

The mode of delivery will depend on the gestation of the patient, with Cesarean section being more likely at early gestations. Epidural analgesia may be considered in patients whose platelet level is above ~80×10^{12}/L. In patients with disordered coagulation or very low platelet counts, fresh frozen plasma or platelet infusions may be required perioperatively or peripartum. However, platelets are usually only required if there is an actual hemorrhagic problem or operative intervention and are not usually required on a prophylactic basis. Transfused platelets are rapidly consumed and the platelet count will recover with disease regression.

Following delivery, these women require high dependency care as their condition may worsen. Blood parameters, fluid balance and observations will need careful monitoring. High dose steroid therapy postnatally to provoke normalization of blood parameters is controversial and unproven.

POSTNATAL CARE

Postnatally, women with chronic hypertension can usually revert to their pre-pregnancy anti-hypertensive medication. Women with PIH or pre-eclampsia can continue anti-hypertensives with careful monitoring of their blood pressure, and reduction of the dosage as necessary. There are no known adverse effects of anti-hypertensives on breastfed infants. However, there can be inadequate milk production with thiazide diuretics, and methyldopa can be associated with maternal depression, and so therefore these two agents are usually avoided. Other agents such as ACE inhibitors and atenolol that are not used in pregnancy are safe for use by breastfeeding mothers, although only enalapril has been studied in breast milk.

Women who have had hypertensive disorders of pregnancy should be reviewed approximately 6 weeks after delivery, when blood pressure should have normalized in 90% of women. Those women who had mild PIH/pre-eclampsia may be seen in primary care. This consultation should be used to measure blood pressure, discuss contraception and the risks of recurrence in future pregnancies.

Women who have had PIH/pre-eclampsia should be reviewed in a specialist obstetric hypertension clinic. Blood pressure should be measured, and medication adjusted accordingly. Women with persistent severe hypertension after delivery should be investigated for underlying causes such as renal disease (renal ultrasound scan) and phaeochromocytoma (24 h urine collection for VMA).

Women who have had severe hypertensive disorders of pregnancy have an increased incidence of subsequent cardiovascular morbidity, especially hypertension. Therefore, the combined oral contraceptive pill may be less suitable for such patients and other methods of contraception should be discussed (e.g. progesterone only preparations, barrier contraception, intrauterine contraceptive devices). Patients who had hypertension in pregnancy, especially if severe, will have had a difficult pregnancy with much medical intervention. This opportunity should be taken to educate the patient about hypertension in pregnancy, and discuss the risks of recurrence if the patient wishes to conceive again. For women who have had severe hypertension in pregnancy, the risk of recurrence is approximately 50%, although this may be reduced by prophylactic aspirin to approximately 42%. The risk of recurrence is greater for women who had early onset or particularly severe disease. It is vital that women who had eclampsia are seen postnatally to fully discuss events. These women also have a recurrence risk. For women that had HELLP syndrome, there may be a recurrence risk of up to 27% of developing HELLP syndrome again, but also a risk of up to 42% of developing pre-eclampsia.

Finally, epidemiological studies have recently demonstrated a relationship between a pregnancy complicated by pre-eclampsia and an increased risk of maternal coronary heart disease in later life. This link between pregnancy complications and risk of vascular disease provides an important opportunity for identifying those individuals at risk. Interventions could start at the routine 6 week postpartum review when these women could be made aware of their potentially increased risk for coronary heart disease and counseled appropriately regarding lifestyle modification, such as diet and exercise.

CONCLUSION

Hypertensive disorders in pregnancy are a significant cause of maternal and perinatal morbidity and mortality worldwide. In pre-eclampsia, the placenta releases circulating factors or placental syncytial debris that cause endothelial cell dysfunction and the subsequent multisystem disorder. The identification of risk factors can determine women at high risk of developing pre-eclampsia. Prophylactic measures in high risk women include prescription of low dose aspirin and calcium. Women with chronic hypertension or pre-eclampsia require increased fetal surveillance through growth scans. At present, the only treatment option for pre-eclampsia is delivery. There is a risk–benefit balance for delivery depending on the gestation. It is vital to control hypertension with pharmacological agents, especially at levels $\geq 160/110$ mmHg. Women with pre-eclampsia require careful immediate postpartum care with particular attention to fluid balance.

Further reading

Attalah A N, Hofmeyr G J, Duley L 2002 Calcium supplementation during pregnancy for preventing hypertensive disorders and related problems. The Cochrane Database of Systematic Reviews, Issue 1

Brown M A, Hague W, Higgins J et al 2000 The detection, investigation and management of hypertension in pregnancy: full consensus statement. Australian & New Zealand Journal of Obstetrics & Gynaecology 40(2):139-155

Chappell LC, Seed PT, Briley AL et al 1999 Effect of antioxidants on the occurrence of pre-eclampsia in women at increased risk: a randomised trial. Lancet 354:810-816

Confidential Enquiry into Maternal and Child Health 2004 Why mothers die 2000-2002. RCOG, London

Duley L, Henderson-Smart D, Knight M et al 2003 Antiplatelet drugs for prevention of pre-eclampsia and its consequences. The Cochrane Database of Systematic Reviews, Issue 4

Greer I A 2005 Pregnancy-induced hypertension. In: Oxford textbook of clinical nephrology 3rd edn. Oxford University Press, Oxford, p 2261-2284

Kenny L, Baker P N 1999 Maternal pathophysiology in pre-eclampsia. Baillieres Best Practice and Research in Clinical Obstetric Gynaecology 13(1): 59-75

Myers J, Brocklesby J 2004 The epidemiology of pre-eclampsia. In: Baker P, Kingdom J (eds) Pre-eclampsia: current perspectives on management. Parthenon, London, p 25-39

Magpie Trial Collaborative Group 2002 Do women with pre-eclampsia, and their babies, benefit from magnesium sulphate? The Magpie Trial: a randomised placebo-controlled trial. Lancet 359:1877-1890

Milne F, Redman C, Walker J, Baker P, Bradley J et al 2005 The pre-eclampsia community guideline (PRECOG): how to screen for and detect onset of pre-eclampsia in the community. British Medical Journal 330:576-580

Poston L, Briley A L, Seed P T, et al 2006 Vitamins in Pre-eclampsia (VIP) Trial Consortium. Vitamin C and vitamin E in pregnant women at risk for pre-eclampsia (VIP trial): randomised placebo-controlled trial. Lancet 367(9517):1119-1120

Rumbold A R, Crowther C A, Haslam R R, et al 2006 ACTS study group. Vitamins C and E and the risks of preeclampsia and perinatal complications. New England Journal of Medicine 354(17):1841-1843

Sattar N, Greer I A 2002 Pregnancy complications and maternal cardiovascular risk: opportunities for intervention and screening? British Medical Journal 325(7356):157-160

Chapter 4

Renal disorders

D. Williams, L. Lightstone

Renal changes during normal pregnancy and acute renal failure

D. Williams

RENAL CHANGES IN NORMAL PREGNANCY

Renal glomerular function during pregnancy

Renal adaptation to pregnancy is anticipated prior to conception, during the luteal phase of each menstrual cycle. Renal blood flow and glomerular filtration rate (GFR) increase by 10-20% before menstruation. If pregnancy is established the corpus luteum persists and these hemodynamic changes continue. By 16 weeks gestation GFR is 55% above non-pregnant levels. This increment is mediated through an increase in renal blood flow that reaches a maximum of 70-80%

above non-pregnant levels by the second trimester, before falling to around 45% above non-pregnant levels, at term. Elegant human studies have confirmed that unlike the hyperfiltration that precedes diabetic nephropathy, gestational hyperfiltration is not associated with a damaging rise in glomerular capillary blood pressure.

The changes to renal physiology in healthy pregnancy can both hide and mimic renal disease. The increased GFR of pregnancy leads to a fall in serum creatinine concentration (SCR), so that values considered normal in the non-pregnant state may be abnormal during pregnancy. Serum creatinine levels fall from a non-pregnant mean value of 73 µmolL^{-1} (0.82 mg/dL) to 60 µmolL^{-1} (0.68 mg/dL), 54 µmolL^{-1} (0.61 mg/dL) and 64 µmolL^{-1} (0.72 mg/dL) in successive trimesters. Serum creatinine is not however linearly correlated with creatinine clearance and is influenced by muscle mass, physical exercise, racial differences and dietary intake of meat. As SCR roughly doubles for every 50% reduction in GFR, a more useful parameter by which to monitor serial changes in renal function is the reciprocal of SCR (1/SCR). Estimates of GFR can be further refined using the Cockcroft–Gault equation, which calculates GFR using SCR, maternal age and pre-pregnancy weight. For women the Cockcroft–Gault equation is:

$$GFR \ (mL/min) = 0.8 \times [140 - age \ (years) \times weight \ (kg)] \ / \ SCR \ (\mu mol/L)$$

(1 mg/dL creatinine = 88.4 µmol/L creatinine)

The gestational rise in renal blood flow also causes the kidneys to swell so that bipolar renal length increases by approximately 1 cm. During the third trimester renal blood flow falls, leading to a fall in creatinine clearance and a rise in SCR. Serum urea levels however continue to fall in the third trimester due to reduced maternal hepatic urea synthesis. This metabolic adaptation ensures that more nitrogen is available for fetal protein synthesis.

The renal pelvicaliceal system and ureters dilate and can appear obstructed to those unaware of these changes, especially on the right side. The right pelvicaliceal system dilates by a maximum of 0.5 mm each week from 6-32 weeks, reaching a maximum diameter of approximately 20 mm (90th percentile), which is maintained until term. The left pelvicaliceal system reaches a maximum diameter of 8 mm (90th percentile) at 20 weeks gestation.

Proteinuria increases as pregnancy progresses, but levels over 200 mg 24 h^{-1} during the third trimester are above the 95% confidence limit for the normal population. A random urine protein : creatinine ratio is a useful guide to 24-h urinary protein excretion, but is not a substitute for either a 12-h or 24-h urine collection, due to the high incidence of both false positive and false negative results. A random urine sample that gives a protein (mg) : creatinine (mmol) ratio of > 0.20 is a good predictor of significant proteinuria and is an indication for more accurate assessment of proteinuria with a 12- or 24-h urine collection.

Serum albumin levels fall by 5-10 gL^{-1}, serum cholesterol and triglyceride concentrations increase significantly and dependent edema affects most pregnancies at term. Normal pregnancy therefore simulates the classic features of nephrotic syndrome.

Renal tubular function during pregnancy

Increased alveolar ventilation causes a respiratory alkalosis to which the kidney responds by increased bicarbonaturia and a compensatory metabolic acidosis. Other renal tubular changes include reduced tubular glucose reabsorption, which leads to glycosuria in approximately 10% of healthy pregnant women, a 250-300% increase in urinary calcium excretion and a first trimester increase in urate excretion that decreases towards term at which time plasma urate levels rise again to non-pregnancy levels.

During healthy pregnancy a mother gains 6-8 kg of fluid, of which approximately 1.2 L is due to an increase in plasma volume. Plasma osmolality falls by 10 mosmol/kg^{-1} by 5-8 weeks gestation due to a fall in both the threshold for thirst and for the release of anti-diuretic hormone (vasopressin). During pregnancy, vasopressin is metabolised by placental vasopressinase, and at term the maternal posterior pituitary produces four times as much vasopressin to maintain physiological concentrations. Failure of the maternal pituitary to keep up with the increased metabolic clearance of vasopressin leads to a transient polyuric state in the third trimester, which is known as transient diabetes insipidus of pregnancy.

Renal endocrine function during pregnancy

The kidney also acts as an endocrine organ that produces erythropoietin, active vitamin D and renin. The production of all three hormones increases during healthy pregnancy, but their effects are masked by other changes. In early pregnancy, peripheral vasodilatation exceeds renin-aldosterone-mediated plasma volume expansion, so diastolic blood pressure falls by 12 weeks. Conversely, plasma volume expansion exceeds the erythropoietin-mediated increase in red cell mass, causing a 'physiological anaemia', which should not normally lead to a Hb concentration of less than 9.5 g dl^{-1}. Similarly, extra active vitamin D produced by the placenta, circulates at twice non-gravid levels, but concomitant halving of parathyroid hormone levels, hypercalciuria and increased fetal requirements, keep plasma ionized calcium levels unchanged.

Urinary tract infection

General

The incidence of asymptomatic bacteriuria (significant growth of a uropathogen in the absence of symptoms) is 2-10%, which is the same during pregnancy as it is in sexually active non-pregnant women.

However, the structural and immune changes to the urothelium of the renal tracts during pregnancy make it more likely that a lower urinary tract infection (UTI) will ascend to cause acute pyelonephritis. During pregnancy, 12.5-30% of women with untreated asymptomatic bacteriuria will develop acute pyelonephritis; a serious infection with significant morbidity to mother and fetus.

Diagnosis of a urinary tract infection

During pregnancy symptoms suggestive of an UTI are dysuria and offensive-smelling urine. Other symptoms, usually associated with an UTI are urinary frequency, nocturia, urge-incontinence and strangury (the urge to pass urine having just done so), but these symptoms are also found in healthy pregnant women.

Microscopy and culture of a freshly voided mid-stream urine sample will allow quantification of pyuria (leucocytes in the urine) and growth of a urinary pathogen. Bacterial UTI is the most common cause of pyuria and is considered significant if microscopy of a sample of un-spun mid-stream urine reveals more than 10 leucocytes per microliter. Urine culture is conventionally recognized as significant if there is growth of more than 10^5 colony forming units per milliliter (cfu/ml) of a single recognized uropathogen, in association with pyuria. Low counts of bacteriuria (10^2-10^4 cfu/ml) may still be significant if symptomatic women have a high fluid intake or are infected with a slow growing organism. If left untreated, most symptomatic women with 'low-count bacteriuria' will have 10^5 cfu/ml 2 days later. During pregnancy, the most common uro-pathogens are bowel commensals, *Escherichia coli* (70-80%), *Klebsiella*, *Proteus*, *Enterobacter* and *Staphylococcus saprophyticus*.

If urine from a symptomatic pregnant woman is cloudy and positive on dipstick testing for nitrite (produced by most uropathogens) and leucocyte esterase (produced by white blood cells), then an UTI is likely and empirical treatment can be started. These urine sticks are not sensitive enough to be used for screening for asymptomatic bacteriuria in early pregnancy, therefore microscopy and culture of a clean catch mid-stream urine sample is necessary. Hematuria and proteinuria are unreliable indicators of an UTI, but are important signs of renal disease (see later).

Asymptomatic bacteriuria – maternal/fetal risks

During pregnancy, untreated asymptomatic bacteriuria will develop into acute pyelonephritis in 12.5-30% of women, but if treated less than 1% of pregnant women develop pyelonephritis. A systematic review of 14 studies confirmed that antibiotic treatment of asymptomatic bacteriuria significantly reduced the incidence of pyelonephritis compared to placebo or no treatment (odds ratio 0.24; 95% CI 0.19-0.32). Following successful treatment of asymptomatic bacteriuria, monthly screening of mid-stream urine is necessary, as about 30% of women will have a relapse of bacteriuria, making them vulnerable to acute pyelonephritis again.

Asymptomatic bacteriuria has also been associated with an increased risk of preterm delivery and low birth weight. Treatment of asymptomatic bacteriuria has been shown to reduce the incidence of preterm delivery and low birthweight babies (odds ratio 0.60; 95% CI 0.45-0.80). Others have not however found the same association between preterm labor and bacteriuria. It has been suggested that the underlying renal pathology, which is commonly associated with bacteriuria, is responsible for poor pregnancy outcomes. Further good quality studies are needed to settle this issue.

Management of asymptomatic bacteriuria

Contrary to much published advice, not all pregnant women need to be screened for asymptomatic bacteriuria. There are two main reasons. First, the prevalence of asymptomatic bacteriuria varies between populations and where it is low (< 2.5%) it is hard to justify the cost-effectiveness of screening. In populations where the prevalence of asymptomatic bacteriuria is > 5% the case for screening is much stronger. Second, approximately 1-2% of the 90-98% of asymptomatic women who test negative for bacteriuria in the first trimester will develop a symptomatic UTI. Therefore a third of all women who develop an UTI in late pregnancy would have been missed on first trimester screening. Women at increased risk of pyelonephritis or renal impairment should be screened for asymptomatic bacteriuria every 4-6 weeks throughout pregnancy (Box 4.1).

Treatment of urinary tract infections

There is no consensus as to the optimal treatment of asymptomatic bacteriuria, nor the empirical treatment of symptomatic UTIs in pregnancy. Most urinary infections during pregnancy (approximately 75%) are caused by *E. coli*, which is usually sensitive to either nitrofurantoin (89%), trimethoprim (with or without sulfamethoxazole) (87%), ampicillin (72%) or

Box 4.1 Screening for asymptomatic bacteriuria (every 4-6 weeks) is recommended for the following groups of pregnant women

- Past history of asymptomatic bacteriuria.
- Previous recurrent UTIs.
- Pre-existing renal disease, especially scarred kidneys due to reflux nephropathy.
- Structural and neuropathic abnormalities of the renal tracts.
- Renal calculi.
- Pre-existing diabetes mellitus but not gestational diabetes.
- Sickle cell disease and trait.
- Low socio-economic group and less than 12 years higher education.

cephalosporins. Therefore until well-structured trials are done, the most cost-effective treatment regimen for either asymptomatic bacteriuria or a first episode of cystitis is either nitrofurantoin monohydrate macrocrystals (100 mg twice daily for 3 days) – or trimethoprim (200 mg twice daily for 3 days). Nitrofurantoin should be avoided after the onset of labour in patients with glucose-6-phosphate dehydrogenase deficiency, although no well-documented case of hemolysis in the neonate has ever been recorded, and trimethoprim is best avoided in the first trimester as it is a folic acid antagonist associated with a possible increased risk of neural tube defect.

Screening for recurrent infections should begin one week after completion of initial treatment and then 4-6 weekly for the rest of pregnancy. Recurrent infections or a first infection in a pregnant woman at high risk of pyelonephritis (Box 4.1) should be treated with a 7-10 days course of an antibiotic that reflects antibacterial sensitivities. Women who have had two episodes of asymptomatic bacteriuria or cystitis should be considered for low dose antibiotic prophylaxis – guided by the sensitivities of the most recent infective organism, for the remainder of pregnancy and until 4-6 weeks postpartum. Suitable agents for long-term antibiotic prophylaxis include nitrofurantoin 50-100 mg nocte, amoxicillin 250 mg nocte, cephalexin 125-250 mg nocte or trimethoprim 100-150 mg nocte. These women should also be investigated for structural abnormalities of the renal tracts or renal calculus, using ultrasonography.

Acute pyelonephritis

General

The same uropathogens that cause asymptomatic bacteriuria and cystitis are responsible for acute pyelonephritis. Therefore the prevalence of asymptomatic bacteriuria in a pregnant population (see above), dictates the incidence of acute pyelonephritis. Screening and treating a high-risk population for asymptomatic bacteriuria (Box 4.1), reduces the incidence of acute pyelonephritis to less than 1%. Unless acute pyelonephritis is treated promptly there is considerable maternal and fetal morbidity.

Maternal symptoms and signs

Most women with acute pyelonephritis present in the second and third trimester. Over 80% of women present with back ache, fever, rigors and costovertebral angle tenderness, while about one-half have lower urinary tract symptoms, nausea and vomiting. Bacteremia is present in 15-20% of pregnant women with acute pyelonephritis and a small proportion of these women will develop septic shock, increased capillary leak, leading to pulmonary edema. It is important however to differentiate the hypotension due to reduced intravascular volume (fever, nausea and vomiting) from that due to septic shock. Women with pyelonephritis at risk of serious complications are those who present with the highest fever (> 39.4 °C), tachycardia (> 110 bpm), at > 20 weeks gestation and who have received tocolytic agents and injudicious fluid replacement.

Fetal risks

Acute pyelonephritis can trigger uterine contractions and preterm labor. Antibiotic treatment of pyelonephritis will reduce uterine activity, but those with recurrent infection or marked uterine activity are at increased risk of preterm labor. As uterine activity is often present in the absence of cervical change and as tocolysis with beta mimetics aggravates the cardiovascular response to endotoxemia, tocolytic therapy should be used with care and only in those with cervical changes.

Management of acute pyelonephritis

Women suspected of acute pyelonephritis from their history, symptoms and signs should be admitted to hospital. Laboratory tests should include full blood count, SCR, electrolytes and urine culture. If there are systemic symptoms and/or septic shock a blood culture may be useful. Pregnant women with pyelonephritis and septic shock need intensive care. In these women, assessment of the state of hydration is critical and often requires invasive hemodynamic monitoring with a central venous pressure line. This will optimize fluid balance, aiming for a urine output greater than 30 ml h^{-1} to minimize renal impairment and reduce the risk of pulmonary edema. Intravenous antibiotics should be started empirically (see below) until sensitivities of blood and urine cultures are known. These women often have transient renal impairment, thrombocytopenia and hemolysis, suggesting that the endothelium is damaged by endotoxin. A blood film and lactate dehydrogenase concentration will diagnose hemolysis.

Trials investigating the outpatient management of pyelonephritis in pregnancy have identified a group of women who can be managed at home. These women should be less than 24 weeks gestation, be relatively healthy and understand the importance of compliance. They should have an initial period of observation in hospital to demonstrate ability to take oral fluids, receive intramuscular cefuroxime/ceftriaxone and following satisfactory laboratory tests can go home to be seen again within 24 h for a second intramuscular dose of cephalosporin. They then start a 10-day course of oral cephalexin 500 mg four times daily, or appropriate antibiotic with regular outpatient follow-up. Following this regimen 90% of women will improve as outpatients and 10% will require hospital admission due to sepsis or recurrent pyelonephritis. Women with acute pyelonephritis over 24 weeks gestation should be admitted for at least 24 h to observe the maternal condition as above and to monitor uterine activity and fetal heart rate.

Choice of antibiotic

Gram-negative bacteria causing pyelonephritis in pregnancy are often resistant to ampicillin, therefore intravenous cefuroxime 0.75-1.5 mg (depending on severity of condition) every 8 h is an effective first choice until sensitivities are known. Women allergic to beta-lactam antibiotics can be given intravenous gentamicin (1.5 mg/kg every 8 h) for the initial treatment of acute pyelonephritis. A single daily protocol dose (7 mg/kg every 24 h) should be used with caution during pregnancy to reduce the very small risk of eighth nerve damage to the fetus. Serum concentrations of gentamicin should be measured and dose adjustments made according to levels. Intravenous antibiotics should be continued until the patient has been afebrile for 24 h. Oral antibiotics should then be given for a further 7-10 days, according to bacterial

sensitivities, or if not available, as if for symptomatic lower UTI (see above).

Failure of these measures to improve the maternal clinical condition within 48-72 h, suggests an underlying structural abnormality. Ultrasonography is an easy, but inconclusive way of excluding stones. If clinical suspicion is high, a plain abdominal X-ray will identify 90% of renal stones and a one shot intravenous urogram (IVU) at 20-30 min will identify the rest. The risk to the fetus from radiation of one or two X-rays is minimal, especially when compared with the clinical benefit of identifying an obstructed, nonfunctioning kidney. Urinary tract obstruction can also be detected using magnetic resonance urography, especially during the second and third trimesters.

Following one episode of pyelonephritis, pregnant women should have monthly urine cultures to screen for a recurrence. The risk of recurrent pyelonephritis can be reduced with low-dose antimicrobial prophylaxis, according to the sensitivities of initial bacterial infection, for example nitrofurantoin 100 mg nocte continued until 4-6 weeks postpartum.

ACUTE RENAL FAILURE IN PREGNANCY

General

Acute renal failure is now a rare, but serious complication of pregnancy. In early pregnancy acute renal failure is associated with septic abortion (a complication now largely confined to the developing world), and dehydration related to hyperemesis gravidarum. Around the time of delivery, acute renal failure is most commonly caused by gestational syndromes such as pre-eclampsia and abruption placentae (Box 4.2). Pregnancy is however a prothrombotic state, associated with heightened inflammation and major changes to the vascular endothelium, in particular the glomerular capillary endothelium. These physiological changes predispose pregnant women to acute glomerular capillary thrombosis. Whereas non-pregnant patients who suffer an acute pre-renal insult, e.g. hemorrhage, dehydration or septic shock, may develop transient acute tubular necrosis if inadequately treated, the same pre-renal insult in pregnancy is more likely to develop into renal cortical necrosis with permanent renal impairment. This is even more likely to occur if a pre-renal insult coexists with a pregnancy-related condition that induces a consumptive coagulopathy and/or endothelial damage e.g. pre-eclampsia.

The principles of management are aimed at identification and correction of the precipitating insult, optimal fluid resuscitation, which is best guided by

Box 4.2 Causes of acute renal failure in pregnancy

Most common causes
- Placental abruption.
- Severe pre-eclampsia/especially with hemorrhage.

Early pregnancy causes
- Septic abortion.
- Hyperemesis gravidarum.
- Ovarian hyperstimulation syndrome.

Rare causes
- Amniotic fluid embolus.
- HUS/TTP.
- Acute fatty liver of pregnancy.
- Acute obstruction of renal tracts.

monitoring the central venous pressure. If oliguria persists despite euvolemia, with deteriorating renal function or fluid overload, then fluid restriction followed by renal replacement therapy is indicated.

Pre-eclampsia and the kidney

General

Pre-eclampsia rarely causes acute renal failure severe enough to require dialysis. In a cohort of South African women with severe pre-eclampsia and renal impairment 7/72 (10%) required temporary dialysis and none developed chronic renal failure. All women who needed dialysis either had hemorrhage due to abruption placentae or Hemolysis, Elevated Liver enzymes and Low Platelets (HELLP syndrome). Pre-eclampsia causing mild transient renal impairment (SCR up to 125 μmolL^{-1}; 1.41 mg/dL) is common, but with appropriate management, there should be complete recovery of renal function (see below).

Women with pre-existing renal disease are more vulnerable to pre-eclampsia, especially when it is associated with chronic hypertension. A meta-analysis of trials investigating the effectiveness of low dose aspirin (50-150 mg/day) in pregnant women with moderate to severe renal disease revealed a significant reduction in the risk of pre-eclampsia and perinatal death.

Conversely, only 2-5% of women with pre-eclampsia have been found to have underlying renal disease when assessed more than 3 months postpartum. Women who have had pre-eclampsia should therefore be checked for persistent postpartum hypertension and proteinuria. Gestational hypertension usually

resolves within 3 months of delivery, but heavy proteinuria due to pre-eclampsia can take up to 12 months to disappear. Women who have had pre-eclampsia are more likely to have persistent microalbuminuria compatible with microvascular disease and an increased risk of cardiovascular disease in later life.

Women who develop high levels of proteinuria (> 10 g/24 h) tend to have earlier onset pre-eclampsia and deliver at an earlier gestational age as compared with pre-eclamptic women who have less marked proteinuria (< 5 g/24 h). It is of note, that after correction for prematurity, however, massive proteinuria (> 10 g/24 h) has no significant effect on neonatal outcome. Increasing proteinuria per se is not therefore an indication for delivery. Pregnant women who develop proteinuria > 1-3 g/24 h, (the threshold influenced by other maternal risk factors for thrombosis), should be started on thromboprophylaxis with dalteparine enoxaparin 40 mg s.c. o.d. or low molecular heparin 5000 units s.c. o.d.

The diagnosis of pre-eclampsia is difficult if there is chronic hypertension and pre-existing proteinuria, especially as these two parameters become more marked in late pregnancy. Furthermore, hyperuricemia and IUGR are common features of both pre-eclampsia and chronic renal impairment, but the presence of raised hepatic transaminases and thrombocytopenia support a diagnosis of pre-eclampsia.

Pre-eclampsia: management of renal impairment and fluid balance

The cure for severe pre-eclampsia is delivery of the baby and placenta. Delivery may halt the general progression of pre-eclampsia, but postpartum maternal renal function usually deteriorates before improving. Dialysis is very rarely necessary, but is most common in pre-eclamptic women who have hemorrhage in association with placental abruption and who double their SCR in the first 24-48 h after admission. Women with pre-eclampsia who have a rise in SCR from around 70 μmol/L (0.79 mg/dL) to greater than 120 μmol/L (1.36 mg/dL) should be delivered to prevent ongoing renal impairment.

Fluid balance is critical to the management of acute renal failure during pregnancy. Too little intravascular fluid leads to pre-renal failure, especially damaging to chronically impaired kidneys, while too much fluid risks pulmonary edema, adult respiratory distress syndrome and maternal death. Furthermore, transient oliguria (less than 100 mL over 4 h) is a common observation in the first 24 h immediately after a healthy pregnancy. If a pre-eclamptic woman is not obviously hypovolemic and has a serum urea

≤ 5 mmol/L and SCR ≤ 90 µmol/L, repeated fluid challenges to increase urine output are unnecessary and will only increase the maternal risk of pulmonary oedema. Women with severe pre-eclampsia and renal impairment (SCR>120 µmol/L; 1.36 mg/dL) should have their fluid balance guided by careful clinical assessment and sometimes a central venous pressure catheter. The rate of fluid replacement should take account of central venous filling pressure, hourly urine output and insensible losses. Once euvolemic, the rate of i.v. fluid replacement should equal the previous hours' urine output plus insensible losses – usually 30 mL/h, if apyrexial. The amount of i.v. fluid replacement can be reduced, once the mother can take oral fluid and her renal impairment starts to improve. Intravenous fluid orders that adhere to a fixed hourly replacement can lead to fluid overload in oliguric women and to reduced intravascular volume in those having a diuresis. Fluid replacement should include blood to replace blood losses, then isotonic sodium chloride or compound sodium lactate (Hartmann's solution). Dextrose solutions are hypotonic and lead to maternal hyponatremia (5% dextrose contains only 30 mmolL^{-1} NaCl, compared with 150 mmolL^{-1} NaCl in 0.9% sodium chloride solution).

Low dose 'renal' dopamine infusion (3 µg/kg/min) was previously used to increase renal blood flow in people with acute renal failure. However, a group of 60 South African women with severe pre-eclampsia and acute renal failure had a similar improvement in urine output and renal function following furosemide infusion (5 mg/h) as compared with dopamine infusion. As furosemide has fewer side effects than dopamine, it is recommended that once hypovolemia has been corrected, as judged by the CVP, pre-eclamptic women with oliguria (< 200 mL/12 h) and a serum urea>14 mmol/l and SCR>500 µmol/L may benefit from a furosemide infusion in an effort to prevent hemodialysis. Despite a combination of furosemide followed by low dose dopamine infusion and vice versa, 13/60 pre-eclamptic women with oliguric renal failure required temporary dialysis.

Once acute tubular necrosis (ATN) is established, with oliguria and a rising SCR, despite adequate intravascular volume and blood pressure, then fluid intake should be restricted to avoid fluid overload. Under these circumstances, renal replacement therapy is indicated (Box 4.3). There are no good studies that have followed up women with acute renal failure related to pre-eclampsia, but those with the most severe renal impairment will undoubtedly be left with a degree of permanent renal impairment that might not become manifest until later life.

> ### Box 4.3 Indications for renal replacement therapy (RRT; dialysis)
>
> Hyperkalemia (K>7.0 mmol/L), refractory to medical treatment.
> Pulmonary edema, refractory to diuretics.
> Acidosis producing circulatory problems.
> Uremia (there is no absolute level of uremia above which dialysis is mandatory for new onset acute renal failure, but a serum urea over 25-30 mmol/L or SCR>500-700 mmol/L (5.65-7.91 mg/dL), usually indicates a need for dialysis.

Hypertension due to pre-eclampsia is usually caused by vasoconstriction around a reduced plasma volume. For this reason and despite the lack of evidence from randomized trials, women with severe pre-eclampsia often receive plasma volume expansion prior to therapeutic vasodilation. Unless there are signs of pulmonary edema, (basal crackles and PO2<95% on air), 500 ml of colloid or crystalloid given over 30-60 min, or 250 ml/h until the pulmonary wedge pressure is 10-12 mmHg can improve both maternal and fetal well-being in severe pre-eclampsia. A vasodilator given alone can cause profound hypotension that may threaten maternal renal, cerebral and utero-placental blood flow.

Hemolytic uremic syndrome/thrombotic thrombocytopenic purpura

Hemolytic uremic syndrome (HUS) and thrombotic thrombocytopenic purpura (TTP) are very similar syndromes (from here on designated HUS/TTP). They are characterized by microangiopathic hemolytic anemia and thrombocytopenia. Both congenital and acquired forms of HUS/TTP are more common in late pregnancy. Women with HUS/TTP develop platelet thrombi attached to von Willebrand factor multimers in end organ micro-vessels. This typically results in a multi-organ disorder with abdominal ischemia and renal and/or neurological impairment. A plasma metalloprotease (ADAMTS13), which normally cleaves von Willebrand factor multimers to prevent micro-thrombi, is deficient in some women with congenital HUS/TTP and antibodies that neutralize ADAMTS13 have been found in women with acquired HUS/TTP.

HUS/TTP is more common in women (approximately 70% of all cases) and more common in association with pregnancy (approximately 13% of all cases). During pregnancy, the levels of ADAMTS13 fall progressively. This may explain why women with a congenital deficiency of ADAMTS13 or with other risk factors for thrombosis (e.g. obesity or a thrombophilia) are predisposed to peripartum HUS/TTP.

HUS/TTP and pre-eclampsia

Pre-eclampsia shares many similarities with HUS/TTP, and both syndromes occur most frequently in the third trimester or immediately postpartum. It is however important to differentiate between them, because their management is different. Women with HUS/TTP often present with gastrointestinal or neurological abnormalities and they are more likely to have severe renal impairment, hemolysis and thrombocytopenia compared with women who have pre-eclampsia. Disseminated intravascular coagulation (DIC) is rare in HUS/TTP, so prothrombin time and kaolin clotting time are usually normal. Women with pre-eclampsia are more likely to have elevated hepatic transaminases, heavy proteinuria and abnormal clotting compared with women with HUS/TTP. However, in many women the distinction between pre-eclampsia and HUS/TTP can only be determined by the course of the illness following delivery, but here again acute renal failure due to pre-eclampsia usually gets transiently worse before improving.

HUS/TTP management

Maternal survival from HUS/TTP has greatly improved since treatment with plasmapheresis – infusion of fresh plasma and removal of old plasma. Until recently it was unclear why plasmapheresis worked, but the recent discovery of antibodies to ADAMTS13 (removed with old plasma) and a congenital deficiency of ADAMTS13 (replenished with infusion of fresh plasma), gives reason to this process. However, a severe deficiency in ADAMTS13, which is not currently a routine laboratory measurement, is not present in all cases of HUS/TTP and plasmapheresis is effective in pregnant women who have milder deficiencies of ADAMTS13.

Steroids are often added to the plasma exchange regimen and are a rational choice for acquired HUS/TTP with an autoimmune pathology, but there are no randomized controlled trials of their use. Antiplatelet therapy with aspirin and dipyridamole, may also be beneficial in conjunction with plasma exchange. Conversely, administration of platelets to thrombocytopenic patients with HUS/TTP can result in a precipitous decline in clinical status.

Acute renal cortical necrosis

In the developed world, acute renal cortical necrosis (ARCN) has become a rare complication of pregnancy.

The reduced incidence of septic abortion and improved management of peripartum obstetric emergencies has prevented pre-renal impairment developing into acute tubular necrosis and then renal cortical necrosis. In the developing world however, obstetric emergencies are still responsible for the majority of cases of ARCN. Acute renal failure following septic abortion or peripartum obstetric emergencies developed into ARCN in 20% of women following a prolonged period of acute tubular necrosis.

ARCN is most commonly caused by abruption of the placenta with hemorrhage, amniotic fluid embolus and sepsis associated with DIC. Following hemorrhage or sepsis with hypotension, pre-renal failure will without adequate resuscitation lead to acute tubular necrosis. If anuria persists for longer than a week, then ARCN should be suspected. A definitive diagnosis can be made with renal biopsy, but is often missed due to the patchy nature of cortical necrosis. Selective renal angiography will also confirm the diagnosis, but introduces another nephrotoxic agent and is usually unnecessary. Due to the serious nature of the precipitating illness and the limited availability of renal replacement therapy in the developing world, maternal mortality is still high. However, for those women who survive the acute illness, renal function usually returns slowly over the next 6-24 months. Long-term renal function depends on the extent of cortical necrosis, which is often incomplete. Hyperfiltration through remnant glomeruli, usually leads to a subsequent progressive decline in renal function.

Acute fatty liver of pregnancy

Acute fatty liver of pregnancy (AFLP) causes reversible peripartum liver and renal impairment in 1:5000 to 1:10000 pregnancies. The diagnosis is made on clinical and laboratory findings of impaired liver, renal and clotting function, rather than on histological or radiological evidence of a fatty liver. Women with AFLP usually present with nausea, vomiting and abdominal cramps. Impaired renal function and reduced plasma antithrombin levels are early findings of AFLP that may precede liver dysfunction. In established cases of AFLP, depressed function of the liver with prolonged prothrombin time, hypoglycemia and DIC are more markedly abnormal than liver transaminases, which may only be moderately elevated. In a series of 28 women with AFLP, other ubiquitous laboratory findings at the time of delivery were elevated serum total bilirubin (mean 7.5 mg/dL), SCR (mean 205 μmol/L; 2.3 mg/dL) and uric acid levels (mean 11 mg/dL).

A recessively inherited fetal inborn error of mito-chondrial fatty acid oxidation may explain up to 20% of AFLP. Mitochondrial fatty acid oxidation is important for both normal renal and liver function and may therefore explain the dual vulnerability of these organs in women with AFLP.

In women with AFLP, maternal renal impairment is aggravated by hypotension secondary to hemorrhage, which is itself most likely to follow an emergency operative delivery. The combination of renal dysfunction, hemorrhage and DIC secondary to liver failure during pregnancy or postpartum, requires intensive care with a multidisciplinary team of hepatologists, nephrologists, intensivists and obstetricians. Management is supportive, aimed at maintaining adequate fluid balance for renal perfusion, replacing blood, correcting the coagulopathy with fresh frozen plasma and possibly with antithrombin concentrate and fresh platelets. Hypoglycemia should be corrected with 10% dextrose solutions. Temporary dialysis may be necessary, but with good supportive care, recovery of normal renal and liver function is usual. Perinatal survival in association with AFLP is improving, but is dependent on the early recognition of the maternal condition, close fetal surveillance, timely delivery and excellent neonatal care.

Nephrotoxic drugs during pregnancy

Non-steroidal anti-inflammatory drugs (NSAIDs), including the more selective COX-2 inhibitors, when given to the mother peripartum, reduce renal blood flow and can cause acute renal impairment, to both mother and fetus. Women with reduced intravascular volume, especially with pre-existing renal impairment and pre-eclampsia, are particularly vulnerable and should be prescribed NSAID only with extreme caution. Aminoglycosides are also nephrotoxic and should be prescribed with care and attention to drug plasma levels in women with mild renal impairment.

Acute renal obstruction in pregnancy

General

Obstruction of the renal tracts during pregnancy may be due to renal calculi (see later), congenital renal tract abnormalities or a gestational over-distension syndrome. Women born with congenital obstructive uropathies at the pelvo- or vesico-ureteric junction (PUJ or VUJ) are at increased risk of urine outflow obstruction in the second half of pregnancy, even if they have had surgical correction in childhood. Congenital abnormalities of the lower urinary tracts including the bladder and urethra are varied and usually require extensive surgical correction in childhood. During pregnancy, these women are at increased risk of recurrent urine infections and less commonly, of outflow obstruction requiring either temporary nephrostomy or ureteric stent.

Women with a single kidney and urological abnormalities are particularly vulnerable to develop post-renal failure in relation to gestational obstruction of their solitary kidney. An incomplete obstruction can cause renal impairment with an apparently good urine output. High back-pressure compresses and damages the renal medulla, leading to a loss of renal concentrating ability and production of dilute urine that is passed through an incomplete obstruction. It is also important for the obstetrician to remember that a congenitally single kidney is often associated with other abnormalities of the genital tracts, such as a unicornuate uterus.

During pregnancy the renal tracts can rarely and spontaneously become grossly over-distended. If untreated, over-distension can occasionally lead to rupture of the kidney or renal tracts. Women with over-distension of the renal tracts initially present with severe loin pain, most commonly on the right side and radiating to the lower abdomen. The pain is positional and inconstant; it is characteristically relieved by lying on the opposite side and tucking the knees up to the chest. A palpable tender flank mass may suggest renal tract rupture. Rupture of the kidney almost always occurs in a previously diseased kidney, usually in association with a benign hamartoma or renal abscess. Urinalysis will reveal either gross or microscopic hematuria. A renal ultrasound will detect a hydronephrotic kidney with a grossly dilated pelvicaliceal system (see above for physiological pelvicaliceal dimensions). Occasionally a urinoma will be evident around the kidney indicating rupture of the renal pelvis that can sometimes seal spontaneously.

The pain from the over-distension syndrome varies from mild to very severe. Women with mild symptoms can usually be managed with advice on positional relief and regular analgesia. Women with severe unremitting pain, hematuria and grossly distended renal tracts on ultrasound, in the absence of structural or infected masses, usually have immediate pain relief following decompression of the system with either a ureteric stent or nephrostomy. Rupture of the kidney necessitates immediate surgery and almost invariably an emergency nephrectomy.

Chronic kidney disease, dialysis and transplant

L. Lightstone

INTRODUCTION

In an ideal world, women with chronic kidney disease (CKD) would be known to their primary care physicians and would be aware of the need for pre-conception counseling about the risks of pregnancy to themselves and their fetus. However, many patients are entirely unaware that they have CKD and importantly even if they are, it may not occur to them that the CKD could have any influence on the outcome of a pregnancy. The following section highlights the key issues in women who have evidence of CKD whether they present pre-conception or when already pregnant.

CKD is now defined either on the evidence of normal estimated glomerular filtration rate (GFR) together with structural damage or abnormalities including proteinuria or albuminuria, or an estimated GFR of less than 60 mL/min 1.73 m^2. The two common methods for estimating GFR in the population are the MDRD (derived from the Modified Diet in Renal Disease Study and taking into account serum creatinine, age, gender and ethnicity; http://www.renal.org/Resources/resources.html) and the Cockcroft – Gault formula (http://www.renal.org/resources/resources.html). In the non-pregnant population, the MDRD is considered the more useful estimate; however it has not been validated in pregnant women. The Cockcroft–Gault formula appears to work well in pregnancy providing a pre-pregnancy weight is available. The emphasis on estimated GFR rather than serum creatinine reflects the acknowledgement that serum creatinine is not only affected by gender, age, ethnicity, muscle mass and diet but also that it does not rise above the normal range until the GFR has dropped to less than ~40 mL/min. Thus, an elevated creatinine is a good indicator of renal impairment whereas a normal creatinine can cover a multitude of sins. However, in the context of published data on renal disease in pregnancy, all studies to date have used serum creatinine rather than estimated renal function.

During the pre-conception session, the woman needs to be informed if her condition is likely to get worse because of a pregnancy and whether it will affect the health of the fetus during and the baby after the pregnancy.

INFLUENCE OF RENAL FUNCTION ON THE OUTCOME OF PREGNANCY

Pregnancy outcome broadly depends on the level of kidney dysfunction, hypertension and proteinuria, as well as on the specific nature of the renal condition. Large series have determined that the key determinant of outcome is the baseline renal function. Until recently most data classified risk according to three levels of serum creatinine – less than 125 μmol/L, 125-250 μmol/L and greater than 250 μmol/L. More recent data suggest that simply categorizing renal function into those with a creatinine of 180 μmol/L or more marks out those women who are most likely to have problems during the pregnancy, are least likely to have a successful outcome and have at least a 1 in 3 chance of being on dialysis within 1 year of pregnancy (Table 4.1). However, there are caveats – as already mentioned normal creatinine does not equate to normal function and a 45 kg vegan Caucasian woman with a creatinine of 100 μmol/L may have half the estimated creatinine clearance of a 95 kg meat-eating African-Caribbean woman with the same creatinine level. It is important to consider whether there is evidence of progressive renal decline – a patient who has suffered an acute renal insult in the past and has been left with a creatinine of 160 μmol/L but normal blood pressure and no proteinuria may be at much less risk than a woman with diabetic nephropathy whose creatinine was 120 μmol/L 1 year ago, is now 140 μmol/L and who has nephrotic range proteinuria.

All women with CKD are at increased risk of pre-eclampsia (PET) and should be considered as having relatively high risk pregnancies. However, a woman with normal renal function, not requiring anti-hypertensives or well-controlled hypertension on a single agent, with less than 1 g proteinuria/24 h (i.e. a protein : creatinine ratio of less than 100), is likely to have a successful obstetric outcome with minimal risk of progression of her renal disease. All women with renal disease who have hypertension and/or proteinuria or with renal impairment, should be regarded as being at a much higher risk and counseled appropriately. As illustrated in Table 4.2, the particular focus needs to be on the high risk of developing hypertension and worsening proteinuria, the difficulties these pose in diagnosing superimposed PET and the requirement for careful foetal monitoring.

FERTILITY AND GENETICS

Fertility can be impaired by prior treatment with cytotoxic agents, such as cyclophosphamide, by the disease itself (e.g. SLE) and by the level of renal impairment. It is pragmatic to consider assisted conception in some cases.

Several renal disorders are inherited – e.g. adult polycystic disease (APKD) and certain forms of glomerulonephritis. Reflux nephropathy has a strong heritable component. Most people would not consider termination for any of these conditions but it is appropriate to ensure women are aware of the risks and the possible need to screen their offspring. Where appropriate, referral to a clinical geneticist should be offered.

INFLUENCE OF MATERNAL MEDICATION

It is critical to discuss medication, both those that will need to be stopped and those that must not be stopped when pregnant. Importantly, contraception needs to be reviewed. All women taking cytotoxic or teratogenic drugs (e.g. cyclophosphamide or methotrexate) must be counseled to use contraception while taking the drugs and to observe a suitable wash out period

after cessation (usually 3-6 months). Women who do become pregnant while on these drugs are usually advised to have a termination. Newer immunosuppressants are increasingly used in autoimmunity as well as transplantation. All, e.g. mycophenolate mofetil (MMF) and sirolimus, are currently contraindicated in pregnancy. However, there is a school of thought that providing women are adequately counseled about the possible risk of birth defects (as have been reported with MMF) then in some instances it may be safer to remain on such immunosuppression rather than risking a flare of the underlying disease by changing or stopping medication. An alternative approach, only possible with preconception counseling, is to plan to change the immunosuppressant in a controlled fashion, to remain on the new medication (usually azathioprine) for about 6 months to ensure stability of the disease and then to try to conceive. Women should be given information on those drugs that have a good safety record in pregnancy and that should not therefore be stopped. Stopping long-term steroids suddenly is dangerous and risks precipitating an Addisonian crisis. Women need to be reassured that oral prednisolone is metabolized by the placenta and does not have adverse effects on the fetus. It is preferable to stay on a stable low dose of safe immunosuppression than stop suddenly and risk a flare or rejection which may require high doses or drugs that are incompatible with pregnancy. Drugs that have a good safety record and do not need to be stopped during pregnancy include oral prednisolone, hydroxychloroquine, azathioprine, ciclosporin A (Neoral) and tacrolimus.

Most women with CKD will be on ACE inhibitors (ACEI) and/or angiotensin 2 receptor blockers (AT2RB) as these significantly protect kidneys from progressive renal impairment particularly in the presence of proteinuria – whatever the underlying cause of kidney disease. However, ACEI cause a serious fetopathy, which is usually manifest in the second or third trimester, but skull abnormalities have been reported after first trimester exposure. Women on ACEI or AT2RB must be advised about the risks of taking these

Table 4.1 Outcome of pregnancies in women with moderate kidney impairment (creatinine >180 µmol/L)

Problems in pregnancy	Successful obstetric outcome	Long–term problems	End stage renal failure
90% (81-97)	84% (65-93)	50% (39-57)	15% (10-23)

Based on 125 pregnancies in 107 women in data from Jones and Haylsett (1996) and Jungers et al (1997).

Table 4.2 Risks of developing problems during pregnancy

Creatinine (µmol/L)	Problems during pregnancy (%)	Successful obstetric outcome (%)	Long–term renal problems (%)	Hypertension (%)	PET (%)	IUGR/premature (%)
Cr<125	26	96	<3	Variable	10-20	Increased
Cr 125-250	47	89	25	30-50	40	30-50
Cr>250	86	46	53	Most	80	57-73

drugs during pregnancy. Although conception is unpredictable and renal protection might be lost for some time, recent data mean women should be advised to stop ACEI or A2RB pre-conception. First trimester exposure to ACEI was shown to be associated with an increased relative risk (RR 2.71, CI 1.72–4.27) of major congenital malformations, particularly of the cardiovascular system (RR 3.72, CI 1.89–7.3) and central nervous system (RR 4.39, CI 1.37–14.02) when compared to unexposed infants. Some women may feel that the risk is justified to preserve renal function. However, they must be advised to stop ACEI or A2RB as soon as they are pregnant and no later than 7/40. Anti-hypertensives with a good safety record in pregnancy are methyl dopa, labetolol, nifedipine and hydralazine. In the non-pregnant patient with CKD, especially in the presence of proteinuria, the target BP would be less than or equal to 130/75 in the clinic. It is inappropriate to allow a woman with renal impairment to have 6-8 months of poorly controlled BP, particularly since ACEI/A2RB cannot be used for added renoprotection. While hypotension is clearly to be avoided it seems reasonable to aim for a clinic BP of no higher than 135/80 through the pregnancy.

Patients with CKD are more likely to die from cardiovascular disease than from end stage renal failure (ESRF). Hence, many women will be on statins to lower cholesterol and it is important for these to be stopped prior to pregnancy as they are teratogenic.

ADDITIONAL DRUGS THAT MAY BE REQUIRED IN PREGNANCY

CKD with a GFR of less than 30-60 ml/min 1.73 m^2 is often associated with a normochromic normocytic anaemia secondary to erythropoietin (EPO) deficiency. Women of childbearing age with CKD may also be iron deficient. In women with known CKD, while the anemia may be mild, it often becomes much more marked during pregnancy and it is increasingly common to prescribe EPO during pregnancy in order to avoid blood transfusion. Women who are given EPO need to be iron replete as judged by an adequate ferritin (> 200). This is achieved rapidly by giving a course of intravenous iron prior to initiating EPO. The aim is to increase Hb by approximately 1 g/month. More rapid reconstitution may be associated with worsening hypertension and should be avoided. If the Hb continues to rise rapidly EPO should be reduced or stopped.

Pregnancy is a procoagulant state. Proteinuria, especially in the nephrotic range, is associated with an increased risk of thrombosis. Hence, the combination of pregnancy and moderate or severe proteinuria

should stimulate a discussion about the need for thromboprophylaxis. Low molecular weight heparin (LMWH) is indicated for all pregnant women with nephrotic range proteinuria unless there is a contraindication. Caution must be used in patients with impaired renal function as LMWH is renally cleared. In most women with significant renal impairment and no contraindications, it is reasonable to prescribe low dose aspirin as prophylaxis for the increased risk of PET.

WHEN TO GET PREGNANT

In all progressive renal conditions it is advisable to get pregnant sooner rather than later for whatever the cause of the CKD, the worse the renal function the worse the outcome. For instance, a woman with APKD will reliably progress to renal failure usually between the age of 40-60 years but may have significant renal impairment in her mid-30s. Many patients are diagnosed early due to awareness of family history and through screening. In the early stages of the disease they will have normal renal function and mild hypertension – this is the ideal time for pregnancy and the risks only accrue with time. In the relatively recent past, women with progressive renal failure were advised to put off pregnancy until transplanted. However, with the advent of renoprotection, and much stricter BP targets, progression to end stage renal failure is often delayed for years. Furthermore, once on dialysis, patients, especially those from ethnic minority groups, can wait years for a cadaveric renal transplant, all of which means they could be menopausal before successfully transplanted and stable enough to contemplate pregnancy. Recently, this has improved with the promotion of live donor (related or unrelated), often pre-emptive, transplantation. Some patients avoid dialysis altogether and to have a well functioning graft much sooner in their renal history.

Some women have relapsing remitting diseases, most notably those with systemic lupus erythematosus. There is clear evidence that pregnancy should be delayed until remission has been maintained for at least 6 months – not least because of the drugs used for remission induction but also because disease activity is more likely to be associated with impaired outcomes.

DISEASE SPECIFIC CONSIDERATIONS

Microscopic hematuria

Patients with isolated microscopic hematuria, which is thought to be glomerular in origin, generally have one of three conditions: (1) thin basement membrane disease (now known to be a collection of inherited disorders of the basement membrane collagen genes); (2) IgA nephropathy; or (3) adult polycystic kidney disease. The latter can be excluded on USS. The former two conditions, in the absence of proteinuria or hypertension, are associated with an excellent renal prognosis and rarely require renal biopsy. Patients known to have isolated hematuria pre-pregnancy or who are diagnosed during pregnancy, should have a renal tract USS to exclude stones, tumor and APKD, renal blood work to exclude SLE, and to ensure normal renal function (see Table 4.3). They can then be reassured that their condition is unlikely to cause any problem during the pregnancy.

Proteinuria

This is a more significant finding with which two mistakes are commonly made. The first is to assume that a woman with proteinuria has a UTI. UTI is rarely a cause of proteinuria and certainly not of significant sustained proteinuria. The second is to not appreciate that proteinuria present from early pregnancy (i.e. <16 weeks) represents underlying renal disease. This leads not only to underestimating the underlying risk to the mother and baby but also to failure to appreciate the need for renal follow up postpartum. It is all too common to meet women in the renal clinic with advanced renal impairment who have been told in each pregnancy that they have proteinuria but have never been tested or monitored after pregnancy. Proteinuria of greater than 1 g per 24 h (nowadays most commonly measured on a spot urine protein : creatinine ratio of > 100) is associated with a worse renal outcome whatever the underlying cause. If a woman has significant proteinuria in early pregnancy (and of course preconception) she needs a renal work up. The minimum dataset required is described in Table 4.3. If the proteinuria is non-nephrotic, not associated with hematuria, the patient has normal renal function and a negative immune screen, then it is reasonable to watch and wait during pregnancy and plan to do a postpartum renal biopsy. However, the presence of abnormal function, a nephritic urinary sediment or nephrotic range proteinuria are indications for a renal biopsy when the patient presents in early pregnancy. This is because blind treatment with high dose steroids is not only dangerous but may not be appropriate. In acute lupus nephritis the choice of medication is likely to be azathioprine and steroids in pregnancy while in idiopathic membranous nephropathy the choice would be ciclosporin A or tacrolimus. In later pregnancy delivery of the baby in order to facilitate proper assessment and treatment of the mother may be appropriate. Where the mother is known to have an underlying glomerulonephritis accounting for her proteinuria then there is rarely an indication for biopsy in pregnancy. Advice about outcome again depends on the level of renal function, hypertension and proteinuria: the more severe these conditions are, the worse the outcome. It is reasonable to advise that all women who become pregnant while proteinuric are likely to develop increasing proteinuria and may well develop de novo or worsening hypertension. Nephrotic syndrome in the first trimester is associated with worse outcomes. Managing nephrotic patients in pregnancy is difficult. The patient's intravascular fluid status – rather than the degree of peripheral edema – needs to be assessed when considering diuretics. Many patients with a low serum albumin may have gross peripheral edema but be intravascularly depleted – aggressive diuresis will lead to worsening intravascular depletion, poor placental perfusion and the risk of acute renal failure. These women often need to be admitted and

Table 4.3 Assessing renal abnormalities in pregnancy

	Imaging	Blood tests	Urine
Isolated microscopic hematuria	Renal USS	Biochemical profile FBC ANA, complement, ACA	Microscopy MSU
Proteinuria (+/− hematuria)	Renal USS	Biochemical profile FBC and clotting ANA, anti-dsDNA ab, ANCA, complement, ACA Hepatitis B and C virology	Microscopy Protein : creatinine ratio MSU
Renal dysfunction	Renal USS If dilated, consider isotope scan with frusemide	As for proteinuria; focus on rate of change and severity	As for proteinuria

occasionally require i.v. salt poor albumin solution to maintain intravascular volume while undergoing diuresis with i.v. diuretics.

Reflux nephropathy

The discovery of evidence of scarred or refluxing kidneys in pregnant women is common and indeed reflux nephropathy is not uncommonly diagnosed in pregnancy. These women may have no prior history but are often hypertensive, often have recurrent UTIs (particularly in pregnancy) and may occasionally have had catastrophic previous pregnancies complicated by severe hypertension and early pre-eclampsia. There is a group of women presenting in their 20s and early 30s who have had ureteric reimplantation as a result of a vogue for reimplantation as a treatment for reflux in the 1980s. Women with a history of recurrent UTIs, or markedly dilated renal tracts, are usually given prophylactic antibiotics through pregnancy. Hypertension should be treated. In women with dilated tracts or previous ureteric surgery, serial renal USS can be used to ensure no progression to obstruction. Reflux nephropathy has a strong heritable component and early treatment with prophylactic antibiotics can prevent scarring and renal damage. Hence women with reflux or found to have evidence of chronic pyelonephritis (scarred irregular kidneys – may be unilateral or bilateral and may be entirely asymptomatic) should be advised to have their offspring screened by a pediatrician in their first year of life.

Systemic autoimmune disease with renal involvement

The commonest condition is SLE, as this is classically a disease of childbearing years. Active lupus nephritis, especially in association with anticardiolipin antibodies, is associated with much worse maternal and fetal outcomes. Women with lupus nephritis need to be counseled about the risks their treatment poses to fertility, the risks of certain immunosuppressants to the fetus and the need to be in a sustained remission prior to embarking on a pregnancy. Similar advice would be given to women with renal vasculitis.

Diabetic nephropathy

Diabetic nephropathy is a growing problem. Previously most women of childbearing age with diabetes would have type 1 diabetes and few would have developed significant renal involvement by the time they were pregnant. However, there has been a rapid rise in the number of women of childbearing age who have type 2 diabetes, many of whom will have advanced complications by the time of conception. Pregnancy in a woman with established diabetic nephropathy and overt proteinuria is a clinical challenge. If the woman has significant proteinuria pre-pregnancy she is likely to become nephrotic and grossly fluid overloaded during pregnancy which in turn will complicate her coexistent hypertension. Additionally, impaired renal function in early pregnancy is associated with a high risk of rapid loss of renal function during and after pregnancy. Women need to be advised about the risks of diabetes to the fetus, the risk of the pregnancy to their eyes and to their renal function and the need for very close monitoring by a multidisciplinary team including obstetricians, diabetologists and nephrologists. PET rates are increased in women with diabetes without renal dysfunction and hugely so in women with diabetic nephropathy. Advising women to get pregnant earlier in the course of their disease is important. An issue that is much harder to discuss even pre-conception is the high rate of morbidity and mortality in diabetes with nephropathy, especially the incidence of blindness, cardiovascular disease and end stage renal failure. However, the patient needs to be aware of the need to make provision for her children lest she becomes increasingly incapacitated while they are still very young. A depressing study from New Zealand highlighted the high rates of morbidity and mortality in this group of women.

ADVICE FOR WOMEN WITH CKD WHO ARE PLANNING A PREGNANCY OR WHO ARE ALREADY PREGNANT

It is important that they know the risks – the worse their renal function, the worse their hypertension and the greater their proteinuria, the more likely they are to have severe hypertension in pregnancy, to develop PET, to have a premature baby and to sustain significant renal decline, often accelerating their path to dialysis. The key factors for safe outcomes are:

- a well-informed patient;
- early booking to optimize medication and assess at baseline;
- management by a multidisciplinary team including nephrologists and obstetricians;
- close monitoring of renal function and proteinuria, tight control of blood pressure, appropriate management of anemia;
- regular fetal scans; and
- timely early delivery where indicated for obstetric indications or deteriorating renal function.

Patients on dialysis

Women on dialysis have impaired fertility, although this has improved with the advent of erythropoietin to treat anemia. First trimester loss is common and often not diagnosed – women usually have irregular periods and may well not notice a missed or late period. Consequently it is important to advise women of childbearing age who are on dialysis to use contraception. Conversely, it is important to remember that women can and do get pregnant on dialysis, that diagnosis is often delayed as the patient is unaware that she can conceive and the physician may simply not consider the possibility. For women established on dialysis, pregnancy is associated with high maternal morbidity, significant maternal mortality and a high rate of fetal loss. In general, especially if a woman already has children, pregnancy on dialysis is discouraged. However, some women will consider it a priority and many will simply fall pregnant unexpectedly and will not consider termination. Plans need to be implemented to optimize the chance of a successful obstetric outcome with minimal risk to the mother. Any dialysis patient who becomes pregnant must be managed at a center able to provide high-risk obstetric care, neonatal intensive care as well as nephrology input. Dialysis prescription should be altered to try to mimic 'normal' biochemistry and fluid status. Hence, women on hemodialysis should be offered daily dialysis and by 16-18 weeks should be having at least 20 h dialysis per week. This is exceptionally demanding both for the patient and the unit providing care. In women with normal renal function, pregnancy is associated with very low urea and a mild acidosis. The increased frequency and duration of dialysis should easily reduce predialysis urea to less than 15 mmol/L. However, the bicarbonate concentration may well need to be reduced to avoid a relative alkalosis. Since rapid ultrafiltration can lead to intravascular depletion and placental compromise, women need to be encouraged to be very careful about fluid balance and to avoid more than minimal interdialytic weight gains. Two areas need very careful attention during pregnancy: hypertension and anemia. Most dialysis patients tend to hypertension and this can be severe and chaotic during pregnancy. In normal pregnancy volume expansion is secondary to renal adaptation to vasodilation and increased cardiac output. It is not clear how volume expansion occurs in pregnancy in dialysis patients but resistant fluid gains are often noted. The normal early trimester fall in blood pressure is rarely seen in pregnant dialysis patients. Gentle fluid removal to within 1-2 kg of expected dry weight can be attempted to reduce hypertension but care must be taken to avoid hypotension. ACEI and A2RB are commonly used in dialysis patients and these agents must be stopped as soon as pregnancy is diagnosed. Consider aspirin, providing not otherwise contraindicated, as prophylaxis against PET. Pre-eclampsia is common but difficult to diagnose in dialysis patients. Most will already have severe hypertension, may be anuric or oliguric, and, if they produce urine, are likely to have persistent proteinuria and hematuria, and may well be edematous from early pregnancy. PET can occur very early and be associated with catastrophic hypertension. Magnesium sulfate should be avoided as this will rapidly accumulate to toxic levels in dialysis-dependent patients.

The majority of dialysis patients will already be on EPO at the time of conception. Requirements can increase dramatically through pregnancy and full blood count and iron stores need to be monitored closely.

Fetal outcomes are poor in dialysis patients with up to 50-60% fetal losses reported. The outcomes are worse in older women, those who have been on dialysis for more than 5 years and those in whom the dialysis prescription is increased late. The outcome is better in those women who start dialysis during pregnancy rather than prior to pregnancy. Prematurity is almost universal and the causes are multifactorial. Polyhydramnios is common in response to the osmotic diuresis imposed on the fetal kidneys. Intrauterine growth retardation is usual and often necessitates early delivery as does the onset of PET or severe resistant hypertension.

4.2.8.2 Renal transplant recipient

Pregnancy in transplant patients has a better outcome if delayed at least 6 months to 1 year post transplant. However, full fertility is restored very rapidly after successful transplantation. Hence, women must be reminded of the need for safe and effective contraception.

Two excellent guidelines published in recent years from the USA and Europe highlight the need for preconception counseling to form part of the transplant work-up, stability of renal function and immunosuppression before conception and for all such pregnancies to be considered high risk. By discussing pregnancy and fertility as part of transplant work-up, i.e. well before the transplant has occurred, the risk of threatening graft function with an early unplanned pregnancy is reduced. The issues of immunosuppression and the possibility it might need changing, and the impact of the condition and the medication on the fetus and the pregnancy on graft function can all be discussed in advance. Recent data suggest that obstetric outcomes are very good in transplant patients and not dissimilar to those in women with other kidney diseases, i.e. the outcome is dependent on the level of renal function, severity of hypertension and degree of proteinuria at the time of conception. However, there is a significant risk of worsening renal function during or after the pregnancy and several studies have reported a stepwise or progressive decline in function that leads to a shortened transplant half-life during and following pregnancy. Hypertension and pre-eclampsia are common and often lead to IUGR and premature delivery.

Newer immunosuppressants pose problems for pregnant patients. There have been thousands of babies born to mothers taking azathioprine, prednisolone and ciclosporin. These drugs are well tolerated and not associated with fetal malformations. Similarly there is a growing experience that tacrolimus is safe. Ciclosporin and tacrolimus levels can vary in pregnancy and need to be monitored carefully. However, mycophenolate mofetil (MMF) has been shown to be teratogenic in animal models and there have been several reports of malformations, some severe, in babies born to women taking MMF. Women must be cautioned not to get pregnant while taking MMF or to be prepared to risk birth defects. There are case reports only on the use of sirolimus in pregnancy though to date no fetal abnormalities have been described.

A rare but recognized complication of pregnancy in transplantation is obstruction of the renal graft by the growing uterus. This may manifest as worsening renal function. Any rise in creatinine should be investigated appropriately. Infection should be excluded by an MSU, obstruction excluded by USS and if rejection is considered likely, then in early pregnancy a renal biopsy should be considered and in more advanced pregnancy delivery may need to be expedited. Rejection can occur during or after pregnancy. During pregnancy there are limited therapeutic options beyond steroids to treat intercurrent rejection.

Many women receiving renal transplants will have been unable to get pregnant earlier due to severe renal disease. They need to be reassured that once the graft is stable the likelihood of a successful pregnancy is high (assuming normal fertility) but in a poorly functioning graft there is a risk to both mother and baby, and to the graft of premature loss of function. All such women should be managed in specialized renal and obstetric centers and considered to be high risk.

CONCLUSION

Overall, renal disease in pregnancy poses a threat to both mother and baby. Any renal disease can increase the risk of hypertension, PET and consequent prematurity but these adverse events are all much more common and predictable the worse the renal function and the worse the hypertension. Meticulous monitoring of fetal growth and maternal well-being are key to successful outcomes as well as effective planning with preconception advice and review.

Further reading

[Anonymous] 2002 European best practice guidelines for renal transplantation. Section IV: long-term management of the transplant recipient. IV.10. Pregnancy in renal transplant recipients. Nephrology, Dialysis, Transplantation 17(suppl 4):50-55

Alwan S, Polifka J E et al 2005 Angiotensin II receptor antagonist treatment during pregnancy. Birth Defects Research. Part A, Clinical and Molecular Teratology 73(2):123-130

Bar J, Ben-Rafael Z et al 2000 Prediction of pregnancy outcome in subgroups of women with renal disease. Clinical Nephrology 53(6):437-444

Chapman A B, Abraham W T, Zamudio S et al 1998 Temporal relationships between hormonal and hemodynamic changes in early human pregnancy. Kidney International 54:2056-2063

Coomarasamy A, Honest H, Papaioannou S et al 2003 Aspirin for prevention of preeclampsia in women with historical risk factors: a systematic review. Obstetrics & Gynecology 101:1319-1332

Cooper W O, Hernandez-Diaz S, Arbogast P G et al 2006 Major congenital malformations after first – trimester expose to ACE inhibitors. New England Journal of Medicine 354:2443-2451

Davison J M 2001 Renal disorders in pregnancy. Current Opinion in Obstetrics & Gynecology 13(2):109-114

de Swiet M, Lightstone L 2004 Glomerular endotheliosis in normal pregnancy and pre-eclampsia. BJOG 111(2):191-192; author reply 193-195; discussion 195

George J N 2003 The association of pregnancy with thrombotic thrombocytopenic purpura-hemolytic uremic syndrome. Current Opinion in Hematology 10:339-344

Haase M, Morgera S et al 2005 A systematic approach to managing pregnant dialysis patients-the importance of an intensified haemodiafiltration protocol. Nephrology, Dialysis, Transplantation 20(11):2537-2542

Jones D C, Hayslett J P 1996 Outcome of pregnancy in women with moderate or severe renal insufficiency. New England Journal of Medicine 335(4):226-232

Jungers P, Chauveau D et al 1997 Pregnancy in women with impaired renal function. Clinical Nephrology 47(5):281-288

McKay D B, Josephson M A et al 2005 Reproduction and transplantation: report on the AST Consensus Conference on Reproductive Issues and Transplantation. American Journal of Transplantation 5(7):1592-1599

Nowicki B 2000 Urinary tract infection in pregnant women: old dogmas and current concepts regarding pathogenesis. Current Infectious Disease Reports 4:529-535

Pertuiset N, Grunfeld J P 1994 Acute renal failure in pregnancy. Baillière's Clinical Obstetrics and Gynaecology 8:333-351

Poston L, Williams D J 2002 Vascular function in normal pregnancy and pre-eclampsia. In: Hunt B J, Poston L, Schachter M, Halliday A (eds) An introduction to vascular biology. Cambridge University Press, Cambridge, p 398-425

Quadri K H, Bernardini J et al 1994 Assessment of renal function during pregnancy using a random urine protein to creatinine ratio and Cockcroft–Gault formula. American Journal of Kidney Diseases 24(3):416-420

Redman C W, Sacks G P, Sargent I L 1999 Preeclampsia: an excessive maternal inflammatory response to pregnancy. American Journal of Obstetric Gynecology 180:499-506

Rossing K, Jacobsen P et al 2002 Pregnancy and progression of diabetic nephropathy. Diabetologia 45(1):36-41

Smaill F 2001 Antibiotics for asymptomatic bacteriuria in pregnancy. Cochrane Database Systematic Review 2:CD000490

Tabacova S, Little R et al 2003 Adverse pregnancy outcomes associated with maternal enalapril antihypertensive treatment. Pharmacoepidemiology and Drug Safety 12(8):633-646

Tomson C 2003 Urinary tract infection. In: Warrell D A, Cox T M, Firth J, Benz E J (eds) Oxford textbook of medicine, 4th edn. Oxford University Press, Oxford, p 420-433

Vazquez J C, Villar J 2003 Treatments for symptomatic urinary tract infections during pregnancy. Cochrane Database Systematic Review 4:CD002256

Williams D J 2003 Pregnancy – a stress test for life. Current Opinions in Obstetrics & Gynaecology 15:465-471

Williams W W Jr, Ecker J L et al 2005 Case records of the Massachusetts General Hospital. Case 38-2005. A 29-year-old pregnant woman with the nephrotic syndrome and hypertension. New England Journal of Medicine 353(24):2590-2600

Chapter 5

Endocrine and metabolic disorders

W. M. Hague, T. T. Lao, N. W. Cheung, B. N. J. Walters, I. A. Greer, C. Nelson-Piercy

Effect of pregnancy on the endocrine system

W. M. Hague

INTRODUCTION

Every woman who has ever been pregnant is aware of the major impact that a small nubbin of embryonic cells can have on her general health and well-being, an effect that is mediated mainly through the endocrine and metabolic systems. The impact is felt right from the very early days of pregnancy as the body adjusts to the new hormonal milieu. In addition, the ability to establish and sustain a healthy pregnancy depends very much on having a maternal endocrine system that is in balance, with a healthy metabolism also making an important contribution. Not only has the pregnant woman to maintain an environment that will allow her fetus (or fetuses) to grow and develop, but she also needs to prepare for first, the drama of parturition and second, for the metabolic demands of lactation. Finally, once delivered and with lactation under way, her body and mind need to return to an endocrine and metabolic homeostasis that will allow the possibility of another pregnancy to be established in due course of time.

Worldwide, the timing of first pregnancy is still most likely to follow soon after the onset of sexual maturity, with teenage pregnancy being a common phenomenon in the developing world. Although the statistics show increased mortality and morbidity among this age group and their offspring, the major causes for this reflect obstetric and socio-economic pathologies (e.g. hemorrhage, infection (including HIV), unsafe abortion, failure or lack of transport and referral systems (see Ch. 1). In the developed world, however, where pregnancy is often now delayed until the fourth or even the fifth decade of life, the increased potential for metabolic disorders, such as diabetes, hypertension and obesity, casts its shadow over reproductive performance.

Normal endocrine and metabolic homeostasis are also important for ovulation to occur effectively as the precursor to a successful pregnancy. Hyperprolactinemia, whether primary or secondary to drug therapy or to hypothyroidism, is an important contributor to anovulation. Hyperinsulinemia, in the setting of polycystic ovary syndrome or with obesity, is associated with infrequent ovulation. Thyrotoxicosis can also be associated with oligomenorrhea, although most cycles are ovulatory, as adjudged by endometrial biopsy. Autoimmune hypoadrenalism (Addison's disease) is often associated with hypogonadism with the presence of steroid cell antibodies.

CHANGES IN ENDOCRINE FUNCTION IN PREGNANCY

Once a pregnancy has been established, there are immediate effects on almost all the endocrine axes. In the pituitary, there is hyperplasia and proliferation of the lactotrophs, causing an increase in prolactin secretion that continues through to the puerperium. Some of the increase has been attributed to a change in hormone secretion by the somatotrophs that switch from producing growth hormone to prolactin, emphasizing the importance of prolactin secretion for human pregnancy and lactation. The enlargement of the pituitary may be sufficient in the presence of a pre-existent microadenoma to impinge on the optic chiasm and cause a bitemporal hemianopia.

Thyroid stimulating hormone

The alpha-subunit of human chorionic gonadotrophin (hCG) is homologous to that of thyrotrophin (TSH). With the onset of pregnancy and the rise in hCG, there is a relative fall in TSH secretion associated with a TSH-like action of hCG on the thyroid gland. The hCG rise may be sufficient to stimulate excess secretion of thyroid hormone, and a clinical picture indistinguishable from thyrotoxicosis may result (Goodwin et al 1992). This is often seen in neoplastic conditions of the placenta (trophoblastic disease), such as hydatidiform mole and choriocarcinoma, where the secretion of hCG is particularly high. In addition to the increased secretion of thyroid hormone, the increase in circulating oestrogen concentration from first the ovary, and later the placenta, stimulates a compensatory increase in production of thyroxine binding globulin (TBG), so that the free thyroid hormone concentrations, both of thyroxine (T4) and tri-iodothyronine (T3), remain relatively stable (Lao 2005). Small changes in free T4 and free T3 are usually of no clinical significance, but it is important to be aware of the differences in various assays for free thyroid hormones.

Corticosteroids and ACTH

A similar increase of binding protein is seen for cortisol binding globulin (CBG), accompanying the rise in cortisol secretion during pregnancy, associated with an increase in adrenocorticotrophin (ACTH) secretion. Free plasma cortisol concentrations are also elevated, with a reduction of the usual diurnal variation, and there is a rise in urine free cortisol excretion. The urine free cortisol excretion is also not suppressible by the administration of dexamethasone, as normally observed outside pregnancy. It has been proposed that these endocrine changes are in part responsible for the common changes seen in human pregnancy of striae, facial plethora, rising blood pressure and impairment of glucose tolerance, as a 'pseudo-Cushing's syndrome'.

The increased secretion of ACTH has been attributed to an effect of corticotrophin releasing hormone (CRH), now recognized to be generated not just from the hypothalamus but also from many other tissues including placenta. CRH also has local inflammatory activity and may well contribute to the inflammatory state of pregnancy. The hypercortisolism of late pregnancy has been attributed in large part to placental CRH release, one of the putative triggers of the onset of labor. Thus, it has been suggested that preterm labor might follow increased secretion of placental CRH in response to maternal signals indicative of a stressful environment (Kalantaridou et al 2004a). The fall in CRH after delivery of the placenta and subsequent maternal hypoadrenalism has been posited as a cause of the 'post partum blues' phenomenon (Kalantaridou et al 2004).

Glucose tolerance

Changes in glucose tolerance in pregnancy result from numerous factors, including increased secretion of cortisol, human placental lactogen and other diabetogenic hormones. In addition, there is increased insulin resistance that has varied ethnic, constitutional and metabolic determinants, in particular maternal obesity and inactivity. Teleologically, these changes may be seen to promote nutrient transfer to the fetus at the expense of the mother. The progressive rise in insulin resistance as pregnancy proceeds may lead in susceptible individuals to relative beta-cell insufficiency and the associated rise in plasma glucose characteristic of gestational diabetes (Kjos and Buchanan 1999). Impairment of maternal glucose tolerance is well recognized to be associated with fetal hyperinsulinemia and adiposity. Recent work demonstrates that this is associated with an alteration of the fetal adipo-insular axis, increased fetal leptin and a reduction in the fetal adiponectin to leptin ratio. There are also long-term effects on the subsequent insulin sensitivity of the offspring, who become more prone to develop diabetes in later life, potentially contributing to the worldwide pandemic of this disorder.

Vasopressin

Another pituitary hormone whose metabolism changes from early pregnancy is arginine vasopressin (AVP). It was recognized in the latter part of the 20th century that there was a change in the osmostat very early in pregnancy, resulting in a reduction in maternal plasma osmolality (the mean falling from about 290 to 280 mosmol/L by 2-4 weeks gestation) and in the osmolar threshold for thirst. This leads to thirst at a lower osmolality than outside pregnancy, and associated polyuria. AVP secretion is maintained, but there is an increased secretion of cystine aminopeptidase (vasopressinase) from the placenta (Durr and Lindheimer 1996). Altered metabolism of the vasopressinase, particularly in maternal liver dysfunction,

may lead to various syndromes of transient diabetes insipidus in late pregnancy. More recently, a family of aquaporin molecules has been identified in the kidney, each expressed in different sites and with differential activity at those sites. The tight modulation of water balance is modified by at least two actions of AVP, first on expression of the aquaporins and second in changing their transport from intracellular vesicles to the surface of the membrane of the collecting ducts.

Calcium and bone

Extraordinary changes in maternal–fetal physiology occur in the area of calcium metabolism and its interaction with the fetal skeleton. Although the mother has a huge reserve of calcium in her own skeleton, it is now realized that the fetal demands for calcium associated with fetal growth are usually met by increasing maternal absorption of calcium rather than mobilizing her bony reserves. This is achieved through the actions of vitamin D and parathyroid hormone (PTH) (Prentice 2000). The fetus then maintains its mineral balance through the production of PTH related protein (PTHrP), derived from both the fetal parathyroid gland and the placenta, and subsequently from the maternal breast (Hosking 1996). Following parturition, there is a change of maternal economy to allow an increase in bone turnover and a fall in calcium excretion to support the demands for calcium in the breast milk. This results in a loss of bone density of up to 7%, which is not modifiable by any increase in maternal calcium intake but which reverts to normal soon after weaning. There appears to be no increase in the frequency of osteoporotic fractures associated with pregnancy and lactation.

Relaxin

Another area of renewed interest to researchers in the endocrine biology of human pregnancy is the complex physiology of relaxin. With close structural homology to insulin, the original understanding was that relaxin was a peptide hormone released from the corpus luteum and involved in changing connective tissue. Its actions allowed for remodeling of the maternal joints as well as the cervix to facilitate both carriage and passage of the fetus through the birth canal, in addition to alteration of the breast tissues to promote lactation (Sherwood 2004). More recently has come the recognition that relaxin effects pituitary hormone secretion, causes renal vasodilation and affects smooth muscle in the heart and gut. It has also been reported to reduce fibrosis and to counteract allergic reactions.

It used to be taught that the pituitary could be seen as the conductor of the endocrine orchestra. In pregnancy, however, there is a case to make for that honor to go to the placenta. In truth, however, the interaction of endocrine, paracrine, intercrine and autocrine molecules in the pregnant woman and her fetus is more reminiscent of the complexity of the World Wide Web with its multiple facets, allowing networking at both the local and universal levels. In the understanding of these complex interrelationships, 'there remains very much land to be possessed'.

Thyroid disorders in pregnancy
T. T. Lao

INTRODUCTION

Thyroid disorders are among the commonest medical disorders complicating pregnancy. While the incidence of overt thyroid dysfunction in pregnant women is often quoted to be 1-2%, recent reports suggest that milder subclinical forms of hyper- and hypothyroidism are more prevalent but remain unrecognized. The incidence of thyroid disorders increases with increasing maternal age, as well as with subfertility. The rising number of pregnancies in older women as well as successful assisted reproduction programs implies that those who provide healthcare for pregnant women should be alert to the possibility of thyroid disorders, especially in subclinical form, as their correction is necessary to optimize the pregnancy outcome.

The thyroid disorders in pregnancy will be considered as follows:

- pregnancy complications and thyroid dysfunction
- goiter in pregnancy
- hyperthyroidism
- hypothyroidism and
- postpartum thyroid dysfunction.

The adverse obstetric outcomes associated with thyroid disorders are summarized in Table 5.1.

PREGNANCY COMPLICATIONS AND THYROID DYSFUNCTION

Normal pregnancy results in increased serum total thyroxine (TT4) and free tri-iodothyronine (fT3) concentrations, and decreased thyrotropin (TSH) concentration. In the absence of clinical features, elevated fT4 (free thyroxine), or free thyroxine index, elevated TT4 with depressed TSH alone do not indicate hyperthyroidism in a pregnant woman. However, certain pregnancy complications may lead to biochemical and even clinical hyperthyroidism, best known in the case of hydatidiform mole, that is attributable to the excessive production of human chorionic gonadotropin (hCG) with high thyrotropic activity. More commonly encountered is hyperemesis gravidarum, the severity of which is correlated with serum hCG concentration. The hyperthyroidism of hyperemesis always subsides

Table 5.1 Adverse obstetric outcome associated with thyroid disorders in pregnancy

Obstetric outcomes	Hyperthyroidism	Hypothyroidism
Hyperemesis gravidarum	+	−
Spontaneous miscarriage	+	+
Preterm labor	+	+
Pre-eclampsia/ hypertension	+	+
Fetal growth restriction	+	+
Intrauterine fetal death	+	−
Fetal distress	+	+
Lactation problems	+	+
Postpartum mood changes and depression	+	+

spontaneously well before the last trimester and usually by 16 weeks. In both situations, the clinical features may be indistinguishable from those of Graves' disease although eye signs provide useful confirmation that true Graves' disease is underlying the hyperthyroidism. Rarely, a short course of antithyroid treatment may be required, usually with rapid and dramatic response.

Biochemical hypothyroidism may be encountered in pre-eclampsia, with decreased TT4, total triiodothyronine (TT3), free thyroxine (fT4) and fT3 and increased TSH concentration. The latter is correlated with the severity of pre-eclampsia. It is important to distinguish this condition from genuine hypothyroidism, as thyroxine replacement should not be given for the 'pseudo-hypothyroidism' that may accompany pre-eclampsia. Spontaneous recovery of the disturbance in thyroid function occurs after delivery. In case of doubt, thyroid function should be monitored in the puerperium.

GOITER IN PREGNANCY

Pregnancy has a goitrogenic effect, and thyroid volume increases from a mean of 20.2 mL at 18 weeks to 24.1 mL at 36 weeks. Pregnancy may also induce the formation of new thyroid nodules, associated with higher urinary iodine excretion. Nodular hyperplasia on fine needle biopsy is seen. These changes are not accompanied by alterations in thyroid hormone levels.

One important consideration in the management of goiter encountered in pregnancy is the exclusion of differentiated thyroid carcinoma (DTC), one of the commonest cancers in women in the reproductive age group. DTC presents as a lump noticed by the patient, or a nodule discovered by the clinician, that may rapidly increase in size during pregnancy. Diagnosis depends on fine needle aspiration. In one of the two reported series of DTC diagnosed during pregnancy, 78% of the patients were in stage 1-2, while in the other series 93% of the patients were in stage 1, and papillary thyroid carcinoma was found in 78% and 93% of patients, respectively. The diagnosis was often made in the first trimester, but deferral of thyroidectomy for 6-7 months or more after diagnosis did not adversely affect the prognosis, which is excellent with long-term survival the rule. Termination of pregnancy because of the diagnosis of thyroid carcinoma is not necessary. Thyroidectomy may be performed in the second trimester if the diagnosis is made in the first trimester, or deferred until after delivery if the diagnosis is made later.

HYPERTHYROIDISM AND PREGNANCY

The commonest cause of hyperthyroidism in pregnancy is Graves' disease (GD). In most cases the diagnosis has been made prior to pregnancy, and the manifestation during pregnancy is either a relapse or the result of inadequate treatment. GD tends to be exacerbated during the first trimester and improves or becomes quiescent during the later trimesters, only to flare up again postpartum. Occasionally, it presents for the first time in pregnancy, often with hyperemesis gravidarum being the presenting feature. Thyroiditis may also present as hyperthyroidism before or during pregnancy, and gestational thyrotoxicosis associated with hyperemesis gravidarum may present with clinical hyperthyroidism. Poorly controlled hyperthyroidism may lead to congestive heart failure, thyroid storm, preterm labor, pre-eclampsia, fetal growth restriction, and increased perinatal mortality, and even maternal mortality. The risk of low birthweight is higher when control of hyperthyroidism is delayed until pregnancy than when control is achieved before pregnancy. Thus hyperthyroidism should be controlled before conception to optimize pregnancy outcome.

Even in clinically euthyroid women, the presence of thyroid autoimmunity is an independent risk factor for adverse pregnancy outcome that includes spontaneous miscarriage. Thyroglobulin (TG) and thyroperoxidase antibodies are found more commonly in non-pregnant women with a history of recurrent miscarriage and in pregnant women in the first trimester who later miscarry. 40% of the offspring of mothers with evidence of thyroid autoimmunity have elevated serum thyroid peroxidase antibody titres at birth, significantly correlated with maternal antibody titers. Proposed explanations for the association between thyroid autoimmunity and miscarriage include a heightened maternal autoimmune state affecting the fetal allograft with the thyroid antibodies serving as a marker, and mild thyroid failure as suggested by the higher TSH concentration.

Many of the clinical features of hyperthyroidism are found in normal pregnancy (tachycardia, tiredness, heat intolerance, dyspnea) and the diagnosis may easily be overlooked. Mothers with a family history of GD should have thyroid function tested even if clinical features are absent. As for women already on antithyroid medications, their condition should be monitored by both clinical progress, e.g. weight gain and fetal growth, and measurement of serum TSH and fT4 at 2- to 4-weekly intervals. As long as fetal growth and maternal symptomatic control are satisfactory, the patient should be maintained at a slightly hyperthyroid state. It is often necessary to adjust the dose of antithyroid medication each trimester. If possible, treatment should be stopped no later than 36-37 weeks if the maternal and fetal condition is satisfactory, but not before euthyroidism has been achieved. For mothers with a relatively short duration of treatment, the dose should not be reduced too rapidly, as relapse may occur in the last trimester even before cessation of treatment.

For mothers who have completed antithyroid treatment, there is a high frequency of relapse within 24 months. Thyroid function should be tested at booking and at least once per trimester. Treatment should be recommenced if necessary. In patients with previous ablation of the thyroid, and those who have been in remission, subclinical hypothyroidism may exist. Maternal TSH should be monitored at least once per trimester. In the presence of a rising TSH concentration, thyroid function should be monitored more frequently, and thyroxine replacement should be prescribed if the TSH concentration has risen above the normal range even if the fT4 is still within the normal range.

Standard medical treatment utilizes thionamides, including propylthiouracil (PTU), methimazole and carbimazole, which prevent organification of iodide and coupling of iodotyrosines to form T4 and T3 so that thyroid hormone biosynthesis is inhibited. There is also a significant immunosuppressive effect of these drugs. In addition, PTU blocks the peripheral conversion of T4 to T3 and suppresses T3 more quickly, perhaps favoring it as the drug of choice for treatment during pregnancy. The commencing dose of PTU is 200 to 450 mg, with a daily maintenance of 50 to 300 mg. As a higher dose of methimazole and carbimazole is associated with an increased rate of side effects such as allegic reactions and skin rash, it is safer to commence with a lower dose, e.g. methimazole 10 mg or carbimazole 15 mg daily. The most serious side effect is agranulocytosis, therefore the blood count should be assessed before and after treatment is commenced. In addition, GD may be associated with immune thrombocytopenia and hemolytic anemia. In areas of borderline iodine supply, women may be more sensitive to treatment and thyroid function should be assessed regularly.

In cases where there is unexpected lack of response to antithyroid therapy, compliance should always be interrogated. Many women will be concerned at potential effects of the treatment on their baby and some may not take the drugs. Careful explanation and reassurance is usually successful and, of course, should accompany prescription of any medication in pregnancy.

Beta-blockers are usually unnecessary as an adjunct to the thionamides, although sometimes a troublesome tachycardia may require a short-course of treatment. Propranolol is the usual agent employed but it requires caution in the third trimester because of potential fetal effects. It may be necessary for 1-3 weeks in a woman with symptomatic tachycardia, until the antithyroid medication takes effect. Radioactive iodine (RAI) is contraindicated in pregnancy because of the risk of fetal thyroid ablation. As the fetal thyroid does not begin to concentrate iodine until 10-12 weeks of gestation, RAI given even early in the first trimester should not affect the fetus. Patients who received RAI for GD up to 36 years earlier do not have any increase in the rate of miscarriage or congenital anomalies in their offspring. It has been recommended that pregnancy should be avoided within one year of RAI treatment to allow for RAI clearance and hormonal stabilization. Irrespective of the interval between RAI treatment and the index pregnancy, it is prudent to screen for hypothyroidism and give thyroxine replacement where necessary.

Subtotal thyroidectomy is seldom considered during pregnancy, except when medical treatment has failed to achieve control by the second trimester. Postoperative hypocalcemia may be a problem due to interference with the parathyroids and maternal serum calcium level must be monitored and appropriate treatment given.

Thyroid stimulating antibodies (TsAb) in the mother cross the placenta and may stimulate the fetal thyroid, resulting in fetal and neonatal thyrotoxicosis in 2.6%, even in infants born to euthyroid or hypothyroid mothers who have been treated by partial thyroidectomy or radioiodine in the past. The TsAb concentrations in maternal and cord blood are similar and the titre is predictive of neonatal thyrotoxicosis in infants born to both treated and untreated mothers. Clinical features of fetal GD include persistent fetal tachycardia, fetal goiter and frontal bossing, premature craniosynostosis, growth restriction and heart failure. Serial fetal ultrasound assessment for fetal tachycardia, goiter, growth and hydropic change is indicated if fetal GD is suspected. Scanning with transvaginal ultrasound before, and transabdominal ultrasound after, 17 weeks of gestation allows the fetal thyroid size to be determined and correlated with maternal status and treatment. This allows the early detection of an enlarged fetal thyroid on which basis the adjustment of maternal drug dosage can be made. A persistently enlarged fetal thyroid despite reduction in maternal dosage would be suggestive of fetal and neonatal thyrotoxicosis due to the transplacental passage of thyroid stimulating antibodies. In case of doubt, the direct assessment of fetal thyroid function may be performed by fetal blood sampling through cordocentesis, that has been shown to be a relatively safe procedure in this situation.

As untreated fetal thyrotoxicosis is associated with increased perinatal mortality, preterm labor and fetal growth restriction, in utero treatment may be necessary, using thionamides which also cross the placenta and are taken up by the fetal thyroid as early as the second trimester. One can start with PTU 50-200 mg daily and the dose adjusted frequently to titrate against the fetal heart rate. This can reverse the features of fetal thyrotoxicosis and enable the pregnancy to continue with an improved outcome. If large doses, e.g. PTU 300 mg or more per day, are given and maintained towards the end of pregnancy, the newborn may have hypothyroidism. All infants born to mothers with a history of GD, regardless of status, should undergo thyroid assessment after birth. As well, methimazole and carbimazole have both been associated with aplasia cutis in the fetus (although very rarely), and the neonate should be examined carefully after birth.

Breastfeeding is safe even in mothers who continue with treatment. In this regard, PTU is the drug of choice since it is excreted in insignificant amounts in the breast milk and neonatal thyroid function is not depressed. Methimazole may also be used if thyroid function in the infant is monitored frequently. The long-term safety of methimazole has been shown in a study on 42 children assessed at age 48 to 86 months, who were breastfed while their lactating mothers received up to 20-30 mg methimazole daily. No differences in the height, weight, serum concentrations of thyroid hormones and thyroid antibodies, or the verbal and functional IQ and their components, were found. Nevertheless, for nursing mothers on a high dose of thionamides, the infant's thyroid function should be assessed as a precaution against undiagnosed neonatal hypothyroidism.

HYPOTHYROIDISM AND PREGNANCY

Hypothyroidism is a common and often undiagnosed condition, which is particularly prevalent in older women due to autoimmune thyroiditis, while insufficient iodine intake or frank deficiency is an important cause worldwide. Asymptomatic gestational hypothyroidism may occur in up to 2.5% of women, and subclinical hypothyroidism increases pregnancy wastage. Normal maternal thyroid function is critical for fetal brain development and normal cognitive

development, and subclinical hypothyroidism is associated with impaired neurological development in the offspring. However in a recent study was, even when the TSH concentration within the reference range, mothers with fT4 concentration below the 10th percentile at 12 weeks of gestation had offspring with significantly lower scores on the mental and motor scales in the Bayley Scales of Infant Development at the age of 1 and 2 years. If the maternal fT4 concentration was increased at 24 and 32 weeks, then the scores of the offspring were similar to those in the controls. While the cost–benefit ratio of routine screening or treatment for subclinical hypothyroidism, as indicated by serum TSH concentration above the reference range despite fT4 and fT3 concentrations being within the reference range, remains a subject of debate, many believe that subclinical hypothyroidism in pregnant women represents a special category for which case finding and treatment is justified.

Hypothyroidism may present with subtle and nonspecific constitutional and neuropsychiatric features, as well as hyperprolactinemia and hyperhomocysteinemia. The commonest cause is inadequate treatment due to non-compliance, early pregnancy vomiting or poor absorption for uncertain reasons. Hypothyroidism should be ruled out if there is excessive fluid retention early in pregnancy, bradycardia, cold intolerance and a low body temperature.

The majority of hypothyroid women have a history of thyroid ablation or antithyroid medications, but the rest may have no apparent history of thyroid disorders. Their hypothyroidism is usually consequent to previously undiagnosed thyroiditis, occurring alone or in association with other underlying medical diseases such as insulin dependent diabetes mellitus, systemic lupus erythematosus, primary Sjögren's syndrome and glomerulonephritis. Therefore in high-risk women with a significant medical history, thyroid function screening should be part of the initial antenatal investigation.

Inadequate treatment as well as undiagnosed subclinical hypothyroidism is associated with miscarriage, pre-eclampsia, anemia, fetal growth restriction, placental abruption, and neonatal morbidity. Replacement therapy should be monitored every 8–12 weeks to ensure an adequate dosage, whilst avoiding overtreatment, because thyroid function may improve due to transplacental transfer of fetal thyroxine even in untreated hypothyroid women. In this situation, the most reliable method of monitoring thyroid function is by serial measurements of serum TSH concentration. Changes in TSH are amplified by minor alterations in T4 and T3 concentrations. This occurs because for each individual, the reference range for thyroid hormones is much narrower than the laboratory reference range. Thus, hormonal concentrations that lie within the laboratory reference range are not necessarily normal for that individual, while TSH concentration is a bioindicator of adequacy of T4 and T3 concentrations.

As maternal thyroid hormone requirement is increased during pregnancy, women already on thyroxine replacement before pregnancy usually require a small increase in the dose from the first trimester. Thyroxine requirement increases by as much as 50% during the first half of pregnancy from as early as the fifth week of gestation although in many cases it does not increase. Some increase the dose by about 30% as soon as pregnancy is confirmed but there is no need to do this when TSH estimation is available within 24 hours, and the dose may be adjusted with reference to it. Those most likely to require more are women with thyroidectomy. It is possible that diminished absorption of thyroxine due to the ingestion of absorption-inhibiting agents like iron and calcium may account for increased requirements. For those diagnosed during pregnancy, replacement usually commences with 0.05 to 0.1 mg daily and the dose adjusted to keep the serum TSH at <3 mIU/L, The usual dose required is 0.1 to 0.2 mg daily. After delivery, thyroxine requirement usually falls in women whose dose increased during pregnancy. Monitoring of thyroid function with progressive adjustment of the replacement dose follows after delivery.

POSTPARTUM THYROID DYSFUNCTION

Irrespective of the thyroid status before delivery, mothers can develop various forms of postpartum thyroid disorder, the reported incidence being 4-9%, specially associated with the presence of maternal thyroid peroxidase antibody. Postpartum thyroid dysfunction may adversely affect lactation, and often leads to mood changes or depression, in addition to later menstrual disturbance. Hyperthyroidism may present for the first time postpartum, or it can represent an exacerbation of Hashimoto's thyroiditis and

GD. Hashimoto's thyroiditis may present with transient and self-limiting hyperthyroidism 2-4 months postpartum, followed by hypothyroidism at 3-8 months. The Postpartum Painless Thyroiditis (PPT) syndrome, an atypical form of hyperthyroidism due to thyroiditis, is associated with high antimicrosomal antibody titers, and is unrelated to such conditions as atypical subacute thyroiditis. It is typically observed 3-6 months after delivery, and is clinically indistinguishable from the non-pregnancy-related form. A phase of transient thyrotoxicosis of abrupt onset is followed by a second phase of transient hypothyroidism, before recovery to euthyroidism. Some women have no proceeding hyperthyroid phase, while the hypothyroid phase may be absent in up to 60% of cases. Thyroiditis may appear within a few weeks or even days after delivery, and presents not only with signs of hyperthyroidism but sometimes also severe hypertension. The administration of thyroxine 0.1 mg can ameliorate the hypothyroid symptoms but does not alter the course, while the use of 0.15 mg iodide daily appears to aggravate the condition. As well, despite the recovery to euthyroidism, a significant proportion of PPT patients develop hypothyroidism 2-4 years postpartum, the risk factors being high antmicrosomal antibody titer during pregnancy, severe hypothyroid phase, multiparity and a previous history of spontaneous abortion. PPT patients should therefore receive long-term follow-up assessment with thyroid function tests every year.

CONCLUSION

Thyroid disorders are among the commonest medical disorders encountered in pregnancy, and may be associated with poor obstetric outcome if unrecognized, difficult to control or managed inappropriately. Screening for underlying thyroid disorders should be performed in women with an adverse reproductive history as well as in those with pregnancy complications. In high-risk women, screening for thyroid dysfunction and autoimmunity before or early in pregnancy would be justified, since prompt treatment may dramatically improve the outcome of their pregnancy.

Parathyroid, adrenal and pituitary disease in pregnancy
W. M. Hague

INTRODUCTION

Parathyroid disease is uncommon in the general community and is equally so in pregnancy. The most common disorder is primary hyperparathyroidism, associated with either a parathyroid adenoma or with parathyroid hyperplasia. Malignant change in the parathyroid gland is very rare. Hyperparathyroidism may also be secondary to renal insufficiency. Hypoparathyroidism may be due to inadvertent removal of the parathyroid glands at the time of thyroid surgery, or to various rare genetic disorders.

The potential importance of parathyroid disorders in pregnancy lies in their effect on calcium balance both in the mother and in the fetus. When a pregnant woman is hypercalcemic, free calcium passes across the placenta and affects the fetal calcium balance. In utero, the fetus adjusts to excess calcium by negative feedback on its own parathyroid glands, which are then down-regulated. Following delivery and reduction of the previous increased calcium load, the normal response of the neonatal parathyroid glands to a lack of calcium (i.e. increasing parathormone secretion) is blunted, and the neonate can become frankly hypocalcemic with seizures and tetany. If, on the other hand, a pregnant woman is hypocalcemic, fetal parathyroid secretion is up-regulated to maintain fetal calcium homeostasis, leading to neonatal hyperparathyroidism and, in severe cases, to profound demineralization and even death.

The most common presentation of primary hyperparathyroidism in pregnancy is asymptomatic accompanying the recognition of hypercalcemia on routine biochemical screening for other disorders. This is most often mild and may go unrecognized, because of an associated fall in serum albumin to which the circulating calcium is bound. Diagnosis of hyperparathyroidism is established by the finding of non-suppressed parathormone in concert with hypercalcemia. Other clinical features may include thirst, vomiting, malaise, bone pain, abdominal pain (associated with renal colic or pancreatitis) and proximal muscle weakness. The maternal syndrome may also be revealed postpartum following the onset of neonatal seizures and the recognition of neonatal hypocalcemia.

This has been described as late as two months after delivery (Ip 2003).

Other biochemical features include hypercalciuria, established on one or more 24-h urine collections, or on a spot urine calcium-creatinine ratio. There may be evidence of bone demineralization, with osteoporosis demonstrated by ultrasound or a DEXA scan of the forearm, as well as increased urine excretion of pyridinium crosslinks.

Imaging with ultrasound may reveal the site of the tumor, but it has a poor sensitivity, as does parathyroid scintigraphy with Technetium-99m-Sestamibi, which of course is contraindicated in pregnancy. Still the best localization is achieved by having an experienced parathyroid surgeon explore the neck to identify whether an adenoma is present or the glands hyperplastic.

The differential diagnosis of hypercalcemia in pregnancy includes granulomatous disease, such as sarcoidosis, malignant disease with bone secondaries, vitamin D toxicity and milk alkali syndrome, associated with excessive use of calcium-containing antacids. There are also disorders of the extracellular calcium sensing receptor, which lead to the conditions of familial hypocalciuric hypercalcemia (FHH) and neonatal severe primary hyperparathyroidism. These have been shown to be due in some cases to genetic mutations of the receptor protein and rarely, in others, to antibodies against the receptor. These abnormalities are associated usually with loss of function (although cases both of increased and of unchanged function have been described.

The only definitive treatment for primary hyperparathyroidism is surgery, preferably performed by an experienced surgeon (see above). Ideally, this will be carried out in the second trimester, at a time when the risks of inducing premature delivery are lowest, and when a beneficial effect on resetting fetal calcium homeostasis can be achieved. Decisions about surgery will depend on the degree of maternal hypercalcemia. In acute hypercalcemia, fluid replacement and intravenous phosphate may be used to stabilize the patient prior to surgery (Molitch 1992). Women with mild primary hyperparathyroid disease (total serum calcium less than 2.6 mmol/L) may be observed expectantly, though their offspring should none the less be checked carefully for changes in calcium balance. In such mild cases, good hydration should be encouraged and phosphate supplements may be prescribed.

ADRENAL DISEASE

Adrenal disease is rare, both in the non-pregnant and pregnant states. Overactivity may be found in either the cortex or the medulla, while underactivity usually reflects adrenal damage, pituitary insufficiency or previous surgical removal. Non-secreting tumors are also found, both primary and secondary.

Adrenal Excess

Overactivity of the adrenal cortex may be seen either in tumors or in hyperplasia of the gland. Benign adenomas are many times more common than malignant tumors, although in pregnancy malignancy is seen in up to 10% of adrenal masses (Pickard et al 1990). This may reflect either a difficulty or a delay in establishing the diagnosis because of the coexisting pregnancy. Hyperplasia may be secondary to corticotrophin (ACTH), whether from pituitary or extra-pituitary lesions, leading to Cushing's syndrome, or may result from a defect within the adrenocortical pathways leading to cortisol synthesis.

Diagnosis of adrenocortical hormone-secreting tumors in the non-pregnant state includes demonstration of ACTH suppression as well as localization with imaging. In pregnancy, however, some of the circulating ACTH is non-pituitary and may not be suppressible, so that the diagnosis may be missed, although confirmed suppression is diagnostic (Lindsay and Nieman 2005). Dexamethasone suppression testing may be useful to establish the diagnosis in borderline cases.

In adrenal hyperplasia due to cortisol biosynthetic defects, inadequate cortisol secretion leads to a negative feedback loop on the pituitary-hypothalamic axis, with increased ACTH elaboration resulting in over-secretion of the precursor hormones, which cannot be metabolized because of the enzyme deficiency. The most common example of this is found in 21-hydroxylase deficiency, with resultant build up of 17-hydroxyprogesterone and its other downstream androgenic metabolites, including androstenedione and testosterone. The phenotype of this enzyme deficiency will vary, depending on the degree of enzyme activity. Severe cases may result in an intersex phenomenon with salt loss at birth. Lesser degrees of block may result in late onset disease, which may be clinically indistinguishable from polycystic ovary syndrome. Hyperplasia may also follow renin hypersecretion with resulting hyperaldosteronism. Finally, it may be idiopathic.

Adenomas and carcinomas may develop within each layer of the adrenal cortex, and the presentation will therefore vary depending on the active hormone that is being generated. Thus, adenomas of the zona reticularis will cause masculinization, with excessive androgen secretion that cannot be suppressed with exogenous dexamethasone administration. Adenomas of the zona fasciculata will cause Cushing's syndrome, again with excessive cortisol secretion that cannot be suppressed in the standard Liddell's test with exogenous dexamethasone. Excess aldosterone production from a tumour of the zona glomerulosa will cause the typical hypokalemic hypertension of Conn's syndrome. Diagnosis may be difficult and referral to a tertiary centre is usually required.

It is rare to find women with adrenal hypersecretion of androgens and/or cortisol becoming pregnant. Rather, such hypersecretion is generally associated with anovulation and amenorrhea. Women with hyperaldosteronism are more likely to conceive, the underlying diagnosis of their secondary hypertension that is often mild having gone unrecognized.

Pheochromocytoma

Tumors of the adrenal medulla include pheochromocytoma, which may also present in other sites within the sympathetic nervous chain. Active secretion of catecholamines may be episodic and cause the characteristic paroxysms of hypertension, with pallor and tachycardia, sweating and anxiety. Occasionally, there may be supine hypotension. Suspicion should be heightened if there is a family history of pheochromocytoma, of von Recklinghausen's syndrome (neurofibromatosis), or of medullary carcinoma of the thyroid or other component of the multiple endocrine neoplasia (MEN) syndromes (Bravo and Tagle 2003). The diagnosis is established by measurement of catecholamines in a 24-h urine collection. More than one sample may be necessary to establish the diagnosis. Mild elevations of urinary catecholamines or of their metabolites (vanillyl-mandelic acid: VMA) may be seen in subjects with chronic hypertension, but markedly increased concentrations of adrenaline (adrenal-derived) and nor-adrenaline (extra-adrenal) are found in active pheochromocytoma. Localization of an extra-adrenal phaeochromocytoma may be difficult in pregnancy, as use of [^{131}I]-*met*-iodo-benzyl-guanidine (MIBG) scintigraphy is contraindicated during gestation because of the risk to the fetal thyroid. Modern techniques of computed tomography and magnetic resonance imaging may be helpfully applied in this life threatening disorder.

Once the diagnosis of adrenal hypersecretion has been made, appropriate treatment can be initiated. For tumors of the adrenal, surgical treatment follows appropriate patient preparation, preferably before the third trimester to minimize the risk of premature labor. If considered safe, surgery is best delayed until postpartum. Women with adrenal Cushing's syndrome may be treated with metyrapone, which has been used successfully in pregnancy in a number of women. There is a risk of increasing hypertension and therefore of pre-eclampsia with this agent, which increases 11β-deoxy-corticosterone (DOC) secretion. Ketoconazole is embryotoxic and teratogenic in animals, but has been used in Cushing's syndrome outside of pregnancy because of its inhibitory action on mitochondrial cytochrome P450 enzymes, such as 11β-hydroxylase. It has antiandrogenic properties, but in two pregnancies where it was used, normal male infants were born. There are also case reports of the use of cyproheptadine, but with limited outcome data. Trilostane, a 3β-hydroxysteroid dehydrogenase blocking agent, is contraindicated in pregnancy because of its effect on inhibition of placental progesterone production. Spironolactone, an antagonist of aldosterone, which is a mainstay of treatment for Conn's syndrome outside of pregnancy, has antiandrogenic effects and is therefore not recommended for use in pregnancy, although successful cases have been reported where no such effect has been seen. In the case of pheochromocytoma in pregnancy, the vasoactive effects of the circulating catecholamines must be inhibited, first with an alpha-adrenergic blocker such as labetalol or phenoxybenzamine, and subsequently with a beta-blocker such as propranolol. Magnesium sulfate has also been recommended to aid control of vascular reactivity.

Adrenal hyperplasia, whether virilizing or salt-losing, is usually suppressed with corticosteroids such as hydrocortisone, cortisone acetate or prednisolone (Hoepffner et al 2004). The more potent and long-acting fluorinated steroids, such as dexamethasone, cross the placenta with potential effects on the fetal pituitary-adrenal axis and immune status, and are therefore in general best avoided in pregnancy. In recent years, however, it has been possible to diagnose congenital adrenal hyperplasia in the fetus. In such cases dexamethasone has been used, because it crosses the placenta, to treat affected fetuses to reduce the risk of in utero virilization.

Adrenal insufficiency

Primary adrenal insufficiency may be due to intrinsic disease, such as autoimmunity or infection (e.g. tuberculosis or meningococcus). Fertility may not be reduced in affected women, who in pregnancy need ongoing corticosteroid and mineralocorticoid replacement therapy (Ambrosi et al 2003). Despite the rise in corticosteroid binding globulin (CBG) during pregnancy, the dose of steroid required does not alter as pregnancy proceeds (Garner 1993). For labor and other situations of acute stress, such as severe infection (especially that associated with fluid loss, e.g. gastroenteritis), increased and/or parenteral doses of steroid supplementation are required.

If the diagnosis of adrenal insufficiency is entertained, a single dose of parenteral tetracosactrin (Synacthen) 250 μg is administered, followed by measurement of the response of plasma cortisol. A post Synacthen cortisol value of > 550 nmol/L excludes adrenal insufficiency in the non-pregnant individual. Normal values for pregnancy are not well documented, as Synacthen is rarely used because of concern that it might stimulate the fetal adrenal and lead to premature labor. In practice, this is very unlikely, and the risk must be weighed against the benefit of diagnosing a serious disorder. A recent review suggests that using a cut-off of 828 nmol/L will reliably identify adrenal insufficiency in pregnant women (Lindsay and Nieman 2005).

PITUITARY DISEASE

The pituitary enlarges during pregnancy with increasing secretion of hormones, particularly from the anterior lobe. This is not accompanied by local pressure effects, unless there is a pre-existing pituitary lesion, such as a macroprolactinoma or a craniopharyngioma, which may grow to impinge on the optic chiasm, with associated visual disturbance.

Investigation of pituitary disorders during pregnancy has been revolutionized by the availability of magnetic resonance imaging (MRI), which allows detailed views of the anatomy of the gland as well as of the associated blood supply, without recourse to ionizing radiation. Serial scans may also be performed to document temporal progression of any lesion.

The use of dynamic pituitary function tests during pregnancy is controversial. Insulin tolerance testing during pregnancy has not been reported. The associated transient hypoglycemia is unlikely to cause serious fetal harm. Dexamethasone 8 mg overnight suppression testing, used outside of pregnancy to distinguish between pituitary-dependent Cushing's disease and ectopic ACTH Cushing's syndrome, has not been validated in pregnancy (Lindsay and Nieman 2005). CRH testing has been recently reported in three cases of Cushing's disease in pregnancy, with substantial rises in plasma cortisol consistent with the surgical diagnosis, and no ill effects identified in mother or fetus.

Cushing's disease

Cushing's disease is rare during pregnancy, making up 40 (33%) of the 122 cases of Cushing's syndrome in pregnancy reported to date in the world literature, compared to the 50-70% proportion in the non-pregnant population. Similarly only 50-60 cases have been reported of acromegaly in pregnancy (Herman-Bonert et al 1998). Prolactinoma, however, is much more common, with many cases described. Of these 72% had microadenomas, with a very small incidence (1.4%) of significant symptomatic enlargement during pregnancy, whether or not there had been preceding ablative therapy (radiation or surgery). On the other hand, 26% of 84 women with untreated macroadenomas (diameter greater than 1 cm) developed symptoms of enlargement, compared with only 3% of 67 women who had surgery or radiation for their tumor prior to pregnancy.

Despite the rarity of Cushing's disease in pregnancy, it is important to consider the diagnosis. Significant perinatal loss has been noted, mainly associated with prematurity (Garner 1993) but only small numbers have been reported. As with non-pituitary disease, maternal complications described include gestational diabetes, hypertension and pre-eclampsia. Initial investigations should include measurement of plasma ACTH, dexamethasone suppression testing and adrenal imaging. In those in whom the diagnosis of adrenal disease seems unlikely, CRH testing and MRI of the pituitary and hypothalamus are the next stage of the work-up. Finally, inferior petrosal sinus sampling with CRH stimulation has been used to establish the diagnosis.

Prolactinoma

Enlargement of macroprolactinomas in pregnancy may cause chiasmal compression and resulting bitemporal hemianopia, as well as headache and raised intracranial pressure symptoms. If the diagnosis of prolactinoma is already established and such symptoms occur, it is reasonable to commence dopaminergic therapy with bromocriptine 2.5 mg daily, without

waiting for imaging confirmation, doubling the dose as rapidly as can be tolerated to 10 mg/day (Molitch 1992). For most patients without symptoms, however, it is reasonable to arrange review in each trimester and enquire as to visual disturbance and headache. Visual fields can be checked clinically, without requirement for formal testing unless symptoms indicate the need. There is no value in following serum prolactin concentrations through pregnancy: the scatter is wide, while even in enlarging tumors no significant increase may be seen. Breastfeeding should not be discouraged, but weaning may well require reinstitution of bromocriptine or cabergoline.

Acromegaly

Pregnancy does not usually exacerbate acromegaly, only 4 out of 24 cases reported showing acceleration of their disease (Herman-Bonert et al 1998). Dopaminergic therapy has been used in a small number of pregnant women with active acromegaly to assist in control of growth hormone release (Bronstein et al 2002). Similarly octreotide and its analogues have also been used successfully in pregnancy to maintain IGF-1 concentrations in the normal range. Despite a potential risk of intrauterine growth restriction because of transfer of drug across the placenta, normal fetal growth has been observed. Trans-sphenoidal resection has also been recommended in pregnancy to manage actively growing growth hormone-secreting tumors. Such surgery has been associated with an increased risk of prematurity, but no difference in abortion or perinatal mortality rates. Acromegaly may worsen glucose tolerance in pregnancy, with diabetes being reported in up to 32% of patients (Berelowitz and Howgo, reported in Herman-Bonert et al 1998). Hypertension may develop in acromegaly, increasing the risk of pre-eclampsia, though no data are available to quantify the risk.

Lymphocytic hypophysitis

Lymphocytic hypophysitis is an autoimmune disorder of the pituitary that has a striking association with pregnancy and the puerperium (Caturegli et al 2005). It can present in a number of ways, including mass effects within the pituitary fossa causing visual disturbance and headache, hormonal deficiency syndromes of both the anterior and posterior pituitary, and hyperprolactinemia secondary to stalk compression. The diagnosis is suggested when MRI displays a homogeneous symmetrical intrasellar mass with avid enhancement after administration of gadolinium, although cystic change has been described. Pituitary antibodies have been found, but the sensitivity and specificity are low (Caturegli et al 2005). Confirmation of the diagnosis can be established histologically. Current approaches to treatment are to reduce the local inflammation with high dose corticosteroid therapy, proceeding to trans-sphenoidal resection if any pressure symptoms do not rapidly respond to such medical therapy. Long-term hormone replacement may be required.

Pituitary apoplexy

The increased vascularity of the pituitary during pregnancy leaves it susceptible to ischemia. Pituitary apoplexy may be seen during or after pregnancy following acute infarction or hemorrhage within the gland. Presentation is usually with sudden headache, symptoms and signs of meningeal irritation, followed by hypotensive collapse. Visual field defects and diplopia may be present. Treatment is with replacement fluids and parenteral glucocorticoids, without waiting for the results of blood hormone assays. If the patient fails to respond rapidly, then neurosurgical advice should be sought with a view to urgent decompression.

Sheehan's syndrome

Sheehan's syndrome is a less acute, but equally serious, form of hypopituitarism seen after major obstetric hemorrhage associated with pituitary ischemia or necrosis. Failure to lactate, amenorrhea, dry skin and fatigue are the classic symptoms, often not appreciated for some months after delivery. Diabetes insipidus may also be seen, and occasionally will present after initiation of glucocorticoid replacement. Because glucocorticoids normally inhibit ADH secretion, their administration may unveil a masked posterior pituitary insufficiency.

Diabetes insipidus

Diabetes insipidus may first present during pregnancy because of the increased clearance of vasopressin by placental cystine aminopeptidase (Durr and Lindheimer 1996). Transient diabetes insipidus has also been described in association with severe liver dysfunction at the end of pregnancy, most typically in acute fatty liver of pregnancy, but also in severe pre-eclampsia (Krege et al 1989) (also see Ch. 9) The vasopressin analogue, dDAVP (desmopressin), is resistant to the action of cystine aminopeptidase, and it can therefore be used effectively as replacement therapy during pregnancy for both the acute and chronic presentations of diabetes insipidus. In the case of transient diabetes insipidus, intranasal doses of 10 μg bd may be sufficient to relieve the polyuria. Attempts should be made to wean the desmopressin every 3-5 days after delivery, following clearance of the active enzyme subsequent to delivery of the placenta.

Chronic hypopituitarism

In women with chronic hypopituitarism in pregnancy glucocorticoid and thyroxine supplements should be maintained, while oestrogen and progesterone are not required once the feto-placental unit is functional. Monitoring of thyroid replacement is difficult in pregnancy when TSH measurement is unreliable, as in hypopituitarism. The dose of thyroxine may be increased empirically by 10-15% each trimester, as is often needed in pregnancy, or the level of free thyroxine may be utilized, despite its shortcomings in pregnancy (see thyroid disorders above) (Lao 2005). Similarly imprecise is the monitoring of glucocorticoid replacement. Clinical judgment may be the best meter of dose adequacy, relying on symptoms and signs in the patient. Growth hormone supplementation is currently controversial, with few data to guide in respect of pregnancy.

Type 1 and type 2 diabetes in pregnancy
N. W. Cheung, B. N. J. Walters

SIGNIFICANCE OF PRE-EXISTING DIABETES IN PREGNANCY

When the mother has pre-existing diabetes (pregestational diabetes), pregnancy is associated with a sig-

nificantly increased risk of miscarriage, congenital malformations, preterm birth, neonatal morbidity and perinatal mortality. Before the discovery of insulin, it was rare for women with diabetes to fall pregnant, and in those who did, the maternal mortality was as high as 50%. Moreover, survival of the child was unlikely. Following the advent of insulin therapy in the 1920s, and then the introduction of home blood glucose testing and intensive insulin therapy, diabetic pregnancy has become much safer for the mother and perinatal outcomes improved dramatically. Even today however, the outcome of diabetic pregnancy remains suboptimal, with perinatal mortality and other complications significantly higher than observed in the background population. The incidence of fetal loss and congenital malformations remain unacceptably high. However, it should be appreciated that the outcome in pregnancy complicated by diabetes is almost entirely dependent on maternal glycemic control. If optimal control is achieved pre-conceptionally and during pregnancy, all measures of outcome for mother and baby approximate those of normal pregnancy. Unfortunately, although we have the medical knowledge and means to optimize conditions, and therefore outcomes for diabetic pregnancy, all too often this is not achieved. Furthermore, we are facing new challenges, such as the increasing incidence of type 2 diabetes in pregnancy.

Type 1 diabetes in pregnancy

Most of the literature regarding pre-existing diabetes in pregnancy is based on women with type 1 diabetes. People with type 1 diabetes are insulin deficient, with an absolute life sustaining requirement for insulin, and are prone to ketoacidosis. They may also have associated autoimmune endocrinopathies which require special attention during pregnancy.

In the vast majority of cases, these women will have had diabetes for some years, and there should have been opportunities to discuss pregnancy planning. However, in some cases, there may have been limited contact with medical care for some time, and it is not until pregnancy occurs that specialist contact is sought again. Studies have shown that the rate of unplanned pregnancy is high in women with type 1 diabetes. This is a frequent precursor of fetal abnormality. It is very important, therefore, that contraception be discussed with every woman with diabetes, so that pregnancy may occur at an optimal time, with good control.

Type 2 diabetes in pregnancy

Type 2 diabetes is by far the more common form of diabetes in the general population and there has been a rapid increase in its prevalence, particularly in the developing world. It is associated with insulin resistance and relative insulin deficiency. It may be managed by diet and exercise alone, oral hypoglyce-

mic agents, insulin therapy alone or in combination with oral agents. Type 2 diabetes is often associated with the metabolic syndrome and women who have polycystic ovary syndrome are also highly likely to develop type 2 diabetes.

With the increasing prevalence of obesity, the age of onset of type 2 diabetes has been falling and it is now not unusual for type 2 diabetes to occur in women of reproductive age. In some countries, pregnant women with type 2 diabetes are more commonly seen than type 1 diabetes. This presents specific problems, not least of which is a common misconception that type 2 diabetes is a more benign condition than type 1 diabetes in the context of pregnancy. In fact, a number of studies have demonstrated that perinatal mortality and major congenital malformation rates are greater in type 2 diabetes than type 1 diabetes.

Congenital malformations

One of the principal concerns of diabetic pregnancy is the risk of congenital malformation. Congenital malformations are much more frequent in diabetic than in normal pregnancies, with a rate 3-5 times that of the background population. The major factors which influence the development of malformation in diabetic pregnancy are the severity of hyperglycemia, and the timing of the poor control. Even mild degrees of hyperglycemia are associated with an increased likelihood of fetal malformation but the risk of malformation clearly rises with increasing HbA1c. Some studies have found major malformation rates of 20-50% at the upper extremes of HbA1c. Malformations are mainly due to exposure to hyperglycemia and occur early in the process of embryogenesis, with most of these having developed by the eighth week of gestation. The major congenital malformations most commonly seen are neural tube defects, congenital heart disease, malformations of the renal and urinary tract, gastrointestinal and skeletal malformations.

Although diabetic malformations are closely related to hyperglycemia, the exact mechanisms for teratogenicity are unclear. Experimental studies conducted on rodent embryos in culture suggest that elevated levels of glucose generate free oxygen radicals which result in reduced antioxidant defense and increased lipid peroxidation. In laboratory studies, antioxidant therapy lowers the rate of malformation induced by hyperglycemia in some species. Other factors which have been found to be related to diabetic embryopathy in vitro include a reduction in levels of arachidonic acid and myoinositol, and elevated levels of β-hydroxybutyrate. There is also evidence from rodent models that elevated glucose levels may alter the expression of regulatory genes involved in cell cycle progression, in both pre- and post-implantation embryogenesis, leading to apoptosis of progenitor cells, and resulting in dysmorphogenesis. Damage to the yolk sac by hyperglycemia may be another contributor to defective fetal morphogenesis.

Fetal loss and perinatal mortality

There is an increased rate of miscarriage among women with pregestational diabetes who have less optimal control. There is a relationship between elevated first trimester HbA1c and spontaneous abortion, and this parallels the rise in malformation rate with HbA1c. In one study, every increase of one standard deviation (equivalent to 0.5% where the normal range is 4.0-6.0%) in a first trimester HbA1c increased the risk of spontaneous abortion by 3%. A recent study also suggested that there is an increased risk of miscarriage with low extremes of blood glucose as well.

Even today, the perinatal mortality rate of diabetic pregnancy is several times that of the background population. A number of recent studies from developed countries have observed a higher perinatal mortality in type 2 diabetes than in type 1 diabetes, as high as 5-10%. In part, this may reflect the confounding effects of obesity or social disadvantage.

Other fetal complications

Macrosomia is a common complication and is associated with shoulder dystocia and brachial plexus palsy. In one study of 1589 diabetic pregnancies, 21% had macrosomia (fetal weight $\geq$ 4000 g), and 3.1% had shoulder dystocia. Other complications include hypocalcemia, hypomagnesemia, hypoxia, polycythemia, hyperbilirubinemia, neonatal hypoglycemia and respiratory distress syndrome. Many of these complications are presumed to occur on the basis of the Pedersen hypothesis, which states that transplacental transfer of glucose leads to fetal hyperinsulinemia. This causes increased fetal growth and fat deposition, resulting in macrosomia. Following birth, fetal hyperinsulinemia persists, but deprived of the maternal source of glucose, hypoglycemia results. In some cases, intrauterine growth restriction may occur, usually associated with maternal vascular disease and/or pre-eclampsia.

Pre-conception counseling and planning

The lack of pre-conception counseling and planning is a major factor contributing to poor outcomes in diabetic pregnancy. A meta-analysis of 16 studies examining preconception care has found that the risk of congenital anomalies in women who attended pre-pregnancy counseling is one third that of those who do not. Its importance is highlighted by the fact that the critical period for the development of malformations is early in the first trimester. For this reason, delay in addressing diabetes-related issues until after conception leaves insufficient time to prevent such complications from occurring.

Pre-conception counseling requires a proactive approach by the medical practitioner to inform the woman of the need to plan for pregnancy, starting from the age that pregnancy is possible. This should be in the teenage years for women with type 1 diabetes, or soon after diagnosis for women found to have type 2 diabetes. Pre-conception counseling should highlight the need to plan for pregnancy. Issues to be covered include the need for good glycemic control and folic acid supplementation even before conception, as well as information regarding the potential dangers of pregnancy without adequate planning and preparation. In many women with type 2 diabetes, time spent attempting weight loss before pregnancy is worthwhile as obesity markedly increases adverse event rates in pregnancy (Box 5.1).

When pregnancy is planned, diabetes management, control and complications should be addressed. There is evidence that outcomes of diabetic pregnancy are better if the patient is managed by

---

Box 5.1 Preconception planning: key points

- Patient education concerning the various pregnancy issues, including the risks of poor control.
- If practical, involve the woman in the care of a multidiscplinary team experienced in the management of diabetes in pregnancy.
- Review by a dietitian to optimize diet and weight control.
- Review by a diabetes educator to ensure adequate self-management skills, in particular in safety issues such as hypoglycemia management.
- Tighten glycemic control with the aim of achieving an HbA1c as close as possible to the normal range.
- Commence folate 5 mg daily.
- Assess for complications and treat where necessary.
- Review medications for safety in pregnancy.
- Discuss the use of contraception until conditions are optimized for pregnancy.

multidisciplinary teams experienced in this area. Members of these teams usually include an obstetrician, diabetologist, diabetes educator and dietitian. The management team should optimize insulin regimens and glycemic control, with the aim of achieving the tighter targets of pregnancy, prior to conception. This includes lowering the glycosylated hemoglobin as close to the normal range as is practicable. In general, women with type 2 diabetes should cease oral hypoglycemic agent therapy and transfer to insulin prior to conception if necessary, although there is controversy regarding the use of metformin.

Women should be commenced on folate supplementation from the time conception is planned. Folate has clearly been demonstrated to reduce the risk of neural tube defects. Because of the high risk in diabetic pregnancy a dose of 5 mg daily is recommended. A review of other medications should also be undertaken. Women with type 2 diabetes are more likely to suffer from hypertension and hyperlipidemia. Women with hypertension should be treated with an antihypertensive drug suitable for pregnancy. Statins have been associated with teratogenicity and should be ceased either before pregnancy or as soon as it is confirmed.

SCREENING AND MANAGEMENT OF DIABETIC COMPLICATIONS

Screening for complications should occur during pregnancy planning, so that these may be evaluated and dealt with prior to pregnancy. Some complications are more likely to progress during pregnancy, and some may increase the risk to the pregnancy.

Retinopathy

Active retinopathy rapidly deteriorates during pregnancy in some women. The risk exceeds 50% in women with existing proliferative retinopathy. During pre-conception planning, ophthalmological review should be organized so that if there is proliferative retinopathy, laser therapy can be undertaken. Further ophthalmological monitoring should also occur during the pregnancy, ideally at least once each trimester. Factors associated with progression of retinopathy during pregnancy are baseline severity of retinopathy, HbA1c and duration of diabetes. Some studies have shown that, in women with poor control, the risk of retinopathy increases for some months after improvement in control. This occurs in some women in pregnancy when control suddenly improves with the fear of fetal consequences of hyperglycemia.

Nephropathy

There is a risk of progression of diabetic nephropathy during pregnancy, particularly if the serum creatinine is above 0.2 mmol/L. Therefore, under such circumstances, pre-conception counseling should include consideration of the likelihood that renal function will deteriorate more quickly if pregnancy is undertaken. Discussion should deal with the later consequences of renal failure, namely dialysis and transplantation. These concepts need to be dealt with in a sensitive manner as they may not have been discussed before with young diabetic women. It must be understood by the physician that some women will proceed with pregnancy against medical advice. Such women may decide that renal failure ultimately is inevitable and that their chance for pregnancy diminishes as the years pass. In these circumstances, paths of communication must be kept open to ensure optimal management of their difficult problems should pregnancy occur. Women with nephropathy are almost invariably taking angiotensin converting enzyme inhibitors or receptor blockers. These are extremely helpful in slowing the rate of progression of diabetic nephropathy, but must be ceased before pregnancy. This provides one of the reasons for renal deterioration during pregnancy.

Even with lesser degrees of diabetic nephropathy, there is increased risk, in particular for the development of pre-eclampsia and this is a major reason for the high rate of preterm delivery in this situation. In general, screening for nephropathy should occur with a timed urine sample for microalbumin. A level > 20 µg/min is considered abnormal. An albumin/creatinine ratio on an early morning specimen is an alternative screening test. If this is > 3.5 mg albumin/mmol creatinine, a timed sample should be collected.

Cardiovascular disease

Evidence of cardiovascular disease should be sought from history and examination. Although a past history of ischemic heart disease presents enormous risk for the pregnant patient with diabetes, minor and well-controlled disease is not necessarily a contraindication to pregnancy. The risk of further ischemia during pregnancy should be evaluated and the risks of stopping protective therapy such as statins and ACE inhibitors requires discussion (see above). A review of myocardial infarction during diabetic pregnancy found a maternal mortality rate of 62% and only 46% of infants survived.

In the situation of women who have one or more children and who have significant medical complications as mentioned above, pregnancy should be particularly strongly discouraged. In this circumstance, the relative risk to benefit ratio is different from that for the nulliparous woman, for whom more risk may be acceptable. It must be appreciated that the significance and perception of risk by the doctor may differ from the patient's, and again, a difficult discussion is sometimes unavoidable.

Screening for co-existent endocrine disorders

It is common for women with type 1 diabetes to have other autoimmune endocrinopathies, in particular hypothyroidism. This should be tested for during pregnancy planning, and again with the routine antenatal screening tests. Other autoimmune disorders which are more common include adrenal insufficiency and celiac disease.

MANAGEMENT OF PRE-EXISTING DIABETES IN PREGNANCY

Diabetic review during pregnancy

Women with diabetes should be reviewed frequently for monitoring of glycemic control, progression of diabetic complications and hypertension in combination with obstetric surveillance including fetal monitoring at the appropriate times. Generally diabetic review should occur every 1-4 weeks early in pregnancy, depending on the adequacy and stability of control. This is often highly variable in early pregnancy as a result of nausea, vomiting, anorexia or overeating (to combat nausea). Towards the end of the second trimester, review should occur every 1-2 weeks, as insulin requirements rise at this time. However, some of these reviews may be conducted over the telephone. In fact, the availability of a physician or diabetes educator for frequent and impromptu telephone or email consultations is invaluable for women with glycemic instability. In some cases, particularly during the late second trimester, adjustments to insulin may need to be made as frequently as every 1-2 days. Ongoing review by the diabetes educator and dietitian is also an important component of care.

Assessment of glycemic control

There are two main methods of assessing glycemic control. All women with diabetes should perform home blood glucose monitoring, but this is particularly important during pregnancy as glucose targets are narrow, and hypoglycemia always a risk. Home blood glucose monitoring enables an evaluation of the daily excursions of blood glucose whereas glycosylated hemoglobin (HbA1c) is a measure of overall long-term control.

Home blood glucose monitoring

The use of blood glucose meters for self-monitoring is mandatory. Self-testing of blood glucose should occur in the fasting state, and 1-2 h after meals. Particularly for women with type 1 diabetes, it is also helpful, if control is proving difficult, to monitor blood glucose levels before meals, and before bed. Where there is a suspicion of nocturnal hypoglycemia, the measurement of an overnight (around 2.00-3.00 a.m.) blood glucose level is useful. Most authorities recommend maintenance of fasting blood glucose levels above 3.5-4.0 mmol/L and below 5.5 mmol/L. The 2-h postprandial readings should be kept above 4.0 mmol/L and below 7.0 mmol/L. Ideally, these levels should be achieved prior to conception and maintained during pregnancy. Attainment of glycemic targets needs to be balanced against the risk of hypoglycemia (see Box 5.2).

Glycosylated hemoglobin

The second means of assessing glucose control is by measurement of glycosylated hemoglobin. Irreversible glycosylation of hemoglobin to HbA1c occurs during erythropoiesis, and the level of glycosylation is dependent on the ambient level of glucose at the time. Hence the HbA1c is an objective measure of the integrated level of glucose over a 2-3 month period. Because of the lower levels of glucose in pregnancy, the normal range for HbA1c is also lower in pregnancy. To minimize the risk to the pregnancy, it is advisable to achieve a HbA1c within the normal (non-pregnant) range prior to conception, if at all possible. During pregnancy, the HbA1c should be measured every 1-2 months, and the closer this is maintained to

---

Box 5.2 Ideal glycemic targets

- Monitor HbA1c preconception and every 2-3 months during pregnancy:
  - maintain within normal non-diabetic range.
- Self-monitoring of blood glucose:
  - maintain fasting blood glucose levels 3.5-5.5 mol/L;
  - 2-h postprandial glucose levels 4.0-7.0 mmol/L.
- Avoid hypoglycemia.
- Avoid sustained or significant ketosis.

the normal range, the lower the risk to the pregnancy. This is most critical in the pre-conception period, and in the first trimester of pregnancy.

The HbA1c should be interpreted in the context of the woman's daily blood glucose readings. In women performing assiduous blood glucose monitoring and where there is no doubt as to the veracity of their glucose record, frequent HbA1c estimations add little to the assessment of progress or management. Day by day adjustment of insulin dosage is based on the home blood glucose record, and does not depend on the level of HbA1c. However, where there is a discrepancy between the HbA1c and the daily blood glucose readings, then inaccuracies of the blood glucose measurement (e.g. uncalibrated meter, old testing strips) or in the recording of the blood glucose levels should be considered. It must also be borne in mind that recent changes in blood glucose readings or instability in glucose control will not necessarily be reflected in the HbA1c.

Ketosis

Pregnancy is a state of accelerated ketosis so pregnant women with type 1 diabetes are particularly prone to ketoacidosis. Moreover, ketones readily cross the placenta. Embryo culture experiments have found that ketones can be teratogenic although there is no evidence for this in vivo. Some studies have suggested that significant ketosis during pregnancy can affect the child's neuropsychological development. It would therefore be prudent to avoid ketosis in pregnancy. Women with type 1 diabetes who fall ill, or have persistent hyperglycemia, should test for ketones, either in blood or urine. Persistent ketosis would be an indication for review and possibly admission to hospital.

Dietary management

Women with pre-existing diabetes should have previously received dietary advice. However, dietary review should occur during pre-conception planning and early in the pregnancy. In general, women with diabetes should receive 50-60% of their caloric intake as carbohydrate, with a focus on foods of low glycemic index. A lower proportion of carbohydrate has been advocated and successfully used by some practitioners in pregnancy. Total fat should comprise < 30% of energy intake, and saturated fat < 10%, with an increase in the proportion of polyunsaturated and monounsaturated fat. Having smaller main meals, and healthy 'snacks' between meals, tends to promote greater stability in blood glucose levels, and may also be better

tolerated especially in early pregnancy when there is nausea or rapid satiety. The energy needs of a pregnant woman will vary depending on body mass index, daily activities and occupation and a number of other factors may need to be taken into consideration. Dietary advice therefore, needs to be individualized.

Oral hypoglycemic agents

The data regarding the safety of metformin in early pregnancy are incomplete and it is best avoided in pregnancy. Research soon to be completed is investigating the role and safety of metformin in later pregnancy in the management of gestational diabetes. When metformin is used to promote ovulation in women with polycystic ovary syndrome, it should be stopped when pregnancy is confirmed.

In one retrospective review of 332 infants born to women with type 2 diabetes, the use of sulfonylurea therapy early in pregnancy was not related to the risk of developing malformations. Nonetheless, for women with type 2 diabetes who are using oral hypoglycemic agents, it would generally be advisable that these be ceased prior to pregnancy, and substituted with insulin therapy if necessary. If control is perfect on the oral agent, however, it is reasonable, after discussion with the woman, to allow continuation of the oral agent until pregnancy is confirmed, then cease it for consideration of insulin. Most women will suspect pregnancy before, or soon after, the first missed period. There is no evidence of harm from the sulfonylureas or metformin at this gestation. Thus, if a woman conceived whilst on oral hypoglycemic agents, this should not engender alarm.

Insulin management

For women with type 1 diabetes, and for those with type 2 diabetes normally requiring hypoglycemic agent therapy, a basal/bolus regimen of insulin provides the best control. This comprises four injections a day, with short acting insulin (e.g. Actrapid®, Humulin R®) given before meals, and intermediate acting insulin (e.g. Protaphane®, Monotard®, Humulin NPH®) before bed. Essentially, the insulin administered before a particular meal is adjusted to maintain blood glucose levels after that meal within the target range, and bedtime insulin is administered to control fasting hyperglycemia. A basal/bolus regime has been shown to achieve better control in pregnancy than twice daily insulin.

Many women with type 1 diabetes receive more insulin pre-conception and early in the pregnancy as they strive to attain good control. In some cases, insulin requirements will decrease late in the first trimester, possibly due to earlier over-insulinization. The requirements then increase steadily from the late second trimester. In the last week or two of pregnancy, a fall in insulin requirements may occur. An earlier decrease in insulin requirement may suggest the development of placental insufficiency (most commonly in association with pre-eclampsia) or the development of a maternal condition which leads to loss of counter-regulatory control, such as adrenal insufficiency.

Because of their greater insulin resistance, women with type 2 diabetes generally require larger doses of insulin. Their insulin requirements also increase markedly in the late second trimester due to the pregnancy-related increase in insulin resistance. In some cases, very large doses of insulin (e.g. several hundred units daily) may be needed.

Insulin analogues

Through additions or substitutions of individual amino acids in the insulin molecule, insulin analogues with altered pharmacokinetic properties have been developed. There are rapid-acting and long-acting insulin analogues. The rapid analogues include Lispro® and Aspart®. The rapid analogues offer an advantage in the treatment of diabetes as they are injected immediately before meals, without the need to wait for 15-30 min as recommended for conventional fast acting human insulins, and they are less likely to cause hypoglycemia as they have a shorter duration of action. Early case reports found an increase in adverse outcomes in women using Lispro insulin through pregnancy. These findings need to be carefully interpreted as diabetes is itself associated with adverse pregnancy outcomes. Subsequent cohort studies have suggested that Lispro is probably safe, and the rate of malformation in patients treated with Lispro is no greater than for the diabetic women on human insulin. Nevertheless, their use in pregnancy should be discussed with the woman. There is limited information regarding the use of Aspart insulin in pregnancy, though there is no evidence to date that suggests that its effect on pregnancy would be any different from that of Lispro. In general, for women who are pregnant, loss of control through a change in insulin from a rapid-acting analogue to conventional human insulin is considered a greater threat to the pregnancy than the potential danger of the insulin analogue itself.

The new long-acting insulin analogues comprise Glargine® and Detemir®. These analogues have proven very useful and effective in the non-pregnant population, particularly where hypoglycemia

is difficult to prevent. There is a little published experience with Glargine in pregnancy, with anecdotal case reports of usage without ill effects. However, there is insufficient data to date to support its general use in pregnancy, and until there is, it would be prudent to discuss its continuation with the patient. In general, most women using Glargine or Detemir have had severe problems with hypoglycemia when using conventional insulins, so safety factors may well favor continuation of the new analogue.

Insulin pump therapy

Continuous subcutaneous insulin infusion (CSII) therapy via an insulin pump offers an alternative to multiple subcutaneous insulin injections. This has been demonstrated to be as effective in controlling HbA1c and blood glucose levels. CSII may offer a specific advantage in patients who have difficulty controlling their overnight blood glucose levels. For example, the rate of insulin infusion can be reduced in the early hours of the morning, but increased at around 5.00-6.00 a.m. when there often is a rise in blood glucose levels. CSII also offers increased flexibility and it is simple to administer corrective boluses of insulin. The advent of continous glucose sensing devices, used in conbination with CSII may further facilitate achievement of glucose length.

Hypoglycemia in pregnancy

Tight glycemic control in pregnancy needs to be balanced against the risk of hypoglycemia. Maternal deaths due to hypoglycemia, either directly, or through motor vehicle and other accidents have been reported. It is therefore critical that the mother is cognizant of hypoglycemia management and undertakes measures to reduce the risk of this potentially devastating complication.

Studies in rats have demonstrated a harmful effect of hypoglycemia to the fetus. In humans it remains unclear if hypoglycemia adversely affects fetal development. Although severe hypoglycemia has been shown to lead to abnormalities in the fetal heart rate, modest maternal hypoglycemia (above 2.5 mmol/L) does not appear to affect fetal well-being. Nonetheless, it is best that hypoglycemia be avoided, for the welfare of both mother and child. In some cases, this may mean acceptance of suboptimal control, and the clinician needs to weigh up the risk of hypoglycemia against the risk of hyperglycemia. Hypoglycemia is more common from the 6th to the 18th week of pregnancy, and again towards the end of the pregnancy, and appropriate insulin adjustments need to be made.

Obstetric care

The need for regular obstetric review is based on the usual indicators for a high-risk pregnancy. There are subsets within the population of women with diabetes who present special risk, either for the fetus, or the mother, and monitoring should be tailored to the particular aspects of each case. In general, the following characteristics identify women and babies at particular risk, who need specially assiduous surveillance:

- long duration of diabetes
- complicated diabetes – including nephropathy, vascular disease, retinopathy, neuropathy
- co-morbidity such as pre-existing hypertension, myocardial infarction, cystic fibrosis
- poor compliance – such as poor attenders;
- recurrent hypoglycemia
- previous adverse pregnancy outcome
- cigarette smoking or substance abuse
- adolescent pregnancy
- obesity.

In these case, the likelihood of complications is high. Prophylaxis against pre-eclampsia should be considered (see Ch. 3), as should more frequent fetal assessment.

Regular assessment of growth and fetal well-being should be undertaken. In diabetic pregnancy, ultrasound examinations are usually performed at least every trimester. In particular, an ultrasound examination for fetal morphology and fetal echocardiography should be performed at 18-20 weeks. Maternal serum screening for aneuploidy is less reliable in the presence of diabetes. Therefore, first trimester screening using nuchal translucency with measurement of β-hCG and PAPP-A should be offered.

Pre–eclampsia and preterm labor

Women with diabetes have an increased risk of the pregnancy complication pre-eclampsia. Those at particular risk are women with existing hypertension, with diabetic nephropathy, with type 2 diabetes (obesity in particular) and those in whom pre-eclampsia complicated a previous pregnancy. For these women, close monitoring of the blood pressure, proteinuria and of fetal growth are important. Prophylaxis against the development of pre-eclampsia by means of low dose aspirin (80-100 mg/day) has been established as safe and moderately effective, reducing the rate by about 15% of the expected rate (see Ch. 3). Aspirin should be considered in diabetic women with the risk factors above, to be commenced in the first trimester.

In a woman with diabetes and threatened preterm labor, or incipient delivery for pre-eclampsia or other complication, antenatal corticosteroids will often be administered to effect fetal lung maturation. This is a potentially dangerous scenario and many cases of ketoacidosis have followed steroid use. Blood sugar monitoring must be assiduous at such times. In some women, an insulin infusion will be necessary to maintain adequate control for a few days.

Delivery and management of labor

The traditional approach included early delivery for women with pre-existing diabetes. This should no longer be considered routine. In the absence of complications and where control has been excellent and all fetal and maternal indicators are favorable, delivery may be at term. Vaginal delivery is preferable unless there are obstetric reasons for Cesarean section. Because 80% of cases of shoulder dystocia in diabetic pregnancy occur where the birthweight exceeds 4250 g, elective Cesarean section is recommended when the estimated fetal weight exceeds this level.

A plan for management of diabetes during labor should be mapped out in advance and should be standardized for each center so that all staff concerned are familiar with the routines and expectations. Generally, women who require insulin will need to be managed with an insulin and dextrose infusion, particularly if they require fasting for any length of time, such as in preparation for Cesarean section. In particular, there is a risk of ketoacidosis in women with type 1 diabetes deprived of insulin. The usual glucose targets will still apply, as maternal hyperglycemia during labor increases the risk of neonatal hypoglycemia.

Postpartum management

Insulin requirements in women with type 1 diabetes usually decrease dramatically following delivery, often to half that of the last weeks of pregnancy. Close monitoring and adjustment of the dose to meet altered insulin requirements and avoid hypoglycemia is necessary. Breastfeeding may further accentuate the tendency to hypoglycemia, and this needs to be taken into account.

Women with type 2 diabetes who did not require insulin before pregnancy, can usually cease insulin therapy immediately postpartum, even if they required substantial doses of insulin during pregnancy. However, if the woman plans to breastfeed, consideration should be given to continuation of insulin therapy, if diet alone is insufficient to maintain adequate glycemic control (bearing in mind that the tighter glycemic targets of pregnancy may now be relaxed a little). Metformin passes through breast milk in small quantities and although there have not been published reports of any adverse effect on the infant, caution is warranted.

Fetal programming effects of diabetes in pregnancy

Freinkel hypothesized that exposure to hyperglycemia (and over-nutrition) in utero may predispose to a diabetic phenotype, giving rise to his theory of 'fuel-mediated teratogenesis'. He suggested that a fetus exposed to excessive metabolic fuels in utero as a consequence of maternal diabetes, may suffer permanent anthropometric-metabolic modifications. This 'programming' predisposes to the development of obesity in teenage and early adult life and a diabetic phenotype. Hence, the offspring of women who have inadequately controlled diabetes in pregnancy, are probably at increased risk of future diabetes.

The strongest data in support of this comes from long-term follow-up studies of the Pima Indians. Amongst the offspring of mothers who were diabetic when pregnant, the risk of having T2DM by the age of 20-24 was 45%. In contrast, where the mothers had not developed diabetes within 5 years of the pregnancy (non-diabetics), the risk was 1.4% at the same age. It is unlikely that the increased incidence of diabetes amongst offspring of women with T2DM in pregnancy is due to genetic influences alone, as the children of prediabetic women (i.e. developed diabetes after the pregnancy) had a risk of diabetes of only 8.6% by age 20-24. Moreover, among sibships discordant for exposure to hyperglycemia, the sibling exposed to hyperglycemia had a much higher risk of subsequent obesity and diabetes.

More recently, data from a number of birth cohort studies have demonstrated that exposure to maternal diabetes in pregnancy is associated with a higher risk of development of obesity, glucose intolerance and other features of the metabolic syndrome by adolescence and young adulthood. There is also epidemiological evidence of an association between birthweight and diabetes in later life both among individuals with low birthweight ('the Barker Hypothesis'), and also at the upper extremes of birthweight, giving rise to a 'U-shaped' curve. It has been proposed that significant numbers of these subjects with high birthweight may have been exposed to maternal diabetes in pregnancy, and thus subjected to the programming effects of hyperglycemia in utero.

Although a programming effect of hyperglycemia in utero has not been proven conclusively, there is now considerable evidence which supports it. It is not known if there is a threshold effect, but good glycemic control in accordance with standard pregnancy guidelines should minimize any effect of fetal programming, with benefit for generations following the index pregnancy.

Box 5.3 summarizes the key points of this section on pregestational diabetes.

Box 5.3 Pregestational diabetes

- Pregestational diabetes is associated with an increased risk of congenital malformation and fetal loss, and this risk is related to diabetes control in the early stages of pregnancy.
- Pre-conception counseling reduces the likelihood of complications of diabetic pregnancy.
- Ideally, care of the pregnant woman with diabetes should be undertaken by an experienced multidisciplinary team.
- The glycosylated hemoglobin should be maintained in the normal range, or as close to this as possible.
- Blood glucose levels in pregnancy should be lower than outside of pregnancy.
- Oral hypoglycemic agents are generally not recommended in pregnancy, or during breastfeeding.
- Insulin requirements change as the pregnancy progresses and frequent review and adjustment are necessary.
- Diabetic complications, particularly retinopathy, may rapidly deteriorate in pregnancy.
- Postpartum, insulin requirements often decline dramatically and there is a heightened risk of hypoglycemia.

Gestational diabetes
N. W. Cheung, B. N. J. Walters

DEFINITION OF GESTATIONAL DIABETES

Gestational diabetes (GDM) is defined as 'carbohydrate intolerance with onset or first recognition during pregnancy'. In some cases, this may encompass women who had pre-pregnancy diabetes, but were unaware of it until it was detected in pregnancy. Depending on the population examined, and the diagnostic criteria used, GDM occurs in 2.2-8.8% of pregnancies (Table 5.2). It is higher in some ethnic groups.

The principal risk factors for GDM are obesity, age above 30 years, family history of diabetes, previous GDM, ethnicity and polycystic ovary syndrome. The ethnic groups at higher risk of GDM are the same as those predisposed to type 2 diabetes. These include people from Asia (especially the Indian subcontinent), the Middle East, Southern Europe, Pacific Islands, Australian aboriginals and other indigenous populations. Essentially, women at risk of type 2 diabetes are at risk of GDM.

Table 5.2 Diagnostic criteria for GDM

Organization	Glucose load	Diagnostic BSL thresholds (mmol/L)	Number of abnormal values required
American Diabetes Association	Either 75 g or 100 g	75 g Test: Fasting ≥5.3, 1-h 10.0, 2-h 8.6 100 g Test: Fasting ≥5.3, 1-h 10.0, 2-h 8.6, 3 h 7.8	2 2
American College of Obstetricians and Gynecologists	100 g	Either Fasting[a] ≥5.8, 1-h 10.6, 2-h 9.2, 3 h 8.0 or Fasting[b] ≥5.3, 1-h 10.0, 2-h 8.6, 3 h 7.8	2 2
Australasian Diabetes in Pregnancy Society	75 g	Fasting ≥5.5 2-h ≥8.0 (9.0 in New Zealand)	1
Royal Australian and New Zealand College of Obstetricians & Gynaecologists	75 g	Fasting ≥5.5 2-h ≥8.0 (9.0 in New Zealand)	1
Canadian Diabetes Association	75 g	Fasting ≥5.3, 1-h 10.6, 2-h 8.9	1
Society of Obstetricians & Gynaecologists of Canada	100 g	Either Fasting[a] ≥5.8, 1-h 10.6, 2-h 9.2, 3 h 8.0 or Fasting[b] ≥5.3, 1-h 10.0, 2-h 8.6, 3 h 7.8	2 2
Royal College of Obstetricians & Gynaecologists		No recommendation	
Diabetes UK	75 g	2-h 7.8-11.0 'impaired glucose tolerance of pregnancy'[c] Fasting ≥7.0 'gestational diabetes' 2-h ≥11.1	1 1

[a]NDDWG Criteria.

[b]Carpenter and Coustan Criteria.

[c]WHO criteria. This divides women with abnormal results into the categories of 'impaired glucose tolerance of pregnancy' and 'gestational diabetes'.

PATHOPHYSIOLOGY OF GESTATIONAL DIABETES

There is an increase in resistance to insulin during normal pregnancy, particularly in the third trimester. Consequently, there is a compensatory increase in insulin secretion to maintain euglycemia. In fact, blood glucose levels are lower in normal women when they are pregnant.

Insulin resistance amongst women with GDM is not markedly different from that of women who have normal glucose tolerance, but the increased insulin resistance is exhibited earlier in pregnancy. In addition, when studied after pregnancy, these women often have persistent insulin resistance. The key factor which results in glucose intolerance appears to be a failure to compensate for this with increased insulin secretion (Fig. 5.1). Hence these women may have underlying reduced pancreatic β cell reserve. The complications of GDM are not however, purely due to maternal hyperglycemia. There may also be contributions from changes in maternal lipid and amino acid metabolism.

In a minority of women with GDM, the underlying pathology is insulin deficiency, and pregnancy has coincided with an early stage in the evolution of their type 1 diabetes. This may be suspected when a woman of normal weight or underweight demonstrates fasting hyperglycemia, particularly in the absence of a family history of diabetes. In these cases it is worth testing for islet cell antibodies. If positive, the rate of progression to non-gravid type 1 diabetes is very high.

DIAGNOSIS OF GESTATIONAL DIABETES

An oral glucose tolerance test (oGTT) is generally required for the diagnosis of GDM, although a high random or fasting sugar may also be diagnostic. The original diagnostic criteria came from seminal studies performed by O'Sullivan and Mahan (1964; O'Sullivan 1991). These were based upon the risk of the woman developing diabetes later in life, rather than on pregnancy outcome. A number of modifications of the O'Sullivan criteria have since been made by various groups, resulting in the current situation where there is an array of diagnostic criteria used in different countries. It is recommended that practitioners follow the criteria of the national bodies in their country (Table 5.2). Even so, there are sometimes differences in recommendations between the various professional bodies caring for women with GDM within individual countries. This lamentable lack of standardization may be at least partially resolved by the Hyperglycemia and Adverse Pregnancy Outcome (HAPO) study, due for publication in 2007.

SCREENING FOR GESTATIONAL DIABETES

There has been debate as to whether all pregnant women should be screened for GDM (universal screening) or if screening should be reserved for women with risk factors. The earlier literature indicates that if screening is reserved only for women with risk factors, then up to one-third of women with

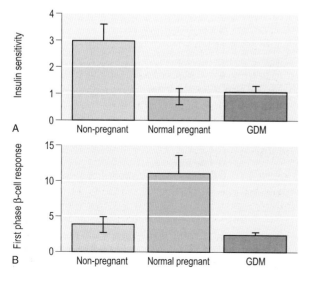

Figure 5.1 Insulin sensitivity and β-cell response in non-pregnant, normal pregnant and GDM women in the third trimester. Adapted from Buchanan et al (1990). The degree of insulin sensitivity is similar between the normal pregnant and GDM women but the latter do not compensate with sufficient insulin secretion.

GDM will be missed. Some authorities have adopted recommendations that all women should be screened, except for those at low risk. Others have made no recommendation, or even recommended against screening until more evidence is available that treating GDM is of benefit.

When biochemical screening is performed, a positive screening test is an indication to proceed to a diagnostic oGTT, A 1-h 50 g oral glucose challenge test (GCT) is the usual screening test for GDM, This test does not require fasting so can be performed during a routine antenatal visit. The lower the glucose threshold adopted on the GCT as the indication to proceed to an oGTT, the more sensitive the test for detection of GDM, but this needs to be balanced against the increased number of women who would need to undergo an oGTT to detect the extra cases.

In Australia, a glucose level of ≥ 7.8 mmol/L after one hour on the GCT is considered a positive result, and indication for an oGTT to be performed. Some groups have adopted the lower GCT threshold of ≥ 7.2 mmol/L. As GDM does not usually occur until the late second trimester, the GCT is performed at around 26-28 weeks. However, if there is a suspicion of hyperglycemia earlier in the pregnancy, then an oGTT should be performed at the time, but repeated at the usual time if the early test was normal. Where GDM is diagnosed early in pregnancy, this should raise the suspicion of pre-existing glucose intolerance or unsuspected diabetes. With the increasing age and adiposity of the pregnant population, diabetes is becoming more prevalent. For this reason, screening for diabetes is justifiable as a pre-conception investigation, or at the booking visit, particularly in high risk women. Even if negative, however, these women require testing again at the usual gestation as stated above.

COMPLICATIONS OF GESTATIONAL DIABETES

The rationale for screening for GDM is based mostly on fetal concerns. The degree of hyperglycemia is usually insufficient to cause maternal morbidity in the short time frame of pregnancy, notwithstanding the long-term implications of the diagnosis. For the baby, the most common complications of GDM are macrosomia and its attendant obstetric problems, preterm birth, neonatal hypoglycemia and the constellation of features implied by the description 'infant of a diabetic mother. These include hyperbilirubinemia, polycythemia, respiratory distress syndrome and hypocalcemia. Women with GDM are more likely to undergo Cesarean section and induced labor. There

is also an association with the development of pre-eclampsia. The likelihood of developing complications of GDM is related to the severity of glucose intolerance.

Evidence of increased perinatal mortality has been demonstrated in large studies. In a retrospective analysis of 78758 pregnancies, from 1971-1994, Beischer et al (1996) found a perinatal mortality rate of 1.0% in women with GDM, 1.31 times that of women with normal glucose tolerance. In another study of 4977 women, the perinatal mortality rate among those with GDM by the World Health Organization (WHO) criteria was 1.59 times that of women who did not have GDM. Some studies have also demonstrated a higher malformation rate, but it is likely that a number of these cases had undiagnosed pre-existing diabetes.

There is also some evidence that even the modest levels of hyperglycemia seen in GDM (lower than in frank diabetes), may result in fetal programming and predispose to later obesity and glucose intolerance in the offspring (see type 1 & type 2 diabetes above). However, there are no data regarding the level and timing of hyperglycemia which may predispose to such effects.

MANAGEMENT OF GESTATIONAL DIABETES

Management of GDM ideally utilizes a team approach. The members of the team comprise the obstetrician, a physician with expertise in the management of diabetes in pregnant women, a dietitian and a diabetes educator/midwife.

In formulating the management plan, attention must be given to the following aspects:

- dietary advice
- education and reassurance
- physical activity
- blood glucose monitoring
- correction of hyperglycemia
- fetal monitoring
- timing and method of delivery
- postnatal care and follow-up.

Dietary management

All women with GDM should receive counseling from a specialist dietitian. Recommendations are individualized after a dietary assessment of each patient. Diet is the cornerstone of treatment of GDM, and for the future, has significance for the patient in reducing her long-term risk of diabetes. In the present pregnancy, the aim is to achieve normoglycemia while providing the required nutrients for normal fetal growth and maternal health. A secondary aim is to prevent excessive maternal weight gain, particularly in women who are overweight or have gained excess weight in pregnancy.

The diet prescription will usually focus on complex carbohydrate in controlled amounts and reduction in simple carbohydrates and fat intake. Carbohydrates with a low glycemic index are favored. The proportion of energy to be taken as carbohydrate is generally between 40 and 50%. Emphasis is given to spreading the dietary intake over six meals daily, with three main meals and three snacks, in order to avoid large food loads at any time.

Calorie restriction for obese patients: In obese women (weight more than 10% above ideal body weight adjusted for gestational age), it is advisable to use modest energy restriction. A dietary caloric content of 1500-1800 kcals is acceptable for use by these women, and has been shown to be safe and effective (in terms of minimizing weight gain, and perhaps macrosomia). Such a diet should also reduce the likelihood of requiring insulin.

The main features of the dietary prescription are as follows:

- avoid sweet foods
- avoid fast foods and take-aways
- small frequent meals
- select high fiber and low glycemic index foods
- reduce fat intake
- liberal intake of 'free' foods, such as salad vegetables.

Physical activity

Exercise has beneficial effects in diabetes care. When there is no medical or obstetric contraindication, the woman should be advised to increase physical activity as this enhances insulin sensitivity and improves weight control. Modest exercise (15-20 min, 3-6 times weekly) in pregnancy may reduce blood glucose, both fasting and postprandial. Vigorous exercise should be avoided, as it is detrimental to fetal growth. It is helpful to reassure women about the safety of activities such as walking for 20-30 min each day, attendance at antenatal exercise classes or water aerobics for pregnancy.

Blood glucose monitoring

Women with GDM should perform home blood glucose monitoring. Blood glucose levels are usually monitored in the fasting state and 1-2 h after meals. Treatment to postprandial targets results in superior

Table 5.3 Blood glucose targets in pregnancy

Time	Plasma glucose (mmol/L)	Capillary glucose (mmol/L)
Fasting	<5.0	<5.5
1 h postprandial	<7.1	<8.0
2 h postprandial	<6.1	<7.0

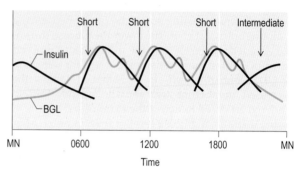

Figure 5.2 Fasting- and meal-related excursions in blood glucose levels in gestational diabetes and the theoretical effect of a basal bolus insulin regimen.

pregnancy outcomes compared to preprandial targets. In some women with mild or well controlled GDM, monitoring need not necessarily be as frequent. Treatment targets are the same as for women with pregestational diabetes (Table 5.3).

Insulin therapy

Lifestyle measures as detailed above can provide adequate control in the majority of cases. When treatment targets are not achieved by dietary means, then insulin is required. A basal/bolus regimen of insulin (short-acting insulin before meals, intermediate-acting insulin before bed) gives the most effective glucose control (Fig. 5.2), and produces better fetal outcomes than a twice daily regime. Unlike women with pre-existing type 1 diabetes, insulin is not necessarily required before every meal. Instead, insulin is given before a particular meal only if monitoring reveals hyperglycemia after that particular meal. The same applies to bedtime intermediate-acting insulin, which is given in response to elevated fasting blood glucose levels.

The required dosage of insulin usually increases gradually over the third trimester of pregnancy. Frequent review and adjustment of the insulin dosage is advisable. In women with marked insulin resistance, substantial doses of insulin, even more than 200 units per day, may be required. Although the woman should be advised regarding appropriate hypoglycemia prevention and management measures, in practice, significant hypoglycemia is uncommon in women with insulin treated GDM.

There are a number of possible reasons for inadequate glycaemic control:

- It may be that the severity of GDM is such that diet alone will be insufficient to accomplish normoglycemia.
- Poor compliance with diet is a common cause of suboptimal control.
- Intercurrent infection, such as a febrile illness or urinary tract infection, should be considered.
- Psychosocial factors are significant and associated with poor glycemic control.
- Exogenous steroids, in particular betamethasone used for fetal lung maturation, are very potent glucocorticoids and usually cause hyperglycemia.

Rather than basing the need for insulin on glycemic parameters alone, some have advocated the combined use of ultrasound assessment of fetal abdominal circumference in combination with blood glucose levels. When the fetal abdominal circumference was < 70th percentile, a higher glucose threshold for initiating insulin therapy did not result in an increase in fetal morbidity or macrosomia. This regimen allowed more women to avoid insulin therapy.

There is controversy regarding the use of oral hypoglycemic agents in the treatment of GDM, As GDM does not develop until later in the pregnancy, it is unlikely that their use would result in fetal malformation. One randomized, controlled trial found no difference in glycemic control and neonatal outcomes between subjects treated with glibenclamide and controls treated with insulin. There is also interest in the use of metformin for the treatment of GDM, and clinical trials are underway. There is growing interest in the potential role of oral agents in GDM, as pharmacologic approaches that enhance insulin sensitivity, at least in theory, are more logical as a therapy than insulin itself. The advantage of oral medication over subcutaneous insulin is obvious. However, until more data regarding their safety is available, insulin, rather than oral hypoglycemic agents should be used in the treatment of GDM.

EVIDENCE THAT TREATMENT OF GESTATIONAL DIABETES IMPROVES PREGNANCY OUTCOMES

The study of Beischer et al (1996) has provided retrospective data that treatment of GDM is of benefit.

In their cohort, there was a perinatal mortality rate of 2.6% in women with 'mild GDM' in the 1970s, when it was untreated, compared to 0.7%, in the 1980s after routine treatment had been introduced. It seems likely that the decreased mortality rate was at least in part a consequence of treatment of GDM, rather than only to other improvements in obstetric outcome. This is suggested by the finding that the perinatal mortality rate of women with mild GDM in the 1970s when it was untreated, was 2.3 times that of women with normal glucose tolerance, but was not different from normal women in the 1980s following the introduction of treatment for GDM.

For many years, there had been reluctance among some practitioners to treat GDM because of the lack of Level 1 evidence that its treatment reduces serious perinatal complications. This should change following the publication of the Australian Carbohydrate Intolerance Study in Pregnant Women in 2005. In this study, 1000 women fulfilling the WHO criteria (1985) for 'glucose intolerance of pregnancy' were randomized to receive either treatment including dietary advice, blood glucose monitoring, and insulin as required, or standard pregnancy care. Women with more severe degrees of carbohydrate intolerance (fasting glucose ≥ 7.8 mmol/L or 2 hour ≥ 11.1 mmol/L were excluded as they satisfied the higher WHO criteria for 'gestational diabetes'. Those receiving standard care were unaware that they had glucose intolerance of pregnancy by WHO criteria, but were informed that they 'did not have GDM'. In the treatment group, there was a 1% incidence of serious perinatal outcomes (death, shoulder dystocia, fracture and nerve palsy) compared to 4% among women provided with standard pregnancy care only (adjusted risk reduction for total adverse events was 0.33 although none individually reached significance). Fewer neonates in the treatment group were large for gestational age, and there was no difference in the incidence of small for gestational age infants. There was no difference in the rate of Cesarean section. Furthermore, treated women scored better on a quality of life scale and lower on a depression questionnaire. This study provides evidence based support for the treatment of GDM, at least by the 1985 WHO criteria.

OBSTETRIC MANAGEMENT

During antenatal care, women with GDM should undergo regular assessments of fetal growth and well-being. There is a higher risk of pre-eclampsia so particular attention should be paid to monitoring of blood pressure and urinalysis.

Fetal monitoring

The aim of monitoring is to avoid stillbirth, to detect evidence of fetal compromise, and to assess efficacy of therapy in terms of fetal growth. Ultrasound gives information about fetal size and amniotic fluid volume. Evidence of macrosomia includes width of the fat layer at certain sites in the baby, abdominal circumference, and amniotic fluid volume. When macrosomia or polyhydramnios is detected in GDM, the inference is that the baby has been exposed to excess nutrient transfer due to maternal hyperglycemia, and is therefore at risk of adverse outcome. Cardiotocography and biophysical profile assessment are used in determining fetal well-being. In some European centers, amniotic fluid insulin estimation has been included in fetal assessment, with high levels indicating fetal compromise.

Timing of delivery

The decision regarding timing and mode of delivery and whether to intervene is difficult and requires assessment of the merits of each case. If there has been a previous adverse outcome, such as stillbirth or severe shoulder dystocia with maternal perineal trauma, the decision is easier as the woman will generally be anxious to avoid any possibility of similar problems and will often desire delivery considerably earlier than term. In cases where fetal monitoring indicates evidence of inadequate glycemic control, the risk to the baby usually justifies intervention earlier than full term, often at 37-39 weeks. Of course if there is an obvious abnormality in the CTG, delivery will be expedited whenever necessary. The presence of comorbid risk factors such as pre-eclampsia, hypertension, bleeding, smoking, previous infertility, multiple pregnancy all influence timing of elective delivery. In the absence of adverse indicators, where the GTT abnormality was mild and insulin was not necessary, it may be possible to allow the pregnancy to continue to term.

During labor, it is prudent to set up an insulin/dextrose infusion for women on large doses of insulin, to ensure glycemic stability. Women on diet therapy alone, or on small doses of insulin, do not require such an infusion for delivery. Postpartum, insulin resistance falls quickly, though may not return to normal levels, and insulin therapy can usually be ceased immediately after delivery of the placenta. Monitoring of the blood glucose, however, should continue for 24 h after resumption of oral intake to confirm that the woman is euglycemic, and that she does not have persistent diabetes.

CONTRACEPTION

After a pregnancy complicated by GDM, family planning is important. First, there is evidence that conversion to permanent diabetes occurs sooner in women who proceed to another pregnancy after GDM. This is not to say that further pregnancy is contraindicated. What is important is that the woman is given all available information to help her make choices that suit her own philosophy. It may be that an increase in the risk of diabetes is enough to lead to a decision to limit the family, or at least to take care with contraception.

Appropriate spacing of pregnancies is also important as it may allow weight control before embarking on another pregnancy. The risk of recurrent GDM is high (at least 70%) but is minimized if ideal body weight is achieved before pregnancy.

In regard to the type of contraception recommended, there is need for caution. One study of Hispanic women in the USA showed that conversion to diabetes after GDM was more frequent in women using progesterone-only contraceptive preparations. Perhaps reasonable advice is to use the progesterone-only pill for the minimum time after GDM pregnancy. There is no serious concern with the modern low dose combined contraceptive pills.

LONG-TERM MATERNAL AND OFFSPRING RISKS OF GESTATIONAL DIABETES

Women who have had GDM are at high risk for the future development of type 2 diabetes. The longest follow-up study has demonstrated a risk of 36% over 25 years. The risk exceeds 50% for many ethnic groups who are predisposed to type 2 diabetes. A meta-analysis has demonstrated that the risk of women with GDM developing type 2 diabetes is six times that of controls. There is a gradation of risk within the population of women with GDM. Those with the highest risk are those who required insulin to achieve control (5-year risk of diabetes exceeds 80%), those with high fasting blood glucose on GTT, those diagnosed before 20 weeks, those with recurrent GDM, and those from the highest risk ethnic groups. For this reason, women who have had GDM should undergo regular screening for diabetes. This will enable early diagnosis and treatment before complications of diabetes develop. Should the woman be planning further pregnancies, early diagnosis of diabetes takes on added importance as it provides the opportunity for optimization of conditions prior to a diabetic pregnancy. Screening is recommended within a couple of months of the GDM pregnancy with a glucose tolerance test, to determine if there is persistent glucose intolerance. Subsequent screening recommendations vary from annually to every 3 years.

It is known that healthy lifestyle measures will reduce the progression to type 2 diabetes among high-risk populations. Women with GDM should therefore be counseled to consume a healthy diet, perform adequate physical activity, and aim for ideal body weight to reduce their risk for the development of diabetes. In addition to diabetes screening, these women should have blood pressure checked at least annually and lipids from time to time, because of the association of GDM with the insulin resistance syndrome and a tendency to atherosclerosis.

In the 21st century, there will be advances in understanding the fetal origins of adult disease. Diabetes in pregnancy was one of the first areas in which this hypothesis was developed. It was shown in animals that diabetes is more prevalent in the offspring of diabetic pregnant mothers, even when the diabetes is induced by surgery or drugs, namely independent of any Mendelian genetic influence. The implication is that if the fetus develops in an abnormal metabolic environment, changes occur in its homeostatic mechanisms and physiology, which may predispose to later diabetes. Of course in the women we have been describing there is often a strong genetic element to the diabetes. The net result of these contributing factors is an increase in the chance of diabetes in the offspring of women with GDM, and it is possible that this is one of the explanations for the apparent explosion in incidence of diabetes in many communities worldwide. Therefore, it is no less important to discuss healthy lifestyle for the children of women with GDM, in the hope, or even expectation, that dietary restraint, exercise and the avoidance of obesity will have beneficial results. Box 5.4 summarizes the key points on gestational diabetes.

Box 5.4 Gestational diabetes

- Gestational diabetes is glucose intolerance first detected in pregnancy, and usually develops late in the second trimester.
- Biochemical screening for GDM is performed with a 50 g glucose challenge.
- An oral glucose tolerance test is required for the diagnosis of GDM.
- GDM is associated with adverse fetal outcomes.
- Women with GDM should undertake self-monitoring of blood glucose levels.
- Most women with GDM can be managed with diet alone, but a proportion will require insulin therapy.
- For the mother, glucose tolerance usually returns to normal postpartum, but there is a substantial risk of future diabetes.

Obesity
I. A. Greer, B. N. J. Walters, C. Nelson–Piercy

INTRODUCTION

Obesity is becoming the most frequent of risk factors in obstetric practice in the developed world and is associated with increased risk of many complications for mother and baby. All who deal with pregnancy have seen the complications of obesity, and their relentless increase over the last 20 years. Indeed, in the UK, 35% of women dying from direct or indirect causes of maternal death were obese. In addition, the number of patients with obesity is growing with rates in young pregnant women doubling in the UK over the last 10-15 years. Obese women may have difficulty in conceiving because of disturbances in ovulation and other factors. However, it is often not appreciated that these women also have a higher rate of miscarriage, and in women treated for anovulatory infertility, those who are obese have around a threefold higher rate of miscarriage. In addition, oocyte donation studies have found that when the recipient had a body mass index >30 kg/m^2, there was a fourfold increased risk of miscarriage. This highlights the need for pre-pregnancy counseling and weight reduction in these women.

FETAL RISK

Women who are obese are also at risk of fetal abnormality. Case control studies have shown a two- to threefold increased risk of spina bifida, omphalocele and heart defects. Pre-conceptional folic acid supplementation is a logical intervention, but, it is noteworthy that the increased risk of neural tube defects in obese women has persisted in populations where flour has been fortified with folic acid. It is important to consider fetal anomaly screening by serum screening and by detailed ultrasound scan, although, this is technically difficult for the sonographer, with overuse injuries now appearing in those who struggle to image the fetus through bulky maternal tissues. In this situation, a transvaginal fetal anomaly scan may be preferable.

There is an increased risk of fetal death in obese women, which increases as gestation advances from around a twofold risk in the latter part of the second trimester to around a fourfold risk after 40 weeks' gestation. This risk appears independent of the specific complications associated with obesity. It may reflect relative placental insufficiency and emphasizes the need for increased fetal surveillance.

PRE-ECLAMPSIA

In later pregnancy, obese women have an increased risk of pre-eclampsia with the risk increasing with body mass index (BMI). Women with a BMI > 30, have around a threefold increased risk of pre-eclampsia, and, thus, should be considered for low dose aspirin prophylaxis. Whether this makes a difference to the incidence of the pre-eclampsia in these women is uncertain. However, as pre-eclampsia has a significant thrombotic component, there is some logic to the use of this agent. As these women are also at increased risk of thromboembolic complications, they may merit prophylactic low molecular weight heparin, and certainly should receive this after Cesarean. There is a three- to four-fold increased risk of gestational diabetes in women who are obese, confirmed in many studies. Again, the risk may be directly related to the level of obesity. The mechanisms underlying these complications reflect not only the metabolic disturbance (with insulin resistance, increased triglycerides and lower HDL cholesterol associated with obesity), but also disturbed microvascular function and a pro-inflammatory phenotype. This metabolic disturbance is already present in obesity and is further exaggerated by pregnancy.

THROMBOSIS

Pregnancy is a well-established risk factor for thrombosis because of increased coagulation, relative venous stasis and pelvic vascular damage at the time of delivery. Thus, all three components of Virchow's triad are present in normal pregnancy and delivery. In the obese patient these effects are all exaggerated. There are few data relating to the risk of VTE and obesity in pregnancy, however, outwith pregnancy an obese woman has almost a threefold increased risk of venous thrombosis. Interestingly, obesity is also a marker for disease progression from deep venous thrombosis to pulmonary embolism with pulmonary embolism being more likely to be associated with DVT in women with significant abdominal obesity.

Every pregnancy should have an assessment for thrombotic risk (see Ch. 8) and significant obesity, itself, must be considered a risk factor. Moreover, the risk of thrombosis in these women rises considerably in the puerperium, notably after Cesarean delivery, but also after vaginal delivery. Many of these women should be considered for low molecular weight heparin and graduated elastic compression stockings, particularly postpartum when the risk will be maximal, but also antenatally for some. It is unclear what the optimal dose of low molecular weight heparin is for prophylaxis in these women and many clinicians will use an intermediate dose rather than the routine prophylactic dose. It is also important to note that dose capping for treatment of deep venous thrombosis should be avoided in these women because of concerns that under-treatment may occur, resulting in extension of the thrombus or recurrent thromboembolic complications which are potentially fatal.

MANAGING OBESITY IN PREGNANCY

In view of these complications, it is important that pre-pregnancy weight loss is encouraged in obese women. However, the clinician must be careful to avoid significant nutritional disturbance in the period leading up to conception and it is best that weight reduction and stabilization of weight occurs before pregnancy is contemplated. Such weight reduction will require significant support from healthcare professionals including dietitians. Ideally, the woman should also receive advice in a program of physical exercise, as diet alone will rarely achieve the desired weight loss.

Increasingly, clinicians are encountering women who are pregnant or considering pregnancy and who have undergone bariatric surgery. There is increasing information on pregnancy in these women. They are at increased risk of internal hernia and small bowel obstruction. In addition, they may have a degree of malabsorption and if so are at risk of anemia, vitamin D deficiency, electrolyte disturbance, intrauterine growth restriction, prematurity and neural tube defects. However, they are at reduced risk of other obesity-related complications, particularly, gestational diabetes. Thus, it is best to delay pregnancy for, at least, a year after bariatric surgery to allow weight and nutritional stabilization. These women should also receive vitamin supplements, before and during the pregnancy, as well as iron supplements. These should be continued postpartum, particularly, if she is breastfeeding.

In summary, in obese women, the emphasis is on pre-pregnancy counseling, weight reduction, nutritional stabilization and vitamin supplementation. During pregnancy, there is a need to screen for fetal abnormality and an awareness of the increased risk of miscarriage. It is also important to monitor maternal and fetal condition for complications such as pre-eclampsia, gestational diabetes and fetal macrosomia which are common in these women. Clinically it is often difficult to estimate fetal growth and it is recommended that assessment of fetal growth by ultrasound scanning should be conducted in women with significant obesity problems. Antenatal weight gain should be minimized. The most reliable way to achieve this is to refer the patient to a dietitian as these women invariably need significant individualized changes in dietary habits. Casual informal advice from a medical practitioner is rarely effective, and a sense of urgency in dealing with the life-threatening problem of obesity should be transmitted to the woman. This is the only way to initiate the psychological determination required to launch the necessary process of behavioral change.

Planning delivery is important in these women. The babies are often macrosomic whether or not there is coexistent gestational diabetes. Indeed, the odds ratio for a macrosomic baby is over two when the BMI exceeds 30 kg/m^2. Shoulder dystocia is also common in obese women, but obesity is not an independent risk factor for shoulder dystocia in contrast to macrosomia. Thus, it is the macrosomia rather than the maternal obesity that is the main factor. Obese women are also at increased risk of dysfunctional labor and have a higher risk of cephalopelvic disproportion, possibly because of fat deposition in the pelvic tissue as well as the larger size of the baby. Because of the increased risk of maternal and fetal complications and problems in labor, the rate of emergency Cesarean section is significantly higher in these women and the primary Cesarean section rate is around 50% for morbidly obese (BMI > 40) patients. These are not Cesarean sections to be taken lightly and performed by junior staff, particularly without supervision, late at night or in emergency situations. Rather, it is impor-

tant to carefully consider the timing and mode of delivery and ensure that experienced personnel are present. As these women are at increased risk of infection and thromboembolism, prophylactic antibiotics and low molecular weight heparin are required. In the obese woman with a previous Cesarean section, successful vaginal delivery may occur in < 15%. Furthermore, vaginal birth after Cesarean section in these women is associated with higher rates of chorioamnionitis, endometritis and puerperal sepsis with no cost saving. Indeed, it has been shown that vaginal birth after Cesarean section is only cost effective if there is a success rate of 40% or more for vaginal delivery. Thus, in the obese woman with a previous Cesarean section, a repeat Cesarean section is usually warranted and, indeed, preferable. Given all these hazards and difficulties, before the second Cesarean is performed it is necessary for the obstetrician to advise the woman that a further pregnancy carries great risks. The woman will be older, often more obese (unfortunately, the prognosis for weight loss is poor with present treatment) and with more likelihood of medical problems, in addition to the major risks of a third Cesarean. For all these reasons, intraoperative sterilization should be considered, and if declined, the matter should again be raised postpartum, in the context of a discussion about reliable long-term contraception. If these steps are not taken, the woman faces considerable medical and surgical risks during the next parlous pregnancy and Cesarean section. The operative risks including placenta accreta and hysterectomy are now well recognized, and prohibitive, particularly for these complex high-risk patients.

When planning delivery, an anesthetic review is critical. These women often pose difficult problems not just for general anesthesia with difficulty in intubation, but, also for neuraxial anesthesia and, thus, the anesthetist must be involved early. Following delivery, there is an increased risk of postpartum hemorrhage, genital infection, urinary tract infection and wound infection.

When all these issues are taken together, it is not surprising that obese women with a body mass index > 30 kg/m^2 spend, on average, between 4-5 more days in hospital during pregnancy. The increased hospital stay along with increased complications and interventions has been shown to add to the cost of antenatal care which may be as much as fivefold higher in these women. There are also implications for neonatal care as there is a substantially higher risk of admission to the neonatal intensive care unit (NICU) in the babies of women who are obese.

There is also an association between obesity and a reduced chance of success at breastfeeding. The reason behind this is not clear. There are often psychosocial disturbances, physical impediments to feeding such as attachment problems, or endocrine factors relating perhaps to disturbances in the hypothalamopituitary ovarian axis. An obese woman is likely, therefore, to need extra support for breastfeeding.

CONCLUSION

Obesity of itself, independent of associated co-morbid conditions such as essential hypertension or diabetes, poses significant challenges for obstetric physicians, obstetricians, anesthetists and neonatologists. Primary prevention will require significant dietary and lifestyle modifications pre-pregnancy. Obese women should be informed of their increased risks preferably prior to pregnancy so that the problem may first be acknowledged by the patient and then approached in an objective, problem directed manner by doctor and patient together, in an attempt to improve pregnancy outcome. In pregnancy, the opportunity for secondary prevention is modest, focusing on appropriate ante-natal care, low dose aspirin, vitamin and iron supple-ments. These women also require careful planning of the timing and mode of delivery with a higher rate of labor and caesarean complications putting both mother and baby at risk.

Further reading

Alexander E K, Marqusee E, Lawrence J et al 2004 Timing and magnitude of increases in levothyroxine requirements during pregnancy in women with hypothyroidism. New England Journal of Medicine 351:241-249

Ambrosi B, Barbetta L, Morricone, L 2003 Diagnosis and management of Addison's disease during pregnancy. Journal of Endocrinological Investigation 26(7):698-702

Andersen S et al 2003 Biologic variation is important for interpretation of thyroid function tests. Thyroid 13:1069-1078

Beischer N A et al 1996 Identification and treatment of women with hyperglycaemia diagnosed during pregnancy can significantly reduce perinatal mortality rates. Australian New Zealand Journal of Obstetrics Gynaecology 36:239-247

Biesenbach G, Stoger H, Zazgornik J 1992 Influence of pregnancy on progression of diabetic nephropathy and subsequent requirement of renal replacement therapy in female type I diabetic patients with impaired renal function. Nephrology, Dialysis, Transplantation 7(2):105-109

Bravo E L, Tagle R 2003 Pheochromocytoma: state-of-the-art and future prospects. Endocrine Reviews 24(4):539-553

Bronstein M D, Salgado L R, de Castro Musolino N R 2002 Medical management of pituitary adenomas: the special case of management of the pregnant woman. Pituitary 5(2):99-107

Bruinse H W, Vermeulen-Meiners C, Wit J M 1988 Fetal treatment for thyrotoxicosis in non-thyrotoxic pregnant women. Fetal Therapy 3:152-157

Buchanan T A et al 1990 Insulin sensitivity and B-cell responsiveness to glucose during late pregnancy in lean and moderately obese women with normal glucose tolerance or mild gestational diabetes. American Journal of Obstetrics and Gynecology 162:1008-1014

Callaway L K et al 2006 The prevalence and impact of overweight and obesity in an Australian obstetric population. Medical Journal of Australia 184(2):56-59

Caturegli P et al 2005 Autoimmune hypophysitis. Endocrine Reviews 26(5):599-614

Cheung N W, Byth K 2003 The population health significance of gestational diabetes. Diabetes Care 26:2005-2009

Chew E Y et al 1995 Metabolic control and progression of retinopathy: The Diabetes in Early Pregnancy Study. Diabetes Care 18:631-637

Chopra I J, Baber K 2003 Treatment of primary hypothyroidism during pregnancy: is there an increase in thyroxine dose requirement in pregnancy? Metabolism: Clinical and Experimental 52:122-128

Clausen T D et al 2005 Poor pregnancy outcome in women with type 2 diabetes. Diabetes Care 28:323-328

Crowther C A et al 2005 Effect of treatment of gestational diabetes on pregnancy outcomes. New England Journal of Medicine 352:2477-2486

de Veciana M et al 1995 Postprandial versus preprandial blood glucose monitoring in women with gestational diabetes mellitus requiring insulin therapy. New England Journal of Medicine 339(19):1237-1241

Durr J A, Lindheimer M D 1996 Diagnosis and management of diabetes insipidus during pregnancy. Endocrine Practice 2(5):353-361

Freinkel N 1980 Of Pregnancy and progeny. Diabetes 29:1023-1035

Garner P R 1993 Disorders of the adrenal cortex in pregnancy. Current Obstetric Medicine 2:183-220

Glinoer D et al 1994 Risk of subclinical hypothyroidism in pregnant women with asymptomatic autoimmune thyroid disorders. Journal of Clinical Endocrinology and Metabolism 79:197-204

Goodwin T M et al 1992 The role of chorionic gonadotropin in transient hyperthyroidism of hyperemesis gravidarum. Journal of Clinical Endocrinology and Metabolism 75(5):1333-1337

Herman-Bonert V, Seliverstov M, Melmed S 1998 Pregnancy in acromegaly: successful therapeutic outcome. Journal of Clinical Endocrinology and Metabolism 83(3):727-731

Hibbard J U et al 2006 National Institute of Child Health and Human Development Maternal-Fetal Medicine Units Network. Trial of labor or repeat cesarean delivery in women with morbid obesity and previous cesarean delivery. Obstetrics and Gynecology 108(1):125-133

Hoepffner, W., et al 2004 Pregnancies in patients with congenital adrenal hyperplasia with complete or almost complete impairment of 21-hydroxylase activity. Fertility and Sterility 81(5):1314-1321

Ip P 2003 Neonatal convulsion revealing maternal hyperparathyroidism: an unusual case of late neonatal hypoparathyroidism. Archives of Gynecology and Obstetrics 268(3):227-229

Jovanovic L et al 2005 Elevated pregnancy losses at high and low extremes of maternal glucose in early normal and diabetic pregnancy. Diabetes Care 28:1113-1117

Kanagalingam M G et al 2005 Changes in booking body mass index over a decade: retrospective analysis from a Glasgow Maternity Hospital. BJOG 112(10):1431-1433

Kalantaridou S N et al 2004 Reproductive functions of corticotropin-releasing hormone. Research and potential clinical utility of antalarmins (CRH receptor type 1 antagonists). American Journal of Reproductive Immunology 51(4):269-274

Kalantaridou S N et al 2004 Stress and the female reproductive system. Journal of Reproductive Immunology 62(1-2):61-68

Kjos S, Buchanan T 1999 Gestational diabetes mellitus. New England Journal of Medicine 341(23):1749-1754

Krege J, Katz V L, Bowes Jr W A 1989 Transient diabetes insipidus of pregnancy. Obstetrical Gynecological Survey 44(11):789-795

Langer O et al 2000 A comparison of glyburide and insulin in women with gestational diabetes mellitus. New England Journal Medicine 343(16):1134-1138

Lao T T 2005 Thyroid disorders in pregnancy. Current Opinion in Obstetrics & Gynecology 17(2):123-127

Lao T T H et al 1986 Transient hyperthyroidism in hyperemesis gravidarum. Journal of the Royal Society of Medicine 79:613-615

Lao T T H et al 1990 Maternal thyroid hormones and outcome of pre-eclamptic pregnancies. British Journal of Obstetrics and Gynaecology 97:71-74

Leung A S et al 1993 Perinatal outcome in hypothyroid pregnancies. Obstetrics and Gynecology 81:349-353

Lindsay J R, Nieman L K 2005 The hypothalamic-pituitary-adrenal axis in pregnancy: Challenges in disease detection and treatment. Endocrine Reviews 26(6):775-799

McElduff A et al 2005 Pregestational diabetes and pregnancy: an Australian experience. Diabetes Care 28:1260-1261

Mills J L et al 1988 Incidence of spontaneous abortion among normal women and insulin-dependent diabetic women whose pregnancies were identified within 21 days of conception. New England Journal of Medicine 319:1617-1623

Molitch M 1992 Endocrine emergencies in pregnancy. Baillière's Clinics in Endocrinology and Metabolism 6:167-191

Nachum Z et al 1999 Twice daily insulin versus four times daily insulin dose regimens for diabetes in pregnancy: randomised controlled trial. BMJ 319:1223-1227

O'Sullivan J B 1991 Diabetes mellitus after GDM. Diabetes 29(2):131-135

O'Sullivan J B, Mahan C B 1964 Criteria for the oral glucose tolerance test in pregnancy. Diabetes 13:278-285

Pettit D J et al 1988 Congenital susceptibility to NIDDM: role of intrauterine environment. Diabetes 37(5):622-628

Pickard J et al 1990 Cushing's syndrome in pregnancy. Obstetrical & Gynecological Survey 45(2):87-93

Pop V J et al 2003 Maternal hypothyroxinaemia during early pregnancy and subsequent child development: a 3-year follow-up study. Clinical Endocrinology 59:282-288

Prentice A 2000 Maternal calcium metabolism and bone mineral status. American Journal of Clinical Nutrition 71(5 suppl):1312S-1316S

Ray J G, O'Brien T E, Chan W S 2001 Preconception care and the risk of congenital anomalies in the offspring of women with diabetes mellitus: a meta-analysis. Quarterly Journal of Medicine 94:435-444

Reece E A, Homko C J 2000 Why do diabetic women deliver malformed infants? Clinical Obstetrics and Gynecology 43(1):32-45

Saravanakumar K, Rao S G, Cooper G M 2006 Obesity and obstetric anaesthesia. Anaesthesia 61(1):36-48

Sermer M et al 1995 Impact of increasing carbohydrate intolerance on maternal-fetal outcomes in 3637 women without gestational diabetes. American Journal of Obstetrics of Gynecology 173(1):146-151

Shah M S, Davies T F, Stagnaro-Green A 2003 The thyroid during pregnancy: a physiological and pathological stress test. Minerva Endocrinologica 28:233-245

Sherwood O D 2004 Relaxin's physiological roles and other diverse actions. Endocrine Reviews 25(2):205-234

Silverman B L et al 1995 Impaired glucose tolerance in adolescent offspring of diabetic mothers. Diabetes Care 18:611-617

Simmons D et al 2004 Metformin therapy and diabetes in pregnancy. Medical Journal of Australia 180(9):462-464

Swaminathan R et al 1989 Thyroid function in hypermesis gravidarum. Acta Endocrinologica 120:155-160

Taylor R et al 2002 Clinical outcomes of pregnancy in women with type 1 diabetes. Obstetrics and Gynecology 99:537-541

Thakker R V 2004 Diseases associated with the extracellular calcium-sensing receptor. Cell Calcium 35(3):275-282

Towner D et al 1995 Congenital malformations in pregnancies complicated by NIDDM: Increased risk from poor metabolic control but not from exposure to sulfonylurea drugs. Diabetes Care 18:1446-1451

Vohr B R, McGarvey S T, Tucker R 1999 Effects of maternal gestational diabetes on offspring adiposity at 4-7 years of age. Diabetes Care 22(8):1284-1291

Chapter 6

Pulmonary disease in pregnancy

R. Powrie

PHYSIOLOGIC CHANGES IN THE RESPIRATORY SYSTEM IN PREGNANCY

Pregnancy is associated with several significant adaptations in maternal respiratory function. Minute ventilation – the volume of gas exchanged over 1 minute – increases by nearly 50% in pregnancy. This is achieved in pregnancy not by increasing the respiratory rate but by increasing the volume of each breath. This increased 'depth' of breathing is an effect of the increased progesterone levels that occur in pregnancy. It causes several important changes in maternal arterial blood gases. The increased ventilation leads to a drop in the normal arterial $PaCO_2$ to 27-32 mmHg. The normal PaO_2 is increased to 95-105 mmHg at sea level. A compensatory renal excretion of bicarbonate occurs in response to the respiratory alkalosis caused by this relative hypocapnia and serum bicarbonate thereby decreases by 4 mEq/L.

Pulmonary function testing and peak expiratory flow rates (PEFR) remain largely unchanged in pregnancy. The main difference is a 20% drop in functional residual capacity (FRC – that portion of a breath that can still be exhaled after normal resting exhalation) due to a decrease in both expiratory reserve volume and residual volume. Although the diaphragm will rise 4 cm above its usual position by the end of gestation this does not have a significant effect on respiratory function as diaphragmatic excursion is not altered.

BREATHLESSNESS OF PREGNANCY

General

Up to 70% of pregnant women will report some level of dyspnea with 5% of women reporting dyspnea with minimal exertion at term. Therefore, the presence of breathlessness in pregnancy does not necessarily indicate cardiorespiratory disease. The most typical description of the 'normal' dyspnea in pregnancy would be 'air hunger' or the feeling that one 'cannot get a deep enough breath'. Patients often report having to pause intermittently while talking to 'catch a deep breath'. Often the breathlessness occurs spontaneously at rest and not in association with exertion. Dyspnea of pregnancy can start during the late first or early second trimester but typically begins between 28 and 31 weeks. The etiology of dyspnea of pregnancy remains unclear although the hormonal effect of progesterone on ventilation and the associated fall in arterial carbon dioxide tension appear to be contributory. It does not appear to be explained by increases in abdominal girth or alterations in diaphragmatic location or function. Some studies have suggested that the presence of dyspnea during pregnancy appears to correlate with a low $PaCO_2$ and that the women most likely to experience it are those with a relatively high baseline non-pregnant $PaCO_2$.

Management

Differentiating the normal dyspnea of pregnancy from the more serious causes such as pulmonary embolism, asthma or cardiomyopathy can be challenging. Some helpful clinical clues based less on evidence and more on a cumulative clinical experience would suggest that dyspnea attributable to pregnancy is generally insidious in onset and should not be associated with any chest discomfort, cough or sudden exacerbation. The ready availability of pulse oximeters makes the measurement of arterial oxygen saturation a useful way to help rule out serious causes of dyspnea in pregnancy. If the oxygen saturation remains normal (> 95%) with moderate exertion (fast walking or climbing a flight of stairs), it is unlikely (although not impossible) that the patient has a major problem. Demonstrating to the patient that oxygenation is maintained despite the feeling of dyspnea can also help alleviate a patient's anxiety about her symptoms.

Asthma is suggested by the presence of cough, wheezing or environmental triggers and this diagnosis can usually be confirmed by a trial of bronchodilators and pulmonary function testing. Pulmonary embolism is suggested by the sudden onset of dyspnea or chest pain and is often accompanied by the presence of tachycardia, tachypnea and/or additional thromboembolic risk factors such as a family history of venous thromboembolism. Cardiac causes are suggested by features such as orthopnea, paroxysmal nocturnal dyspnea, tachypnea, tachycardia, an elevated jugular venous pulse, a concerning murmur and respiratory crackles on auscultation. When any of these features are present a chest X-ray and electrocardiogram (ECG) can be very helpful in looking for evidence of a cardiac cause. Evidence of a cardiac cause should be further evaluated with transthoracic echocardiography.

All relevant diagnostic imaging procedures for investigating other causes of dyspnea can be performed safely during pregnancy.

ASTHMA

General

Asthma is a chronic inflammatory disease of the airways with episodic reversible airway narrowing due to airway hyper-responsiveness that is characterized clinically by coughing, wheezing and shortness of breath. Asthma presently affects at least 4% of pregnant women and is therefore one of the most common potentially life-threatening medical disorders to complicate pregnancy.

Maternal risks

Present data with respect to the effect of pregnancy on the course of asthma are limited and poor. The most robust study indicated that bronchial hyper-responsiveness to methacholine decreased between preconception and pregnancy in 69% of the women, although it deteriorated in 31% of the women. Further, this improvement peaked in the second trimester, reverted after delivery and was greatest among those women who were most hyper-responsive initially.

When women with asthma do deteriorate in pregnancy, the usual reason is the mistaken belief on the part of patients or their healthcare providers that treatment for asthma is harmful to the fetus. The 2004 National Institute of Health (NIH) Working Group report on managing asthma during pregnancy emphasizes that inadequate control of asthma is a greater risk to the fetus and mother than asthma medications and that proper control of asthma should enable a woman with asthma to expect a normal pregnancy with little or no risk to her or her fetus. Pregnancy-related gastroesophageal reflux disease and postnasal drip from 'pregnancy rhinitis' (seen in up to 30% of pregnant women) may also cause some women's asthma to worsen in pregnancy. These common pregnancy-related complaints should be treated when asthma control worsens.

Fetal risks

In general, well-controlled asthma is not associated with a higher risk of adverse pregnancy outcomes. A recently published well-designed, multicenter, prospective, observational cohort study in the United States suggested that there were very few significant differences in neonatal or maternal outcomes between women with asthma and those without it. Therefore, asthma should in no way be considered a contraindication to pregnancy.

Maternal asthma does double the risk of asthma being diagnosed in her offspring, although paternal factors appear to be equally important, as is the presence of eczema, allergic rhinitis, early exposure to environmental antigens and smoking.

Pre-pregnancy care

Women with asthma considering a pregnancy can be reassured that pregnancy is usually well tolerated if asthma is well controlled and that the vast majority of pregnant women with asthma can expect a good pregnancy outcome. Ideally, asthma care should be optimized prior to conception. Patients should receive education about how to monitor and control their disease as described below. Women should be specifically told not to stop or decrease their asthma medications when they find out they are pregnant and that medication use and a strong therapeutic relationship with a trained team of healthcare professionals ensures the best possible outcome for both mother and child.

Antenatal care

Asthma management: general principles

Present asthma management strategies focus on treating the airway inflammation that leads to symptoms by avoiding triggers and using inhaled corticosteroids. While the use of short-acting bronchodilators is still a part of asthma care, it is now perceived as a way of obtaining short-term symptomatic relief rather than disease control. The goal of therapy is to achieve (1) minimal or no chronic symptoms during the day or night, (2) minimal use of short-acting bronchodilators, (3) minimal or no exacerbations, (4) no limitations on activities and (5) minimal or no adverse effects from medications. Most agents commonly used to treat asthma can be safely used during pregnancy with a few exceptions to be discussed below. Whenever possible, treatment should be by inhalation rather than oral agents, since this reduces systemic effects. It also reduces any possible effects on the fetus.

Asthma management: prevention and patient education

The likelihood of successful pharmacologic management of asthma is greatly increased by an intensive effort on the part of healthcare providers to make sure the woman is well educated about her disease. This education may be most effective if initiated prior to pregnancy. Key concepts emphasized by present clinical guidelines are as follows:

1. Patients should be taught to measure peak etpiratory flow rate (PEF) twice daily to allow early detection of deterioration in pulmonary function before they become symptomatic. PEF is best measured upon awakening and approximately 12 hours later. PEFs can be especially helpful to pregnant women with asthma in determining if their dyspnea is due to breathlessness of pregnancy or an exacerbation of asthma. In general the patient should be told to interpret her status on the basis of its variance from her previous personal best PEF. Normal PEF can be found in age- and height-based normograms. (A typical 'normal' PEF for a 25-year-old non-pregnant 163-cm woman would be 540 L/minute.)

2. Patients should have their inhaler technique reviewed regularly. Correct use includes using a spacer to improve delivery of any aerosolized medication to the lungs, help avoid local side effects of inhaled steroids (such as oral thrush) and decrease unnecessary systemic absorption of medication through the buccal mucosa. Patients should be told to rinse out their mouths after use of inhaled steroids to further decrease the risk of oral thrush.

3. Patients should be given a written asthma management plan that directs the patient in adjusting their medication according to their PEF and provides clear guidance on when to seek medical advice. Typical action plans would tell a patient to 'step-up' therapy for transient PEF drops of 20% and that sustained drops should prompt review by a doctor. A sustained PEF drop > 50% from the previous personal best warrants either an urgent call to the doctor or a trip to the emergency room.

4. Patients should be taught to avoid triggers. This advice includes the use of impermeable pillow and mattress covers to minimize contact with dust mites, removal of pets from home (or at least the bedroom), removal of carpets in bedroom and avoidance of cigarette smoke.

5. Smoking cessation should be particularly addressed as this has been shown to have benefits in pregnancy even in patients without asthma. Adverse effects of smoking in pregnancy are extensive and discussed later in this chapter.

6. Patients should be informed clearly of present evidence that well-controlled asthma does not appear to increase pregnancy risk, while poorly controlled asthma may do so. This information may help enhance compliance and

alleviate patients' fears about medication use in pregnancy.

Asthma management: specific asthma medications

Asthma medications are classified as either 'rescue/ reliever agents' or 'maintenance/preventer agents'. 'Rescue/reliever agents' (short-acting inhaled beta-agonists) are medications that are used to treat acute bronchospasm. They provide symptomatic relief but do not treat the underlying inflammation. 'Maintenance/preventer agents' are medications that treat the underlying inflammation and thereby the hyper-reactivity, of the airway. The data regarding the effectiveness and safety in pregnancy of the commonly used rescue/reliever and maintenance/preventer agents are reviewed in Table 6.1.

Asthma management: daily asthma management with stepwise plan

The US National Asthma Education and Prevention Program and the British Thoracic Society both recommend that asthma be managed in a 'stepwise' manner. Adjustments in medication should be made either 'upwards' or 'downwards' in intensity in response to the severity of the individual patient's asthma at that particular point in time. Figure 6.1 reviews the criteria for classification of asthma into four separate classes of severity and summarizes the treatment recommended during pregnancy for each classification.

Once control has been established and is maintained for several months, the treatment regimen should be 'stepped-down' to the next lower level of asthma severity. However, if asthma fails to be controlled or worsens, 'stepping-up' a treatment level is

Table 6.1 Summary of pregnancy and breastfeeding data about medications commonly used to treat asthma. Adapted from Powrie (2001).

Class	Pregnancy effects	Breastfeeding
Short-acting inhaled beta 2 adrenergic agonists (e.g. albuterol/salbutamol, levalbuterol, bitolterol, pirbuterol, metaproelenol)	Published experience with these drugs in animals and humans suggests that beta-sympathomimetics do not increase the risk of congenital anomalies. Albuterol/salbutamol is the most studied of these agents in pregnancy. Metaproterenol is the second most studied.	Inhaled beta-agonists when used in pharmacologic doses are unlikely to be transferred to any significant degree to the neonate via breast milk
Long-acting inhaled beta 2 adrenergic agonists (e.g. salmeterol, formoterol)	Animal data about intravenously administered salmeterol have not been reassuring but this agent is still felt likely to be safe in humans when administered by inhalation. However, no human data about this agent have been published at this point and therefore the use of this agent should be reserved for women in whom inhaled steroids alone have failed. Formoterol has very limited human pregnancy data but animal data have been reassuring.	There are no data regarding breastfeeding and salmeterol. The manufacturer states that milk levels are likely to be low because plasma levels are low. It is generally accepted that, if indicated, the maternal benefits of salmeterol justify its use in breastfeeding mothers.
Inhaled anticholinergic (e.g. Ipratropium)	There are reassuring animal studies about ipratropium use in pregnancy but no published human pregnancy data. This agent is poorly absorbed by the bronchial mucosa so fetal exposure is likely to be minimal.	Given its structure, ipratropium is unlikely to be excreted into breast milk at more than exceedingly small doses and it is also unlikely that there is significant gastrointestinal

Table 6.1 *Continued*

Class	Pregnancy effects	Breastfeeding
	Efficacy in acute asthma attack presenting to the emergency room makes its short-term use seem justifiable. It has no role in the management of asthma except for acute exacerbations.	absorption in the infant. It is generally felt therefore that the use of ipratroprium when indicated in breastfeeding mothers is justifiable.
Inhaled corticosteroids (e.g. beclometasone dipropionate, triamcinolone acetonide, fluticasone propionate, budesonide, flunisolide, mometasone furoate)	Inhaled corticosteroids are the most important pharmacologic agents in maintaining asthma control in and out of pregnancy. Only 4% of 257 patients taking inhaled glucocorticoids from the start of pregnancy had acute attacks of asthma during pregnancy by contrast with 17% of 177 patients who were not. Although the specific data vary from agent to agent, they are considered generally safe for use in pregnancy. Beclometasone and budesonide are the most widely studied of the inhaled corticosteroids in pregnancy and should be considered the preferred inhaled steroids in pregnancy. Relatively little of these agents is absorbed and human data have not suggested any teratogenic effects of these agents. Triamcinolone is the next most studied inhaled steroid in pregnancy with limited experience suggesting no adverse pregnancy effects. Fluticasone, mometasone furoate and flunisolide have not been studied in human pregnancies, however minimal systemic absorption and the safety of the other steroids in pregnancy make their use in pregnancy generally felt to be justifiable.	Because of the minimal plasma levels in mothers, inhaled corticosteroids are unlikely to produce clinically significant levels in breastfeeding infants and are generally felt to be 'safe' to use with breastfeeding.
Mast cell stabilizers (e. g. disodium cromoglicate (cromolyn), sodium nedocromil)	Human and animal data suggest that these agents are not teratogens. These agents are virtually not absorbed at all through mucosal surfaces and the swallowed portion is largely excreted in the feces. Fetal exposure can be deemed to be minimal. Unfortunately, these agents are not particularly effective and are therefore best reserved for mild cases of asthma in which there has been a decision not to use inhaled steroids for some reason. Cromolyn has been better evaluated in human pregnancy	No harmful effects of cromolyn on breastfeeding infants have been reported but there are few data. The pharmacologic properties of cromolyn suggest that there should be extremely low penetrance of this agent into breast milk. Subsequent gastrointestinal absorption of any cromolyn present in breast milk would likewise be minimal.

Table 6.1 *Continued*

Class	Pregnancy effects	Breastfeeding
	than nedocromil and should be considered the preferred agent of this class.	
Leukotriene antagonists (e.g. zafirlukast, montelukast, zileuton)	The leukotriene antagonists represent an important exception to the general rule that asthma treatment is largely unchanged in pregnancy. Zafirlukast and montelukast both have favorable animal data but data about their safety in human pregnancy are extremely limited at this point. The use of zafirlukast and montelukast should therefore be limited in pregnancy to those unusual cases in which asthma control was not obtainable through the use of other agents. In most cases, leukotriene inhibitors will not add significantly to asthma control already obtained with inhaled corticosteroids. Zileuton should not be used in pregnancy because of concerning animal data.	The manufacturer recommends against the use of all of these agents in breastfeeding. Zafirlukast is found in breast milk at levels approaching 20% of maternal serum levels but its absorption when taken with food is generally poor and therefore the infant is unlikely to absorb significant levels from breast milk. Montelukast and zileuton levels in breast milk appear not to have been studied to date.
Sustained-release methylxanthines (e.g. theophylline)	Theophylline and its intravenous form aminophylline do not appear to be human teratogens. The safety of theophylline therapy in the second and third trimester has been demonstrated in a large cohort of 212 gravidas in Finland. Physicians prescribing theophylline in pregnancy should be aware that the clearance of theophylline is increased in pregnancy in a rather variable way. Any patient who is taking more than 700 mg of theophylline per day should have blood measurements made for optimal dosing. The present role of these agents in treating asthma is generally felt to be as a second- or third-line agent and these agents do not appear to be of benefit in an acute exacerbation. A randomized control trial has demonstrated that theophylline is not more effective and is less well tolerated than inhaled corticosteroids in the management of chronic asthma in pregnancy.	The American Academy of Pediatrics considers theophylline to be compatible with breastfeeding but does note that it may cause irritability in the infant.
Systemic steroids (e.g. oral: prednisone; intravenous: methylprednisolone, hydrocortisone)	Most data suggest that systemic steroids do not present a significant teratogenic risk in human pregnancy. In doses equivalent to prednisone 25 mg per day,	The American Academy of Pediatrics considers prednisone and methylprednisolone to be compatible with breastfeeding.

Table 6.1 *Continued*

Class	Pregnancy effects	Breastfeeding
	they do not cross the placenta because of placental metabolism (the same is not true for betamethasone or dexamethasone). Even in higher doses, the effect of hydrocortisone or prednisone on the fetus in terms of suppression of the hypothalamus-pituitary-adrenal axis is minimal. However, a recent case-control study found a significant association with first trimester use of corticosteroids and oral clefts (OR=6.55, 95% CI=1.44-29.76). However, even if this association is real, the importance of controlling a life-threatening disease makes steroid use in the first trimester readily justifiable. Women should be screened for corticosteroid-related hyperglycemia.	The use of other systemic steroids in breastfeeding mothers is also generally felt likely to be justifiable.
Immunotherapy (e.g. administering of gradually increasing quantities of an allergen extract to an allergic subject to down-regulate response.)	Human data from small trials suggest the safety of continuing immunotherapy in pregnancy. Traditional practice has been to avoid the initiation or escalation of immunotherapy in pregnancy because of fear of provoking anaphylaxis. However, There is no reason to believe that immunotherapy cannot be safely escalated or initiated during pregnancy.	Immunotherapy, although not specifically studied for safety during breastfeeding, is not felt to be contraindicated during breastfeeding.

then advisable. A rescue course of 3-10 days of 40-60 mg of oral prednisone may be used at any time in any class of severity to gain control from a prolonged or severe exacerbation. This may be particularly helpful in the setting of an upper respiratory tract infection (URTI)-related exacerbation. Gastroesophageal reflux disease, vasomotor rhinitis of pregnancy and non-compliance should also always be considered as possible contributing factors when asthma is difficult to control during pregnancy.

Asthma management: treatment of an acute asthma exacerbation

Patients with worsening asthma at home should be instructed to assess their severity and begin initial treatment as outlined in Figure 6.2. Patients whose distress is severe and non-responsive to initial home management should proceed to the emergency department. Treatment in the emergency department and subsequent hospital-based care is reviewed in Figure 6.3. On this flow chart, it is suggested that patients who have an 'incomplete' (but not 'poor') response to initial treatment have an individualized decision made regarding whether they can go home or should be admitted to hospital. In cases of doubt, clinicians should err on the side of admitting patients since patients with asthma can deteriorate very quickly. General guidelines for admission to hospital include a sustained drop in PEFR to less than 50% of baseline, a $PaO_2 < 70$ at sea level, a $PaCO_2 > 35$, a heart rate of > 120/minute or a respiratory rate > 22/minute. It is important to remember that a $PaCO_2$ > 40 mmHg in a pregnant women with an asthmatic exacerbation suggests impending respiratory failure as the normal $PaCO_2$ in pregnancy is 32-34 mmHg. Most experts also feel that maternal PaO_2 should be maintained at > 95% to ensure fetal well-being and

Classify severity: Clinical features before treatment or adequate control			Medications required to maintain long-term control
	Symptoms/day Symptoms/night	PEF or FEV, PEF variability	Daily medications

Step 4
Severe persistent
	Continual
	Frequent
		≤60%
		>30%
			• Preferred treatment:
			  – High dose inhaled corticosteroid*
			  and
			  – Long-acting inhaled beta-agonist
			  and, if needed,
			  – Corticosteroid tablets or syrup long term (2 mg/kg per day, generally not to exceed 60 mg per day). (Make repeat attempts to reduce systemic corticosteroid and maintain control with high-dose inhaled corticosteroid.*)
			
			• Alternative treatment:
			  – High dose inhaled corticosteroid.*
			  and
			  – Sustained release theophylline to serum concentration of 5–12 mcg/mL.

Step 3
Moderate persistent
	Daily
	>1 night/week
		>60% – <80%
		>30%
			• Preferred treatment:
			  Either
			  – Low dose inhaled corticosteroid* and long-acting inhaled beta-agonist
			  or
			  – Medium dose inhaled corticosteroid.*
			  If needed (particularly in patients with recurring severe exacerbations):
			  – Medium dose inhaled corticosteroid* and long-acting inhaled beta-agonist
			
			• Alternative treatment:
			  – Low dose inhaled corticosteroid* and either theophylline or leukotriene receptor antagonist.†
			  If needed:
			  – Medium dose inhaled corticosteroid* and either theophylline or leukotriene receptor antagonist.†

Step 2 Mild persistent	>2 days/week but <daily >2 nights/month	≥80% 20–30%	• Preferred treatment: – Low dose inhaled corticosteroid.* • Alternative treatment (listed alphabetically): cromolyn, leukotriene receptor, antagonist† or sustained release theophylliac to scrum concentration of 5–12 mcg/mL.
Step 1 Mild intermittent	≤2 days/week ≤2 nights/month	≥80% <20%	• No daily medication needed. • Severe exacerbations may occur, seperated by long periods of normal function and no symptoms. A course of systemic corticosteroid is recommended.
Quick relief All patients			• Short-acting bronchodilator: 2–4 puffs short-acting inhaled beta₂-agonist‡ as needed for symptoms. • Intensity of treatment will depend on severity of exacerbation: up to three treatments at 20-min intervals or a single nebulizer treatment as needed. Course of systemic corticosteroid may be needed. • Use of short-acting inhaled beta₂-agonist‡ >2 times a week in intermittent asthma (daily, or increasing use in persistent asthma) may indicate the need to initiate (increase) long-term control therapy.

Step down
Review treatment every 1–6 months; a gradual stepwise reduction in treatment may be possible.

Step up
If control is not maintained, consider step up. First, review patient medication technique, adherence, and environmental control.

Goals of therapy: Asthma control

- Minimal or no chronic symptoms day or night
- Minimal or no exacerbations
- No limitations on activities; no school/work missed
- Maintain (near) normal pulmonary function
- Minimal use of short-acting inhaled beta-agonist‡
- Minimal or no adverse effects from medications

Notes:

- The stepwise approach is meant to assist, not replace, the clinical decision making required to meet individual patient needs.
- Classify severity: assign patient to most severe step in which any feature occurs (PEF is percent of personal best; FEV is percent predicted).
- Gain control as quickly as possible (consider a short course of systematic corticosteroid), then step down to the least medication necessary to maintain control.
- Minimize use of short-acting inhaled beta-agonist‡ (e.g. use of approximately one canister a month even if not using it every day indicates inadequate control of asthma and the need to initiate or intensify long-term control therapy.
- Provide education on self-management and controlling environmental factors that make asthma worse (e.g. allergens, irritants).
- Refer to an asthma specialist if there are difficulties controlling asthma or if Step 4 care is required. Referral may be considered if Step 3 care is required.

* There are more data on using budesonide during pregnancy than on using other inhaled corticosteroids.
† There are minimal data on using leukotriene receptor antagonists in humans during pregnancy, although there are reassuring animal data submitted to FDA.
‡ There are more data on using albuterol during pregnancy than on using other short-acting inhaled beta-agonists.

Figure 6.1 Stepwise approach for managing asthma during pregnancy and lactation.
Source: NAEEP Working Group Report on Managing Asthma during Pregnancy (2004).

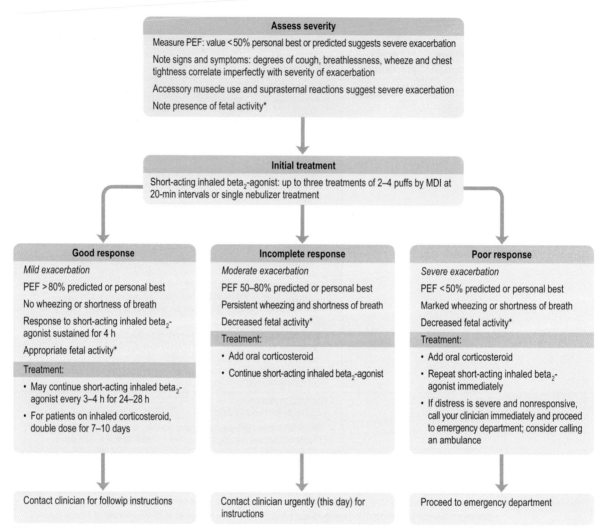

MDI, metered-dose inhaler, PEF, peak expiratory flow.
*Fetal activity is monitored by observing whether fetal kick counts decrease over time.

Figure 6.2 Management of asthma exacerbations at home during pregnancy and lactation.
Source: NAEEP (2004).

failure to maintain this level of oxygenation with ambulation should generally be viewed an indication for admission to hospital.

Clinical predictors of mortality from asthma should also be taken into account when deciding whether a patient with an asthma exacerbation can be sent home. These include marked circadian variation in lung function, a large bronchodilator response, psychosocial instabilities, use of three or more medications, frequent visits to the emergency department, recurrent hospitalizations and previous life-threatening exacerbations.

Asthma exacerbation is not an indication for elective delivery, although if there are other maternal or fetal indications, an asthmatic exacerbation is not a reason to delay a delivery.

Labor and delivery

Asthma exacerbations during labor are relatively rare, presumably due to the natural outpouring of endogenous steroids and epinephrine associated with the stress of delivery. When a peripartum exacerbation

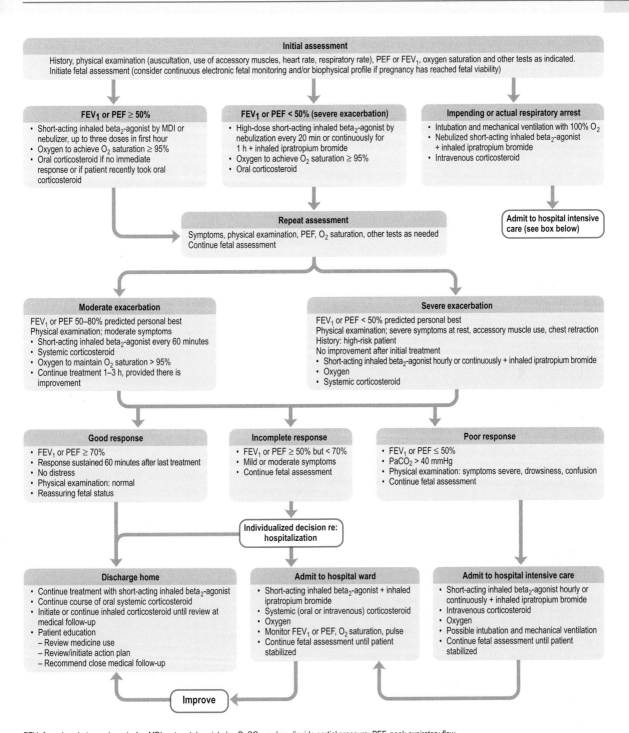

FEV$_1$ forced expiratory volume in 1 s; MDI metered-dose inhaler; PaCO$_2$, carbon dioxide partial pressure; PEF, peak expiratory flow.

Figure 6.3 Management of asthma exacerbations in the emergency department and hospital during pregnancy and lactation. Source: NAEEP (2004).

does occur, a differential diagnosis that includes pulmonary edema (from cardiac causes or non-cardiac ones such as pre-eclampsia, tocolysis and sepsis), pulmonary embolism and aspiration should be considered.

15-methyl prostaglandin F_2-alpha should be used with extreme caution in asthmatic patients because it can cause bronchoconstriction. Ergometrine and other ergot derivatives should also be used with extreme caution as they too have caused severe bronchospasm in patients with asthma, particularly in association with general anesthesia. Oxytocin and prostaglandin E_2 compounds can be safely used. Morphine and pethidine (meperidine) are commonly used analgesic drugs in labor. Both drugs may theoretically cause bronchoconstriction through histamine release, however in practice this is not generally a problem and many women with asthma are given morphine and pethidine (meperidine) in labor without harm. Nonetheless, some experts recommend the use of butorphanol or fentanyl as alternatives because these agents are less likely to cause histamine release. These agents also have shorter half-lives and are less likely to lead to neonatal respiratory suppression. If anesthesia is required, an epidural is preferable to general anesthesia because of the risks of chest infection and atelectasis with general anesthesia. For those patients who do require general anesthetic, bronchodilatory agents such as ketamine and halogenated anesthetics are preferred.

It is known that daily doses of systemic steroids given for as little as 3 weeks may suppress the hypothalamic-pituitary-adrenal (HPA) axis for up to 1 year and thereby blunt the normal physiologic outpouring of adrenal corticosteroids that occurs with stressors such as illness and surgery. To avoid precipitating an adrenal crisis, it is recommended in the USA that patients undergoing general surgery who have received more than 5 mg of prednisone per day for more than 3 weeks in the preceding year should be given stress-dose steroids unless a low-dose adrenocorticotrophic hormone (ACTH) stimulation test has documented intact HPA axis function. The relevance of this recommendation to labor and delivery is not established but in the absence of pregnancy-specific data (and recognizing that there is no way to know in advance who will require a Cesarean delivery), stress-dose steroids are generally provided to this group of women in the peripartum period. One recommended regimen is to instruct patients to take their usual daily dose of steroids on the day of delivery and then give additional empiric stress-dose steroids (hydrocortisone 50 mg i.v. beginning with well-established labor or induction of anesthesia and then continue with hydrocortisone 25 mg every 8 hours for 24-48 hours postpartum). If stress dose steroids are not given, it is advisable to watch the patient for signs of adrenal insufficiency (anorexia, nausea, vomiting, weakness, hypotension, hyponatremia and hyperkemia) postpartum.

Post-pregnancy care

Patients should have their medications continued postpartum and their peak flow monitored in the days following delivery. Breastfeeding is not contraindicated in patients taking any form of asthma treatment including oral prednisone. Mothers should be encouraged to breastfeed and to do so exclusively for the first 6 months as well as to maintain a smoke-, pet- and dust-free environment in their home as evidence exists that these interventions may not only be of benefit to the mother but will also help to prevent the onset of atopy and asthma in her child. There are no disease specific recommendations for birth control in patients with asthma.

CYSTIC FIBROSIS

General

Cystic fibrosis (CF) is a potentially fatal autosomal recessive disorder caused by mutations of the cystic fibrosis transmembrane conductance regulator (CFTR) gene located on chromosome 7. CF usually presents with the symptoms and signs of persistent pulmonary infection and pancreatic insufficiency in association with elevated sweat chloride levels. The incidence of CF is 1/2000-3000 among whites; 1 in 20 whites are heterozygous for the CF gene.

Because of the complex nature of this disease, care for patients with cystic fibrosis is best accomplished by a multidisciplinary team experienced in the care of cystic fibrosis.

Maternal risks

Fertility may be decreased among women with CF. This is likely due both to the production of abnormally tenacious cervical mucus and to anovulation related to malnutrition. Data from the USA and the UK suggest a pregnancy rate for women with CF over the age of 16 of 40/1000 per year (compared with 80/1000 in healthy women in the UK) although some of this difference may be due to personal choice and physician advice. Up to 70-80% of pregnancies in patients with CF will result in a delivery. In those pregnancies that continue beyond the first trimester, the likelihood of delivering a live infant is high.

Early reports of poor outcome in mothers with CF have been discounted by more recent studies demonstrating the good pregnancy outcomes of many women. Pregnancy does not appear to affect the decline in forced expiratory volume in one second (FEV_1) or subsequent maternal survival as compared to the entire adult female CF population. Important predictors of a poor pregnancy outcome include a pre-pregnancy FEV_1 that is less than 50% of the predicted value, colonization with *Burkholderia cepacia,* presence of pancreatic insufficiency and the presence and degree of pulmonary hypertension.

Pregnancy does put an additional nutritional demand on the mother with CF. Women who enter a pregnancy underweight may become emaciated if they are unable to keep up with the nutritional demands of the fetoplacental unit.

Diabetes is also associated with an increased risk of adverse pregnancy outcome in women with CF consistent with the risk of diabetes itself. In those patients with CF who have not been diagnosed with diabetes prior to pregnancy, pregnancy may unmask impaired glucose tolerance and the risk of gestational diabetes may be high.

Fetal risks

Well-nourished mothers with reasonably preserved lung function can generally expect a good pregnancy outcome. The pregnancy should still be considered high risk however; fetal growth restriction, premature labor and pregnancy loss can all result from chronic hypoxia, malnutrition and pneumonias. Although most medications used to treat CF are safe for use in pregnancy, infection with some multidrug-resistant organisms may require use of agents with less extensive pregnancy data.

Pre-pregnancy care

Medical care of both pulmonary infection and malabsorption should be optimized before conception. This is best done in a multidisciplinary setting with a special expertise and focus on CF. Patients who are already significantly malnourished should be warned of the further weakness and emaciation that pregnancy may cause. A BMI < 18 kg/m^2 should also be considered a relative contraindication to pregnancy. Patients with diabetes should aim for a normal hemoglobin A1c prior to conception.

Patients with an FEV_1 of < 50% of predicted should be made aware of the increased risk of prematurity, infant complications and maternal death. These patients should also have an echocardiographic esti-mation of pulmonary artery pressure as the presence of moderate-to-severe pulmonary hypertension should lead the clinician to strongly discourage pregnancy.

Antenatal screening for CF should be offered to all women with CF and their partners but not all couples will choose this option. If a mutation is identified in both mother and father, antenatal diagnosis with chorionic villous sampling or amniocentesis can be offered. Because antenatal diagnosis does carry a small risk of pregnancy loss, parents should be aware that it should only be performed either to help them prepare emotionally or to guide them towards termination if the fetus is found to be affected.

In addition, the fact that a future child is at risk of being left without a mother at a relatively young age needs to be raised tactfully and future childcare issues considered. The 10-year mortality rate among pregnant women with CF is 20%. Although heart and lung transplantation may be possible for some patients with cystic fibrosis, it will not be possible for the majority, if only because of the shortage of donors.

Antenatal care

Management of patients with cystic fibrosis during pregnancy means optimizing their pulmonary and nutritional status. Patients with severe lung impairment and/or pulmonary hypertension should be informed of the substantial personal risk to their own health of a pregnancy and offered a termination of pregnancy. Patients who are continuing with pregnancy should ideally be seen at CF units on a bimonthly basis for sputum culturing, evaluation and treatment. Extended lung function testing should be performed and regular adjustments made in the patient's individualized treatment regimens that may include chest physiotherapy, antibiotics (oral, intravenous and/or aerosolized), inhaled beta-agonists, ipratropium, steroids and/or endonuclease DNase (used to decrease the viscosity of expectorated sputum). Consideration of medication interactions, teratogenicity and embryotoxicity should occur but be guided by the principle that fetal well-being is dependent on maternal well-being.

Pulmonary exacerbations increase the risk of preterm delivery. There should therefore be no hesitation about hospital admission to treat either exacerbations of respiratory infection or malnutrition. Antibiotic dosing typically needs adjustment because of the altered pharmacokinetics of both CF and pregnancy. Use of penicillins, cephalosporins, aminoglycosides and when necessary fluoroquinolones and/or trimethoprim sulfamethoxazole (TMP/SMX) are generally justifiable in these patients.

Pancreatic insufficiency is common in CF, leading to malabsorption of fat and protein. These problems can often be reversed with oral supplementation of pancreatic enzyme extracts. However, many patients may remain significantly underweight. A healthy weight gain in pregnancy is 10-12 kg but this can be a challenge for the pregnant woman with CF. Even non-pregnant women with CF need to eat 120-150% of the routine recommended daily requirements to maintain their body weight. Normal pregnancy weight gain requires them to eat a further 300 kcal/day. Significantly underweight women may therefore become emaciated in pregnancy. Malnutrition in turn, may be a cause of intrauterine growth restriction. Even for patients who enter the pregnancy with a normal weight, pregnancy-related dyspepsia, reflux, nausea and vomiting and constipation may hinder appropriate weight gain. In some cases supplemental enteral feeding may be required.

Patients with CF who also have diabetes will require the usual tight control of their blood glucose to optimize pregnancy outcome. Women with CF who have not previously been identified as diabetic should undergo early screening for gestational diabetes. The majority of patients with CF identified to have gestational diabetes will require insulin therapy.

Intrauterine growth deficiency, decreasing maternal weight and deteriorating respiratory function despite optimal medical treatment in hospital should lead to consideration of early delivery.

Labor and delivery

A vaginal delivery is desirable in patients with CF to decrease the risk of postoperative pneumonia associated with surgery. The patient should be encouraged to receive an epidural to decrease maternal oxygen requirements associated with pain and avoid the need for general anesthesia should an urgent Cesarean delivery be needed. Forceps or vacuum delivery may be considered to prevent a prolonged second stage causing maternal exhaustion. Medical treatment and chest physiotherapy should be continued throughout the puerperium. Patients with pulmonary hypertension will require intensive management in this period and the days following delivery as discussed in Chapter 2.

Postnatal care

Patients with cystic fibrosis who are not severely underweight should be encouraged to breastfeed. The breast milk of mothers with CF has normal electrolyte content but a slightly lower fat content than normal, specifically for essential fatty acids, although it has enough to nourish the child.

Most medications needed for the treatment of CF are compatible with breastfeeding. Breastfeeding is not advisable however where maternal nutrition is a problem or the mother's general health is very poor.

Infants of mothers with CF should be screened by their pediatrician for CF.

SARCOIDOSIS

General

Sarcoidosis is a disease most commonly seen in women of reproductive age. The prevalence is estimated to be 10-20 per 100 000 population with a lifetime risk of 0.85% among whites. It is three to four times more common in blacks. It is characterized by non-caseating granulomas that typically affect the lung with bilateral hilar adenopathy and/or pulmonary infiltrates. Its etiology and pathogenesis remain unknown. When symptomatic, sarcoidosis may present as cough, dyspnea, chest pain, fatigue, malaise, weakness, fever and weight loss. However, over half of all cases are detected incidentally on routine chest X-rays that reveal either the classic bilateral hilar adenopathy and/or interstitial or alveolar infiltrates.

Other organ systems that may be affected include skin (maculopapular eruptions, skin nodules and erythema nodosum), lymphatic system (lymphadenopathy), eye (iridocyclitis, chorioretinitis and keratoconjunctivitis) and liver. Less commonly manifestations can occur in the spleen (splenomegaly), the neurologic system, the salivary glands, the bone marrow, the ear nose and throat, heart, kidneys, bone, joint or muscle. Calcium homeostasis (leading to hypercalciuria and hypercalcemia) can also be affected in sarcoidosis.

Treatment for sarcoidosis is reserved for those with significant symptoms (particularly ocular disease) or pulmonary compromise. Systemic steroids are the cornerstone of treatment for sarcoidosis. Whether the risks of long-term corticosteroids in patients with more mild or asymptomatic disease are worth the modest benefit remains unclear. Chloroquine, hydroxychloroquine, methotrexate, azathioprine, pentoxifylline, thalidomide, cyclophosphamide, ciclosporin and infliximab have all also been used to treat chronic or steroid-unresponsive sarcoidosis in non-pregnant patients with variable success.

Maternal risks

Although sarcoidosis of the endometrium, ovary and leiomyoma has been reported, sarcoidosis rarely involves the female reproductive organs. In the absence of significant cardiopulmonary compromise, sarcoidosis does not appear to affect fertility or increase the incidence of fetal or obstetric complications.

Few studies of sarcoidosis in pregnancy have been published. However, most experts believe that pregnancy does not influence the natural history of sarcoidosis. In some cases it will improve during pregnancy, possibly due to increases in maternal free cortisol.

Some patients with severe pulmonary sarcoidosis will develop pulmonary fibrosis with an associated hypoxemia that can progress to cor pulmonale and pulmonary hypertension. Pulmonary hypertension is associated with a significant risk of maternal mortality. Patients with severe disease should therefore have a formal evaluation for pulmonary hypertension and patients with moderate-to-severe pulmonary hypertension should be informed frankly of the risks of pregnancy.

Fetal risks

Sarcoidosis does not appear to represent any significant risk to the fetus aside from the uncommon circumstance where a mother has severe systemic disease that is a threat to maternal health and thereby leads to fetal compromise. Sarcoid granulomas have been found in the placenta but not in the fetus. Although use of steroids in pregnancy is generally felt to be readily justifiable and 'safe' for the fetus, severe sarcoidosis that is unresponsive to steroids may lead to consideration of treatments with pharmacologic agents with unknown or adverse fetal effects. Untreated maternal hypercalcemia from sarcoidosis could theoretically lead to neonatal hypocalcemia and tetany. However, the hypercalcemia associated with sarcoidosis is usually mild and unlikely to cause neonatal problems.

Pre-pregnancy care

Pre-pregnancy counseling that incorporates the above information should be given to all patients with sarcoidosis. Advice and management will be aided by obtaining a baseline complete blood count, liver function tests, creatinine, blood urea nitrogen and serum calcium. These blood tests should be supplemented by an oxygen saturation (both resting and with exercise), pulmonary function testing (including a diffusing capacity for carbon monoxide – a 'DLCO' – as a measurement of gas exchange that is very sensitive to the presence of interstitial lung disease) and a chest X-ray. Patients with asymptomatic disease or minor extra-pulmonary manifestations can anticipate a good outcome. Patients with more severe disease should be warned that their disease progression and treatment may complicate the course of their pregnancy but will not usually have direct adverse effects on the fetus.

Antenatal care

Breathlessness is common in the normal pregnancy but can also be seen due to progression of sarcoidosis. Women with sarcoidosis who complain of increased dyspnea should have their oxygen saturation measured (both resting and with exercise) and undergo a chest X-ray and pulmonary function testing (including a DLCO) and have these results compared to those obtained prior to the pregnancy. In some circumstances a high-resolution computed tomography (CT) scan may be needed to define the extent of disease and there is no reason why this investigation cannot be carried out during pregnancy.

Painful joints and erythema nodosum are also manifestations of sarcoidosis that may be seen in normal pregnancy. These symptoms need to be interpreted cautiously as they do not necessarily represent a manifestation of disease progression in the setting of pregnancy.

Symptomatic disease attributable to sarcoidosis is generally treated with systemic steroids and this should be undertaken under the supervision of a respiratory physician with experience in treating this disease. Patients who require steroids should be reassured about the use of these agents in pregnancy. (See discussion above on asthma.) Patients on other agents may want to consider the risks and benefits of continued use of these medications or consider delaying a pregnancy in the hope that the disease will go into remission.

Patients with sarcoidosis can develop hypercalcemia. This is particularly true in the setting of vitamin D supplementation. Even when the calcium levels are normal, sarcoidosis-associated hypercalciuria can cause nephrocalcinosis. Pregnant patients with sarcoidosis should therefore generally avoid both vitamin D and calcium supplementation and the ingredients of their antenatal vitamins should be reviewed.

Angiotensin-converting enzyme has been advocated by some experts as an index of disease activity in sarcoidosis but should not be used in this manner in pregnancy when angiotensin-converting enzyme levels appear to change independently of sarcoid activity.

Labor and delivery

Epidural blocks are generally preferable over general anesthesia in pregnancy but this is particularly true for patients with pulmonary disease. Women who have received greater than the equivalent of 5 mg of prednisone for more than 3 weeks in the year prior to surgical stress should be given stress-dose steroids around the time of labor and delivery as discussed in the section on asthma above.

Postnatal care

There are no specific recommendations for the postpartum management of the patient with sarcoidosis. The data as to whether 'flares' of sarcoidosis are more common in the postpartum period are conflicting but these appear to be most likely to occur in those women who already have symptomatic disease while pregnant.

KYPHOSCOLIOSIS

General

Kyphosis refers to spinal anteroposterior angulation of the spine, while scoliosis refers to its lateral displacement or curvature. Most cases begin in childhood and are idiopathic. The degree of lung function impairment correlates well with the degree of spinal deformity. A restrictive pattern is seen on pulmonary function testing, with decreased total lung capacity (TLC), vital capacity (VC) and preserved residual volume (RV). With time the chest wall compliance decreases and the work of breathing increases. Persistent hypoxemia can lead to pulmonary hypertension in some patients.

Surgical treatment has little if any role for adults with kyphoscoliosis. Mild kyphoscoliosis with relatively preserved lung function has a good prognosis and requires supportive care only. Patients with severe restrictive disease, hypoxemia and subsequent cor pulmonale have a greatly shortened life expectancy. Medical therapy including supplemental oxygen, noninvasive ventilation and pulmonary rehabilitation is the mainstay of management.

Kyphoscoliosis should not affect pregnancy outcomes unless there is a significant degree of respiratory impairment and/or pulmonary hypertension

and thankfully such circumstances are relatively rare.

Maternal risks

The risks to the mother are those of cardiac failure and cor pulmonale in those very few patients with pulmonary hypertension. For pulmonary hypertension to develop, the restrictive lung disease has to be severe enough to produce hypoxemia at rest. This is most likely if the vital capacity is less than 1.5 L, and especially so if it is less than 1 L. This level of restriction also places the patient at increased risk of pulmonary infection following Cesarean delivery.

Fetal risks

Despite significant deformities that appear to greatly foreshorten the abdominal cavity, babies can and do grow normally in these adverse surroundings as long as pulmonary function is preserved. The fetus, however, is at risk from preterm delivery and, if the mother is hypoxemic, from intrauterine growth restriction. Many preterm deliveries in these patients are elective because of concern about maternal well-being with the expanding uterus.

Pre-pregnancy care

Pre-pregnancy counseling should be provided to the patient after an assessment of pulmonary function and an evaluation for pulmonary hypertension. If vital capacity is greater than 2 L, patients will generally tolerate pregnancy and delivery. If it is less than 2 L, patients will be at increased risk for pulmonary complications with pregnancy. An arterial blood gas should also be obtained in all patients with a vital capacity of less than 2 L. If the resting PaO_2 is decreased, then the fetus is at risk of growth deficiency. If the $PaCO_2$ is increased, the risk of pulmonary complications is very high.

In the setting of significant compromise in pulmonary function testing, hypoxia or hypercapnia, Doppler echocardiography should be performed as a non-invasive screening test that can detect pulmonary hypertension, although it may be imprecise in determining actual pressures. Moderate-to-severe pulmonary hypertension is an absolute contraindication to pregnancy. However, before such a drastic recommendation is made, the physician may want to perform a direct assessment of pulmonary vascular resistance by measurement of pulmonary artery pressure and cardiac output by formal right-sided cardiac catheterization.

Antenatal care

Patients who have significantly severe pulmonary hypertension should be offered termination because of the maternal risk. All other patients should receive medical care for any intercurrent respiratory infection, bronchospasm and cardiac failure. Supplementary oxygen therapy and non-invasive ventilation should be provided to those patients who are hypoxemic.

Patients with marked kyphoscoliosis may require hospital admission in the final months of pregnancy either because of concern about impending respiratory failure or simply because they get so tired. Nasal positive-pressure ventilation has been used to help some patients.

Obstetric antenatal care should be focused on detecting intrauterine growth deficiency. Elective preterm delivery may be necessary for increasing hypoxemia or frank respiratory failure in the mother or because of intrauterine growth deficiency.

Labor and delivery

Many patients with severe kyphoscoliosis will be delivered by Cesarean section because of associated pelvic deformity. Because the defect in kyphoscoliosis is often in the upper part of the spine, epidural catheterization is often possible and when it is possible it is the preferred modality, as is the case for any patient with respiratory disease.

Postnatal care

No special measures are necessary after delivery apart from a continuation of optimal medical and obstetric care, including early mobilization and physiotherapy. Patients who have undergone Cesarean delivery may benefit from use of incentive spirometry, chest physiotherapy and/or intermittent positive-pressure breathing that help decrease the risk of postoperative atelectasis and thereby pneumonia. In more severe cases, use of non-invasive positive-pressure ventilation may be advisable.

TUBERCULOSIS

General

Worldwide there are still 8 million new cases of tuberculosis (TB) and 2 million deaths caused by TB each year. Up to one-third of the world population has been infected with TB. Even in the resource-rich nations, there remain a large number of unidentified latent and active cases of TB among inner-city minority populations and immigrants from countries with a high prevalence of tuberculosis. Pregnancy can represent an important opportunity for identification and treatment of tuberculosis that will be of benefit to a mother, her child and the general public.

Maternal risks

Pregnancy is not associated with an increased risk of tuberculosis nor does the course of tuberculosis appear to be affected by pregnancy. Some concern exists that the hepatotoxicity of isoniazid – one of the key agents in anti-tubercular agents – is increased in pregnancy and warrants increased monitoring (see below).

Fetal risks

Pulmonary tuberculosis or TB lymphadenitis generally poses little risk to the fetus. Untreated pulmonary and extra-pulmonary disease may be associated with some increased risk of adverse fetal outcomes such as intrauterine growth retardation (IUGR) and low birthweight. True congenital infection with TB is exceptionally uncommon, though granulomas have been found in the placenta and bacilli have been retrieved from the decidua, amnion and chorioinic villi. On the rare occasions that congenital infection occurs, it is usually in the setting of endometrial or miliary TB. Criteria for congenital tuberculosis include demonstration of either a primary focus in the fetal liver or documentation of the presence of infection in the first few days of life. In practice the real risk to the fetus is the very questionable teratogenicity of anti-tuberculosis drugs (see below). Far more common than congenital infections with TB are neonatal infections that occur due to exposure to an infected mother or other family member. Active identification and then treatment of TB during the pregnancy is the best way to prevent this unfortunate outcome.

Pre-pregnancy care

Pre-pregnancy counseling may be given, incorporating the information given above. The main problem concerning the management of tuberculosis in pregnancy is concerns about the possible teratogenicity of some anti-tuberculosis drugs. Present data suggest that the most commonly used agents are safe in pregnancy, but women undergoing treatment for active TB might want to consider delaying pregnancy until their treatment course is completed. Previously treated tuberculosis is no contraindication to pregnancy and tuberculosis is no more likely to be reactivated in pregnancy than at any other time.

Antenatal care

Screening and diagnosis

Routine screening of all pregnant women for TB is not justifiable. However, targeted screening among high-risk populations may be appropriate. In the USA it is customary for minority women living in inner cities and patients who have recently emigrated from an area of the world with a high prevalence of tuberculosis to be offered tuberculin skin testing (TST) unless documentation of recent TST status is available. TST is both safe and reasonably sensitive throughout pregnancy. Many experts in the UK however do not recommend routine screening among at-risk populations and would only perform TST if there were clinical evidence of active TB, recent close contact with an infected individual or in patients with immunosuppression. The standard TST is a Mantoux test of 5 tuberculin units (TU) injected into the skin and reviewed by an experienced clinician at 48-72 hours by measuring the maximum area of induration.

Positive skin test reactors and any woman with symptoms suggestive of tuberculosis regardless of their TST results should have a chest X-ray. If the chest radiograph is suggestive of tuberculosis, three separate morning sputum collections should be made and tested for Mycobacterium by both smear and culture (and often now with polymerase chain reaction (PCR)). If any of the sputum tests are positive, treatment should be initiated. Because of increasing rates of multidrug-resistant TB, susceptibility testing for isoniazid, rifampin and ethambutol should be performed on a positive initial culture. Baseline measurements of serum aminotransferases, bilirubin, alkaline phosphatase, serum creatinine and a platelet count should be obtained. HIV testing of all TB patients is critical to guiding therapy. Use of ethambutol can affect visual acuity and red–green color discrimination. Patients should be told to report any changes in vision promptly. Some experts recommend baseline visual testing followed by monthly testing if the patient is on ethambutol for more than 2 months or if they are on a higher than standard dose.

Treatment of active tuberculosis

Active TB can be treated successfully in pregnancy. The benefits of treatment dramatically outweigh any concerns about potential drug toxicity. Due to the challenging nature of the emergence of multidrug-resistant TB it is advisable that all tubercular infections be managed in conjunction with a physician experienced in the care of tuberculosis. Directly observed therapy (in which patients are observed to ingest each dose of anti-tuberculosis medications), is also highly recommended. The current recommendation in the UK and by the World Health Organization (WHO) and the International Union against Tuberculosis and Lung Disease (IUATLD) for uncomplicated tuberculosis in a pregnant individual calls for two phases of treatment with a total treatment course of 6 months. The first or 'initial phase' is a 2-month course of ethambutol, pyrazinamide, rifampicin and isoniazid. The second or 'continuation phase' is a further 4 months of rifampicin and isoniazid. A sputum specimen for microscopic examination and culture should be obtained at a minimum of monthly intervals until two consecutive specimens are negative on culture. The initial four-drug regimen is important because of the increasing prevalence of multidrug-resistant TB. Although this standard regimen described above is effective in most cases, treatment may need to be adjusted once formal antibacterial susceptibility patterns are established. There are several second-line anti-tubercular drugs that should be avoided in pregnancy except for in special circumstances. These include ethionamide, amikacin, kanamycin and the fluoroquinolones.

Anti-tubercular therapy can be given in various regimens from a program of 7 days a week therapy in both phases of therapy or a modified regimen of 5 days a week in the initial phase and either 2 or 5 days a week in the continuation phase. Less-frequent dosing makes directly observed therapy more feasible.

Pregnancy data about the commonly used antimycobacterial agents are reviewed in Table 6.2. Streptomycin has been shown to cause both vestibular and auditory eighth nerve damage leading to deafness in the newborn and is therefore the only commonly used anti-tubercular drug clearly contraindicated in pregnancy. Although detailed human pregnancy safety data for pyrazinamide are still evolving, most official recommendations now support its use in pregnancy. When pyrazinamide is not included in the initial treatment regimen, anti-tubercular therapy should be continued for 9 months.

Isoniazid is associated with a risk of neuropathy and this risk can be minimized by concurrent prescription of pyridoxine 25-50 mg daily. Most antenatal vitamins provide less than this dose. Vitamin K 10 mg daily from 36 weeks gestation onwards is also commonly recommended to decrease the risk of hemorrhagic disease of the newborn. The most common serious adverse effect of isoniazid is drug-induced hepatitis. Isoniazid therapy should be discontinued

Table 6.2 Pregnancy data regarding commonly used anti-mycobacterial agents.

Agent and usual dose	Adverse effects in general	Pregnancy data*	Additional notes
Isoniazid • 5 mg/kg up to a maximum of 300 mg daily • Dispensed in the USA as 50, 100 and 300 mg tabs and 50 mg/5 mL syrup	• Hepatitis • Gastrointestinal distress • Peripheral neuropathy • Drug interaction with many agents especially anticonvulsants • Seizures • Cutaneous hypersensitivity	• FDA pregnancy classification C • High lipid solubility and therefore passes easily into fetal circulation • Fair data to suggest this agent is safe in human pregnancy and any risk is outweighed by potential benefit. However, concerns about potential increase in isoniazid hepatotoxicity in pregnancy makes its routine use for prophylaxis in pregnancy in low-risk cases inadvisable	• Always administer with 25-50 mg per day of pyridoxine (vitamin B6) to decrease the risk of neurotoxicity in the mother • Give vitamin K to mother near birth (10 mg orally daily from 36 weeks onwards) and infant at birth to decrease risk of postpartum hemorrhage and hemorrhagic disease of the newborn. Because of concern about possible increased hepatotoxicity in pregnancy, it has become routine for pregnant women on isoniazid to undergo hepatic transaminase testing at initiation of treatment and at monthly intervals thereafter. Consider discontinuing if the enzymes rise above three times normal
Rifampin • 10 mg/kg up to a maximum of 600 mg daily. • Dispensed as 150 and 300 mg scored tablets in the USA	• Fever • Nausea • Hepatitis • Purpura • Flu-like symptoms at high doses • Orange secretions • Increased metabolism of many agents	• FDA pregnancy classification C • Limited data suggest no adverse fetal effects	• Give vitamin K to mother near birth (10 mg orally daily from 36 weeks onwards) and infant at birth to decrease risk of postpartum hemorrhage and hemorrhagic disease of the newborn
Ethambutol • 15-25 mg/kg up to a maximum of 1600 mg daily. Dispensed as 100 mg and 400 mg tablets in the USA	• Retrobulbar neuritis occurs in 1% of patients • Peripheral neuropathy • Skin reactions	• FDA pregnancy classification B • Limited data suggest no adverse fetal effects	• At each monthly visit patients taking ethambutol should be questioned regarding possible visual disturbances including blurred vision or scotomata; monthly testing of visual acuity and color discrimination is recommended for

Table 6.2 *Continued*

Agent and usual dose	Adverse effects in general	Pregnancy data*	Additional notes
			patients receiving the drug for longer than 2 months
Pyrazinamide • 15–30 mg/kg orally daily up to a maximum of 1600 mg daily	• Thrombocytopenia • Hepatotoxicity • Interstitial nephritis	• FDA pregnancy classification C • Human data extremely limited	• Use in pregnancy supported by international recommendations in all pregnant patients with active TB after the first trimester and particularly essential for multidrug-resistant TB and HIV-positive patients
Streptomycin Dose varies	• An aminoglycoside with nephro- and oto-toxicitiy	• FDA pregnancy classification D • Reports of fetal ototoxicity	• Use in pregnancy avoided

*US Food and Drug Adminitration (FDA) classification explained in Appendix A.

and the medication regimen altered in the setting of nausea, abdominal pain and hepatic tenderness occurring in association with hepatic transaminase elevations greater than three times the normal range or in asymptomatic patients with transaminases greater than five times the normal range. There is some evidence to suggest that pregnant women are at a higher risk of developing isoniazid-related hepatotoxicity and therefore it has become routine that pregnant women on isoniazid undergo hepatic transaminases testing at initiation of treatment and at monthly intervals thereafter.

Management of HIV-related tuberculosis is complex and requires expertise in the management of both HIV disease and tuberculosis. Discussion of its management is beyond the scope of this chapter but the most recent guidelines for its treatment can be found at the AIDSinfo website sponsored by the US department of Health and Human Services at http://aidsinfo.nih.gov/guidelines.

Tuberculosis prophylaxis

Patients who have positive TST but show no evidence of active infection often warrant prophylactic treatment of latent tubercular infection (LTBI) with a 6-month course of isoniazid 5 mg/kg to prevent future development of active TB. Because of concerns about isoniazid toxicity in pregnancy, it may be justifiable to delay prophylactic treatment in some women while they are still pregnant. Although some controversy exists around this issue, the pregnant woman with a normal immune status and a positive TST who has not been previously treated should probably only receive prophylaxis during pregnancy if there has been a recent contact with an active TB case and the patient has a TST that is > 5 mm. Otherwise prophylaxis for tuberculosis in the asymptomatic immunocompetent pregnant woman can generally be delayed until the postpartum period.

This is not true for immunocompromised patients and in particular all HIV infected women with a tuberculin skin test result > 5 mm or who have even been exposed to an active case of TB should receive prophylactic therapy during pregnancy.

Labor and delivery

The only issue with tuberculosis that warrants special consideration during labor and delivery is maintenance of excellent infection control. TB-specific precautions for healthcare workers should be employed if the mother is untreated and has not been demonstrated to have smear negative sputum prior to delivery. Initiation of treatment and documentation that the sputum is no longer infective prior to delivery will reassure both mother and staff.

Postnatal care

Neonatal infection can occur if the baby is in close contact with a mother or other family member who has active tuberculosis. In addition to treating active TB during pregnancy, it is important to ensure that all family members in the household are also screened and if necessary, treated for TB.

If the mother has had 3 months of treatment with negative sputum, the neonate can simply be examined monthly for evidence of TB and have tuberculin skin testing done at 6, 12 and 24 weeks of life. Administration of Bacillus Calmette-Guérin (BCG) is encouraged. Infants of mothers believed to have sterile sputum but who have not had 3 months of documented bacilli-negative sputum should be considered for isoniazid prophylaxis in addition to the BCG.

After delivery, patients with untreated sputum-positive tuberculosis (i.e. tubercular bacilli in their sputum) should be separated from their babies until they are no longer overtly infective. Since pyrazinamide generally renders the sputum sterile in 10 days, this situation should be short-lived. In addition, the neonate should be given isoniazid and BCG.

Breastfeeding should be encouraged for women being treated with isoniazid, pyrazinamide, ethambutol and/or rifampin. These agents are found in only small concentrations in breast milk and are not known to produce toxicity in the nursing newborn. These concentrations however are not significant enough to provide any protection to the nursing infant from infection with TB.

Antimycobacterial agents can theoretically decrease the efficacy of some oral contraceptive pills and the use of an additional method of birth control in postpartum women receiving these agents may be advisable.

RESPIRATORY INFECTIONS

Respiratory infections (the common cold, bronchitis, sinusitis and community-acquired pneumonia) are the most common reasons that patients present to healthcare providers, and their management in pregnancy is an important part of obstetric care.

The common cold

Etiology and clinical features

The average adult has two to three colds per year. They generally last from 3 to 7 days but may persist for up to 2 weeks in 25% of patients. It is a benign and self-limited illness, most commonly caused by rhinoviruses, coronaviruses and the respiratory syncytial virus. Symptoms of the common cold include rhinitis, nasal congestion, rhinorrhea, sneezing, sore throat and cough, typically with none of these symptoms predominating. Examination is usually normal. Between 0.5 and 2.5% of cases of the common cold are complicated by acute sinusitis and the common cold is said to be responsible for 40% of asthma exacerbations.

Treatment

Despite their widespread use, no study has shown any benefit of treatment with antibiotics for uncomplicated upper respiratory tract infections even if the nasal discharge is purulent. Symptomatic therapy is therefore the mainstay of treatment. Unfortunately the efficacy of most common cold therapies is limited. Some of the more commonly used agents are reviewed and the data regarding their safety in pregnancy summarized in Table 6.3.

Acute bacterial sinusitis

Definition and etiology of acute sinusitis

Acute sinusitis is an infection of the paranasal sinuses which usually occurs as a complication of the common cold. The organisms responsible for community-acquired sinusitis include *Streptococcus pneumoniae*, *Haemophilus influenza*, *Moraxella catarrhalis* and Group A *Streptococcus*, anaerobes, viruses and *Staphylococcus aureus*.

Distinguishing the common cold from bacterial sinusitis

It can be a challenge to distinguish the acute viral rhinosinusitis of the common cold from an acute bacterial sinusitis. There are no signs and symptoms that are both sensitive and specific in making this distinction. It is therefore recommended that the clinical diagnosis of acute bacterial rhinosinusitis be reserved for those patients whose symptoms persist without improvement (or worsen) beyond 7 days who have purulent nasal secretions and maxillary, tooth or facial pain or tenderness.

Treatment of acute sinusitis

In sharp distinction from the common cold, antibiotic treatment for acute bacterial sinusitis helps to eradi-

Table 6.3 Efficacy and safety of medications used to treat the common cold in pregnancy. Adapted from Powrie (2001).

Agent	Dose	Effect in randomized control trials	Pregnancy data*
Ipratropium bromide 0.06% nasal spray	Two sprays per nostril three or four times daily for 4 days.	Mild improvement in rhinorrhea and sneezing.	FDA pregnancy category B. Data on human effects have not been published but it is presumed that the agent can be used nasally in pregnancy because of the small systemic absorption and reassuring animal data.
Cromolyn as dry powder (20 mg per inhalation in spincaps) OR aqueous nasal spray (5.2 mg per dose)	Intranasally every 2 hours during waking hours on days 1 and 2, and then four times daily on days 3-7	Mildly shortens the duration and severity of cold symptoms.	FDA pregnancy category B Less than 10% of an inhaled dose of cromolyn is absorbed systemically. Animal data are reassuring. The published data with respect to the use of this agent to treat asthma in pregnancy are very reassuring.
Acetaminophen/ paracetemol (paracetamol)	325-1000 mg orally every 4-6 hours. Not more than 3 g per day	Antipyretic and symptomatic relief of associated myalgias, headaches and sore throat.	FDA pregnancy category B Extensive animal data and population-based studies are very reassuring regarding the safety of this agent in pregnancy.
Non-steroidal anti-inflammatory drugs (NSAIDs)	Different dosing for each agent	Reductions in headache, malaise, myalgia with a 29% reduction in the total (5-day) symptom score. Has no effect on nasal symptoms.	Most NSAIDs are FDA pregnancy category B in first trimester and D in second and third trimester These agents do not appear to cause malformations but have been associated with oligohydramnios, pulmonary hypertension and an increased risk of intracranial hemorrhage and necrotizing enterocolitis in infants born prematurely. Their use in pregnancy, although perhaps justifiable in some circumstances, is not appropriate for the treatment of common cold symptoms during pregnancy. Acetaminophen/paracetemol (paracetamol) will likely offer similar relief in this setting without placing the fetus at increased risk.
Decongestants: intranasal and oral	Different dosing for each agent	Short-lived mild relief of obstruction with single use. No evidence of sustained effects. Spray decongestants associated with rebound effects upon withdrawal.	All FDA pregnancy classification C. Most commonly used decongestants are in need of further study before they can be definitively considered safe in pregnancy. Present data are variable but these agents probably represent a low risk Oxymetazoline is the preferred intranasal decongestant but its use for mild symptoms should be discouraged in pregnancy. There is no clear human teratogenic effect and no effect on uterine blood flow in the setting of normal nasal mucosa but concerns exist about its possible effects on

Table 6.3 *Continued*

Agent	Dose	Effect in randomized control trials	Pregnancy data*
			uterine blood flow in the setting of overuse, inflamed nasal mucosa and in cases where poor placental perfusion is already suspected. Pseudoephedrine is probably the preferred oral agent among the oral decongestants. Two studies have suggested an increased risk of gastroschisis. However, this agent is less likely to raise blood pressure than the other oral decongestants. Ephedrine is teratogenic in chicks even at small doses. No evidence of human teratogenesis but data are limited. Phenylephrine has been associated with a wide range of congenital anomalies in humans and dramatic effects on uterine blood flow in sheep. This agent should be avoided at all stages of pregnancy.
Antihistamines	Different dosing for each agent	No antihistamine affects total symptom score or duration for the common cold. Clemastine and brompheniramine (and loratadine in conjunction with pseudoephedrine) decrease sneezing and nasal discharge but have no effect on sore throat, cough, headache and malaise.	FDA pregnancy classification B and C. Most of the older antihistamines are not considered to increase the incidence of congenital malformations in humans. Although some antihistamines have been associated with oral clefts in retrospective studies, others have found no significant increase in the incidence of major or minor malformations, and one study even found that significantly fewer infants with malformations were exposed to antihistamines while in utero than were controls. Chlorpheniramine and diphenhydramine have mostly reassuring pregnancy data and should be considered the preferred antihistamines in pregnancy. The newer antihistamines fexofenadine, cetirizine, and loratadine have limited published human pregnancy data and should not be considered first-line agents in pregnancy. Use of antihistamine with women in preterm labor was associated in one study with an increased risk of retrolental fibroplasias and should be avoided in this setting.
Cough medicine: codeine, dextromethorphan, guaifenisin, benzonatate, hydrocodone	Different dosing for each agent	Uniformly ineffective in the setting of cough from common cold	All FDA pregnancy classification C. Animal data for codeine, dextromethorphan and hydrocodone conflicting. Human data for all these agents are poor but no clear teratogenic effects have been identified except for guaifenisin, which was associated with inguinal hernias in one study only. Neonatal withdrawal has been reported in babies born both to addicted and non-addicted women

Table 6.3 *Continued*

Agent	Dose	Effect in randomized control trials	Pregnancy data*
			who took codeine in the days prior to delivery. Codeine ingestion near the time of labor can produce respiratory depression in the newborn. The lack of efficacy of these agents suggests their use is not justifiable in pregnancy for the common cold especially given questions about the safety of some of these agents in pregnancy.
Zinc gluconate	Varying doses. Tablets for the common cold usually contain 12 mg per tablet	The evidence of zinc efficacy for treating the common cold is inconclusive at best, and any beneficial effect is minor.	The noxious taste of zinc lozenges limit their usefulness particularly in pregnant patients. Animal experiments and human case reports have produced variable but frequently concerning results regarding the safety of high-dose zinc supplementation in pregnancy.
Vitamin C	Varying doses	Current extensive literature does not appear to support the routine use of vitamin C therapy for the common cold.	Little pregnancy data available, however there is concern that large doses of this vitamin may lead to an excessively rapid metabolism of vitamin C that can cause scurvy in the newborn period.
Echinacea	Varying doses	No evidence to support efficacy	Recent data reporting on 206 exposed pregnancies found no increased incidence of anomalies compared with controls.

*US Food and Drug Adminitration (FDA) classification explained in Appendix A.

cate infection and to reduce the duration of symptoms. The antibiotic chosen should be the most narrow spectrum agent that still has activity against the most likely pathogens. The emergence of beta-lactamase-producing *H. influenzae* and *M. catarrhalis* and of multiple antibiotic resistant *S. pneumoniae* warrants consideration when prescribing for acute sinusitis, particularly in patients who have had antibiotic treatment in the past month, are exposed to children in day care or live in an area where the incidence of multiple antibiotic resistant *S. pneumoniae* is greater than 30%.

If the patient is at low risk for antibiotic-resistant bacteria, the use of amoxicillin 1 g orally three times a day for 10 days is still considered adequate by most experts. Other authorities recommend regimens that cover the possibility of resistant *Pneumococcus* and *Haemophilus*. One such regimen that is acceptable in

pregnancy is amoxicillin clavulanate extended release 2000/125 mg every 12 hours for 10 days. Clarithromycin, trimethoprim sulfamethoxazole and fluoroquinolones should not generally be used for this indication in pregnancy. Cefpodoxime, cefuroxime or cefprozil may be used for patients who have a penicillin allergy that manifests only as a skin rash. For patients with more significant penicillin reactions, azithromycin may be used.

The role of symptomatic treatments of sinusitis as adjuncts to antibiotic therapy is unclear. The use of pseudoephedrine to aid drainage in the nasal passages is logical, widespread and probably safe in pregnancy. Antihistamines are not recommended because they may thicken mucus secretion and thereby impair drainage. No evidence exists for a role for nasal steroids in the treatment of acute sinusitis.

VASOMOTOR RHINITIS OF PREGNANCY

Vasomotor rhinitis of pregnancy is defined as nasal congestion present during the second half of pregnancy without other signs of respiratory tract infection and with no known allergic cause, which disappears completely within a few weeks after delivery. It is present in over 20% of pregnant women. It is caused by hormonal effects upon the nasal mucosa and is more common among smokers. In and of itself it does not warrant treatment. If a patient's discomfort with this common pregnancy symptom leads her to seek treatment, saline nasal sprays, nasal ipratropium, nasal steroids (preferably beclometasone or budesonide) or pseudoephedrine may be tried. Nasal decongestant sprays can be effective but run the risk of causing rhinitis medicamentosa if used for more than a few days. The efficacy of these agents in pregnancy rhinitis has not been studied and is purely anecdotal. Reassurance is probably the most important intervention.

ALLERGIC RHINITIS

Allergic rhinitis is another important cause of a stuffy nose in pregnancy. It generally presents as a chronic or recurrent complaint of nasal congestion with prominent nasal itching and sneezing but no purulent nasal discharge. Patients are reasonably accurate at distinguishing allergic rhinitis from other causes of stuffy nose. Nasal symptoms in pregnant women with a history of allergic rhinitis tend to improve in 34%, worsen in 15% and remain unchanged in the remainder.

The most important intervention to treat allergic rhinitis is avoidance of allergens. When necessary however, a wide range of pharmaceutical options are available for use in pregnancy.

Chlorphenamine or diphenhydramine are the preferred first-line antihistamines during pregnancy given the considerable data that exist to support the safety of these agents. Among the newer less-sedating antihistamines loratadine and desloratadine have the best pregnancy data although it remains inferior to that established for the older agents. There are fewer published data documenting human safety of the other newer antihistamines such as cetirizine and fexofenadine and routine use should therefore be avoided in pregnancy.

Nasal cromolyn has excellent pregnancy safety data that support its use as another first-line agent in the treatment of allergic rhinitis in pregnancy. Oral and intranasal decongestants such as pseudoephedrine and oxymetalozine may be considered reasonable second-line agents in pregnancy, but more data are needed before they should be considered a first-line treatment (see Table 6.3 for comments on the use of decongestants in pregnancy). Patients should be cautioned against overuse of intranasal decongestants.

No studies have examined the safety of intranasal steroids in pregnancy but the studies of the use of inhaled steroids for the treatment of asthma in pregnancy suggest that these agents are not teratogens. Of the available inhaled nasal steroids, beclometasone and budesonide can therefore be considered first-line agents. Other nasal steroids such as triamcinolone and fluticasone are almost certainly also safe but there are few published data about these particular agents in pregnancy.

Immunotherapy ('allergy shots') has a proven role in the control of severe allergic rhinitis. Present evidence suggests this therapy can be continued safely during pregnancy. It has generally not been initiated during pregnancy however because of an understandable unwillingness among physicians to expose an expectant mother to the risk of anaphylaxis.

ACUTE BRONCHITIS

Five per cent of adults suffer an episode of acute bronchitis each year. Acute bronchitis is an inflammation of the bronchi that presents as a persistent productive cough that lasts for up to 3 weeks. 90% of cases are viral in origin. In the absence of fever, tachycardia, tachypnea and crackles on pulmonary auscultation, the presence of pneumonia can be confidently ruled out and a chest X-ray is not routinely necessary. The presence of purulent sputum has no role in making a clinical distinction between pneumonia and bronchitis.

Only *Mycoplasma pneumoniae*, *Chlamydia pneumoniae* (TWAR) or *Bordetella pertussis* have been identified as bacterial causes of acute bronchitis and these organisms account for less than 10% of all cases. Unless a specific exposure is reported, these organisms should only be considered in cases of acute bronchitis that lasts beyond 21 days.

Role of antibiotics in treating acute bronchitis

Most cases of acute bronchitis require no more than reassurance and symptomatic treatment. Patients with acute bronchitis do not benefit from antibiotics because bacteria are rarely responsible. Although patients expect antibiotics for acute bronchitis, research suggests that they do so because they have received antibiotics for this indication in the past. Research also suggests that patient satisfaction can readily be achieved without antibiotics by referring to the illness as a 'chest cold' rather than 'bronchitis', emphasizing that it will last 10-14 days and pointing out the danger that antibiotic resistance may represent for the patient in the future.

On the rare occasion that bronchitis persists beyond 21 days and *Mycoplasma pneumoniae, Chlamydia pneumoniae* (TWAR) and *Bordetella pertussis* are identified as the etiology, treatment with a 14-day course of erythromycin 500 mg four times a day can be considered. However, antibiotic therapy will only mildly shorten the course of these illnesses in adults.

Symptomatic treatment

There is evidence that some patients experience symptomatic relief from cough with inhaled albuterol/ salbutamol (one or two puffs every 4 hours) and it can be used safely in pregnancy. However, evidence exists that cough suppressants such as dextromethorphan, guaifenisin or codeine are not generally useful in the cough associated with bronchitis. Supportive care and reassurance that the cough will eventually resolve are often the best treatment measures.

PNEUMONIA

General

Pneumonia is the sixth leading cause of death in the United States but is relatively infrequent in pregnancy. The incidence of pneumonia requiring hospitalization in pregnancy is between 2.6 and 15.1 per 10 000 deliveries, which is a similar rate to that seen in non-pregnant women of a similar age. Mothers who develop pneumonia are more likely to have coexisting medical problems including drug abuse, anemia and HIV infection.

Perhaps the most important role for physicians who are treating pneumonia in pregnancy is to review carefully the differential diagnosis. Pulmonary embolism can present identically to an acute pneumonia with dyspnea, cough, chest pain, fever and chest X-ray infiltrates and remains the leading direct cause of maternal mortality in the USA and the UK. Aspiration chemical pneumonitis, amniotic fluid embolism and pulmonary edema related to

sepsis, tocolysis or pre-eclampsia can also present in a similar fashion.

Rigorous investigation into the specific etiology and treatment of pneumonia in pregnancy has not occurred. The pathogens responsible for community-acquired pneumonia in pregnancy are likely similar to those in non-pregnant patients and include *Streptococcus pneumoniae, Haemophilus influenzae, Staphylococcus aureus,* Gram-negative bacilli, legionella, mycoplasma, chlamydia and viruses. Importantly, the reduction in cell-mediated immunity associated with pregnancy does place women at an increased risk of severe pneumonia and disseminated disease from some atypical pathogens such as herpes virus, influenza, varicella and coccidioidomycosis.

Maternal and fetal risks

Gravid women with pneumonia are at significant increased risk of preterm labor and they are more likely to develop pulmonary edema. While there does not appear to be an increase in perinatal mortality, there is a doubling of the frequency of low birthweight in babies born to mothers with pneumonia versus controls. In addition, some organisms, such as varicella, may present specific risks to the fetus. However, most cases of pneumonia in pregnancy are caused by organisms that do not affect the fetus except through their effects on maternal status. The fetus may also be at risk from maternal conditions which predispose to pneumonia (e.g. HIV infection) and all women who present with pneumonia in pregnancy should be offered HIV testing.

Pre-pregnancy care

Pre-pregnancy counseling is usually not relevant, since pneumonia presents as an acute event without warning. However, HIV-infected individuals with low CD4 cell counts should be counseled to continue *Pneumocystis carinii* prophylaxis during pregnancy. Additionally, the Centers for Disease Control (CDC) and the American College of Obstetricians and Gynecologists advise that women should routinely receive influenza vaccination if they will be in the second and third trimester during influenza season. Pneumococcal vaccine is also recommended before or during pregnancy for women with diabetes mellitus, asthma, chronic cardiac or pulmonary disease, chronic hypertension or immune compromise disease. It is mandatory post-splenectomy and in women with functional hyposplenism (e.g. sickle cell disease). It is also recommended for women living in prisons or long-term care facilities. The CDC recommends that all non-pregnant women of childbearing age who are not immune to varicella be vaccinated against it. However, varicella vaccine is a live vaccine and should not be given during pregnancy.

Antenatal care

General

The patient with community-acquired pneumonia typically presents with cough, sputum production, dyspnea and pleuritic chest pain. Physical examination shows fever, tachycardia, tachypnea and bronchial breath sounds and/or crackles on lung auscultation. However, any of these features may be absent at the time of presentation. Traditional teaching emphasized the different presentations of typical and atypical pneumonias but the clinical utility of these observations is questionable as all etiologies may present either acutely or subacutely.

The presence of an infiltrate on chest X-ray is considered the 'gold standard' for diagnosing pneumonia. There should be no hesitation performing chest radiography in pregnancy. The X-ray appearance cannot be used to reliably differentiate bacterial from non-bacterial pneumonia, nor does the presence of an infiltrate preclude pulmonary embolism as its cause. Routine Gram stains and cultures of sputum may be obtained but cultures lack specificity and sensitivity and an etiologic agent is found in less than half of cases investigated. Blood cultures should also be obtained but are positive in less than 15% of cases. Urine studies for legionella and pneumococcal antigen and rapid testing for influenza antigens may be warranted for severe cases.

HIV status should be reviewed for all pregnant women with pneumonia and testing should be offered if it has not previously been done. Testing for *Pneumocystis carinii* infection should occur in all HIV positive women who present with pneumonia.

Pneumonia should generally be treated on an inpatient basis in pregnancy to help monitor fetal and maternal well-being and to ensure adequate oxygenation (an O_2 saturation of > 95%). Discriminatory features that identify a population of pregnant women with pneumonia who can be successfully managed as outpatients have not been determined. In patients who present with high fever, purulent sputum, chest pain and clinical and radiological signs of consolidation, the clinician should feel comfortable proceeding with empiric therapy for pneumonia. However, in patients who only have modest pyrexia, no sputum

and indeterminate physical and radiological signs a radioisotope ventilation perfusion lung scanning or CT angiography should be obtained to rule out the diagnosis of pulmonary infarction.

Treatment

Several recommendations for the empiric treatment of community-acquired pneumonia exist. These recommendations support the use of a macrolide (erythromycin – in any form aside from the estolate ester – azithromycin and, although there is some question about its safety in pregnancy, clarithromycin) in conjunction with a beta lactam (cefotaxime, ceftriaxone or ampicillin–sulbactam) for most inpatients with pneumonia. Although levofloxacin and doxycycline are often recommended for the treatment of pneumonia in the non-pregnant population, these drugs should be avoided in pregnancy. Use of amoxicillin alone is supported in some European recommendations for non-pregnant outpatients but high doses (3-4 g a day) are now required to achieve activity in > 90% of strains of *S. pneumoniae* and may still be ineffective for many strains.

With appropriate antibiotic therapy, some improvement in the patient's clinical course should be seen within 72 hours. Patients initially treated with intravenous antibiotics can be switched to oral agents (erythromycin/azithromycin with cefprozil or cefpodoxime) once the patient is afebrile for 24-48 hours. Continuation of therapy for a total of 10-14 days is recommended.

Dosage of antibiotics in pregnancy should be towards the upper range of therapeutic doses because of increased renal clearance. Maternal oxygen saturation should be maintained at > 95%. Patients should receive paracetamol as an antipyretic. Respiratory failure is one of the leading reasons for admission of pregnant patients to the intensive care unit and pneumonia is responsible for some of these cases. Those who are very sick may require assisted ventilation as judged by deteriorating blood gas status.

Influenza pneumonia

Data from the influenza pandemics of 1918 and 1957 suggest that influenza may be particularly virulent in pregnant women. In 1918 the mortality for all infected pregnant women was 27% and for those infected in the last month of pregnancy, the mortality rate was over 60%. Mortality rates from influenza have improved greatly with modern healthcare and the emergence of less virulent strains of the virus. However, influenza remains a common occurrence in pregnancy. Up to 11% of women in one UK study had serologic evidence of a new influenza infection during pregnancy and another study found that 25 out of 10000 pregnant women in the third trimester will require hospitalization for influenza.

The fetal effects of influenza infection during pregnancy are less clear. Reports of increased congenital anomalies, stillbirths, and prematurity occurred with the pandemics. More recently, a US study found no significant increase in adverse perinatal outcomes associated with respiratory hospitalizations during the influenza season.

Pregnant women with influenza should be cared for supportively with rest, fluids and acetominophen/paracetamol. Close observation of respiratory rate and oxygen saturation are critical. The antiviral agents amantadine and rimantidine cannot be recommended for use in pregnancy because of animal studies showing teratogenicity and embryotoxic effects. There is no information on the use of the newer influenza agents in pregnancy. Antibiotics (a beta lactam such as amoxicillin clavulanate, cefpodoxime, cefprozil or cefuroxime) should be used for bacterial super-infections.

The best way to prevent influenza morbidity and mortality in pregnancy is to routinely immunize women who will be pregnant during the season for influenza. This intervention is recommended by the American College of Obstetrics and Gynecology (ACOG) and the Centers for Disease Control and Prevention (CDC) and is safe for the fetus.

Varicella pneumonia

Varicella is another cause of pneumonia that appears to be particularly virulent in pregnancy. Fulminant pneumonia will develop in 10-20% of women who develop primary varicella infection in pregnancy. Maternal mortality may be as high as 40%. Varicella embryopathy may occur as a result of maternal infection, particularly in the first half of pregnancy with an incidence of 1-2%. Varicella of the newborn is a life-threatening illness that may occur when a newborn is delivered within 5 days of the onset of maternal illness or exposed to a new infection after delivery. Because of these concerns, the CDC recommends that all non-pregnant women of childbearing age who are not immune to varicella be vaccinated prior to pregnancy. (Varicella vaccine is a live vaccine and should not be given during pregnancy.) If exposure to varicella in pregnancy occurs in a woman without immunity, Varicella zoster immune globulin (VZIG) should be administered within 96 hours in an attempt to prevent maternal infection. Parenteral aciclovir should also be given to all varicella non-immune patients who develop respiratory symptoms within 10 days of exposure to varicella.

Aspiration syndromes: Mendelson's syndrome and bacterial aspiration pneumonia

Despite much progress in modern obstetric and anesthetic management, acute aspiration pneumonitis still occurs in up to 1 in 1500 Cesarean deliveries and 1 in 6000 vaginal deliveries and remains an important cause of pneumonia in pregnancy. Its prevalence is likely due to a combination of pregnancy-related delayed gastric emptying and decreased lower esophageal sphincter pressure. Although aspiration usually occurs in association with a difficult intubation or during the post-anesthetic period when the gag reflex may be depressed, it may also occur de novo in pregnant women. Gastric juice in the lungs leads to intense pulmonary inflammation over 8-24 hours. The patient becomes tachypneic, hypoxic and febrile and chest X-ray can show a complete 'white-out'. Despite this rapidly deteriorating course, this picture resolves without antibiotics within 48-72 hours unless bacterial super-infection intervenes.

Bacterial aspiration pneumonia usually has a more insidious onset than described above for acute bacterial pneumonitis. Clinical manifestations typically begin 48-72 hours after aspiration with persistent fever, sputum and leukocytosis. In this syndrome, chest X-ray findings are typically localized to the basilar segments (if the patient aspirated while upright) or to the posterior segment of the upper lobe or the superior segment of the lower lobe (if the patient aspirated while supine). The bacterial infection is generally polymicrobial with mouth anaerobes predominating, and antibiotic treatment with penicillin or clindamycin is necessary.

PULMONARY EDEMA, ACUTE LUNG INJURY AND ACUTE RESPIRATORY DISTRESS SYNDROME

General

Pregnant women are known to develop pulmonary edema more frequently than non-pregnant women. The incidence of pulmonary edema in pregnancy is estimated to be between 80 and 500 cases per 100 000 and is responsible for 25% of transfers of obstetric patients to intensive care units. The average time to resolution of non-cardiogenic pulmonary edema in pregnancy is between 2 and 3 days and although half of all cases will need intensive care monitoring, only a small minority will need endotracheal intubation and mechanical ventilation.

Both the normal decrease in serum oncotic pressure that occurs in pregnancy (due to a physiologic dilutional hypoalbuminemia) and changes in maternal endothelium may explain this pregnancy-related propensity to pulmonary edema.

Despite these physiologic changes, the occurrence of pulmonary edema still requires an inciting agent or event to 'tip the balance' and allow fluid to move into the interstitial spaces of the lung. The typical precipitating factors are discussed below. While pulmonary edema can be cardiogenic or non-cardiogenic only the non-cardiogenic causes will be discussed here. Cardiogenic pulmonary edema is discussed in Chapter 2.

In all cases, the presence of excessive crystalloid administration, anemia and/or multi-fetal gestations can significantly increase the risk that a particular precipitating factor will lead to pulmonary edema. In fact, many experts believe that excessive fluid administration in and of itself can cause pulmonary edema in pregnancy without any other precipitating cause.

Causes of pulmonary edema in pregnancy

Tocolysis

A previously common cause of pulmonary edema in pregnancy is the use of beta-adrenergic agonists (such as terbutaline) for tocolysis. The proposed mechanism by which these agents might be able to cause pulmonary edema includes beta-mimetic effects on capillary permeability and plasma colloid osmotic pressure and/or a primary cardiogenic component related to beta-mimetic induced myocardial fatigue. The fluids routinely given in association with tocolytics are also likely responsible. This is less common since the advent of new therapies for tocolysis such as atosiban and nifedipine.

Pre-eclampsia

Pre-eclampsia is another important precipitant of pulmonary edema, which develops in 3% of patients with the condition. 30% of these cases occur antepartum and 70% occur in the 72 hours after delivery. Pulmonary edema often occurs in women with the severest forms of pre-eclampsia or eclampsia so maternal and fetal morbidity and mortality is high. Pre-eclampsia related pulmonary edema can be multifactorial. Pre-eclampsia related drops in plasma colloid oncotic pressure and alterations in endothelial permeability are important non-cardiogenic precipitants. In some cases there is a cardiogenic contribution to the pulmonary edema in pre-eclampsia. A stiff left ventricle with significant diastolic dysfunction working against a high systemic vascular resistance may contribute. In others, pre-eclampsia related vasospasm and endothelial effects may induce a transiently stunned myocardium that manifests as ventricular systolic dysfunction.

Sepsis

Sepsis is another important risk factor for pulmonary edema in pregnancy. Pneumonia is a direct insult to the lungs that can precipitate secondary pulmonary edema. However, any systemic bacterial infection can lead to pulmonary edema in pregnant women. Again, alterations in plasma colloid oncotic pressure, capillary permeability and sensitivity of pregnant women to endotoxins are all likely contributory factors. Pyelonephritis, chorioamnionitis and appendicitis may all lead to acute respiratory compromise in some pregnant patients.

Clinical findings in pulmonary edema in pregnancy

Patients with pulmonary edema may present with increasing dyspnea, orthopnea and/or cough/hemoptysis in association with tachypnea and tachycardia. The chest may initially be clear to auscultation, but eventually diffuse crackles and/or wheezing develop.

Arterial blood gases in patients with pulmonary edema typically initially show a decrease in both PaO_2 and $PaCO_2$. As the condition worsens, PaO_2 will decrease further but $PaCO_2$ may increase if the patient is no longer able to maintain adequate ventilation and respiratory failure ensues. The chest radiograph in pulmonary edema may initially be normal but eventually pulmonic infiltrates and often pleural effusions develop. Classically, pulmonary edema is associated with diffuse chest X-ray changes. However, in some cases of pulmonary edema the damage may be patchy or unilateral, particularly if a patient has spent prolonged periods in the left lateral decubitus position or in the Trendelenburg position.

Management of pulmonary edema in pregnancy

Pulmonary edema in pregnancy is a medical emergency. The first and immediate goal is to maintain adequate maternal oxygenation ($PaO_2 > 70$ mmHg) through the use of oxygen supplementation to avoid hypoxia in the fetus. A maternal oxygen saturation of 95% is generally aimed for.

The second step is to carefully consider the full differential diagnosis. Presence of fever, a history of any infectious exposures and any infectious prodrome may suggest the need for empiric antibiotics. If in doubt, it is often worth beginning a course of antibiotics for pneumonia until the clinical picture becomes clearer. An inquiry should also be made into any history suggestive of aspiration such as an episode of choking occurring in the setting of altered mental status. A review of the patient's risk factors for thromboembolic disease should also occur and if the onset of the patient's dyspnea was acute and the chest X-ray is not typical for pulmonary edema, a CT angiogram, ventilation perfusion scan or pulmonary angiogram should be considered. A review of the patient's history for any recent transfusions or drug use should also be carried out.

Differentiating non-cardiogenic pulmonary edema from cardiogenic pulmonary edema caused by peripartum cardiomyopathy, ischemic heart disease or occult valvular heart disease begins with a careful history, cardiac examination and ECG. When doubt exists an echocardiogram is indicated to exclude or confirm a cardiac cause. Unsuspected cardiac abnormalities are not unusual in cases of pulmonary edema even in the setting of pre-eclampsia or tocolytic therapy.

Patients presenting with suspected pulmonary edema in pregnancy should have the following blood tests performed: (1) complete blood count (CBC), (to look for anemia as a contributing factor), (2) creatinine and blood urea nitrogen (to look for renal failure as a contributing factor), (3) PTT, fibrinogen and fibrinogen degradation products (FDP) (to look for evidence of amniotic fluid embolism), (4) 'pre-eclampsia bloods' (AST, uric acid and urinalysis in addition to the above-mentioned CBC and creatinine) in any patient greater than 20 weeks gestation, (5) blood and urine cultures in all patients with a fever and (6) a urine drug screen (to look for evidence of cocaine or narcotics as a cause).

The third step in managing acute pulmonary edema in pregnancy, if the other causes of respiratory failure appear unlikely, is to address any possible underlying precipitating cause. If the pulmonary edema is due to tocolytics, they should generally be discontinued. If pre-eclampsia is the presumed cause, maternal blood pressure should be controlled below 160/100 mmHg and consideration given to

delivery. Magnesium, if necessary for the pre-eclampsia, should be given in the smallest volume possible. A careful examination for evidence of any underlying infection should be carried out with particular consideration of pyelonephritis, appendicitis and chorioamnionitis/endometritis. Appropriate treatment for any suspected infection should be initiated.

Since intravenous fluids are often important contributors to pulmonary edema in pregnancy, careful monitoring of fluid balance is essential. Minimizing intravenous fluids and aiming for a neutral or negative fluid balance is critical. Although some of these patients will not be volume overloaded, use of a diuretic to try to achieve the lowest possible pulmonary artery occlusive pressure that will still support normal blood pressure is advisable. Data from the treatment of acute respiratory disease syndrome in non-pregnant patients suggest that lowering the pulmonary artery wedge pressure by 25% with diuretics and fluid restriction can improve pulmonary function and perhaps outcome. It is our experience that most patients with pulmonary edema in pregnancy will respond dramatically to doses of furosemide as low as 10 mg i.v. Use of such a low dose has an additional importance in the setting of pre-eclampsia because many pre-eclamptic patients are relatively volume-contracted intravascularly despite having massive amounts of peripheral edema and pulmonary edema. Overdiuresis of a pre-eclamptic patient can lead to intravascular hypovolemia that might impair placental perfusion and cause fetal distress. Despite the need for careful fluid restriction and gentle diuresis, there is little evidence for a role for central hemodynamic monitoring in these patients and the vast majority of these women can be successfully managed without pulmonary artery catheterization.

Endotracheal intubation

If oxygenation cannot be maintained above a PaO_2 of 70 mmHg or the patient shows evidence of becoming tired (by either subjective evidence based on the findings of accessory muscle use, intercostal indrawing and abdominal breathing, or on the basis of a rising $PaCO_2$), a trial of spontaneous breathing with supplemental oxygen and positive end expiratory pressure administered through a tightly fitting mask should be attempted. Non-invasive nasal intermittent positive pressure ventilation (NIPPV) may also be used but a theoretical concern about the possibility of aspiration with NIPPV has limited its use in critical care obstetrics.

Intubation is generally required if the patient is unresponsive to therapy and has signs of respiratory failure (a PaO_2 less than 70 mmHg or $PaCO_2$ greater than 45 mmHg on 100% oxygen administered through a tightly fitting mask and a non-rebreathing mask). Intubation of the pregnant woman should always be performed by the most experienced person available. Intubation and mechanical ventilation of pregnant women is discussed in Chapter 18 – Anesthesia and critical illness in pregnancy.

PNEUMOTHORAX AND PNEUMOMEDIASTINUM

Pneumomediastinum is the presence of free air in the mediastinum. It is rare in pregnancy but when it does occur this is most often in the setting of hyperemesis or labor and delivery. Both situations are associated with intense increases in intra-alveolar pressure that cause rupture of marginal alveoli. Air from these marginal alveoli is released into tissue planes along the microvasculature and tracks towards the mediastinum and subsequently dissects tissue planes towards the face, causing subcutaneous emphysema. Pneumomediastinum can present with sudden onset of dyspnea and chest pain that may radiate to the shoulder and arm and be worse with swallowing, coughing and deep breaths. Hamman's sign – a crackling sound that occurs with each heartbeat – may be present. Subcutaneous emphysema may take hours to develop. A chest X-ray may show a radiolucent stripe outlining the left heart border or adjacent to the thoracic aorta. Lateral films may show either retrosternal air or increased definition of the mediastinal structures. This condition usually resolves spontaneously. In patients who have had hyperemesis, esophageal rupture should be considered as an alternative diagnosis but these patients generally have a rapidly deteriorating course with progressive evidence of sepsis.

Primary spontaneous pneumothorax is the presence of free air in the pleural space that occurs without a significant precipitating event in a person with no clinical lung disease. It can occur at any time in pregnancy but again is particularly common in the setting of hyperemesis or the Valsalva maneuver in labor. Patients who have spontaneous pneumothoraces are believed to have previously unrecognized subpleural blebs. Smoking is also a risk factor. Primary spontaneous pneumothorax typically presents with sudden onset of dyspnea and chest pain. Physical findings may include decreased chest excursion on the affected side, diminished breath sounds, and hyper-resonant percussion. The diagnosis is confirmed by demonstration of a pleural line on the standard chest radiograph.

If the pneumothorax is less than 15% of the hemithorax, treatment options include observation with supplemental oxygen or simple aspiration. Larger or persistent pneumothoraces warrant either thorascopy (with instillation of a pleurodesis agent, stapling of blebs and/or pleural abrasion) or tube thoracostomy with or without a pleurodesis agent. All of the above procedures may be carried out in pregnancy if indicated. Since this tends to be a recurrent condition, consideration of corrective intervention is warranted for many patients.

SMOKING

The association between cigarettes and cancer, chronic obstructive pulmonary disease (COPD) and coronary artery disease is well established. In the last decade considerable advances have been made into understanding the effects of smoking on the fetus.

Between 15 and 29% of pregnant women smoke. Pregnancy seems an ideal time for clinicians to intervene and help women to stop smoking both for the benefit of their fetus and their own long-term heath. An important part of assisting women to quit smoking while pregnant is to inform them clearly of the risks that cigarettes represent to the pregnancy. The facts as we presently understand them are as follows:

1. Smoking may increase the risk of birth defects including cleft lip/palate, terminal transverse limb defects and urinary tract anomalies.
2. Smoking is associated with a decrease in birth weight that is independent of gestational age.
3. Smoking is associated with a higher perinatal mortality rate likely because of its association with an increased risk of abruptio placentae, placenta previa, premature rupture of membranes, preterm birth and intrauterine growth restriction.
4. Smoking is associated with an increased risk of sudden infant death syndrome (SIDS).
5. Smoking appears to be associated with an increased risk of childhood cancers, childhood asthma, infant respiratory infections and a decrease in long-term growth in lung function that appears to be somewhat independent of exposure to second-hand smoke after birth.

Interventions to aid smoking cessation in pregnancy appear to be both effective in decreasing smoking and in preventing the adverse outcomes associated with it. Group programs coupled with a smoking cessation aid such as bupropion and or nicotine replacement therapy achieve the best quit rates. However, bupropion is not generally regarded as an appropriate drug for this indication in pregnancy, and use of nicotine replacement therapy – while in this author's opinion clearly a better choice than continued smoking – has not yet gained general acceptance. Group counseling should be strongly encouraged but for many women the time and cost involved is prohibitive. For most women the most important help will come in the form of her own desire to quit and the informed support of her healthcarers. After informing the patient of the risks of smoking and exploring with the patient what she can expect to go through when she does quit, a follow-up doctor's appointment 3-7 days after a 'quit date' chosen by the patient and her doctor should be scheduled. This simple intervention has been shown to significantly increase the patient's likelihood of success in quitting. A useful online resource for both patients and their providers can be found at www.helppregnantsmokersquit.org.

Further reading

Barnardo P D, Jenking J G 2000 l. Failed intubation in obstetrics: a 6-year review in a UK region. Anaesthesia 55:685-694

Baughman R B, Lower E E, du Bois R M 2003 Sarcoidosis. Lancet 361:1111-1118

British Thoracic Society 2001 Guidelines for the Management of Community Acquired Pneumonia in Adults. 2001 Guidelines. Thorax 56(suppl IV):1-64. http://www.brit-thoracic.org.uk/c2/uploads/MACAP2001gline.pdf

Dombrowski M P, Schatz M, Wise R, et al 2004 Asthma during pregnancy. Obstetrics and Gynecology 103(1):5-12

Gilljam M, Antoniou M, Shin J, et al 2000 Pregnancy in cystic fibrosis. Fetal and maternal outcome. Chest 118(1):85-91

Gorospe L, Puente S, Madrid C, et al 2002 Spontaneous pneumothorax during pregnancy. Southern Medical Journal 95(5):555-558

Incaudo G A 2004 Diagnosis and treatment of allergic rhinitis and sinusitis during pregnancy and lactation. Clinical Reviews in Allergy and Immunology 27(2):159-177

King T E Jr 1992 Restrictive lung disease in pregnancy. Clinics in Chest Medicine 13(4):607-622

Kwon H L, Belanger K, Bracken M B 2004 Effect of pregnancy and stage of pregnancy on asthma severity: a systematic review. American Journal of Obstetrics and Gynecology 190(5):201-210

Laibl V R, Sheffield J S 2005 Influenza and pneumonia in pregnancy. Clinics in Perinatology 32(3):727-738

Laibl V R, Sheffield J S 2005 Tuberculosis in pregnancy. Clinics in Perinatology 32(3):739-747

Lumley J, Oliver S S, Chamberlain C, et al 2004 Interventions for promoting smoking cessation during pregnancy. Cochrane Database Systematic Review Oct 18;(4):CD001055

Mabie W C, Hackman B B, Sibai B M 1993 Acute pulmonary edema associated with pregnancy: Echocardiographic insights and implications for treatment. Obstetrics and Gynecology 81:227-234

Mandell L A, Bartlett J G, Dowell S F, et al 2003 Update of practice guidelines for the management of community-acquired pneumonia in immunocompetent adults. Clinical Infectious Diseases 37(11):1405-1433.

NAEEP Working Group Report on Managing Asthma During Pregnancy 2004 Recommendations for pharmacologic treatment update 2004. NIH Publication no. 05-3279. Online. Available: http://www.nhlbi.nih.gov/health/prof/lung/asthma/astpreg.htm 26 Apr 2006

Ormerod P 2001 Tuberculosis in pregnancy and the puerperium. Thorax 56:494

Powrie R O 2001 Drugs in pregnancy. Respiratory disease. Best Practice and Research. Clinical Obstetrics and Gynaecology 15(6):913-936.

Sciscione A C, Ivester T, Largoza M, et al 2003 Acute pulmonary edema in pregnancy. Obstetrics and Gynecology 101(3):511-515

Selroos O 1990 Sarcoidosis and pregnancy: a review with results of a retrospective survey. Journal of Internal Medicine 227:221

To W W, Wong M W 1996 Kyphoscoliosis complicating pregnancy. International Journal of Gynaecology and Obstetrics 55(2):123-128

Appendix A US Food and Drug Administration (FDA) classification of drug risk in pregnancy

US FDA Drug Risk in Pregnancy category	Definition
Category A	Controlled studies in women fail to demonstrate a risk to the fetus in the first trimester (and there is no evidence of a risk in later trimesters), and the possibility of fetal harm appears remote.
Category B	Either animal-reproduction studies have not demonstrated a fetal risk but there are no controlled studies in pregnant women, or animal-reproduction studies have shown an adverse effect (other than a decrease in fertility) that was not confirmed in controlled studies in women in the first trimester (and there is no evidence of a risk in later trimesters).
Category C	Either studies in animals have revealed adverse effects on the fetus (teratogenic or embryocidal or other) and there are no controlled studies in women, or studies in women and animals are not available. Drugs should be given only if the potential benefit justifies the potential risk to the fetus.
Category D	There is positive evidence of human fetal risk, but the benefits from use in pregnant women may be acceptable despite the risk (e.g. if the drug is needed in a life-threatening situation or for a serious disease for which safer drugs cannot be used or are ineffective).
Category X	Studies in animals or human beings have demonstrated fetal abnormalities, or there is evidence of fetal risk based on human experience or both, and the risk of the use of the drug in pregnant women clearly outweighs any possible benefit. The drug is contraindicated in women who are or may become pregnant.

Chapter 7

Hematological disorders

I. D. Walker

INTRODUCTION

The demands of the developing uterus and fetus pose a major challenge to maternal hematological systems. This is due to the increase in maternal plasma volume (see Ch. 2) and a rising red cell mass and hemoglobin mass. Among women not on iron supplements, the red cell mass may increase by only 15-20%, but, in women taking iron supplements the red cell mass rises 20-30% above non-pregnant levels by the end of pregnancy. The increased blood volume and hemoglobin mass provide a reserve against the blood loss at parturition.

Anemia is common in pregnancy, particularly in underdeveloped countries and in women whose nutritional status is compromised by poverty or lifestyle. In many of the world's poorer regions other factors such as infestation or infection further increase the risk of anemia. Inherited abnormalities of globin are prevalent in many areas, and with increasing population mobility they are of increasing relevance in areas where they were previously seen rarely. Underlying hematological disorders such as polycythemia and essential thrombocythemia are uncommon in young women and may be asymptomatic. These disorders are frequently first recognized on a routine full blood count ordered from the antenatal clinic.

ANEMIA

Anemia is defined arbitrarily as a reduction in peripheral blood hemoglobin concentration, red cell count or hematocrit to below the levels in the 'normal' population. The World Health Organization has suggested that in the non-pregnant adult female, the lower limit of the normal range for hemoglobin concentration is 12 g/dL and defined anemia during pregnancy as a hemoglobin of less than 11 g/dL. The Centers for Disease Control and Prevention have modified the definition to include hemoglobins of less than 11.0 g/dL in the first and third trimesters and less than 10.5 g/dL in the second trimester.

The clinical effects of anemia depend on its severity and rapidity of onset as well as other general health factors such as infection or heart disease. In acute blood loss, the symptoms and signs are related to falling blood volume. In more slowly developing anemia, the total blood volume may be only slightly reduced as plasma volume increases to compensate. The effects of chronic anemia are due to the decreased ability to deliver oxygen to the tissues and the compensatory changes in the cardiovascular system.

Physiological anemia of pregnancy

Low hemoglobin concentrations are part of the normal physiologic response to pregnancy. The greater increase in plasma volume than in red cell mass results in a dilutional anemia. Hemoglobin concentration falls from early pregnancy to reach a nadir at 36 weeks gestation 2.0-2.5 g/dL below the pre-pregnancy concentration. The maternal hematocrit similarly falls from early pregnancy to reach its nadir about 6.5% lower than the pre-pregnancy hematocrit at 36 weeks gestation. Following delivery about 500 mL of blood sequestered in uteroplacental vessels is autotransfused into the maternal circulation. In healthy women, 3 months after a normal delivery, mean hemoglobin and hematocrit levels have returned to their pre-pregnancy values and the vast majority of women who enter pregnancy non-anemic are again non-anemic.

HEMATINIC DEFICIENCY

Iron deficiency

The iron content of the body is the result of a balance between the amount of iron absorbed and the amount lost. Non-pregnant women require around 1300 µg of iron per day to replace normal physiological losses including menstrual iron loss. The fetus requires about 280 mg of iron and a further 400-500 mg is required for the expansion of the maternal red cell mass. About 200 mg of iron are lost with the placenta and bleeding at delivery. Each normal pregnancy and delivery therefore requires around 1 g of iron. In spite of increased absorption of iron during pregnancy and reduced iron loss with the cessation of menstruation, as pregnancy progresses most women develop falling serum iron levels, rising total iron binding capacity and a mild hypochromic, microcytic anemia. A third to a half of all pregnant women who do not use iron supplements will have a hemoglobin of less than 11 g/dL (Department of Health 1992). In women eating an adequate diet, the decrease in hemoglobin concentration is seldom great enough to pose a serious clinical problem. The risk of symptomatic iron deficiency anemia is increased in women of low socio-economic status or limited education, in those with poor nutrition, in multiparae, in women with multiple gestations and in women with a history of menorrhagia. In developing countries the prevalence of iron deficiency anemia is increased and dietary iron may be inadequate to meet the added demands placed on maternal iron stores by her increasing red cell mass and the growing fetus and placenta.

What are the risks associated with iron deficiency?

Although there is no doubt that iron supplementation in pregnancy raises maternal hemoglobin concentration, there is a lack of evidence that maternal iron supplementation has a consistent effect on the hematologic status of the fetus or neonate. Among the postulated maternal risks of iron deficiency anemia are fatigue, cardiovascular stress, impaired resistance to infection and poor tolerance of blood loss. Anemic mothers have an increased risk of requiring blood transfusion (with its attendant risks) and perhaps of an operative delivery although supportive data is lacking. The postulated risks to the conceptus and placenta relate to the impaired delivery of oxygen. Whilst providing consistent evidence that anemia during pregnancy increases the risk of adverse pregnancy outcome (preterm birth, low birth weight, stillbirth and neonatal death), the published observational studies have limitations. Many lack statistical power and interventions vary widely from study to study. Few have report clinical outcomes: most have used changes in hematologic indices as markers of effect. In some studies, women were given not only iron but folate and/or other vitamins. A randomized trial carried out in Scotland in the 1960s noted no difference in the incidence of adverse pregnancy outcomes between women randomized to placebo and those randomized to daily iron supplements. Most published studies do not control for other factors, such as smoking, known to be associated with adverse pregnancy outcome. Studies from developing countries have often failed to recognize that factors associated with endemic anemia, such as malaria, may be more directly responsible than iron deficiency for poor pregnancy outcomes.

Iron-deficient infants score relatively poorly on tests of psychomotor development but it is not clear whether iron supplementation during pregnancy lowers the incidence of iron deficiency in children or improves results in these tests. Except in severe maternal iron deficiency, protective mechanisms allow the fetus to achieve proper hemoglobin and iron stores regardless of maternal values. Most published evidence suggests that iron-deficient mothers are no more likely to give birth to an iron-deficient child than are women with replete iron stores.

Routine iron supplementation

Routine iron supplementation in pregnancy raises or maintains the maternal serum ferritin above 10 µg/L and reduces the number of women with hemoglobin below 10 or 10.5 g/dL in late pregnancy. The previous practice of administering iron supplements to all pregnant women has been criticized on the grounds that it may increase blood viscosity, impairing placental circulation and fetal growth. It has been suggested that where there are facilities for routine hemoglobin monitoring and where antenatal attendance is regular, iron supplements should be offered only to those who demonstrate evidence of iron deficiency anemia. The largest trial of selective versus routine iron supplements in pregnancy reported a reduced risk of stillbirth and neonatal death in the selective supplementation group but there was also a significantly increased likelihood of Cesarean section (OR 1.36, 96% CI 1.04-1.78) and postpartum blood transfusion (OR 1.68, 95% CI 1.05-2.67), possibly because attendant clinicians were made nervous by the lower hematocrits in this group.

From the limited number of evaluable trials, no clear conclusions can be drawn about the effects, beneficial or harmful, of iron supplementation on either maternal or fetal outcomes. Thus there is no evidence to proscribe a policy of offering iron supplements to all pregnant women. Indeed, routine supplementation is justifiable in populations where there is a high background prevalence of iron deficiency anemia.

Folate deficiency

Folic acid is a water-soluble B complex vitamin found in leafy green vegetables, liver, nuts and fruits. It is required for the synthesis of DNA and RNA. In the absence of folate or vitamin B_{12} the conversion of homocysteine to methionine is impaired and homocysteine levels rise. During normal pregnancy, folate requirement increases to around 400 µg per day, partly due to transfer of folate to the fetus but mainly due to increased folate catabolism. As a result of hemodilution and a negative folate balance, there is a gradual fall in serum folate levels as pregnancy progresses. Deficiency of this vitamin during pregnancy may result in maternal megaloblastosis and red cell macrocytosis and an increased risk of a low birthweight baby. Without folate supplementation during pregnancy, about a third of women will have subnormal folate levels in the puerperium and around 10% of them will develop a macrocytic anemia. Folic acid demands are increased in patients with hemolytic anemia (including sickle cell disease) and in areas where malaria is endemic.

Folic acid supplementation to prevent neural tube defects

Serum and red cell folate and serum vitamin B_{12} levels are lower and plasma homocysteine levels are higher in women who have a fetus with a neural tube development defect than in women carrying an unaffected fetus. Periconceptional ingestion of folic acid reduces the risk of fetal neural tube defects. The effect is seen in all women, not just those with a previously affected pregnancy. Deficiency of folate or vitamin B_{12} alone probably does not directly cause neural tube defects, but women who have affected infants may have an underlying abnormality in their homocysteine metabolic pathway. Folic acid supplementation during pregnancy results in lower homocysteine levels. UK national guidelines recommend that women with a previous fetus with a neural tube defect attempting to conceive should take 4 mg of folic acid orally daily until the 12th week of pregnancy. For primary prevention, increased dietary intake plus a daily supplement of 400 µg of folate (until the 12th week) is recommended.

Folic acid supplementation to prevent anemia

The value of routine folic acid supplementation throughout the whole of pregnancy remains unclear. Supplementation reduces the risk of having a hemoglobin of less than 10.0-10.5 g/dL and of macrocytic anemia. There is no evident benefit in reducing other adverse obstetric events. However, there is no evidence of adverse effects and folate supplementation should be given where nutrition is compromised, such as with hyperemesis and inflammatory bowel disease, celiac disease, etc.

Vitamin B_{12} levels in pregnancy

Deficiency of vitamin B_{12} (cobalamin) results in megaloblastosis and macrocytic anemia with potential neurological problems and reduced fertility. Cobalamin is synthesized solely by micro-organisms and its only source is food of animal origin. Vegans and those with grossly inadequate diets for any reason are at risk of deficiency.

Maternal cobalamin stores in healthy women are about 3000 µg, more than adequate for the developing fetus whose requirement is around 50 µg. During late pregnancy, serum cobalamin levels fall as a result of hemodilution and active transport across the placenta, with reduced levels seen in up to a third of uncomplicated pregnancies. Some of the fall in serum levels is caused by hormonally induced changes in transcobalamin binder production. After delivery levels return rapidly to normal without supplementation.

HEMOGLOBINOPATHIES

Inherited disorders of hemoglobin are worldwide the commonest single-gene disorders, affecting about 7% of the world population as carriers. Population migration has resulted in these conditions being seen with increasing frequency in countries where they had not previously occurred.

Structure of hemoglobin

The embryo, the fetus and the adult have different hemoglobins adapted for their particular oxygen requirements. Human hemoglobins are all tetramers consisting of two pairs of globin chains, each of which is attached to one heme molecule. In adults, the major hemoglobin, hemoglobin A (HbA) consists of two pairs of α chains and two pairs of β chains: $\alpha_2\beta_2$. A second, minority, adult hemoglobin hemoglobin A_2 (HbA$_2$) consists of two pairs of α chains and two pairs of δ chains: $\alpha_2\delta_2$. Normally, the ratio of production of α to non-α globin chains is very close to unity. In the fetus the major hemoglobin, hemoglobin F (HbF) consists of two pairs of α chains and two pairs of γ chains: $\alpha_2\gamma_2$. A number of different hemoglobins are produced as the embryo develops – α-like chains called ζ chains combine with γ chains to form hemoglobin Portland ($\zeta_2\gamma_2$) or with ε chains to form hemoglobin Gower 1 ($\zeta_2\varepsilon_2$) and α chains combine with ε chains to form hemoglobin Gower 2 ($\alpha_2\varepsilon_2$).

Thalassemia

The thalassemias are single-gene disorders (with many different mutations) characterized by impaired production of normal globin peptide chains. They occur widely throughout the world reflecting heterozygote protection against malaria.

β-Thalassaemia

The β-thalassemias are prevalent in a wide belt from the Mediterranean and parts of North and West Africa through the Middle East and Indian subcontinent to South-east Asia. The high incidence zone includes the former Yugoslavia, Romania, the southern part of the former USSR, southern regions of China, Thailand, the Malay Peninsula, Indonesia and some Pacific island populations but β-thalassemia can occur sporadically in any racial group.

The β-globin gene cluster is on chromosome 11. Impaired production of β-globin chains leads to a relative excess of α-globin chains which cannot form soluble tetramers on their own, and precipitate within the cell. The degree of α-globin chain excess determines the severity of clinical manifestations, with homozygous patients experiencing severe clinical manifestations and heterozygotes having only minimal or mild anemia.

Homozygous β-thalassemia

β-Thalassemia major (homozygous β-thalassemia – Cooley's anemia) is characterized by markedly ineffective erythropoiesis and severe hemolysis. Clinical manifestations are seen in many organ systems. Patients suffer simultaneously from the effects of severe and chronic anemia, from chronic hemolysis, and from the local and systemic effects of a rapidly expanding mass of erythroid bone marrow progenitors. Transfusion therapy causes iron overload with end-organ damage. Folic acid deficiency may develop due the high rate of cellular turnover. Cardiac hemosiderosis is a feared complication of repeated transfusion. Without early institution of iron chelation therapy patients develop a sterile pericarditis, arrhythmias, and restrictive cardiomyopathy. Sexual development is delayed and fertility is often reduced due to anovulation subsequent to hemosiderin deposits. Prior to the introduction of hypertransfusions and chelation therapy in the late 1970s, pregnancy was rare in patients with thalassemia major, however within the past decade favorable perinatal outcomes have been reported in women with β-thalassemia major, although the Cesarean section rate is high.

Heterozygous β-thalassemia

The terms β-thalassemia minor and β-thalassemia trait describe heterozygotes with one normal β-globin allele and one β-thalassemic allele. Heterozygotes are usually symptom-free except in periods of excess stress such as pregnancy when they tend to become anemic. Hemoglobin values are in the 9-11 g/dL range and the red cells are hypochromic and microcytic, sometimes erroneously diagnosed as iron deficiency anemia. The microcytosis is however more profound than in iron deficiency. Characteristically hemoglobin A_2 levels are raised to 4-6% with a slight rise in HbF to 1-3% in 50% of cases. The bone marrow shows erythroid hyperplasia. Splenomegaly is rare. β-Thalassemia is commonly co-inherited with other structural hemoglobin variants

α-Thalassemia

α-Thalassemias are due to impaired production of α-globin chains, with resultant relative excess of β-globin chains that seem less toxic on the red cell memberane than the excess α-globin chains in β-thalassemia. α-Thalassemia is caused by mutations or deletions on chromosome 16 affecting one, two, three or four α-globin genes leading to decreased production of α-globin chains.

α^+-Thalassemia trait (inactivation or deletion of a single α-globin gene) is usually asymptomatic. As a population, the mean of the mean corpuscular volume (MCV) may be less than that in a normal population but individual patients rarely fall below the normal range for MCV.

α^0-Thalassemia trait (two α-globin genes are deleted or inactivated) usually leads to mild anemia. The peripheral blood film shows hypochromia, microcytosis and target cells. The MCV is often less than 80 fL, but hemoglobin electrophoresis is normal.

Hemoglobin H disease (inactivation or deletion of three α-globin genes) is associated with moderate anemia, marked microcytosis and hypochromia. Such marked impairment in α-globin production results in accumulation of excess unpaired β-globin chains which form β_4 tetramers known as hemoglobin H (HbH). Hemoglobin H exhibits a dramatically left-shifted oxygen dissociation curve. It is therefore ineffective for oxygen transport. Patients suffer chronic hemolysis, due to the formation of inclusion bodies in circulating red cells as HbH precipitates, easily seen in the blood film, with hypochromia and microcytosis. Typically patients with hemoglobin H disease exhibit the signs of chronic hemolytic anemia, including hepatosplenomegaly, indirect hyperbilirubinemia, elevated LDH, reduced haptoglobin, leg ulcers and premature biliary tract disease. Transfusion support is usually necessary from the second or third decade of life and iron overload is a significant issue. Because HbH is readily oxidized, exacerbation of hemolysis may occur with exposure to oxidant stressors, such as infection or oxidizing drugs. Aplastic or hypoplastic crises are also possible.

Hemoglobin Barts is the presence of four α-globin gene defects. α-Globin is essential for the production of both adult HbA ($\alpha_2\beta_2$) and HbF ($\alpha_2\gamma_2$). When none of the four α-globin gene loci is functional, γ_4 tetramers form in the fetal red cells (Hb Barts). Affected fetuses have deficient oxygen transport capabilities. Most develop severe hydrops and die in utero during the second or third trimester or shortly after birth. Occasional live births have been reported. Affected neonates require massive total exchange transfusions. Mothers of fetuses with hydrops fetalis are at risk for the development of polyhydramnios, and associated obstetric complications.

Genetic counseling and prenatal diagnosis of thalassemia

With two parents each heterozygous for β-thalassemia, the chance of producing a child with heterozygous β-thalassemia are 1 in 2, a homozygous child are 1 in 4, and a normal child 1 in 4. Such couples should be referred to a center with special expertise in the management of thalassemia and access to a hemoglobinopathy reference laboratory.

The potential risks, benefits and availability of prenatal diagnosis should be discussed with them prior to pregnancy. Within individual populations β-thalassemia mutations have been thoroughly characterized and categorized. Using polymerase chain reaction (PCR) techniques and allele-specific oligonucleotide hybridization probes designed to detect the most prevalent mutations, diagnosis of homozygous β-thalassemia, β-heterozygous thalassemia, compound heterozygous states and normal hemoglobin genotypes is generally possible on a chorion villous sample or on amniocytes.

Couples in whom a fetus homozygous for β-thalassemia is identified may choose pregnancy termination, an individual decision that depends on personal, cultural and religious beliefs. The considerable burden of disease morbidity must be weighed against the potential for long-term survival. One study has raised the possibility of early stem cell transplantation for homozygous β-thalassemia. In some regions of the world, such as Cyprus, Sardinia, Northern Italy and parts of Greece, genetic counseling, DNA-based prenatal diagnosis and selective abortion has led to a nearly complete eradication of new cases of severe β-thalassemia. In other areas the uptake of prenatal diagnosis and selective termination of pregnancy is lower.

α-Thalassemia possesses more complex genetics (see Fig. 7.1) than β-thalassemia. Since uncomplicated α^+ and α^0 thalassemia traits (single or two α-globin gene defects) are usually asymptomatic, the likelihood of foreknowledge of families at risk is less than in families with β-globin defects. Women in whose families hemoglobin H or hydrops fetalis (due to defects in three or four α-globin genes) have previously occurred are at risk of giving birth to further affected infants. In these patients the principles of genetic counseling and prenatal diagnosis are similar to those outlined above for β-thalassemia.

Sickle cell disease

Sickle cell disease refers to a group of genetic disorders characterized by the presence of hemoglobin S (HbS). The clinical manifestations of the disease are due to the tendency of HbS to polymerize and deform red cells into a characteristic sickle shape. This property is due to the substitution of valine for glutamic acid at position 6 of the β-globin chain ($\beta^{6glu} \rightarrow {}^{val}$ or β^S). Included within the group are homozygous HbS (sickle cell anemia), double heterozygote states, e.g. HbS with hemoglobin C disease, HbS with β-thalassemia, HbS with α-thalassemia, and HbS with high fetal hemoglobin.

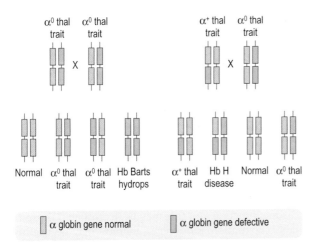

Figure 7.1 Genetics of α-thalassemia.

Clinical features of sickling disorders

Hemoglobin concentrations of 6-8 g/dL, macrocytosis, reticulocytosis and the presence of many sickled cells on the peripheral blood film are typical of homozygous (SS) sickle cell anemia. Patients with heterozygous HbS in combination with another heterozygous hemoglobin disorder like hemoglobin C have higher hemoglobin levels. Microcytosis would suggest the patient either has an associated thalassemia or is iron deficient. Because HbS releases oxygen more readily than HbA, patients with sickle cell anemia often tolerate anemia remarkably well.

Patients with sickle cell disease (SS) may suffer episodes of localized or generalized pain due probably to microscopic tissue infarctions. Clinically they present with fever, leukocytosis and mild elevations of liver enzymes with, or occasionally without, pain. These events may occur spontaneously but frequently they have an identifiable precipitant such as dehydration, infection or physical exertion. Treatment includes hydration and analgesia. Patients with sickle cell disease are at increased risk of infection due to their impaired splenic function, deficiency of opsonin and overloading of the reticuloendothelial system with sickled red cells. Patients with sickle cell disease have a delayed puberty but there is no evidence that they are prone to gynecological problems, nor, as has been suggested, is there evidence that they are relatively infertile.

Management of sickling disorders

Until the mid 1990s, treatment of patients with sickling disorders was limited to supportive care – prevention of infection, folic acid supplementation, hydration and management of pain – with no clinically useful agents available to reduce the risk of HbS polymerization. Since 1995, however, hydroxycarbamide has been increasingly and successfully used in a variety of sickle cell disease situations. The principle rationale for its use is its ability to induce fetal hemoglobin (HbF: $\alpha_2\gamma_2$). Increased HbF levels interfere with HbS polymerization. Hydroxycarbamide also seems to modify red cell–endothelial interactions and to alter the rheological properties of HbS-containing red cells. Hydroxycarbamide is teratogenic and, where appropriate, men and women using this agent should be advised to use effective contraception.

Risk of adverse pregnancy outcome in sickle anemia

Pregnancy increases the risks for women with sickle cell disease but in general the increased risks are not so great as to indicate a routine policy of pregnancy termination. Vascular complications of pregnancy are increased in women with sickle cell disease. Maternal anemia results in poor oxygen delivery to the fetus. Maternal sickled cells plug decidual arterioles causing placental hypoperfusion and hypoxia with subsequent placental injury. Spontaneous miscarriage rates in women with homozygous sickle cell disease have been reported to be between 9% and 24% but may be higher because in many surveys very early pregnancy losses have been overlooked. The risk of intrauterine growth restriction is increased. Pre-eclampsia and intrauterine growth restriction are more common in women with homozygous sickle cell anemia. An increased incidence of placenta previa and abruption has been reported. Preterm labor and premature delivery commonly occur in women with sickle cell disease – perhaps as a result of increased prostaglandin production. Maternal and perinatal morbidity and mortality rates reflect the availability of antenatal services, level of expertise amongst healthcare providers and patient compliance with advice offered.

Preconception counseling

Women with sickle cell disorders should be referred to a unit with special expertise in the diagnosis and management of sickling disorders. Pre-pregnancy they should receive genetic counseling and be informed about the availability of prenatal testing. The advisability of early booking should be stressed. Knowledge of the hemoglobin type of her partner is useful. In couples wishing to conceive, where either partner is using hydroxycarbamide, this should be discontinued 3-6 months ahead of switching to unprotected intercourse. Despite strict instructions to both men and women taking hydroxycarbamide that contraceptive precautions should be taken, a number of successful pregnancies, resulting in healthy live-born infants without congenital malformations, have been reported.

Management during pregnancy

The management of pregnancy in women with sickle cell disease requires input from a multidisciplinary team with expertise in dealing with patients with sickle cell disease – including obstetricians, midwives, hematologists, neonatologists and anesthetists. At the booking antenatal visit a comprehensive assessment is indicated to allow evaluation of factors which may influence pregnancy outcome. Prenatal diagnosis by chorionic villous sampling should be offered early in pregnancy if the partner is a carrier for sickle cell disease. The pre-pregnancy sickling status of the woman usually predicts the antenatal course. Mothers with sickle cell anemia are prone to a range of complications including pain crises, splenic sequestration, left ventricular dysfunction, pyelonephritis and pregnancy hypertension. Folic acid supplements should be given, penicillin prophylaxis continued, and the patient reminded of the importance of maintaining good hydration. The intrauterine growth rate should be monitored as pregnancy progresses.

Women with sickle cell disease experience worsening anemia during pregnancy. Indications for blood transfusion include a reduction in hemoglobin concentration greater than 20% from baseline, a hemoglobin of less than 5 g/dL, anticipated surgery (including cesarean section), acute chest syndrome or septicaemia. If the hemoglobin is less than 5 g/dL and the reticulocyte count less than 3%, simple top-up transfusion with packed red cells is indicated. Partial exchange transfusion is required however if the hemoglobin is 8-10 g/dL and transfusion is indicated – to obtain a post-transfusion hemoglobin concentration of 10-11 g/dL and an HbS level of around 50%.

Acute cholecystitis, presenting with fever and right upper quadrant pain, can occur during pregnancy. Ultrasound assessment of the right upper quadrant may assist in the differential diagnosis. Acute chest syndrome during pregnancy presents with pleuritic pain, tachypnea, fever, cough, leukocytosis and pulmonary infiltrates. The common etiologic agents are mycoplasma, *Haemophilus influenza*, *Streptococcus pneumonia*, staphylococci and Gram-negative organisms. Treatment includes hydration, antibiotics, analgesics and oxygen. The risk of acute chest syndrome increases with decreasing hemoglobin levels. Simple or partial exchange transfusion to reduce HbS to about 50% with a hemoglobin concentration of 8-11 g/dL may be required. It is reported that over 55% of pregnancies in women with sickle cell anemia are complicated by one or more vaso-occlusive events. Achieving adequate pain relief with opiate analgesia if required is important, as in the non-pregnant.

Management of delivery

Chronic anemia and hypoxemia may compromise cardiac function and this may be accentuated during labor. Hydration and oxygen therapy may be useful to minimize the risk of intravascular sickling during labor. Epidural analgesia provides effective analgesia and reduces circulating catecholamine concentrations, lessening the risk of sickling. Regional analgesia also avoids potential airway complications and the depressant effect of anesthetic agents on the neonate. The operative delivery rate is high in women with sickle cell anemia. Following delivery early ambulation is important and the wearing of graduated compression stockings should be encouraged.

Doubly heterozygous disease

Women with sickle hemoglobin C disease or sickle β-thalassemia may be asymptomatic and diagnosed only when they present at antenatal clinic. Patients with these disorders however may suffer pain crises during pregnancy. The majority of patients with sickle hemoglobin C disease or sickle β-thalassemia have splenomegaly and splenic sequestration, with abdominal pain, increasing splenomegaly and pancytopenia, may occur during pregnancy. Blood transfusion to maintain a hemoglobin level between 10-11 g/dL usually reverses the process.

AUTOIMMUNE HEMOLYTIC ANEMIA

Autoimmune disorders are relatively common in young women. In the age range 20-50 years autoimmune hemolysis occurs at a rate of around 5 per million, and in pregnant women, around 20 per million. During pregnancy the antibodies are mainly IgG warm-reacting autoantibodies that do not bind complement but cause hemolysis via antibody-dependent cell-mediated cytotoxicity and phagocytosis. The antibodies can cross the placenta and cause hemolysis in the fetus.

Steroids (initial daily dose 1-2 mg/kg early pregnancy weight) are usually effective in controlling IgG-mediated hemolysis presenting in pregnancy. Intravenous immunoglobulin (0.4 mg/kg early pregnancy weight daily for 4-5 days) has been used but the response rate in autoimmune hemolysis is lower than that in autoimmune thrombocytopenia.

Occasionally IgM cold- or warm-reacting antibodies may be associated with pregnancy autoimmune hemolysis. These do not cross the placenta but they can bind complement and cause intravascular hemolysis which does not usually respond significantly to steroid therapy.

Women with autoimmune hemolysis diagnosed prior to pregnancy or with underlying associated disease (such as systemic lupus erythematosus) generally have more severe hemolysis which is refractory to treatment. In these women maternal and perinatal morbidity and mortality may be significantly increased.

APLASTIC ANEMIA

Aplastic anemia is a life-threatening disorder of the pluripotent stem cell, characterized by absent or severely decreased hematopoietic precursors in the bone marrow. Affected patients have evidence of pancytopenia in the absence of splenomegaly. The peripheral blood and bone marrow are virtually devoid of stem cells bearing the CD34 antigen, measured by flow cytometry. The reduced telomere length noted in patients with aplastic anemia is consistent with hematopoiesis under extreme stress. The classification of aplasia as severe aplastic anemia (SAA – with a neutrophil count below 0.5×10^9/L) and very severe aplastic anemia (VSAA – with a neutrophil count below 0.2×10^9/L) remains useful despite major treatment advances.

Etiology and clinical presentation of aplasia

The stem cell failure may be induced by a variety of disorders but immune mechanisms with local activation of interferon-γ may be a common etiologic path. It is suggested that in most cases bone marrow failure results from immunologically mediated tissue-specific organ destruction. After exposure to an inciting agent, cells and cytokines of the immune system attack and destroy marrow stem cells. The immune mediated causes include transfusion associated graft-versus-host disease, hepatitis associated disease and the aplasia associated with pregnancy.

Typically patients present with a history of recurrent infections, due to neutropenia, and bleeding, secondary to thrombocytopenia. Occasionally the presenting complaint is fatigue due to anemia. The bone marrow is profoundly hypocellular with a decrease in the precursors of all cell lines. The residual hematopoietic cells are morphologically normal and there is no infiltrate of malignant or fibrotic cells. The prognosis is directly related to the quantitative reduction in the peripheral blood cells – particularly the neutrophils.

Management of aplasia

Marrow or peripheral blood stem cell transplantation from a histocompatible donor usually cures the aplasia. Allogeneic transplant however is available to a minority only. Patients without a suitable matched donor have to rely on immunosuppressive therapy using antilymphocyte globulin often combined with ciclosporin. Most patients with aplastic anemia respond favorably to immunosuppressive therapy. Anemia and thrombocytopenia can be corrected by transfusion. Careful oral hygiene and avoidance of minor injuries to skin and mucosae are important. Neutropenic fever must be treated aggressively with parenteral broad-pectrum antibiotics. Fungal infections, in particular aspergillosis, can be difficult to detect early. Antifungal therapy should therefore be introduced in any patient who is persistently febrile.

Aplastic anemia and pregnancy: prognosis and management

Aplastic anemia in pregnancy may be viewed as a chance coincidence or pregnancy may be etiological. The possible association between pregnancy and aplastic anemia has important implications with respect to the risk of relapse in future pregnancies. Pregnancy-associated aplastic anemia was first defined as a clinical entity in 1888 by Ehrlich in a pregnant woman who had died after a brief catastrophic illness. Since then other authors have described cases of hypoplastic anemia in pregnant women. The relationship is however a matter of speculation – some authors holding that the association is coincidental and that the stress of pregnancy merely uncovers a pre-existing disorder. Other authors suggest that relapse of aplasia in pregnancy and recovery with delivery indicates a causal relationship, at least in some. Others have suggested that increased estrogen levels suppress erythropoiesis.

Whether the association is causal or coincidental, there is general agreement that pregnancy has a detrimental effect on the disease as it either worsens or becomes overt during pregnancy. Both mother and fetus are at risk; the fetus because maternal anemia may lead to intrauterine growth restriction and intrauterine death. Maternal neutropenia may result in chorioamnionitis and preterm labor. The maternal mortality associated with aplastic anemia diagnosed in pregnancy has been as high as 20% – mainly due to infection and hemorrhage. Women who have a history of pre-existing aplastic anemia appear to have a better prognosis than those first presenting in pregnancy.

Termination of pregnancy is generally advised in women with severe aplasia. Women who decline pregnancy termination require intensive hematological support during their pregnancy. Repeated platelet transfusion may result in platelet refractoriness. The risk of platelet refractoriness may be minimized by limiting platelet transfusions to situations of overt bleeding, and, ideally, by the use of human leukocyte antigen (HLA)-matched platelets.

PAROXYSMAL NOCTURNAL HEMOGLOBINURIA

Paroxysmal nocturnal hemoglobinuria (PNH) is a rare disorder (1-10 per million) resulting from an acquired defect of one or more lineages of hemopoietic stem cells. The disorder arises from a variety of coding mutations in the phosphotidylinositol glycan (PIG-A) gene with resultant deficiency of specific cell surface proteins which regulate complement activation, and lysis of clonal red cells, white cells and platelets. The cause of the clonal expansion in PNH is unclear.

Clinical presentation of paroxysmal nocturnal hemoglobinuria

Classically PNH presents as nocturnal hemolysis with the passage of dark-colored early morning urine. More often the presentation is insidious with episodes of acute on chronic hemolysis. Serious complications include major intra-abdominal or intracerebral thrombosis, infection and hemorrhage. Major thrombosis is the leading cause of mortality in patients with PNH.

Risks associated with pregnancy in paroxysmal nocturnal hemoglobinuria

Although it is a disease predominantly of young adults only a few cases of pregnancy in women with PNH appear in the literature. Women with PNH are

at risk of obstetric hemorrhage – 14% of 66 women with 88 pregnancies in one study, but they (even those who are thrombocytopenic) are also at increased risk of venous thromboembolism. In a review published in 1999, preterm labor was recorded in half of the 33 pregnant women with PNH. There was a 9% perinatal mortality and 21% maternal mortality. In this review 12% (4 of 33) suffered a major thrombotic event; three of which were fatal.

Management of pregnancy in paroxysmal nocturnal hemoglobinuria

In pregnancy the aim is to maintain maternal hemoglobin concentration above 10 g/dL. Folate supplements should be given but iron supplements should be used with caution as they may provoke a hemolytic episode. Steroids may attenuate an acute hemolytic event but are not generally indicated in chronic hemolysis. In some cases erythropoietin may be helpful. Since many patients are neutropenic, infection control is a priority. Although there is a lack of evidence, prophylactic anticoagulation with a low molecular weight heparin, from the first trimester until 4-6 weeks after delivery, has been recommended. Thrombocytopenia may make regional analgesia during labor or for a Cesarean section inappropriate. If general anesthesia is necessary, measures to maintain normothermia, normovolemia and acid–base homeostasis are important. Provocation of stress responses and the use of agents which may result in complement activation should be avoided. If transfusion is required, irradiated leukocyte-depleted cells are preferable.

MYELOPROLIFERATIVE DISORDERS

The myeloproliferative disorders include essential thrombocythemia, polycythemia vera, myelofibrosis and chronic myeloid leukemia.

Essential thrombocythemia

Essential thrombocythemia was considered to be a disease of middle or old age but is increasingly recognized in young people, particularly women. Cytoreduction and treatment with antiplatelet agents is controversial in young patients with essential thrombocythemia. Hydroxycarbamide is frequently used for cytoreduction in myeloproliferative disorders but is teratogenic. If it is prescribed, advice about effective contraception should be offered. In couples where either partner is using hydroxycarbamide, this should be discontinued 3-6 months prior to cessation of contraception.

Essential thrombocythemia in pregnancy

The main clinical features of essential thrombocythemia are thrombosis (both arterial and venous), hemorrhage and, in a few, transformation to a myelofibrotic or leukemic phase. Many patients remain asymptomatic. The published literature contains accounts of spontaneous remissions and uncomplicated pregnancies but also reports of an increased risk of recurrent pregnancy loss, abruption, intrauterine growth restriction, pre-eclampsia, premature labor and stillbirth. In a review of over 200 published cases the live birth rate was around 60%. About 30% suffered a first-trimester miscarriage. Adverse events in the second and third trimesters were less common. Maternal complications are uncommon but include thrombotic events and an increased risk of postpartum hemorrhage.

Management of essential thrombocythemia in pregnancy

Neither a previous history of thrombotic event nor the pre-conception platelet count nor treatment with aspirin during the pregnancy seem to significantly influence pregnancy outcome. However some authors advocate the use of aspirin and prophylactic doses of a low molecular weight heparin during pregnancy in a regimen similar to that which has been used in pregnant women with antiphospholipid syndrome.

The use of cytotoxic drugs should be avoided during pregnancy if possible, but if necessary the agent of choice currently is interferon-α. Rebound thrombocytosis and thrombotic complications have been reported following delivery in women with essential thrombocythemia. Extra caution postpartum with the use of graduated compression stockings and consideration of prophylactic thromboprophylaxis seem appropriate. Non-surgical postpartum bleeding presents a particular problem. ε-Aminocaproic acid (50 mg/kg four times a day) or tranexamic acid (25 mg/kg three times a day) may be administered with caution. Both carry a potential risk of thrombosis in patients with an underlying prethrombotic state.

Polycythemia

Absolute erythrocytosis may be primary (polycythemia vera) or secondary; rarely as the result of a congenital abnormality, commonly secondary to hypoxia and occasionally secondary to abnormal production of erythropoietin. Women with a hematocrit persistently above 0.48 require investigation but full investigation is not usually appropriate during pregnancy.

Whatever the underlying etiology, persistent erythrocytosis increases the risk of maternal thrombosis and may increase the risk of placental dysfunction and poor pregnancy outcome.

Polycythemia vera

Polycythemia vera (PV) is a clonal disorder which results in the overproduction of phenotypically normal erythroid cell lines independent of physiological stimulus. Complications of PV include thrombosis, hemorrhage and hypertension and about a third of patients with PV or essential thrombocythemia have markedly higher homocysteine levels compared to age-matched healthy controls.

Polycythemia vera and pregnancy
Given that the median age at diagnosis is around 60 years, PV is rarely associated with pregnancy. There is a very limited published literature about the management of PV in pregnancy. The risks of pregnancy in women with PV are probably similar to the risks of pregnancy in women with essential thrombocythemia – an increased risk of adverse events. As in essential thrombocythemia, in PV the clonal hematopoiesis may remit during pregnancy. Pre-conception counseling is important so that anagrelide or hydroxycarbamide may be gradually withdrawn 3-6 months prior to conceiving. If necessary interferon-α may be substituted, but maintenance with venesection would be generally preferable.

Management of pregnancy in polycythemia vera
Management strategies have to be decided on an individual basis depending on the patient's obstetric history and current disease status. Risk to the mother and/or the fetus is increased if there is a previous history of thrombosis (venous or arterial), or if her platelet count rises above 1000×10^9/L. Risk is also increased if the pregnant woman has a history of polycythemia-related hemorrhage, associated with pregnancy or not. A poor obstetric history – recurrent first-trimester pregnancy loss, a later pregnancy loss, intrauterine growth restriction or severe pre-eclampsia also significantly increase risks for both mother and fetus.

It is suggested that during pregnancy in women with PV, the hematocrit should be kept below 0.36. In some women the pregnancy associated physiological decrease in platelet count and hematocrit may obviate the need for active intervention to control blood cell counts. If necessary, venesection is immediately effective and generally safe. Maintenance of the red cell mass at a physiological level reduces the risks associated with the hypercoagulability of PV. Control of the hematocrit should also reduce the risk of hemorrhage and hypertension. Iron supplementation is contraindicated but folic acid supplementation is advised.

Extrapolating from experience in women with essential thrombocythemia, an elevated platelet count is not a significant predictor of adverse pregnancy outcome. Some authors suggest that asymptomatic thrombocytosis requires no intervention but others suggest that, providing there is no contraindication, aspirin (75 mg per day) may be useful throughout pregnancy and for around 6 weeks following delivery. Low molecular weight heparin (LMWH) in prophylactic doses has been used safely in women at high risk of thrombosis or with a history of recurrent fetal loss. LMWH use in women with polycythemia and a history of thrombosis or fetal loss is anecdotal but may be considered on an individual basis.

Leukocytosis is usually mild and requires no intervention. If at all possible, cytoreduction should be avoided during pregnancy – particularly during the first trimester. If cytoreduction does become necessary – because the patient cannot tolerate venesection, or splenomegaly requires correction, the agent of choice appears to be interferon-α. There are no published reports of teratogenicity with interferon-α but it may reduce maternal fertility. Hydroxycarbamide should be avoided during pregnancy because animal teratogenicity has been reported. There is insufficient data on the use of anagrelide during pregnancy to recommend its use.

As in women with essential thrombocythemia, extra care postpartum with the use of graduated compression stockings and consideration of prophylactic thromboprophylaxis is appropriate. Antifibrinolytics should be used with extreme caution as they may provoke a thrombotic event.

Further reading

Aessopos A, Karabatsos F, Farmakis D, et al 1999 Pregnancy in patients with well-treated beta-thalassemia: outcome for mothers and newborn infants. American Journal of Obstetrics & Gynecology 180(2 Pt 1):360-365

Ball S E 2000 The modern management of severe aplastic anaemia. British Journal of Haematology 110(1):41-53

Bangerter M, Guthner C, Beneke H, et al 2000 Pregnancy in essential thrombocythaemia: treatment and outcome of 17 pregnancies. European Journal of Haematology 65(3):165-169

Benraad C E, Scheerder H A, 1994 Autoimmune haemolytic anaemia during pregnancy. European Journal of Obstetrics, Gynecology & Reproductive Biology 55(3):209-211

Bourantas K, Makrydimas G, Georgiou I, et al 1997 Aplastic anemia. Report of a case with recurrent episodes in consecutive pregnancies. Journal of Reproductive Medicine 42(10):672-674

Browne I, Byrne H, Briggs L 2003 Sickle cell disease in pregnancy. European Journal of Anaesthesiology 20(1):75-76

Charache S, Terrin M L, Moore R D, et al 1995 Effect of hydroxyurea on the frequency of painful crises in sickle cell anemia. Investigators of the Multicenter Study of Hydroxyurea in Sickle Cell Anemia. New England Journal of Medicine 332(20): 1317-1322

Czeizel A E, Dudas I 1992 Prevention of the first occurrence of neural-tube defects by periconceptional vitamin supplementation. New England Journal of Medicine 327(26):1832-1835

Daskalakis G J, Papageorgiou I S, Antsaklis A J, et al 1998 Pregnancy and homozygous beta thalassaemia major. [See comment]. British Journal of Obstetrics & Gynaecology 105(9):1028-1032

Dilek T U, Oktem M, Yildiz A 2004 Polycythemia vera and pregnancy. International Journal of Gynaecology & Obstetrics 85(2):161-162

Department of Health Expert Advisory Group 1992 Folic acid and the prevention of neural tube defects. Department of Health, London

Harrison C N 2002 Current trends in essential thrombocythaemia. British Journal of Haematology 117(4):796-808

Hemminki E, Rimpela U 1991 A randomized comparison of routine versus selective iron supplementation during pregnancy. Journal of the American College of Nutrition 10(1):3-10

Hemminki E, Merilainen J 1995 Long-term follow-up of mothers and their infants in a randomized trial on iron prophylaxis during pregnancy. American Journal of Obstetrics & Gynecology 173(1):205-209

Kathirvel S, Prakash A, Lokesh B N, et al 2000 The anesthetic management of a patient with paroxysmal nocturnal hemoglobinuria. Anesthesia & Analgesia 91(4):1029-1031

Koshy M 1995 Sickle cell disease and pregnancy. Blood Reviews 9(3):157-164

McMullin M F, Bareford D, Campbell P, et al 2004 Guidelines for the diagnosis, investigation and management of polycythaemia/erythrocytosis. Online. Available: http://www.bcshguidelines.com/pdf/polycythaemia.pdf

McPartlin J, Halligan A, Scott J M, et al 1993 Accelerated folate breakdown in pregnancy. Lancet 341(8838):148-149

Mahomed K 2005 Folate supplementation in pregnancy. The Cochrane Database of Systematic Reviews 2

Mahomed K 2005 Iron supplementation in pregnancy. Cochrane Database of Systematic Reviews 1

Mills J L, McPartlin J M, Kirke P N, et al 1995 Homocysteine metabolism in pregnancies complicated by neural-tube defects. Lancet 345(8943):149-151

Oosterkamp H M, Brand A, Kluin-Nelemans J C, 1998 Pregnancy and severe aplastic anaemia: causal relation or coincidence? British Journal of Haematology 103(2):315-316

Orofino M G, Argiolu F, Sanna M A, et al 2004 Fetal HLA typing in beta thalassaemia: implications for haemopoietic stem-cell transplantation. Lancet 362(9377):41-42

Paech M J, Pavy T J 2004 Management of a parturient with paroxysmal nocturnal haemoglobinuria. International Journal of Obstetric Anesthesia 13(3):188-191

Pardo J, Gindes L, Orvieto R 2004 Cobalamin (vitamin B12) metabolism during pregnancy. International Journal of Gynaecology & Obstetrics 84(1):77-78

Ray J G, Burows R F, Ginsberg J S, et al 2000 Paroxysmal nocturnal hemoglobinuria and the risk of venous thrombosis: review and recommendations for management of the pregnant and nonpregnant patient. Haemostasis 30(3):103-117

Serjeant G R, Loy L L, Crowther M, et al 2004 Outcome of pregnancy in homozygous sickle cell disease. Obstetrics & Gynecology 103(6):1278-1285

Sun P M, Wilburn W, Raynor B D, et al 2001 Sickle cell disease in pregnancy: twenty years of experience at Grady Memorial Hospital, Atlanta, Georgia. American Journal of Obstetrics & Gynecology 184(6):1127-1130

Walker M C, Smith G N, Perkins S L, et al 1999 Changes in homocysteine levels during normal pregnancy. American Journal of Obstetrics & Gynecology 180(3PartI):660-664

Whittaker P G, Macphail S, Lind T 1996 Serial hematologic changes and pregnancy outcome. Obstetrics & Gynecology 88(1):33-39

Wright C A, Tefferi A 2001 A single institutional experience with 43 pregnancies in essential thrombocythemia. European Journal of Haematology 66(3):152-159

Chapter 8

Thrombosis and hemostasis

I. A. Greer, I. D. Walker

Thrombosis
I. A. Greer

INTRODUCTION

Pulmonary thromboembolism (PTE) remains a major cause of direct maternal mortality. PTE arises from deep venous thrombosis (DVT). DVT is associated with a significant risk of recurrent venous thrombosis and deep venous insufficiency, while PTE carries a risk of subsequent pulmonary hypertension. The Confidential Enquiries into Maternal and Child Health (CEMACH) (2004) in the UK have shown that while the overall incidence of fatal PTE has fallen substantially in the last 50 years, significant concerns remain. Many deaths are associated with substandard care, including a failure to recognize risk factors for venous thromboembolism (VTE), a failure to provide appropriate thromboprophylaxis for those at risk, a failure to objectively diagnose VTE and a failure to provide appropriate treatment. The incidence of antenatal and postnatal DVT has been estimated at 0.615/1000 and at 0.304/1000 maternities respectively in women under 35 years of age, and these risks approximately double for women over 35 years of age. The event rate is higher in the puerperium making it the time of greatest risk. A recent study from the UK obstetric surveillance system has found a reported rate of antenatal PTE of 0.16/1000 maternities. Almost 40% of postpartum VTE present following the woman's discharge from hospital, but complete data on postpartum DVT are difficult to obtain as many cases present to non-obstetric services. In addition PTE is more likely to occur postpartum than antepartum and is strongly associated with Cesarean section in epidemiological studies. Almost half of antenatal VTE occur before 15 weeks gestation emphasizing the need for risk assessment pre-pregnancy and prophylaxis in early pregnancy.

Interestingly, almost 90% of pregnancy-associated DVT occur on the left side in contrast to the non-pregnant situation, where only 55% of DVT occur on the left. This may reflect some compression of the left common iliac vein by the right iliac artery and the ovarian artery, which cross the vein on the left side only. More importantly, perhaps, around 70% of gestational DVT are ileo-femoral in their location. This contrasts with around a 9% rate of ileo-femoral DVT in the non-pregnant, where calf vein DVT predominate. As ileo-femoral DVT are more likely to embolize than calf vein thrombosis, this is an important consideration.

PHYSIOLOGICAL CHANGES OF PREGNANCY RELEVANT TO THROMBOSIS

Virchow's triad of hypercoagulability, venous stasis and vascular damage, all occur in the course of uncomplicated pregnancy and delivery. The physiological changes in the hemostatic system in pregnancy result in an acquired thrombophilic state due to increased concentrations of coagulation factors, reduced endogenous anticoagulants and suppression of fibrinolysis. Physiologically this acts as preparation for the hemostatic challenge of delivery, but may also predispose the woman to thrombosis. The changes in the hemostatic system are shown in Box 8.1. Relative venous stasis, measured by ultrasound, also occurs in pregnancy with a 50% reduction in venous flow velocity by 25-29 weeks' gestation, reaching a nadir at 36

Box 8.1 Summary of hemostatic changes in pregnancy

- Concentrations of factors I (fibrinogen), V, VII, VIII, IX, X, XII and von Willebrand factor increase.
- The endogenous anticoagulants protein C and antithrombin levels remain within the normal non-pregnant range, but protein S falls substantially from early in pregnancy while protein Z is thought to increase.
- Fibrinolysis is suppressed due to an increase in endothelial derived plasminogen activator inhibitor-1 (PAI-I) and placentally derived plasminogen activator inhibitor-2 (PAI-II). Thrombin activatable fibrinolysis inhibitor (TAFI) is not altered in pregnancy.

---

weeks and taking up to 6 weeks to return to normal non-pregnant flow rates after delivery. Finally, some degree of endothelial damage to pelvic vessels is inevitable during vaginal or abdominal delivery.

THROMBOPHILIA

Heritable thrombophilic conditions are found in over 15% of Caucasian populations and around 50% of gestational VTE. They act by disrupting the endogenous anticoagulant systems or via procoagulant effects. This can be through deficiencies of endogenous anticoagulants (antithrombin, protein C and protein S) or through genetic mutations in procoagulant factors such as factor V Leiden (FVL), and prothrombin G20210A. Other relatively common thrombophilias with a combination of both heritable and acquired components include elevated factor VIIIc concentrations, hyperhomocysteinemia and acquired activated protein C (aPC) resistance (see below). The prevalence of several thrombophilias in Europeans and their association with VTE is shown in Table 8.1. There are significant differences between populations, for example in the Taiwan Chinese, only 0.2% are heterozygous for factor V Leiden and a similar number heterozygous for prothrombin G20210A. Interestingly, the risk of VTE associated with factor V Leiden is largely due to DVT. Outwith pregnancy, the prevalence of underlying factor V Leiden in PTE is around half of that for DVT. This differs from other thrombophilias such as prothrombin G20210A where there is no difference in the underlying prevalence between DVT and PTE. The mechanism is not clear. It has been

Table 8.1 Typical prevalence of thrombophilia and association with gestational VTE in European populations

Thrombophilia	Population prevalence (%)	Approximate prevalence in women with gestational VTE (%)	Typical estimate of odds ratio of VTE in women with specific thrombophilias
Factor V Leiden heterozygous	2–7	20–40	8 (NB Homozygote OR 34)
Prothrombin G20210A heterozygous	2	6 (increasing to 20% with strong family history)	2–7 (NB Homozygote OR 26)
Antithrombin deficiency	0.25–0.55	< 10	Type 1 280 Type 2 28
Protein C deficiency	0.20–0.33		4–5
Protein S deficiency	0.03–0.13		3

Note: Combined defects substantially increase risk with an odds ratio estimated at 107 for factor V Leiden and prothrombin G20210A compound heterozygotes.

proposed that factor V Leiden is associated with a more adherent and stable thrombus, possibly due to increased local thrombin generation, so reducing the likelihood of embolization. Whether this applies in pregnancy to women with factor V Leiden is not yet clear.

FVL is functionally manifest as resistance to aPC due to a single point mutation in the factor V gene at the cleavage site where aPC acts, but there are other causes of aPC resistance. Of particular interest in pregnancy is acquired activated protein C resistance which is found in around 40% of pregnant women. Interestingly, the acquired aPC resistance of pregnancy correlates directly with thrombin generation and indirectly with birthweight, suggesting potential involvement of the coagulation system in perinatal outcome. This acquired aPC resistance may reflect, at least in part, gestational increases in factors V and VIII. In the non-pregnant state high levels of factor VIII and activated protein C resistance are associated with an increased risk of VTE independent of factor V Leiden and this may also be relevant for pregnancy. Activated protein C resistance is also found with antiphospholipid antibodies (which should be assessed in any pregnant woman with activated protein C resistance), and other genetic defects in factor V such as factor V Cambridge or the HR2 haplotype. Although factor V Cambridge is rare, the HR2 haplotype is relatively common and has been reported to carry an excess risk of VTE in high risk patients.

Homozygosity for methylene-tetrahydrofolate reductase (MTHFR) C677T is associated with hyperhomocysteinaemia. This genotype predisposes to arterial and venous thrombosis outwith pregnancy where there is concomitant B vitamin deficiency. About 10% of individuals in Western European populations are homozygous for this genetic variant. However, such homozygotes do not appear to be at increased risk of gestational VTE, which may reflect physiological reductions in homocysteine levels and/or the effects of folic acid supplementation in pregnancy. In any event there is no indication to screen for this genotype in women with gestational VTE.

Antiphospholipid antibodies are a heterogeneous collection of autoantibodies that react with negatively charged phospholipid components of cell membranes. The prevalence of antiphospholipid autoantibodies (lupus anticoagulant [LA] and anticardiolipin antibodies [aCL]) in the general obstetric population is around 2% but is higher in selected populations with fetal loss. Antiphospholipid syndrome describes the clinical syndrome associated with these antibodies but, this is a misnomer as the clinically relevant autoantibodies are not directed against phospholipid antigens but rather the phospholipid-binding proteins, or conformation epitopes involving the binding proteins. Thus, many antiphospholipid antibodies require β_2-glycoprotein-I (β_2-GP-1), a phospholipid-binding plasma protein with weak anticoagulant activity, for binding to phospholipids. The clinical manifestations of this acquired thrombophilia include arterial and venous thrombosis, recurrent miscarriage and other pregnancy complications (Box 8.2).

Box 8.2 Diagnosis of the antiphospholipid syndrome

At least one of the clinical criteria and one of the laboratory criteria below must be met for a diagnosis to be made

Clinical criteria

1. Vascular thrombosis:
   One or more clinical episode(s) of objectively confirmed arterial, venous or small vessel thrombosis in any tissue or organ. For histological confirmation, thrombosis should be present without significant evidence of inflammation in the vessel wall.

2. Pregnancy morbidity:
   one or more unexplained death(s) of a morphologically normal fetus at or beyond the 10th week of pregnancy; or
   one or more premature birth(s) of a morphologically normal baby before the 34th week of pregnancy because of: (i) eclampsia or severe pre-eclampsia or (ii) recognized features of placental insufficiency; or
   three or more unexplained consecutive spontaneous miscarriages before the 10th week of gestation, with maternal anatomic or hormonal

abnormalities and paternal and maternal chromosomal causes excluded.

Laboratory criteria

1. Lupus anticoagulant (LA) present in plasma, on two or more occasions at least 12 weeks apart; or
2. anticardiolipin (aCL) antibody of IgG and/or IgM isotype in serum or plasma, present in medium or high titer on two or more occasions, at least 12 weeks apart; or
3. anti-β2 glycoprotein-1 antibody of IgG and/or IgM isotype in serum or plasma (in titer > the 99th percentile), present on two or more occasions, at least 12 weeks apart.

Note: it is important to note that acute infections can cause transient antibody positivity particularly for anticardiolipin antibodies, which are not associated with thrombosis, hence the need for repeated testing. Furthermore persistently positive tests for antiphospholipid antibodies may occur in association with infections including syphilis, hepatitis C, HIV, chronic malaria and *Helicobacter pylori* without associated thrombosis. Finally it should be noted that there is considerable interassay variation in identifying those positive and negative for anticardiolipin antibodies and lupus anticoagulant.

RISK FACTORS FOR GESTATIONAL VENOUS THROMBOEMBOLISM AND THROMBOPHILIA SCREENING

Specific thromboprophylaxis depends on identifying the level of risk for individual women. Ideally, such risk assessment should be made pre-pregnancy or in early pregnancy. The common risk factors for VTE in pregnancy are: age over 35 years; obesity; operative delivery; thrombophilia; and a family or personal history of thrombosis suggestive of an underlying thrombophilia (Box 8.3). With regard to thrombophilia the likelihood of thrombosis depends on the thrombophilia (Box 8.3), whether more than one thrombophilia is present or the woman is homozygous for FV Leiden or prothrombin G20210A, whether previous VTE have occurred, and additional risk factors, such as obesity. At present, there is no evidence to support universal screening for thrombophilia in pregnancy. The natural history of many of these thrombophilias, particularly in asymptomatic kindred, is not yet established, appropriate intervention is unclear, and screening is not cost effective. Selective screening of women with VTE in pregnancy, or who have a personal or family history of, ideally, objectively confirmed, VTE, may be of value

as around 50% of such women will have a heritable thrombophilia.

Screening for thrombophilia in patients with problems such as recurrent miscarriage, intrauterine death, intrauterine growth restriction, abruption and severe pre-eclampsia, which may all be associated with an underlying thrombophilia and, therefore, risk of VTE, should also be considered. However, apart from recurrent miscarriage associated with antiphosphlipid antibody syndrome, effective intervention for these pregnancy complications is not established. Nonetheless, if these women have a thrombophilia that is symptomatic in relation to a pregnancy complication, they may also be at risk of venous thrombosis due to the presence of multiple risk factors including a thrombophilia, or a severe thrombophilia such as antithrombin deficiency, conditions which would, themselves, merit specific thromboprophylaxis. As in any screening situation, appropriate counseling should be offered.

Venous thromboembolism and ovarian stimulation

Often overlooked is the risk of VTE associated with ovarian hyperstimulation, which is associated with procoagulant changes in the hemostatic and fibrino-

Box 8.3 Common risk factors for VTE in pregnancy

Patient-related factors
- Age over 35 years.
- Obesity (BMI ≥30 kg/m^2) in early pregnancy.
- Thrombophilia.
- Past history of VTE (especially if idiopathic or thrombophilia associated).
- Gross varicose veins.
- Significant current medical problem (e.g. nephrotic syndrome, heart failure).
- Current infection or inflammatory process (e.g. active inflammatory bowel disease or urinary tract infection).
- Immobility (e.g. bed rest or lower limb fracture).
- Paraplegia.
- Recent long-distance travel.
- Dehydration.
- Intravenous drug abuse.
- Ovarian hyperstimulation.

Pregnancy/obstetric-related factors
- Cesarean section particularly as an emergency in labor.
- Operative vaginal delivery.
- Major obstetric hemorrhage with blood or blood product transfusion.
- Hyperemesis gravidarum.
- Pre-eclampsia.

lytic systems. Up to 1-2% of IVF conceptions are complicated by severe hyperstimulation. Both venous and arterial thrombosis can occur, but the absolute rate is low. Interestingly, when VTE occurs with hyperstimulation, it is usually located in the internal jugular vein presenting with neck pain and swelling. Subclavian, axillary and brachiocephalic vein thrombosis can also occur with slight preponderance in the right-sided vessels. Bilateral thrombosis can occur. The reason for the location of the thrombosis is unclear, but anatomic change in the upper extremity veins associated with a rapidly developing hyperdynamic circulation, and hyperestrogenism resulting from fertility treatment up-regulating the coagulation cascade and possibly interacting with a pre-existing thrombophilia have been proposed. The average gestation at diagnosis is around 7 weeks. Thrombophilia can be identified in around 50% of cases. Thus, a risk assessment for thrombosis should be undertaken in women undergoing assisted reproduction therapy and appropriate thromboprophylaxis offered to those at risk. The

thrombotic problem can be substantial in these women and sequelae, including PTE and extension of the DVT, can develop despite thromboprophylaxis and therapeutic anticoagulation while undergoing fertility treatment. If ovarian hyperstimulation syndrome develops, graduated elastic compression stockings (GECS) and prolonged anticoagulant therapy are key components of the management.

LONG-TERM MORBIDITY FROM GESTATIONAL VENOUS THROMBOEMBOLISM

Previous VTE is associated with an increased risk of future VTE. The post-thrombotic syndrome is a common complication following DVT. Mild to moderate post-thrombotic syndrome can be found in over 60% of cases within 5 years. It is characterized by chronic persistent leg swelling, pain, a feeling of heaviness, dependent cyanosis, telangiectasis, chronic pigmentation, eczema, associated varicose veins and in some cases lipodermatosclerosis, and chronic ulceration. Almost 4% of patients with DVT develop ulceration within 20 years of the primary event. Symptoms are made worse by standing or walking and improve with rest and recumbancy. It reflects damage to the vein by the thrombus itself and associated inflammation. The syndrome is more common where there is a recurrent DVT, with obesity and where there has been inadequate anticoagulation. The risk of developing venous insufficiency after DVT is greater than with PTE. This may be due to the clot clearing from the leg veins in those with PTE leading to less extensive damage to the deep venous system. This is a significant problem and up to 21% of women with a treated DVT in pregnancy require a compression bandage and 6% have venous ulcers at a median time of follow-up of 10 years. Historical data show rates for venous ulceration following untreated DVT to be 19-28% on follow-up periods ranging from 6-31 years. Recently the risk of pulmonary hypertension after PTE has been estimated at 3-4%.

ANTITHROMBOTIC THERAPY IN PREGNANCY

Warfarin

Management of VTE in pregnancy centers on the use of low molecular weight heparin (LMWH), or occasionally unfractionated heparin (UFH), due to the fetal hazards of warfarin. The use of warfarin in pregnancy is restricted to only a few situations where heparin is considered unsuitable. Although warfarin is not secreted in breast milk in clinically significant amounts and is safe to use during lactation, it crosses the placenta and is a known teratogen. Warfarin embryopathy consists of midface hypoplasia, stippled chondral calcification, scoliosis, short proximal limbs and short phalanges. It may occur with exposure to the drug between 6 and 9 weeks' gestation. It is during this period that the nasal septum more than doubles in length. In a rat model, ectopic calcification occurs in the septal cartilage, causing a reduction in the longitudinal growth of the nasal septum and associated maxillo-nasal hypoplasia, so illustrating the causative link. The characteristic nasal hypoplasia can be corrected with plastic surgery techniques. The incidence of this condition has been estimated at 5%. This problem is potentially preventable by substitution of heparin for warfarin during the first trimester. The risk of embryopathy may be dose dependent, as an increased risk has been reported when the dose of warfarin is greater than 5 mg/day. In addition to warfarin embryopathy, problems may arise due to fetal bleeding. As the fetal liver is immature and levels of vitamin K dependent coagulation factors low, maternal warfarin therapy maintained in the therapeutic range, may be associated with excessive anticoagulation of the fetus and, therefore, potential hemorrhagic complications. Furthermore, recent data show that prenatal exposure to coumarins is associated with an increased risk of disturbance in development manifest as minor neurological dysfunction, or a low intelligence quotient in school-age children, with a relative risk of greater than seven for two or more of these minor abnormalities. Warfarin should be avoided around the time of delivery because of maternal and fetal bleeding risk, and therefore, is usually stopped at around 36 weeks' gestation, or earlier, if preterm delivery is planned or expected.

Heparin

Neither UFH nor LMWH cross the placenta as determined by measuring anti-Xa activity in fetal blood, and there is no evidence of teratogenesis or risk of fetal hemorrhage. On systematic review, LMWHs appear safe for the mother and fetus. Heparins are not secreted in breast milk and can be used during breast feeding. Prolonged use of UFH is associated with symptomatic osteoporosis, with a 2% incidence of osteoporotic fractures, allergy and heparin-induced thrombocytopenia (HIT). However, LMWHs appear to have a substantially lower risk of osteoporosis. Trials of LMWH in pregnancy that measured bone mineral density in the lumbar spine for up to 3 years after delivery found no osteoporosis with LMWH. HIT is an idiosyncratic immune reaction associated with extensive venous thrombosis. It usually occurs between 5 and 15 days after starting heparin. The risk is around 1-3% with UFH but is negligible, with LMWH. Local allergic reactions to heparin usually take the form of itchy, erythematous lesions at the injection sites. Changing the heparin preparation may be helpful but cross reactivity is common. Skin reactions can be associated with HIT and therefore the platelet count should be checked. Allergic reactions should be distinguished from faulty injection technique with associated bruising. LMWH is now the heparin of choice in pregnancy because of a better side effect profile, good safety record for mother and fetus and convenient once daily dosing for prophylaxis. The risk of recurrent venous thrombosis with LMWH used for thromboprophylaxis in pregnancy is < 1%. These data confirm that LMWHs provide effective thromboprophylaxis in pregnancy.

One of the advantages of LMWH over UFH is the potential reduced risk of bleeding. This is of particular relevance in obstetric practice where postpartum hemorrhage remains the commonest cause of severe obstetric morbidity. LMWHs are not associated with an increased risk of severe bleeding peripartum. The observed rate of major bleeding in a systematic review was < 2% which compares favorably with the rate of massive hemorrhage (0.7%), (defined as blood loss > 1500 mL) from one prospective study without the use of LMWH. In most cases of postpartum hemorrhage with LMWH, there is a primary obstetric cause for the bleeding, such as uterine atony or vaginal lacerations, although the blood loss may have been increased by the concomitant use of LMWH.

Hirudin

Hirudin is a direct thrombin inhibitor, used in the non-pregnant for treatment of HIT, and has also been used successfully for postoperative thromboprophylaxis as an alternative to heparin. As it crosses the placenta, it is probably best avoided in pregnancy, although there are case reports of its use in women with HIT without adverse effects. It has also been used in a lactating mother because of HIT and hirudin was not detectable in breast milk. As it is a protein of non-human origin, it is potentially immunogenic and antihirudin antibodies have been reported in over 40% of patients with HIT who received lepirudin as parenteral anticoagulation for 2 to 10 days. Development of these antibodies is related to the duration of treatment. Further, they will enhance the activity of lepirudin and so, during prolonged treatment with lepirudin, anticoagulant activity should be monitored to avoid bleeding complications.

Fondaparinux

Fondaparinux is a synthetic pentasaccharide. It has been shown to be at least as effective as LMWH in thromboprophylaxis after orthopedic surgery. It has also been successfully in trials of thromboprophylaxis in medical patients. It is not associated with HIT, and because it is synthetic, concerns about using bovine or porcine products are avoided. In an ex vivo model using dually perfused human cotyledons transplacental passage was not found. However, fondaparinux concentration in umbilical cord blood measured after maternal administration of 2.5 mg fondaparinux daily was approximately one-tenth of the concentration of maternal plasma. While these limited data suggest it may be reasonably safe in the second and third trimester, its use at present should probably be restricted to women with previous HIT or heparin allergy, or postpartum.

Dextran

Dextran has been used for peripartum thromboprophylaxis, particularly, during Cesarean section. There is a significant risk of maternal anaphylactoid reactions, which have been associated with uterine hypertonus, profound fetal distress, and a high incidence of fetal death or profound neurological damage. Thus, Dextran for thromboprophylaxis should be avoided prior to delivery.

Low dose aspirin

Aspirin inhibits platelet function. It irreversibly acetylates platelet cyclo-oxygense so preventing thromboxane formation, which is important for primary haemostasis by promoting platelet aggregation and vasoconstriction. Unlike endothelial cells, the anucleate platelet cannot synthesize new enzyme and so the effect persists. Platelets are pivotal in arterial thrombosis, but play a much more modest role in venous thrombosis. Aspirin has been found in meta-analysis to have a beneficial effect in the prevention of DVT. Its effectiveness for VTE prophylaxis in pregnancy, in comparison with heparin, remains to be established, but it is likely to offer some benefit. Its effectiveness is likely to be substantially less than that of heparin, reflecting the different mechanism of action of these agents. In women who are unable to take heparin or, in whom the balance of risk is not considered sufficient to merit heparin, low dose aspirin may be useful. Low dose (60-75 mg daily) aspirin is not associated with adverse pregnancy outcome in the second and third trimesters.

Graduated elastic compression stockings

Graduated elastic compression stockings (GECS), which exert maximum pressure at the ankles and less pressure above, are effective in the prevention and treatment of DVT in the non-pregnant. In view of the pregnancy-related changes in the venous system, GECS should be of value in pregnancy and postpartum. While full-length stockings are usually used in pregnancy where ileo-femoral thrombosis is more common and indeed are recommended in high risk situations for prophylaxis, most data on efficacy in the non-pregnant come from below knee stockings. Compliance may be better with the below knee stockings. The mechanism of action of GECS is uncertain but they may act by preventing over-distension of the leg veins so preventing endothelial damage and exposure of sub-endothelial collagen with subsequent activation of the coagulation system. The classification of GECS depends on the level of compression at the ankle. To complicate matters, classification differs in Europe and the USA. In Europe class II compression stockings exert a pressure of 20-30 mmHg at the ankle, but in the USA a pressure of 30-40 mmHg. For this reason, and to avoid confusion, it is advisable to prescribe stockings by indicating the target pressure rather than the compression class. Antiembolism stockings for prophylaxis have a pressure of around 20 mmHg at the ankle, however after a DVT, GECS with an ankle pressure of 30-40 mmHg should be used.

Other mechanical techniques, such as intermittent pneumatic compression, are of value for prophylaxis during Cesarean section and immediately postpartum.

THROMBOPROPHYLAXIS IN PREGNANCY

The management of the woman with a single previous VTE has been controversial until recently. This was because of the wide variation in risk that has been reported (1-13%) and concerns about the hazards of long-term UFH therapy, particularly, osteoporosis. The higher estimate of risk led many clinicians to employ pharmacological prophylaxis with heparin during pregnancy and the puerperium. However, these estimates of risk have significant limitations. For example, objective testing was not used in all cases, some of the studies were retrospective and the prospective studies had relatively small sample sizes. In a recent Canadian report of a prospective study of 125 pregnant women with a single previous objectively diagnosed VTE, no heparin was given antenatally but anticoagulants, usually warfarin following an initial short course of heparin or LMWH, was given for 4 to 6 weeks' postpartum. The overall rate for recurrent antenatal VTE was 2.4% (95% CI 0.2 to 6.9). Interestingly, none of the 44 women (95% CI 0.0 to 8.0) who did not have an underlying thrombophilia and whose previous VTE had been associated with a temporary risk factor, developed a VTE, while 5.9% (95% CI 1.2-16%) of the women who were found to have an underlying thrombophilia or whose previous VTE had been idiopathic, had a recurrent event. As pregnancy is associated with hyper-estrogenism, this should probably be considered a recurrent risk factor in women with a previous VTE on the 'pill' or in pregnancy.

Thus, in a woman with a previous VTE that was not pregnancy-related, associated with a risk factor that is no longer present and with no additional risk factor or underlying thrombophilia, antenatal LMWH should not be routinely prescribed, but this strategy must be discussed with the woman and her views taken into account, especially in view of the wide confidence intervals reported (95% CI 0-8.0%). Graduated elastic compression stockings and/or low dose aspirin can be offered antenatally in these women. Postpartum, she should receive anticoagulant therapy for at least 6 weeks (e.g. 40 mg enoxaparin or 5000 IU dalteparin daily or warfarin (target INR 2-3) with LMWH overlap until the INR is > 2.0.) ± GECS (Table 8.2).

In those women with a single previous VTE and an underlying thrombophilia, or where the VTE was idiopathic or pregnancy- or 'pill'-related, or where there are additional risk factors such as obesity or nephrotic syndrome, there is a stronger case for LMWH prophylaxis. Antenatally, these women should be considered for prophylactic doses of LMWH (e.g. 40 mg enoxaparin or 5000 IU dalteparin daily) ± GECS. This should be started as soon as possible following the diagnosis of pregnancy. More intense LMWH therapy is indicated in the presence of antithrombin deficiency (e.g. enoxaparin 0.5-1 mg/kg 12-hourly or dalteparin 50-100 IU/kg 12-hourly), although many women with previous VTE and antithrombin deficiency will be on long-term anticoagulant therapy (see below). Postpartum anticoagulant therapy for at least 6 weeks (e.g. 40 mg enoxaparin or 5000 IU dalteparin daily or warfarin (target INR 2-3) with LMWH overlap until the INR is > 2.0.) ± GECS is recommended (Table 8.2).

The suggested management of thromboprophylaxis in the various situations encountered in pregnancy is described in Table 8.2.

When prophylactic doses of LMWH are used, the dose may need adjustment in women with very low or very high bodyweight. At low body weight (< 50 kg or BMI less than 20 kg/M^2), lower doses of LMWH may be required (e.g. 20 mg enoxaparin daily or 2500 IU dalteparin daily). In very obese patients higher doses of LMWH may be required. There are no data to guide practice on this issue and thus clinical judgment of risk is required after individual assessment. Empirically in women with morbid obesity the author uses an intermediate dose of 40 mg enoxaparin or 5000 IU dalteparin bid or for those considered at greater risk but with a lower level of obesity 60 mg of enoxaparin or 7500 IU daltaparin once daily.

Traditionally the platelet count was checked before, and one week after, the introduction of LMWH, then on around a monthly basis to detect HIT. However, where a woman has not previously received UFH then the risk of HIT with exclusive use of LMWH is so low that the ACCP recommend that there is no need to monitor platelet routinely in this situation.

There has been concern with regard to LMWH and epidural hematoma, through post marketing reports to the FDA largely from the USA. These events have mostly been in elderly women (median age 75 years) undergoing orthopedic surgery. Additional factors such as concomitant non-steroidal anti-inflammatory agent use (which can enhance bleeding risk particularly in the elderly) or multiple puncture attempts at spinal or epidural have also been implicated. The true incidence of epidural hematoma is impossible to determine due to lack of denominator data. In addition, practice in North America and Europe may differ, particularly, with regard to LMWH use. In Europe, enoxaparin is used in a dose of 20 mg or 40 mg daily, while in North America, 30 mg twice daily is the standard dosage regime. Such differences in patients and practice make it difficult to extrapolate the information in these reports to obstetric practice. A degree of caution must, nonetheless, be exercised in the concomitant use of LMWH and neuraxial anesthesia. In general terms, neuraxial anesthesia is not used until at least 12 h after the previous prophylactic dose of LMWH. When a woman presents whilst on a therapeutic regimen of LMWH, regional techniques should not be employed for at least 24 h after the last dose of LMWH. LMWH should not be given for at least three hours after the epidural catheter has been removed and the cannula should not be removed within 10-12 h of the most recent injection. Planning management of anticoagulation around delivery requires prior involvement and discussion with obstetric anesthetists. LMWH may preclude urgent regional analgesia and anesthesia and assessment of general anesthetic risk may influence timing and route of delivery.

Table 8.2 Suggested management strategies for various clinical situations

Clinical situation	Suggested management
Single previous VTE (not pregnancy or 'pill' related) associated with a transient risk factor and no additional current risk factors, such as obesity.	Antenatal: surveillance *or* prophylactic doses of LMWH (e.g. 40 mg enoxaparin or 5000 IU dalteparin daily), ± graduated elastic compression stockings. Discuss decision regarding antenatal LMWH with the woman. Postpartum: anticoagulant therapy for at least 6 weeks (e.g. 40 mg enoxaparin or 5000 IU dalteparin daily or warfarin (target INR 2-3) with LMWH overlap until the INR is ≥ 2.0.) ± graduated elastic compression stockings.
Single previous *idiopathic* VTE or single previous VTE with underlying thrombophilia or positive family history and not on long-term anticoagulant therapy, or single previous VTE and additional current risk factor(s) (eg morbid obesity, nephrotic syndrome).	Antenatal: prophylactic doses of LMWH (e.g. 40 mg enoxaparin or 5000 IU dalteparin daily) ± graduated elastic compression stockings. NB: there is a strong case for more intense LMWH therapy in antithrombin deficiency, homozygotes or compound heterozygotes for FV Leiden and prothrombin 20210A (e.g. enoxaparin 0.5-1 mg/kg 12-hourly or dalteparin 50-100 IU/kg 12 hourly). Postpartum: anticoagulant therapy for at least 6 weeks (e.g. 40 mg enoxaparin or 5000 IU dalteparin daily or warfarin (target INR 2-3) with LMWH overlap until the INR is ≥ 2.0.) ± graduated elastic compression stockings.
More than one previous episode of VTE, with no thrombophilia and not on long-term anticoagulant therapy	Antenatal: prophylactic doses of LMWH (e.g. 40 mg enoxaparin or 5000 IU dalteparin daily) + graduated elastic compression stockings. Postpartum: anticoagulant therapy for at least 6 weeks (e.g. 40 mg enoxaparin or 5000 IU dalteparin daily or warfarin (target INR 2-3) with LMWH overlap until the INR is ≥ 2.0.) + graduated elastic compression stockings.
Previous episode(s) of VTE in women receiving long-term anticoagulants (e.g. with underlying thrombophilia)	Antenatal: switch from oral anticoagulants to LMWH therapy (e.g. enoxaparin 0.5-1 mg/kg 12 hourly or dalteparin 50-100 IU/kg 12-hourly) by 6 weeks gestation + graduated elastic compression stockings. Postpartum: resume long-term anticoagulants with LMWH overlap until INR in pre-pregnancy therapeutic range + graduated elastic compression stockings.
Thrombophilia (confirmed laboratory abnormality) but no prior VTE.	Antenatal: surveillance *or* prophylactic LMWH ± graduated elastic compression stockings. The indication for pharmacological prophylaxis in the antenatal period is stronger in AT deficient women, homozygotes or compound heterozygotes for FV Leiden and prothrombin 20210A than the other thrombophilias, in symptomatic kindred compared to asymptomatic kindred and also where additional risk factors are present. Postpartum: anticoagulant therapy for at least 6 weeks (e.g. 40 mg enoxaparin or 5000 IU dalteparin daily or warfarin (target INR 2-3) with LMWH overlap until the INR is ≥ 2.0.) ± graduated elastic compression stockings.
Following Cesarean section or vaginal delivery.	Carry out risk assessment for VTE. If additional risk factors such as emergency Cesarean section in labor, age over 35 years, high BMI, etc. present then consider LMWH thromboprophylaxis (e.g. 40 mg enoxaparin or 5000 IU dalteparin) ± graduated elastic compression stockings.

Note: specialist advice for individualized management of patients is advisable in many of these situations.

Antiphospholipid syndrome

In view of the range of presentation and severity, antiphospholipid syndrome (APS) merits separate consideration. The diagnostic features are described above. While recurrent pregnancy loss is perhaps the most common clinical feature and is often the only manifestation of the syndrome, thrombosis can also involve arteries, veins, and the microvasculature. In particular thrombosis may occur in unusual sites such as intracranial and retinal veins, and visceral veins, including hepatic and portal veins. Ischemic stroke and transient cerebral ischemic attacks are the most common arterial occlusive events. Embolization from sterile endocardial and heart valve vegetations is also a recognized feature. Additional clinical features in APS include thrombocytopenia (usually with platelets of $50-100 \times 10^9/L$ and no bleeding tendency), livedo reticularis, transverse myelopathy, multifocal central nervous system lesions resembling multiple sclerosis, pulmonary hypertension, and skin necrosis and ulceration. Catastrophic antiphospholipid syndrome is used to describe the phenomenon, in which renal, pulmonary, central nervous system, cardiac and skin microvascular thrombosis occur acutely with multiorgan dysfunction.

The treatment of acute thrombosis in APS is similar to other acute VTE in pregnancy (see below) but the lupus anticoagulant may result in prolongation of the APTT. Thus the APTT, which is an unreliable test in pregnancy due to coagulation changes, may be even less useful for monitoring the dose of UFH and so LMWH is usually preferred.

Women with APS are often on warfarin outwith pregnancy. In addition the target INR is often set higher at 3 to 4 in order to provide optimal secondary prophylaxis due to the high risk of recurrence, and combined treatment of warfarin and low dose aspirin has been recommended. Both the higher target INR and the combination with aspirin are associated with an increased bleeding risk (The risk of life-threatening bleeding on warfarin therapy with target INR 2-3 is > 1% annually). Recently, two randomized clinical trials comparing these different INR targets in APS patients, with mostly VTE rather than arterial events, found that the lower intensity treatment was equivalent in preventing thrombosis recurrence. Thus the target INR for warfarin therapy in APS of 2-3 should be satisfactory in most cases, increasing to 3-4 if recurrent thrombosis occurs whilst in the lower target range. There may be a stronger case for the higher range in arterial thrombosis in APS. When these women enter pregnancy there is a need to switch them from oral antocoagulants by 5 weeks' gestation, to heparin and usually this will be LMWH. An intermediate dose of 5000 IU dalteparin or 40 mg enoxaparin twice daily is usually satisfactory and this is usually combined with low dose aspirin.

More commonly these women with APS have a history of a pregnancy complication such as recurrent pregnancy loss or severe IUGR or pre-eclampsia. They are usually treated with LMWH in a prophylactic dose (e.g. 40 mg enoxaparin or 5000 IU dalteparin) once daily, combined with low dose aspirin, starting from the time of pregnancy diagnosis and continued throughout pregnancy. The basis of the use of heparin and low dose aspirin for recurrent pregnancy loss comes from two studies that compared aspirin/ heparin with aspirin alone and reported benefit from the combined treatment. Both used UFH rather than LMWH. One of these studies was not randomized and excluded women with lupus anticoagulant making it difficult to interpret and apply. However a more recent randomized trial found no benefit from combined LMWH/low dose aspirin therapy over aspirin alone. This has brought the use of combined therapy into question and particularly raises the issue of whether the type of heparin used explains the different results. Meantime because of the better safety profile of LMWH for long-term use in pregnancy this is usually preferred for these women in combination with low dose aspirin. While further large randomized trials are needed in this area, they are difficult to perform as these patients are often reluctant to accept a placebo or no treatment especially given the favorable safety profile of LMWH and low dose aspirin in pregnancy and the emotional trauma of recurrent pregnancy complications. Steroid therapy is not recommended in treatment of pregnancy complication in APS as trials have shown that it is no more effective than aspirin and heparin regimes, and it is associated with significant maternal morbidity from steroid related side effects.

Diagnosis of venous thromboembolism in pregnancy

The subjective, clinical assessment of DVT and PTE are unreliable and much less than half of women with clinically suspected VTE have the diagnosis confirmed when objective testing is employed. Acute VTE should be suspected during pregnancy in women with risk factors for VTE (see above), and symptoms and signs consistent with possible VTE.

The symptoms and signs of VTE are:

- DVT: leg pain or discomfort, (especially in the left leg), swelling, tenderness, increased temperature and edema, lower abdominal pain and elevated white cell count.
- PTE: dyspnea, collapse, chest pain, hemoptysis, faintness, raised JVP, tachycardia, tachypnea, reduced PaO2 and/or PaCO2, focal signs in chest, abnormalities on X-ray (particularly plate-like atelectasis) and symptoms and signs associated with DVT.

In women with clinical features consistent with VTE, anticoagulant treatment should be employed until an objective diagnosis is made (see below). The vast majority of DVTs in pregnancy are ileo-femoral, with a higher likelihood of pulmonary embolism than calf vein thrombosis, and will therefore require treatment. Isolated below knee DVT is uncommon but, if identified, treatment should be given, although at present there is insufficient evidence to determine the optimal treatment or indeed whether specific pharmacological treatment is required for isolated below knee DVT in pregnancy.

Deep venous thrombosis

If ultrasound (compression or Duplex scanning), which is the first line diagnostic test for DVT in pregnancy, confirms the diagnosis of DVT, anticoagulant treatment should be commenced or continued. In non-pregnant patients, the pre-test clinical probability of DVT strongly modifies both the positive predictive value and the negative predictive value of objective diagnostic tests. Extrapolating this to the pregnant situation, if ultrasound is negative and there is a low level of clinical suspicion, anticoagulant treatment can be discontinued. If ultrasound is negative and a high level of clinical suspicion exists, the patient should be anticoagulated and ultrasound repeated in one week or an alternative test such as X-ray venography should be considered. If repeat testing is negative, anticoagulant treatment should be discontinued.

Pulmonary thromboembolism

With suspected PTE bilateral Doppler ultrasound leg studies and a V/Q scan or spiral CTPA should ideally be performed sequentially as required. Treatment should be continued when the ultrasound venogram is positive or the V/Q scan reports a 'medium' or 'high' probability of PTE or the spiral CT is positive. When the V/Q scan reports a 'low' probability of PTE or negative spiral CT and (Doppler) ultrasound studies of the leg are positive, anticoagulant treatment should be continued. When the V/Q scan reports a low risk of PTE or spiral CT is negative and leg Doppler ultrasound studies are negative, yet there is a high degree of clinical suspicion, continue anticoagulant treatment, and perform alternative test (V/Q, spiral CTPA or MRI) or repeat testing in one week.

If the chest X-ray has abnormalities which lead to difficulties in the diagnosis of PTE, then imaging techniques other than V/Q scan are warranted. Spiral CT is now commonly used for diagnosis of PTE, but its sensitivity and specificity is not substantially better than a V/Q scan and in particular can provide a false negative result with peripheral emboli below the level of the segmental vessels. However, this may be overcome with multi detector row CTPA. Thus there is a role for both tests in contemporary practice and particularly when practical limitations are considered such as

allergy to contrast medium. The average fetal radiation dose with helical CT is less than that with ventilation-perfusion lung scanning during all trimesters of pregnancy. A survey of North American radiology departments found that most respondents already perform CT angiography in pregnant patients suspected of having PTE. However, while helical CT scanning is associated with a lower risk of radiation for the fetus, this must be offset by the relatively high radiation dose (2.0-3.5 rads) to the mother's thorax and in particular breast tissue which is especially sensitive to radiation exposure during pregnancy. The delivery of 1 rad of radiation to a woman's breast has been calculated to increase her lifetime risk of developing breast cancer by up to 14%. Thus there are increasing concerns regarding the risk of radiation exposure to the mother with CTPA especially as the majority of tests will be negative in pregnancy as there is an appropriately low threshold for objective testing as clinical diagnosis of this potentially fatal condition is unreliable. This emphasizes the continued role for V/Q scans in pregnancy.

Further, with helical CT angiography there have been concerns over the safety of iodinated contrast medium, as this can potentially alter fetal or neonatal thyroid function. There is no evidence of this posing a significant problem in clinical practice. Any alteration in thyroid function can be detected by screening in the neonatal period if there are such concerns. Indeed, current guidelines developed by the Contrast Media Safety Committee of the European Society of Urogenital Radiology, state that iodinated contrast media may be given to a pregnant patient when radiographic examination is essential, and that following administration of iodinated agents to the mother during pregnancy, thyroid function should be checked in the neonate. In the context of the risks flowing from failure to treat a PTE, the balance of risk of thrombosis against transient neonatal thyroid dysfunction are clear and the use of contrast medium need not be avoided in the pregnant woman with a suspected PTE.

Additional alternative techniques include pulmonary angiography and magnetic resonance imaging; the latter has substantial potential but currently is expensive with limited access, there are fewer data available and the age of thrombus may be difficult to determine. Nonetheless its safety makes it an appealing tool in pregnancy.

D-dimer for screening for venous thromboembolism prior to objective diagnosis

D-dimer, a degradation product of cross-linked fiber is now used as a screening test for VTE in the non-pregnant situation, where it has a high negative predictive value. Outwith pregnancy, a low level of D-dimer suggests the absence of VTE and further objective tests are not performed. An increased level of D-dimer suggests that thrombosis may be present and an objective diagnostic test for DVT and/or PTE should be performed. In pregnancy, D-dimer can be elevated due to the physiological changes in the coagulation system and levels become 'abnormal' at term and in the postnatal period in most healthy pregnant women. Furthermore, D-dimer levels are increased if there is a concomitant problem such as pre-eclampsia. Thus a 'positive' D-dimer test in pregnancy is not necessarily consistent with VTE and objective testing is required. However, a low level of D-dimer in pregnancy is likely, as in the non-pregnant, to suggest that there is no VTE. It is important to note however that in the non-pregnant even with a high pre-test probability and a highly sensitive D-Dimer assay, 4% of DVTs will not be identified by the D-dimer test, increasing to 17% with a moderately sensitive D-dimer assay. Thus in patients with a moderate or high pretest probability (which accounts for the majority of pregnant patients), it would be inappropriate to rely on D-dimer to exclude VTE in pregnancy.

Initial treatment of venous thromboembolism

The pharmacokinetic properties of LMWHs allow fixed-dose, subcutaneous LMWH to be used in the initial treatment of VTE minimizing or avoiding the need for monitoring. When combined with the compelling safety and efficacy data from systematic review and the problems associated with monitoring UFH and the increased risk of side effects with UFH, LMWH is now the treatment of choice for acute VTE in pregnancy. With massive PTE and hemodynamic compromise, there may be a place for management with intravenous UFH and thrombolysis.

There is an increasing realization that activated partial thromboplastin time (APTT) monitoring of UFH is frequently poorly performed and is technically problematic, particularly in late pregnancy when an apparent heparin resistance occurs due to increased fibrinogen and factor VIII which influence the APTT. This can lead to unnecessarily high doses of heparin being used with subsequent hemorrhagic problems. Where such problems are considered to exist it may be useful to determine the anti-Xa level as a measure of heparin dose (target range 0.35-0.7 U/mL). RCTs of UFH in acute DVT showed that failure to achieve the lower limit of the target therapeutic range of the APTT ratio (1.5), was associated with a 10-15-fold increase in the risk of recurrent VTE. These monitoring problems emphasize the benefits of LMWH in pregnancy.

Low molecular weight heparin

Meta-analyses of RCTs indicate that LMWHs are more effective, are associated with a lower risk of haemorrhagic complications and are associated with lower mortality than UFH in the initial treatment of DVT in non-pregnant patients and have shown equivalent efficacy of LMWH to UFH in the initial treatment of PTE. With regard to safety, there is substantial accumulating evidence with the use of LMWHs, both in pregnant and non-pregnant patients, for the prevention and treatment of VTE. Systematic reviews and large series of cases have concluded that LMWH is a safe alternative to UFH as an anticoagulant during pregnancy. Further, there is evidence that LMWHs do not cross the placenta. A large systematic review demonstrated a risk of recurrent VTE of 1.15% when treatment doses of LMWH were used to manage VTE in pregnancy. This compares favorably with recurrence rates of 5-8% reported in trials carried out in non-pregnant patients treated with LMWH or UFH followed by coumarin therapy who are followed up for 3-6 months and confirms that LMWHs are effective in the treatment of acute VTE in pregnancy.

In non-pregnant patients, different therapeutic doses of LMWHs are recommended by different manufacturers (enoxaparin 1.5 mg/kg once daily; dalteparin 10 000-18 000 IU once daily depending on body weight; tinzaparin 175 IU/kg once daily). In view of recognized alterations in the pharmacokinetics of dalteparin and enoxaparin during pregnancy, a twice daily dosage regimen for these LMWHs in the treatment of VTE in pregnancy is recommended, (enoxaparin 1 mg/kg twice daily; dalteparin 100 IU/kg twice daily) (Table 8.3). These doses have also been used to treat VTE outwith pregnancy. Preliminary data from a relatively small number of patients suggest that once daily administration of tinzaparin

Table 8.3 Typical initial doses of a LMWH used for treatment of acute VTE in pregnancy

Early pregnancy weight (kg)	Initial dose of enoxaparin (mg twice daily)
< 50	40
50-69	60
70-89	80
≥ 90	100

(175 IU/kg) may be appropriate in the treatment of VTE in pregnancy. However, at present there are substantially fewer published data on the safety and efficacy of tinzaparin compared with dalteparin and enoxaparin and further data on this LMWH in pregnancy is required. In obese patients it is recommended that dose capping is *not* used and if concerns exist for dose in these women anti-Xa monitoring should be used.

If the diagnosis of VTE is confirmed, treatment should be continued. Experience indicates that satisfactory anti-Xa levels are obtained using this weight-based regimen and monitoring of anti-Xa is not routinely required in patients with VTE on therapeutic doses of LMWH, particularly as there are concerns over the accuracy of anti-Xa monitoring. There may be a case for monitoring levels at extremes of body weight or in the presence of renal impairment. It has been recommended that the peak anti-Xa activity (3 h post-injection) should be measured by a chromogenic substrate assay. The target therapeutic range is 0.5-1.2 U/mL for peak levels. If the peak anti-Xa level is > 1.2 U/mL, the dose of LMWH should be reduced, (e.g. for enoxaparin 100 mg bd to 80 mg bd, and 80 mg bd to 60 mg bd), and peak anti-Xa activity reassessed. As with prophylaxis, guidelines recommend that routine platelet count monitoring is not required in obstetric patients who have received only LMWH. If UFH is employed, or if the obstetric patient is receiving LMWH after first receiving UFH, or if she has received UFH in the past, the platelet count should ideally be monitored every 3 days from day 4 to day 14, or until heparin is stopped, whichever occurs first.

Intravenous unfractionated heparin

Intravenous UFH is the traditional method of heparin administration in acute VTE and remains the preferred treatment in massive PTE because of its rapid effect and extensive experience of its use in this situation. The regimen for the administration of intravenous UFH is:

1. loading dose of 5000 IU, followed by continuous intravenous infusion of 1000-2000 IU/h adjusted by at least daily laboratory results (see below);
2. an initial infusion concentration of 1000 IU/mL should be employed;
3. measure APTT level 6 h after the loading dose, then at least daily. The dose should be adjusted to achieve a therapeutic target range within 24 h. Protocols for heparin dose adjustment according to APTT ratio results should be employed since they improve the achievement of therapeutic target ranges. The therapeutic target APTT ratio

is usually 1.5-2.5 times the average laboratory control value. Each laboratory should standardize its own target range for the APTT ratio. The target range for the anti-Xa level in this situation is 0.35-0.70 IU/ml (note this is different for the target used with LMWH due to differences in action of UFH).

Subcutaneous unfractionated heparin

In a meta-analysis of RCTs, 12-hourly subcutaneous UFH has been shown to be as effective, and at least as safe as intravenous UFH, in the prevention of recurrent thromboembolism in non-pregnant patients with acute DVT. The regimen for the administration of subcutaneous, UFH includes an initial intravenous bolus of 5000 IU and then subcutaneous injections of 15 000-20 000 IU, 12 hourly. UFH treatment should be monitored by the APTT, with the mid-interval APTT maintained between 1.5-2.5 times the control.

Women receiving therapeutic-dose UFH should have their platelet count monitored (see above). Pregnant women who develop HIT and require ongoing anticoagulant therapy, should be managed with the heparinoid, danaparoid sodium or possibly fondaparinux. Warfarin may also be justified in this situation.

Additional therapy for venous thromboembolism

Pain and swelling in the affected leg are debilitating symptoms of DVT. There is evidence that compression stockings (30-40 mmHg), along with maintaining mobility, can reduce pain and swelling as well as reduce clot progression. This approach can also prevent the development of post-thrombotic syndrome (see below). Short-term studies with proximal DVT, found that pain and swelling improved significantly faster in those wearing compression hosiery and who were mobile, than in those resting in bed without any compression. Studies in the non-pregnant have shown that early mobilization, with compression therapy, does not increase the likelihood of developing PTE. Thus there is no requirement for bed rest in a stable patient on anticoagulant treatment with acute DVT, and no other contraindication to mobilizing, such as a large fresh free floating thrombus in the vena cava.

Where DVT threatens leg viability through venous gangrene, the leg should be elevated, anticoagulation given and consideration given to surgical embolectomy or thrombolytic therapy.

Eaval filters are not usually required and in the author's experience are rarely necessary.

MASSIVE LIFE THREATENING PULMONARY THROMBOEMBOLISM WITH HEMODYNAMIC COMPROMISE

In massive life threatening PTE with hemodynamic compromise there is a case for considering thrombolytic therapy as anticoagulant therapy will not reduce the obstruction of the pulmonary circulation. Data are limited in pregnancy and, at least, initially, there was some reluctance to use thrombolytic agents, because of concerns for maternal bleeding and adverse fetal effects. Currently, the two thrombolytic agents used are streptokinase and recombinant tissue plasminogen activator (rtPA). rtPA is more specific than streptokinase in that it has a high affinity for plasminogen, which is linked to fibrin contained within the clot. This, at least theoretically, will result in a more localized breakdown of the clot, and, so avoid, a generalized coagulation disturbance. rtPA is a large molecule that does not cross the placenta, and, thus, has no direct effect on the fetus. In contrast with streptokinase, the patient may receive repeated doses of rtPA. While streptokinase does not cross the placenta, it does cause a reaction in the mother, sensitizing her to this substance, and, thus, she cannot receive further administration for six months after its use.

Several randomized trials using thrombolytic agents for pulmonary thromboembolism have established that thrombolytic therapy is more effective in reducing clot burden and improving hemodynamics more rapidly compared to heparin therapy. These studies, however, have not shown any impact on long-term survival over and above that of conventional therapy with heparin or LMWH, and, no thrombolytic agent has been shown to be superior to any of the others. Because of this, current recommendations suggest that thrombolytic therapy should be reserved for patients with severe pulmonary thromboembolism with hemodynamic compromise. There are now a large number of case reports in the literature with regard to the use of thrombolytic therapy in pregnancy. Over 172 women have been reported after treatment with thrombolytic therapy – 164 with streptokinase, 3 with urokinase and 5 with rtPA. Problems associated with treatment included five non-fatal maternal bleeding complications (2.9%), and three fetal deaths (1.7%). These data suggest that the maternal bleeding complication rate is in the range of 1-6%, which is consistent to that in non-pregnant patients, receiving thrombolytic therapy. Most bleeding events occur around catheter and puncture sites, and, in pregnant women, there have been no reports in the literature of intracranial bleeding.

More recently, catheter-directed thrombolytic therapy has been employed, as thrombolytic therapy can then be given at a lower dose down the catheter and also with a lower risk of bleeding complications. However, there is no evidence that catheter-directed thrombolytic therapy is superior to systemic thrombolytic therapy and even standard heparin. This technique also requires specialized facilities and expertise.

BASELINE ASSESSMENT BEFORE INITIATING ANTICOAGULANT THERAPY

Before anticoagulant treatment is commenced, blood should be taken for a full thrombophilia screen, a full blood count and a coagulation screen. Blood should also be sent for urea, electrolytes and liver function tests, to exclude renal or hepatic dysfunction, which are cautions for anticoagulant therapy. Although the results of a thrombophilia screen will not influence immediate management, it can provide information that can influence the duration and intensity of anticoagulation, such as when antithrombin deficiency is identified. It is important to be aware of the effects of pregnancy and thrombus on the results of a thrombophilia screen. For example, protein S levels fall in normal pregnancy, making it extremely difficult to make a diagnosis of protein S deficiency during pregnancy. Activated protein C (aPC) resistance is found with the aPC sensitivity ratio test in around 40% of pregnancies, due to the physiological changes in the coagulation system. This effect can be overcome by repeating the test using the modified aPC sensitivity ratio, where the test plasma is diluted with factor V-deficient plasma to increase the sensitivity and specificity of the test. Anticardiolipin antibodies can also influence the result of the test for aPC resistance. Antithrombin may be reduced when extensive thrombus is present. Other factors can also influence the results of a thrombophilia screen. In nephrotic syndrome and pre-eclampsia (conditions associated with an increased risk of thrombosis) antithrombin levels are reduced and in liver disease protein C and S will be reduced. Genotyping for factor V Leiden and prothrombin G20210A will not be influenced by pregnancy or current thrombosis. It is important, therefore, that thrombophilia screens are interpreted by clinicians with specific expertise in the area.

MAINTENANCE TREATMENT OF VENOUS THROMBOEMBOLISM

Following initial heparinization in patients with VTE, maintenance of anticoagulation with oral anticoagulants is recommended in non-pregnant patients. The hazards of warfarin discussed above make such treatment unsuitable in pregnancy. Thus oral anticoagulants are generally avoided for maintenance therapy in pregnancy. Women with antenatal VTE can be managed with subcutaneous LMWH (or an adjusted-dose regimen of subcutaneous UFH) for the remainder of the pregnancy. Subcutaneous LMWH has many advantages over APTT-monitored UFH in the maintenance treatment of VTE in pregnancy (see above). The simplified therapeutic regimen for LMWH is convenient for patients and facilitates outpatient treatment. Women should be taught to selfinject and can then be managed as outpatients until delivery. Arrangements should be made to allow safe disposal of needles and syringes.

Therapeutic doses of heparin should be used for maintenance treatment. The rationale for this is based on the ongoing risk of recurrent venous thromboembolism. However, in certain clinical situations outwith pregnancy, notably patients with contraindications to warfarin and patients with malignant disease, the dose of LMWH has been successfully reduced to an intermediate dose after initial full-dose anticoagulation in an attempt to reduce the risks of anticoagulant-related bleeding and heparin-induced osteoporosis. This type of modified dosing regimen may be useful in pregnant women who require prolonged periods of anticoagulation with heparin although there have been no comparative studies investigating these strategies in pregnancy. Furthermore the compelling safety data on LMWH in pregnancy are reassuring with regard to continued use of a therapeutic rather than an intermediate dose.

The duration of therapeutic anticoagulation treatment in the non-pregnant situation is usually 6 months for VTE provoked by major transient risk factor with thrombophilia, or ongoing risk factors or unprovoked VTE. Pregnancy itself is associated with ongoing risk factors, and most thombi are ileo-femoral, therefore 6 months therapy is appropriate. If VTE occurs early in pregnancy consider LMWH at prophylactic or intermediate doses after 6 months (but take into account any thrombophilia and risk factors for recurrent thrombosis). Following delivery, treatment should continue for at least 6-12 weeks. Warfarin can be used following delivery and it does not cross into breast milk.

ANTICOAGULANT THERAPY DURING LABOR AND DELIVERY

In order to avoid an unwanted anticoagulant effect during delivery, it is suggested that heparin be discontinued 24 h prior to elective induction of labor or Cesarean section. If spontaneous labor occurs in women receiving adjusted-dose subcutaneous UFH, careful monitoring of the APTT is required. If it is markedly prolonged near delivery, protamine sulfate may be required to reduce the risk of bleeding. Although bleeding complications appear to be very uncommon with LMWH, the same approach to women receiving 'therapeutic doses' of LMWH as in those receiving adjusted-dose UFH, namely administering the last dose of LMWH 24 h prior to elective induction of labor is suggested.

For delivery by elective Cesarean section, the treatment doses of heparin should be omitted on the evening prior to surgery and on the morning of surgery (i.e. heparin should be omitted for 24 h prior to surgery). A thromboprophylactic dose of LMWH should be given by 3 h post-operatively (> 4 h after removal of the epidural catheter, if appropriate), and the treatment dose recommenced that evening. There is an increased risk of wound hematoma following Cesarean section with both UFH and LMWH of around 2%. In patients receiving therapeutic doses of LMWH, wound drains (abdominal and rectus sheath) should be considered at Cesarean section, and the skin incision should be closed with staples or interrupted sutures to allow drainage of any hematoma.

In women at risk of thrombosis and with concurrent high risk of hemorrhage, such as those with major antepartum hemorrhage, coagulopathy, progressive wound hematoma, suspected intra-abdominal bleeding and postpartum hemorrhage, UFH is often preferred as it has a shorter half-life than LMWH and its activity is more completely reversed with protamine sulfate.

POSTNATAL ANTICOAGULATION

Anticoagulant therapy (either warfarin or subcutaneous heparin) should be continued for at least 6 weeks postpartum and longer to allow a total duration of treatment of 6 months if applicable. Before discontinuing treatment the ongoing risk of thrombosis should be assessed. Warfarin is not contraindicated in breastfeeding. There are no published data on whether LMWHs are secreted in breast milk, although extensive experience of enoxaparin in the puerperium reports no problems during breastfeeding and other heparins are known not to cross the breast. Furthermore, neither UFH nor LMWH are orally active and no effect would therefore be anticipated in the fetus.

If the woman chooses to commence warfarin postpartum, this can usually be initiated on the third postnatal day. Switching from LMWH to warfarin can be associated with secondary PPH and so warfarin administration should be delayed further in women with risk of PPH. Thus, the time to start warfarin will depend on the individual patient. The regimen for commencing warfarin should be based on local protocols developed with hematologists; usually 7 mg/day for the first 3 days is used with the INR checked thereafter and dose adjusted. The international normalized ratio (INR) should be checked on day two of warfarin treatment and subsequent warfarin doses titrated to maintain the INR between 2.0-3.0. Heparin treatment should be continued until the INR is > 2.0 on two successive days.

PERSISTENT ABNORMALITIES ON IMAGING INVESTIGATIONS

It is not unusual for persistent abnormalities to be seen on follow up imaging after PTE or DVT. Clot resolution can take a considerable time. This is important as persistent obstruction of flow by thrombus will lead to pulmonary arterial or venous hypertension for PTE and DVT respectively. Studies of repeated ultrasound examinations after a first popliteal or femoral DVT have shown show that after 9 months, just over 50% of patients have normal features. A study examining resolution of PTE found 50% of patients still had residual thrombus after around 11 months. Thus, many patients will have residual thrombus after 6 months of anticoagulant therapy. Clot resolution may continue after anticoagulant therapy is discontinued. Whether prolonged anticoagulant therapy is worthwhile in those patients with persistent residual obstruction is uncertain. However, there is a case for prolonging anticoagulant therapy in such patients by around 3 months. LMWH may be preferable as it is associated with lower recurrent VTE rates than oral anticoagulants in cancer patients and antagonizes activated coagulation factors rather than depleting them. Further LMWH is likely to offer better anticoagulation than warfarin where around 20% of the time the patient may be under anticoagulated. Clearly these patients should also have GECS where DVT has occurred. There is no controlled clinical trial evidence to support the use of such persistent anticoagulation and this must be discussed with the patient when this strategy is employed.

PREVENTION OF POST-THROMBOTIC SYNDROME

GECS will improve the microcirculation by assisting the calf muscle pump, reducing swelling and reflux, and reducing venous hypertension. A randomized trial reported that mild to moderate post-thrombotic syndrome decreased from 47% to 20%, and severe post-thrombotic syndrome decreased from 23% to 11% with use of GECS over 2 years. Thus women should be advised to continue with GECS (30-40 mmHG ankle pressure) use for 2 years after DVT in pregnancy.

THROMBOSIS AND ADVERSE PREGNANCY OUTCOME

Activation of the hemostatic system at the level of the placenta can potentially disrupt placentation or affect placental function adversely through thrombosis and placental infarction. Recurrent fetal loss is common, with three or more successive losses affecting 1-2% of women of reproductive age and two or more successive losses affecting around 5%. A small number of such pregnancy losses are due to identifiable anatomical, chromosomal, endocrinological or immunological problems in the mother or fetus. However, in the majority of cases no cause is identified. Recent data show that both acquired and inherited thrombophilias are associated with a substantial proportion of these fetal losses. This association with fetal loss extends to the second trimester and was stronger for both factor V Leiden and prothrombin 20210A heterozygosity. The most compelling evidence is derived from studies in women with antiphospholipid antibodies, which show that anticardiolipin antibodies and lupus anticoagulant are associated, not only with increased thrombin generation but also with increased risk of early fetal loss. Furthermore prevention of fetal loss in these women is achievable by anti-thrombotic therapy, in particular heparin and low dose aspirin (see above). It is not just early pregnancy loss that is important. Women with antiphospholipid syndrome who progress beyond the first half of pregnancy are at substantial risk of pre-eclampsia, intrauterine growth restriction (IUGR), abruption and fetal loss. For example, gestational hypertension complicates 17% of such ongoing pregnancies, antepartum hemorrhage 7%, preterm delivery 24% and 15% of the infants are small for gestational age. The association with pre-eclampsia is perhaps not surprising as widespread vascular damage associated with endothelial dysfunction, enhanced coagulation and fibrin deposition suggests a role for thrombophilia as a potentially modifiable risk factor. IUGR is also associated with thrombosis and placental infarction on the maternal side, again implicating the hemostatic system.

There is therefore growing interest in the association between inherited and acquired thrombophilias and adverse pregnancy outcome and whether this

Table 8.4 Risk of adverse outcome in women with thrombophilia

Thrombophilic defect	Risk of early fetal loss OR (95% CI)	Risk of pre-eclampsia OR (95% CI)	Risk of IUGR OR (95% CI)	Risk of abruption OR (95% CI)
Factor V Leiden homozygous	2.71 (1.32-5.58)	1.87 (0.44-7.88)	4.64 (0.19-115.68)	8.43 (0.41-171.20)
Factor V Leiden heterozygous	1.68 (1.09-2.58)	2.19 (1.46-3.27)	2.68 (0.59-12.13)	4.70 (1.13-19.59)
Prothrombin G20210A heterozygous	2.49 (1.24-5.00)	2.54 (1.52-4.23)	2.92 (0.62-13.70)	7.71 (3.01-9.76)
MTHFR homozygous	1.40 (0.77-2.55)	1.37 (1.07-1.76)	1.24 (0.84-1.82)	1.47 (0.40-5.35)
Antithrombin deficiency	0.88 (0.17-4.48)	3.89 (0.16-97.19)	n/a	1.08 (0.06-18.12)
Protein C deficiency	2.29 (0.20-26.43)	5.15 (0.26-102.22)	n/a	5.93 (0.23-151.58)
Protein S deficiency	3.55 (0.35-35.72)	2.83 (0.76-10.57)	n/a	2.11 (0.47-9.34)
Anticardiolipin antibodies	3.40 (1.33-8.68)	2.73 (1.65-4.51)	6.91 (2.70-17.68)	1.42 (0.42-4.77)
Lupus anticoagulants	2.97 (1.03-9.76)	1.45 (0.70-4.61)	n/a	n/a
Acquired APCR	4.04 (1.67-9.76)	3.49 (1.21-10.11)	n/a	1.25 (0.36-4.37)
Hyperhomocysteinaemia	6.25 (1.37-28.42)	1.87 (0.44-7.88)	n/a	2.40 (0.36-15.89)

Note: Data derived from Robertson et al (2006).

can be ameliorated by anti-thrombotic therapy. These associations based on a recent systematic review and meta-analysis are summarised in Table 8.4. However, retrospective studies often overestimate risk and prospective cohort studies are required to confirm these associations.

Given the associations described above, clinicians are increasingly using anti-thrombotic therapy in women considered at risk of such complications, despite limited evidence of benefit in heritable thrombophilia. The use of anti-thrombotic therapy, in particular aspirin and heparin, has been evaluated in fetal loss related to antiphospholipid syndrome. Only UFH combined with aspirin has been shown to reduce the incidence of pregnancy loss when compared with aspirin alone. When LMWH and UFH studies are pooled there is a 35% reduction in pregnancy loss or premature delivery. No direct comparison of LMWH and UFH have been performed, but the superior properties of LMWH compared to UFH in pregnancy have led to LMWH being preferred by clinicians.

Anti-thrombotic therapy in women with heritable thrombophilia and recurrent pregnancy loss has been examined in small and predominantly uncontrolled trials or observational studies. When the data from these studies are combined, there is significant circumstantial evidence that LMWH may improve the pregnancy outcome in women with thrombophilia and pregnancy loss. Therefore, until results from randomised controlled trials are available clinicians may consider the use of prophylaxis with LMWH, such as 40mg enoxaparin daily, throughout gestation, in women with thrombophilia and a previous adverse pregnancy outcome.

Hemostasis

I. D. Walker

INHERITED COAGULATION DEFICIENCY

Hemophilia

Hemophilia A and B are sex-linked recessive disorders. Hemophilia A is due to deficiency of coagulation factor VIII (FVIII). Hemophilia B is due to coagulation factor IX (FIX) deficiency. Affected males have reduced or no detectable clotting FVIII or FIX; heterozygous female carriers usually have FVIII or FIX levels around 50% of normal. Unexpectedly low levels of clotting factor activity in hemophilia carriers may be the result of extreme Lyonization of the normal chromosome or of coincidence with a chromosomal abnormality such as Turner's syndrome (XO). The prevalence of hemophilia is approximately 13-18 per 100 000 males. The ratio between hemophilia A and hemophilia B is about 4:1.

Plasma coagulation factor levels are used to classify hemophilia. Patients with < 1 iu/dl are classified as severe; 1-5 iu/dl as moderate; and 5-40 iu/dl as mild hemophilics. About 50% of hemophilics are severely affected, 10% moderately affected and 30-40% mildly so.

The most common genetic abnormality in hemophilia A – affecting about 40% of patients with severe hemophilia A (about 20% of all patients with hemophilia A) – is the result of homologous intrachromosomal recombination of one of two repeats of a segment of intron 22. Mutations in the other 80% of patients are predominantly single nucleotide changes, small deletions or insertions of one or a few base pairs. In hemophilia B the FIX mutations are of the same types as the non-inversion mutations in the FVIII gene.

The degree of bleeding in hemophilia A and B correlates inversely and closely with the degree of deficiency of FVIII and FIX respectively. Patients with severe hemophilia have spontaneous severe muscle and joint bleeds. Those with moderate or mild disease, bleed usually only after trauma. Carriers are usually asymptomatic and unless specifically sought, risk remaining undetected until they produce an affected son. Affected males are readily detected with standard coagulation tests but, the detection of carrier females is more difficult.

Detection of hemophilia carriers

The daughters of males with hemophilia A or B are obligate carriers who have a 50:50 chance of passing the disorder to a son and a 50:50 chance of passing the carrier state to a daughter. Sons of hemophilia carriers have a 50:50 chance of inheriting the abnormal gene and therefore having hemophilia. Daughters of carriers have a 50:50 chance of inheriting the abnormal gene and being carriers themselves (Fig. 8.1).

Confirmation of carrier status depends on previous identification of the mutation in an affected male relative. Over recent years hemophilia centers have strived to ensure that, as far as possible, the mutation responsible for the disorder is identified in each hemophilic kindred. Genetic testing of potential hemophilia carriers may take several weeks.

Because genetic testing may reveal unsuspected non-paternity, its role in confirming carriership in women whose father has hemophilia A or B is controversial. Genetic testing of minors raises ethical and legal problems. Education and counseling of potential

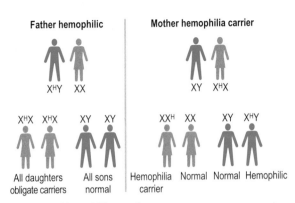

Figure 8.1 Hemophilia genetics.

carriers is useful from very early puberty but in general DNA testing should be delayed until the girl is able to understand the reasons for testing and competent to consent herself. Confirmation (or exclusion) of carrier status facilitates appropriate counseling and where appropriate should be offered prior to the first pregnancy. In women with genetic proof of carriership, prenatal diagnosis becomes possible. Although the availability of preimplantation genetic diagnosis (PGD) services is very limited, identification of a DNA marker makes PGD theoretically possible for those willing to undergo an in vitro fertilization procedure.

Von Willebrand disease

Von Willebrand disease (VWD) is the commonest heritable bleeding disorder, affecting as many as 1-2% of some populations. It is autosomally inherited. Both men and women are affected. It is due to a quantitative or qualitative deficiency of von Willebrand factor (VWF), a high molecular weight (HMW) glycoprotein which serves as a carrier for FVIII and has essential platelet dependent functions in primary hemostasis. Deficiency of VWF results in FVIII deficiency. Von Willebrand factor is synthesized by endothelial cells and megakaryocytes. The primary product undergoes considerable post-translational modification resulting in the formation of dimers, tetramers and ultimately large VWF multimers. Lack of large HMW multimers results in excessive bleeding.

Patients with VWD have a combined platelet and coagulation defect, characterized by mucosal bleeding and a prolonged bleeding time. Affected women frequently report a life dominated by menorrhagia and other bleeding episodes.

Classification of von Willebrand disease

Inherited VWD is classified into three types (Box 8.4). Type 1 and type 3 VWD represent respectively a

Box 8.4 Classification of von Willebrand disease

Type 1 VWD
- partial quantitative deficiency of vWF;
- VWF activity:VWF antigen ratio ≥0.7.

Type 2 VWD
- qualitative deficiency of VWF;
- VWF activity:VWF antigen <0.7.

Type 2A VWD
- qualitative variants with decreased platelet-dependent function due to absence of high molecular weight multimers.

Type 2B VWD
- qualitative variants with increased affinity for platelet GP1b.

Type 2M VWD
- qualitative variants with decreased platelet-dependent function not due to absence of high molecular weight multimers.

Type 2N VWD
- qualitative variants with markedly decreased affinity for factor VIII.

Type 3 VWD
- virtually total deficiency of VWF.

partial or virtually complete quantitative deficiency of qualitatively normal VWF. Type 2 VWD is the result of a qualitative defect in VWF. Type 2 VWD is subclassified into 4 subtypes (2A, 2B, 2M and 2N) according to phenotypic features. Type 1 VWD is the most prevalent accounting for 60%-80% of patients; type 2 variants account for 15-30% of VWD patients, while type 3 accounts for only 5%-10% of patients.

Type 1 VWD is characterized by concordantly reduced levels of VWF antigen and activity. Multimer studies reveal normal VWF multimers. The clinical presentation of type 1 VWD is heterogeneous but the bleeding tendency is usually mild to moderate. With the exception of patients with type 2N VWD, patients with type 2 VWD have a discordantly severe reduction in VWF activity with normal or only slightly reduced levels of VWF antigen. Type 2A is the most prevalent subtype. Patients with type 2A VWD have an abnormal VWF multimer pattern with loss of HMW multimers and display reduced ristocetin induced platelet aggregation. Type 2B VWD is

characterized by an increased platelet aggregation response to ristocetin and an absence of large VWD multimers from the plasma. Patients with type 2B VWD typically have mild thrombocytopenia with increased mean platelet volume, a prolonged bleeding time, and normal or low levels of FVIII. Type 2M VWD includes variants with impaired platelet binding but normal VWF multimer distribution. Type 2N VWD is characterized by normal levels of VWF antigen and activity with normal VWF multimers but a low level of FVIII due to impaired binding of FVIII to VWF. The phenotype resembles hemophilia A but it is autosomally transmitted. Type 3 VWD is characterized by undetectable VWF antigen and activity in both plasma and platelets. Plasma FVIII levels are very significantly reduced (1-5 IU/dL). Affected patients have a severe bleeding tendency with joint and muscle bleeding as well as mucocutaneous bleeding. Inheritance is autosomal recessive.

Genetic diagnosis of VWD involves either direct mutation detection or linkage analysis; both are difficult and neither is at present considered a first-line investigation in the diagnosis of VWD but may be considered in the prenatal diagnosis of severe VWD or to identify heterozygous carriers in recessive forms of VWD.

Treatment of inherited coagulation factor deficiency

The risk of bleeding is minimal when clotting factor levels exceed 50 IU/dL. Desmopressin (1-deamino-8-D-arginine vasopressin: DDAVP) is a synthetic analogue of vasopressin. DDAVP increases the plasma levels of endogenous VWF and FVIII in patients with mild hemophilia A, in carriers of hemophilia A and in many (but not all) patients with VWD. DDAVP is usually administered as a 30 min intravenous infusion at a dose of 0.3 mg/kg^{-1} diluted in 50 ml of saline. This dose usually increases FVIII and VWF 3-5-fold within 30 min. In general, the elevated levels of FVIII and VWF last for 6-8 h. Depending on the type and severity of bleeding, DDAVP infusions may be repeated every 12-24 h. Most patients become less responsive with repeated DDAVP doses. DDAVP may cause mild tachycardia, headache and flushing due to its vasomotor effect. It has been reported rarely to cause hyponatremia and volume overload due to its antidiuretic effect. DDAVP does not pass into breast milk and may be used by breastfeeding mothers.

DDAVP is most effective in type 1 VWD, with increases in VWF and FVIII and shortening of the bleeding time. In type 2 VWD, FVIII levels are usually corrected but the bleeding time usually remains prolonged. DDAVP is contraindicated in type 2B VWD because of the theoretical risk of provoking significant thrombocytopenia however there are reports of its clinical usefulness in some type 2B patients. In type 2N relatively high levels of FVIII may be recorded after DDAVP infusion but the response is usually transient due to the lack of the stabilizing effect of normal VWF. Type 3 VWD patients are generally unresponsive to DDAVP.

The preferred treatment for patients or carriers with moderate or severe hemophilia A and patients or carriers with hemophilia B to raise their coagulation factors is recombinant clotting factor concentrate. Recombinant FVIII and recombinant FIX are both now widely available and the only deterrent to their universal use is cost. Young patients with hemophilia and female carriers should be given priority in the allocation of resources. The safety of plasma derived clotting factor concentrates has improved dramatically and there is no longer significant risk of transmission of HIV or hepatitis agents. However the evidence that the highly thermoresistant B19 parvovirus may still be transmitted warns that other blood borne viruses could be transmitted. In addition it is feared that abnormal prion proteins associated with new variant Creuzfeldt-Jakob disease (nvCJD) could be transmitted by plasma coagulation factor concentrates or albumin. Where a patient with VWD is unresponsive to DDAVP or immediate increases in VWF and FVIII are required, virus inactivated, intermediate purity plasma-derived FVIII concentrate may be transfused. These concentrates may not however correct the bleeding time.

Antifibrinolytic amino acids are synthetic drugs that interfere with the lysis of newly formed clots. Epsilon aminocaproic acid (50 mg/kg four times a day) and tranexamic acid (25 mg/kg three times a day) are the most frequently used. Either may be administered orally or intravenously. They carry a potential risk of thrombosis in patients with an underlying prethrombotic state.

Management of pregnancy

Preconception counseling

Pregnancy planning should be encouraged and patients with heritable bleeding disorders should be offered the opportunity to discuss with their hematologist and with an obstetrician experienced in the management of patients with hemorrhagic disorders, the reproductive choices available. The availability (or unavailability) of prenatal diagnosis should be discussed. Immunization against hepatitis B should, if possible, be completed prior to conception.

Prenatal diagnosis

Chorion villous sampling (CVS) is the principle method currently used for prenatal diagnosis of hemophilia – preferable to amniocentesis since it permits testing in the first trimester. Mothers should be aware that CVS carries a measurable risk of pregnancy loss and that it is not necessary to know the status (affected or unaffected) of a fetus for the purposes of planning the management of the pregnancy or delivery. In order to minimize the risk of fetal limb abnormalities, CVS should not be undertaken prior to 11 weeks' gestation.

If DNA based tests are not possible or produce non-informative results, fetal blood sampling from fetal umbilical vessels for measurement of clotting factors may be considered. This technique requires considerable expertise and is not widely available. It is usually delayed until at least 18 weeks' gestation. Prior to CVS or fetal blood sampling the maternal level of FVIII or FIX (as appropriate) must be checked and if necessary clotting factor replacement given to raise the level to at least 50 IU/dL. Anti-D immunoglobulin should be given to those women who are rhesus (D) negative.

Several studies have reported that only a small minority of hemophilia carriers opt for termination of pregnancy if they are found to be carrying a child with hemophilia. The reasons for this are complex but reflect the unacceptability of termination of the pregnancy to some women and the recognition that the management of hemophilia has been greatly improved recently with the introduction of recombinant coagulation factors. In hemophilia carriers wishing to avoid invasive prenatal testing or in whom it would be uninformative, ultrasound fetal sexing is strongly recommended. Ultrasound determination of the fetal sex is difficult in the first trimester, but by 20 weeks' gestation fetal sex can be accurately determined on ultrasound. An alternative non-invasive method of determining fetal sex is by assessing free fetal DNA in the maternal circulation for the presence or absence of SRY loci.

Antenatal care

Women with heritable bleeding disorders, including women with VWD and confirmed or potential carriers of hemophilia A or B, require review by a hemophilia center during pregnancy. Maternal levels of FVIII and VWF normally rise significantly during pregnancy, particularly during the third trimester. Coagulation factor activity and VWF levels however show little change during the first trimester and no significant improvements in clotting factor levels occur in carriers of hemophilia B or in patients with type 3 VWD.

Hemophilia A carriers and women with type 1 VWD seldom require treatment during normal pregnancy. When bleeding does occur it happens most frequently after delivery and usually only after operative delivery or if there has been significant trauma or tearing of the perineum or genital tract. Serious maternal bleeding unless the levels of coagulation factor activity exceed 50 IU/dL however may complicate spontaneous abortion, pregnancy termination, surgery or other invasive procedures during pregnancy. In some patients prophylactic administration of clotting factor concentrate or DDAVP may be required. Carriers of hemophilia B and women with type 2 VWD seldom require treatment during pregnancy but may need factor replacement at and following delivery. In patients with type 2B VWD, thrombocytopenia may be aggravated during pregnancy but it is not clear whether thrombocytopenia exacerbates clinical bleeding. Women with type 3 VWD need factor replacement at delivery and postpartum. They may also require treatment antenatally.

Management of delivery and the puerperium

The risk of serious fetal or neonatal bleeding in conjunction with normal vaginal delivery is small, but if the fetus has a proven or potential inherited bleeding disorder, interventions such as vacuum extraction, rotational forceps, fetal scalp electrodes and fetal scalp blood sampling should be avoided. Although spontaneous vaginal delivery is usually safe if there is no obstetric contraindication, recourse to elective Cesarean section to avoid the risks of an emergency section or an instrumental delivery may be preferred.

In women with heritable bleeding disorders, a clotting factor activity level greater than 50 IU/dL is usually safe for either vaginal delivery or Cesarean section. Reported experience of the use of epidural anesthesia at delivery in hemophilia carriers or patients with VWD is limited, but it has been suggested that providing the coagulation screen is normal, the (relevant) coagulation factor activity greater than 50 IU/dL and the platelet count greater than 80×10^9/L there should be no hematological contraindication to a regional block. In order to minimize the risk of primary and secondary postpartum hemorrhage, the (relevant) clotting factor activity should be monitored daily and maintained above 50 IU/dL for 3-4 days following uncomplicated vaginal delivery or 4-5 days following an operative delivery.

Care of the neonate

A cord blood sample should be collected from all male offspring of proven or potential hemophilia carriers and sent for clotting factor assay. Because VWF is elevated in the neonate, it is generally recommended that testing for VWD is delayed until the infant is around six months old. The usefulness of routinely performing ultrasound or computed tomography heads scans on all neonates at increased bleeding risk is debated but should be performed if there is any suspicion of intracranial bleeding. A traumatic or instrumental delivery, overt bleeding or suspicion of intracranial bleeding or any other internal bleeding, usually demands immediate treatment with clotting factor concentrate to raise the neonate's plasma factor level to greater than 100 IU/dL. Intramuscular injections should be avoided in neonates with proven or potential severe inherited bleeding disorders. To avoid delay awaiting coagulation test results, it is frequently most practical to give an initial oral dose of vitamin K. If the neonate is proven to have an inherited bleeding disorder, follow-up oral doses of vitamin K must be given. If on testing, an inherited bleeding disorder is excluded, intramuscular vitamin K may be administered.

ACQUIRED BLEEDING DISORDERS

Compared with inherited bleeding disorders acquired coagulation defects present different and often more challenging problems.

Acquired hemophilia

Rarely acquired hemophilia A due to an inhibitor against FVIII presents in association with pregnancy in a healthy young woman. Postpartum inhibitors of FVIII usually persist for a few months to several years. Further pregnancies in patients with prior postpartum inhibitor against FVIII do not provoke reappearance of the inhibitor. The effectiveness of immunosuppressive therapy in patients with postpartum FVIII inhibitors is debatable. Treatment options include high dose recombinant factor VIII, FEIBA (FVIII inhibitor bypassing agent) or recombinant FVIIa. DDAVP is of no clinical use because it induces no or little increase in FVIII levels and what is produced is rapidly neutralized by the FVIII inhibitor.

Disseminated intravascular coagulation

Disseminated intravascular coagulation (DIC) is an acquired disorder secondary to underlying pathology including a variety of obstetric complications (Box 8.5). It is characterized by intravascular coagulation throughout the microcirculation resulting in thrombin generation and intravascular fibrin formation. Massive continuing activation of coagulation results in consumption of clotting factors and platelets.

Box 8.5 Obstetric complications predisposing to acute or chronic DIC

Acute DIC
- Amniotic fluid embolism
- Abruptio placentae
- Septic abortion
- Acute fatty liver
- Uterine rupture
- Septicemia
- Extensive surgery

Chronic DIC
- Pre-eclampsia
- HELLP syndrome
- Retained dead fetus

Box 8.6 Features of acute and chronic DIC

Early acute DIC or chronic DIC
- No symptoms.
- No measurable consumption of components:
  - PT, APTT, TT: within normal;
  - platelet count: within normal.
- Activation markers increased:
  - F_{1+2}, TAT: elevated;
  - soluble fibrin may be increased.
- Inhibitor levels may be reduced:
  - antithrombin slightly reduced.
- Peripheral blood film:
  - occasional RBC fragments.

Acute DIC
- Increased bleeding and decreased organ function (kidneys, lungs, liver).
- Consumption of coagulation factors:
  - PT and APTT prolonged;
  - TT normal or prolonged;
  - fibrinogen normal or reduced.
- Consumption of platelets:
  - platelet count reduced.
- Activation markers increased:
  - FDPs, F_{1+2}, TAT: elevated;
  - soluble fibrin increased.
- Inhibitor levels reduced:
  - antithrombin reduced.
- Peripheral blood film:
  - Frequent RBC fragments.

APTT = activated partial thromboplastin time; PT = prothrombin time; TT = thrombin time, FDP = fibrin degradation product; TAT = thrombin antithrombin complex; F_{1+2} = prothrombin fragment 1+2; RBC = red blood cell.

Clinical presentation

The clinical presentation of disseminated intravascular coagulation is variable. If the initiating event causes explosive activation of coagulation, the clinical picture is dominated by the effects of rapid depletion of coagulation factors and platelets. Patients present with petechiae and bruising. Frequently also there is oozing from venepuncture sites, wound sites and mucosal surfaces. The bleeding may become life threatening if it involves the gastrointestinal tract, lungs, central nervous system, the placental bed or operative sites. Acute renal failure due to microthromboses of afferent arterioles may develop.

If the activation of coagulation is slow, providing the liver can compensate for the consumption of clotting factors and the bone marrow maintains an adequate platelet count, severe bleeding is unlikely. Patients with chronic compensated DIC may be asymptomatic or manifest signs of venous or arterial thrombosis. Some may have minor skin or mucosal bleeding. Obstetric complications such as placental abruption, amniotic fluid embolism and septic abortion are associated with acute decompensated DIC, while others such as pre-eclampsia, the HELLP syndrome (hemolysis, elevated liver enzymes, and low platelet count) and retained dead fetus may cause a more chronic low-grade compensated DIC.

The diagnosis of DIC requires an appreciation of the underlying disorders in which DIC can develop. Because acute DIC requires urgent intervention, DIC must always be considered where a complex coagulation disorder is noted in a woman with an underlying disorder potentially associated with DIC. The diagnosis of acute DIC is suggested by the history and clinical presentation. The woman is usually moderately to severely thrombocytopenic and there is evidence of red blood cell fragmentation on the peripheral blood film. Chronic DIC may be more difficult to diagnose but the clinical history and examination should raise the suspicion and lead to appropriate investigation. Box 8.6 summarizes the laboratory findings in women with DIC.

Diagnosis

There is no single stand-alone test for DIC. A low threshold of suspicion in clinical situations that predispose to DIC is paramount. Investigation relies on the platelet count in conjunction with classic global screening tests of coagulation – the activated partial thromboplastin time (APTT), the prothrombin time (PT) and the thrombin time (TT) (Box 8.6). The APTT measures components of the intrinsic coagulation path and is sensitive to deficiencies of factors XII, XI, IX and VIII. Prolongation of the PT reflects reduced activity of the components of the extrinsic and final common coagulation paths including factors VII, X and V. These tests are non-specific but are rapid, simple to perform and widely available. Their usefulness in the diagnosis of DIC is enhanced when combined with measurement of fibrinogen and fibrin degradation product (FDP) or D-dimer levels. Normal APPT or PT results do not exclude DIC. Similarly, the TT and fibrinogen levels may be within normal 'non-pregnant' ranges in some patients with DIC. Isolated thrombocytopenia is not specific for DIC and, since FDPs and D-dimers are raised in many conditions, they cannot be regarded as specific for DIC. Changes in global screening tests, platelet counts, fibrinogen levels and FDPs and D-dimers do not occur at the same rate and repeat testing to detect trends is often necessary. Furthermore these tests are of limited value in patients with chronic DIC where little abnormality in their results may be observed. Markers of coagulation or fibrinolytic activation such as thrombin – antithrombin complexes, prothrombin fragment 1+2 and soluble fibrin monomers may be helpful in the diagnosis of low grade chronic DIC but the availability of these tests is very limited. Depletion of naturally occurring anticoagulants such as antithrombin or protein C have been related to clinical outcome and have been the focus of replacement therapy in clinical trials. Their sensitivity in the diagnosis of early DIC is unclear.

Management

The cornerstone of management of DIC is treatment of the underlying cause. Replacement of platelets and/or clotting factors would seem rational in patients who have reduced levels. Theoretically replacement therapy may 'add fuel to the fire' but this has not been demonstrated either clinically or in studies. Plasma and platelet replacement therapy should not be based on laboratory results but offered only to patients who are already bleeding or in danger of bleeding. Coagulation factor concentrates should be avoided since they are potentially thrombogenic.

The safety of anticoagulant therapy in patients with DIC is debatable. The administration of heparin or LMWH is generally limited to women with low grade chronic compensated DIC who have predominantly thrombotic manifestations such as thrombophlebitis or who are at risk of VTE. The use of antifibrinolytic agents is not generally recommended in women with DIC because fibrin deposition, which is in part due to reduced fibrinolytic activity, is an important feature of DIC.

A number of controlled trials of antithrombin concentrates have been reported in patients with DIC. All showed some benefits in terms of improved laboratory results and shortening of the duration of DIC. Some showed a modest reduction in DIC mortality in antithrombin treated patients but the effect did not reach statistical significance in individual trials. It is not clear which patients may benefit from antithrombin treatment and currently the availability of antithrombin concentrate is limited. In a randomized, double-blind trial, women with severe sepsis received recombinant activated protein C (aPC) or placebo. A statistically significant favorable result was observed in the recombinant aPC treated group.

Further reading

Ahearn G S, Hadjiliadis M D, Govert J A, et al 2002 Massive pulmonary embolism during pregnancy successfully treated with recombinant tissue plasminogen activator. Archives in Internal Medicine 162:1221-1227

Azzi A, Morfini M, Mannucci P M 1994 The transfusion-associated transmission of parvovirus B19. Transfusion Medicine Reviews 13(3):194-204

Bates S M et al 2004 Use of antithrombotic agents during pregnancy: the Seventh ACCP Conference on Antithrombotic and thrombolytic therapy. Chest 163:627S-644S

Batlle J et al 2002 Advances in the therapy of von Willebrand disease. Haemophilia 8(3):301-307

Bernard G R et al 2001 Efficacy and safety of recombinant human activated protein C for severe sepsis. New England Journal of Medicine 344(10):699-709

Blättler W, Partsch H 2003 Leg compression and ambulation is better than bed rest for the treatment of acute deep vein thrombosis. International Angiology 22:393-400

Brandjes D P et al 1997 Randomised trial of effect of compression stockings in patients with symptomatic proximal-vein thrombosis. Lancet 349:759-62

Brenner B et al 2005 Efficacy and safety of two doses of enoxaparin in women with thrombophilia and recurrent pregnancy loss: the LIVE-ENOX study. Journal of Thrombosis and Haemostasis 3(2):227-229

CEMACH 2004 Why mothers die 2000-2002. RCOG, London 2004

Chan W S et al 2002 Suspected pulmonary embolism in pregnancy: clinical presentation, results of lung scanning, and subsequent maternal and pediatric outcomes. Archives of internal medicine 162:1170-1175

Clark P et al 1998 Activated protein C sensitivity, protein C, protein S and coagulation in normal pregnancy. Thrombosis & Haemostasis 79(6):1166-1170

Farquharson R G, Quenby S, Greaves M 2002 Antiphospholipid syndrome in pregnancy: a randomized, controlled trial of treatment. Obstetrics and Gynecology 100(3):408-413

Federici A B, Castaman G, Mannucci P M 2002 Italian Association of Hemophilia Centers (AICE). Guidelines for the diagnosis and management of von Willebrand disease in Italy. Haemophilia 8(5):607-621

Gherman R B et al 1999 Incidence, clinical characteristics, and timing of objectively diagnosed venous thromboembolism during pregnancy. Obstetrics and Gynecology 94(5 Pt 1):730-734

Greer I A, Nelson-Piercy C 2005 Low-molecular-weight heparins for thromboprophylaxis and treatment of venous thromboembolism in pregnancy: a systematic review of safety and efficacy. Blood 106:401-407

Greer I A, Thomson A J 2001 Management of venous thromboembolism in pregnancy. Best Practice & research Clinical Obstetrics and Gynaecology 15:583-603

Gris J C et al 2004 Low-molecular-weight heparin versus low-dose aspirin in women with one fetal loss and a constitutional thrombophilic disorder. Blood 103(10):3695-3699

Hauser I, Schneider B, Lechner K 1995 Post-partum factor VIII inhibitors. A review of the literature with special reference to the value of steroid and immunosuppressive treatment. Thrombosis & Haemostasis 73(1):1-5

Kadir R A et al 1997 The obstetric experience of carriers of haemophilia. British Journal of Obstetrics & Gynaecology 104(7):803-810

Kirtava A et al 2003 Medical, reproductive and psychosocial experiences of women diagnosed with von Willebrand's disease receiving care in haemophilia treatment centres: a case-control study. Haemophilia 9(3):292-297

Levi M, Ten Cate H 1999 Disseminated intravascular coagulation. New England Journal of Medicine 341(8):586-592

Ludlam C A 1997 New-variant Creutzfeldt-Jakob disease and treatment of haemophilia. Executive Committee of the UKHCDO. United Kingdom Haemophilia Centre Directors' Organisation. Lancet 350(9092):1704

Mannucci P M 2003 Hemophilia: treatment options in the twenty-first century. Journal of Thrombosis & Haemostasis 1(7):1349-1355

Mannucci P M 2005 Use of desmopressin (DDAVP) during early pregnancy in factor VIII-deficient women. Blood 105(8):3382

Mazurier C et al 2001 Type 2N von Willebrand disease: clinical manifestations, pathophysiology, laboratory diagnosis and molecular biology. Bailliere's Best Practice in Clinical Haematology 14(2):337-347

McColl M D et al 2000 Prevalence of the post thrombotic syndrome in young women with previous venous thromboembolism. British Journal of Haematology 108:272-274

Michiels J J et al 1997 Acquired haemophilia A in women postpartum: management of bleeding episodes and natural history of the factor VIII inhibitor. European Journal of Haematology 59(2):105-109

Nijkeuter M et al 2004 Diagnosing pulmonary embolism in pregnancy: rationalizing fetal radiation exposure in radiological procedures. Journal of Thrombosis and Haemostasis 2(10):1857

Nijkeuter M, Huismand M V 2005 More on: diagnosing pulmonary embolism with helical computed tomography during pregnancy: what about exposure to iodinated contrast agents? Journal of Thrombosis and Haemostasis 3:814

Pettila V et al 2002 Postpartum bone mineral density in women treated for thromboprophylaxis with unfractionated heparin or LMW heparin. Thrombosis and Haemostasis 87(2):182-186

Rai R et al 1997 Randomised controlled trial of aspirin and aspirin plus heparin in pregnant women with recurrent miscarriage associated with phospholipid antibodies (or antiphospholipid antibodies). British Medical Journal 314(7076):253-257

Robertson L et al 2006 Thrombophilia in pregnancy: a systematic review. British Journal of Haematology 132(2):171-196

Rosendaal F R, Smit C, Briet E 1991 Hemophilia treatment in historical perspective: a review of medical and social developments. Annals of Hematology 62(1):5-15

Sadler J E 1994 A revised classification of von Willebrand disease. For the Subcommittee on von Willebrand Factor of the Scientific and Standardization Committee of the International Society on Thrombosis and Haemostasis. Thrombosis & Haemostasis 71(4):520525

Sadler J E 1997 Appendix II: A revised classification of Von Willebrand disease. Haemophilia 3(suppl. 2)

Scarsbrook A F et al 2006 Diagnosis of suspected venous thromboembolic disease in pregnancy. Clinical Radiology 61:1-12

Scottish Intercollegiate Guidelines Network (SIGN) 1999 Antithrombotic therapy. SIGN, Edinburgh

Tabor E 1999 The epidemiology of virus transmission by plasma derivatives: clinical studies verifying the lack of transmission of hepatitis B and C viruses and HIV type 1. Transfusion 39(11-12):1160-1168

Varekamp I et al 1990 Carrier testing and prenatal diagnosis for hemophilia: experiences and attitudes of 549 potential and obligate carriers. American Journal of Medical Genetics 37(1):147-154

Warkentin T E, Greinacher A 2004 Heparin-induced
thrombocytopenia: recognition, treatment, and
prevention: the Seventh ACCP Conference on
Antithrombotic and Thrombolytic Therapy. Chest 126(3
suppl):S311-S337

White G C et al 2001 Definitions in hemophilia.
Recommendation of the scientific subcommittee on
factor VIII and factor IX of the scientific and
standardization committee of the International Society
on Thrombosis and Haemostasis. Thrombosis &
Haemostasis 85(3):560

Wu O et al 2005 Screening for thrombophilia in high-risk
situations: a meta-analysis and cost-effectiveness
analysis. British Journal of Haematology 131(1):80-90

Chapter 9

Gastrointestinal and hepatic disorders

C. Nelson-Piercy, C. Williamson

Gastrointestinal disorders

C. Nelson-Piercy C. Williamson

INTRODUCTION

Nausea, vomiting, gastroesophageal reflux and constipation are among the commonest symptoms in normal pregnancy. They are usually mild but can cause much distress and in more severe forms lead to significant morbidity. Inflammatory bowel disease and irritable bowel syndrome are the commonest gastrointestinal diseases to pre-date pregnancy. Peptic ulceration is unusual in pregnancy.

PHYSIOLOGICAL CHANGES IN PREGNANCY

The general relaxation of smooth muscle accompanying pregnancy is associated with decreased lower esophageal pressure, decreased gastric peristalsis and delayed gastric emptying. This is especially so in late pregnancy and intrapartum. Gastrointestinal motility is reduced with increased small- and large-bowel transit times.

NAUSEA, VOMITING AND HYPEREMESIS

Nausea and vomiting are experienced by over half of pregnant women. The onset of symptoms is usually early in the first trimester at around 5-8 weeks gestation. 'Morning sickness' is a misnomer since symptoms may occur at any time of day.

Hyperemesis is less common (< 1%) but causes much morbidity, repeated hospital admissions and can be dangerous if inadequately or inappropriately treated. There is no widely accepted definition of hyperemesis but most would apply the term when, the woman is unable to maintain adequate hydration and nutrition, either because of severity or duration of symptoms. Epidemiological data indicate that hyperemesis gravidarum is commoner in women with pre-existing diabetes mellitus, psychiatric illness, hyperthyroidism, gastrointestinal disorders, asthma and previous molar pregnancy. Several studies have also indicated that seropositivity for *Helicobacter pylori* infection is associated with the condition and smoking appears to be protective. Hyperemesis is associated with marked weight loss and muscle wasting, and a requirement for hospital admission with intravenous therapy. A common associated symptom is ptyalism; the inability to swallow saliva which leads to constant spitting and drooling.

On examination there is often dehydration with a sinus tachycardia, postural hypotension and ketonuria. Investigation commonly reveals electrolyte disturbance including hypokalemia, hyponatremia, a low serum urea and a metabolic hypochloremic alkalosis (due to loss of hydrochloric acid from the stomach). Other findings may include a raised hematocrit level, increased specific gravity of the urine, abnormal liver enzymes (usually transaminases, and found in up to 50% of cases), and abnormal thyroid function tests (see below).

Hyperemesis is a diagnosis of exclusion requiring a careful clinical evaluation for other causes and there is no single confirmatory test. It is important to consider other causes of nausea and vomiting in pregnancy (Table 9.1) such as reflux esophagitis, urinary tract infection, hypercalcemia, diabetic ketoacidosis, and more rarely Addison's disease (insidious onset with some features predating the pregnancy), peptic ulceration, pancreatitis or cholecystitis (abdominal pain is not a prominent symptom in hyperemesis). Vomiting beginning after week 12 of amenorrhea should not be attributed to hyperemesis unless other causes have been excluded. Hyperemesis tends to recur in subsequent pregnancies, so a previous history makes the diagnosis more likely. The natural history of hyperemesis is gradual improvement with increasing gestation, although in a minority of women symptoms may persist beyond 20 weeks' gestation.

Pathophysiology

The pathophysiology of hyperemesis is poorly understood. Various hormonal, mechanical and psychologi-

Table 9.1 Coexisting pathology that should be considered in a woman with hyperemesis gravidarum

System	Diagnosis	Investigation/initial assessment
Genitourinary	Urinary tract infection	Mid-stream urine specimen
	Uremia	U&E
	Molar pregnancy	Ultrasound of the uterus
Gastrointestinal	Gastritis/peptic ulceration	*Helicobacter pylori* antibodies
	Gastroesophageal reflux and ulcerative esophagitis	Endoscopy or empirical proton pump inhibitor therapy
	Pancreatitis	Amylase, blood glucose, calcium
	Bowel obstruction	Plain supine abdominal X-ray
Endocrine	Addison's disease	U&E, early morning cortisol, short Synacthen test with ACTH
	Hyperthyroidism	Surveillance for symptoms and signs of hyperthyroidism, TFTs, thyroid autoantibodies
	Diabetic ketoacidosis	Blood glucose, urinary dipstick for ketones, glucose tolerance test
CNS	Intracranial tumour	CNS examination, brain imaging
	Vestibular disease	CNS examination
Respiratory	Asthma	Chest examination, peak expiratory flow rate

cal factors have been implicated. There is a direct relationship between the severity of hyperemesis and the degree of biochemical hyperthyroidism (see below), and it has been suggested that the raised thyroxine levels or suppressed TSH may be causative. The level of human chorionic gonadotropin (hCG), which shares a common αsubunit with TSH, is directly correlated with the severity of vomiting and free thyroxine concentrations, and inversely correlated with TSH levels. hCG probably acts as a thyroid stimulator in patients with hyperemesis. There is structural homology not only in the hCG and TSH molecules but also in their receptors, and this suggests the basis for the reactivity of hCG with the TSH receptor.

The positive correlation between severity of hyperemesis and hCG levels explains the increased incidence of this condition in multiple pregnancy and hydatidiform mole. The theory is also supported by the fact that the peak in hCG levels (in weeks 6-12) coincides with the presentation of hyperemesis. Other hormonal deficiencies or excesses, involving follicle-stimulating hormone (FSH), progesterone, cortisol and adrenocorticotrophic hormone (ACTH), have been proposed as etiological factors, but never proven.

The physiological changes in esophageal pressure, gastric peristalsis and gastric emptying may well exacerbate the symptoms of hyperemesis, but are unlikely to be causative in isolation. Many psychological and behavioral theories have been suggested to explain hyperemesis, usually involving hyperemesis as an expression of rejection of the pregnancy. There is often a psychological component to the condition, but this may be a result of symptoms and recurrent admissions rather than causal. Separation from family, inability to work, anger at being unwell, and guilt when this anger is turned inwards towards the fetus and resentment of the pregnancy may result in severe psychological morbidity. Psychological factors do play a role in a proportion of cases and this is often suggested by the rapid improvement on admission to hospital and consequent removal from a stressful home environment. It is however extremely dangerous to assume psychological or psychiatric factors are solely responsible for the clinical picture in cases of severe hyperemesis. Maternal deaths have been reported following inappropriate transfer to a psychiatric ward.

Gestational pseudo-thyrotoxicosis

This may be found in up to 66% of cases of hyperemesis and is seen more often in Asians compared to Europeans. There is biochemical hyperthyroidism with a raised free thyroxine and/or suppressed thyroid-stimulating hormone (TSH). Women with these abnormalities are clinically euthyroid (although may have weight loss and a tachycardia) and it is important to establish the absence of symptoms prior to pregnancy. The abnormal thyroid function tests do not require treatment with antithyroid drugs and resolve as the hyperemesis improves.

Of course, true thyrotoxicosis may present in early pregnancy. Discriminatory features to distinguish this from a gestational syndrome include the presence of a tremor, signs of thyroid eye disease such as exophthalmos, a goiter, particularly if associated with a bruit, and the presence of thyroid stimulating antibodies.

Complications of hyperemesis

The risks associated with severe hyperemesis include fetal growth restriction, maternal hypokalemia causing lethargy and muscle weakness, hyponatremia leading to central pontine myelinolysis and thiamine deficiency leading to Wernicke's encephalopathy (Box 9.1). Markers of severity include weight loss > 10%, abnormal thyroid function tests and abnormal liver enzymes with raised transaminases.

Hyponatremia (plasma sodium, < 120 mmol/L) causes lethargy, seizures and respiratory arrest. Central pontine myelinolysis (osmotic demyelination syndrome) is a rare complication of hyperemesis and may result from severe hyponatremia or from over rapid correction of hyponatremia. This is associated with symmetrical destruction of myelin at the center of the basal pons and causes pyramidal tract signs, spastic quadraparesis, pseudobulbar palsy and impaired consciousness.

Box 9.1 Complications of hyperemesis gravidarum

Fetal
- Growth restriction
- Fetal death

Maternal
- Hypokalemia
- Hyponatremia + central pontine myelinolysis
- Wernicke's encephalopathy
- Vitamin B_6/B_{12} deficiency
- Malnutrition
- Mallory–Weiss esophageal tears
- Venous thromboembolism
- Psychological morbidity

Hypokalemia may result in cardiac dysrhythmias and skeletal muscle weakness.

Wernicke's encephalopathy results from vitamin B_1 (thiamine) deficiency and is also rare. It is characterised by ophthalmoplegia, diplopia, ataxia and confusion. The typical ocular signs are a sixth nerve palsy, gaze palsy or nystagmus. A recent review of 45 reported cases established that the commonest presenting symptoms are ocular signs (82%), confusion (71%) and ataxia (69%). Wernicke's encephalopathy may be precipitated by i.v. fluids containing high concentrations of dextrose. There is an increased incidence of abnormal liver tests in women with hyperemesis complicated by Wernicke's encephalopathy compared with the incidence in other cases of hyperemesis. As in alcohol abuse, the liver disturbance of hyperemesis may participate in the development of Wernicke's encephalopathy by decreased conversion of thiamine to its active metabolite thiamine pyrophosphate and by a decreased capacity to store thiamine.

Diagnosis of Wernicke's encephalopathy may be confirmed by the finding of a low red cell transketolase, a thiamine-dependent enzyme. Enhanced magnetic resonance imaging (MRI) in acute Wernicke's encephalopathy may reveal symmetrical lesions around the aqueduct and fourth ventricle, which resolve after treatment with thiamine. Although institution of thiamine replacement may improve the symptoms of Wernicke's encephalopathy, if Korsakoff psychosis develops manifest by retrograde amnesia, impaired ability to learn and confabulation, the recovery rate is only about 50%. Wernicke's encephalopathy is associated with a 40% incidence of fetal death.

Central pontine myelinolysis and Wernicke's encephalopathy may coexist during pregnancy and thiamine deficiency may render the myelin sheaths of the central pons more sensitive to changes in serum sodium.

Protein and calorie malnutrition results in weight loss, which may be profound (10-20%), and muscle wasting with consequent weakness. Other vitamin deficiencies occur in hyperemesis, including cyanocobalamin (vitamin B_{12}) and pyridoxine (vitamin B_6) causing anemia and peripheral neuropathy. If total parenteral nutrition (TPN) is required, this is usually given via a central venous catheter, and this has its own potential problems (e.g. infection, pneumothorax).

Prolonged vomiting in hyperemesis may lead to Mallory–Weiss tears of the esophagus and episodes of hematemesis.

The psychological problems resulting from severe hyperemesis are often underestimated. Certain problems such as eating disorders may pre-date the onset of hyperemesis, but others result from the condition itself. Requests for termination of pregnancy should not be assumed to indicate or confirm that the pregnancy was not wanted, but rather this should be an indication of the degree of desperation felt by the patient.

Since hyperemesis may result in profound dehydration and prolonged periods of bed rest and immobility, it constitutes an important risk factor for venous thromboembolism.

Previously it was thought that hyperemesis was not associated with any adverse fetal outcome and there is indeed no increase in the risk of congenital malformations for affected individuals. Studies have also suggested improved fetal outcome in women who suffer nausea and vomiting in pregnancy. However, it has been shown that infants of mothers with severe hyperemesis (associated with abnormal biochemistry and weight loss > 5%) have significantly lower birthweights and birthweight percentiles compared to infants of mothers with mild hyper-emesis and those of the general antenatal population.

Women admitted repeatedly for hyperemesis have a more severe nutritional disturbance, associated with a significantly reduced maternal weight gain and their infants have significantly lower birth-weights than infants of mothers requiring only a single admission.

Management

Investigation to exclude other causes of nausea and vomiting as well as to establish the severity of the hyperemesis and any associated electrolyte derangement is important. An ultrasound scan of the uterus is important to exclude hydatidiform mole, and to diagnose multiple pregnancy both of which increase the risk of hyperemesis (Box 9.2).

Drugs that may cause nausea and vomiting should be temporarily discontinued. The commonest example is iron supplements. Any woman who is ketotic and unable to maintain adequate hydration should be admitted to hospital. With the advent of emergency gynecology/early pregnancy units, it should be possible to manage women with less severe degrees of hyperemesis as day cases by short admission and administration of intravenous fluid therapy and antiemetics as required. All women with hyperemesis require emotional support with frequent reassurance and encouragement from nursing and medical staff. Because of the increased risk of thromboembolism, women admitted with hyperemesis should receive thromboprophylaxis with low molecular weight heparin.

Box 9.2 Protocol for the management of hyperemesis gravidarum

Investigations
- U+E, FBC, LFTs and calcium, TFTs;
- MSU;
- US scan uterus.

Fluid therapy
- normal saline 1 L + 40 mmol KCL, 8 hourly.

Vitamin therapy
- thiamine orally 25-50 mg t.d.s.; or
- thiamine intravenously 100 mg in 100 mL normal saline weekly; or
- Pabrinex® (contains 250 mg thiamine per pair of ampules) weekly.

Antiemetic therapy (possible regimens include)
- cyclizine 50 mg p.o./i.m./i.v. t.d.s.;
- promethazine 25 mg po nocte;
- stemetil 5 mg po tds; 12.5 mg i.m./i.v. t.d.s.; 5 mg p.r. t.d.s. or 25 mg o.d.;
- metoclopramide 10 mg p.o./i.m./i.v. t.d.s.;
- domperidone 10 mg p.o. q.d.s.; 30-60 mg p.r. t.d.s.;
- chlorpromazine 10-25 mg p.o.; 25 mg i.m. t.d.s.

Thromboprophylaxis
- low molecular weight haparin (LMWH) e.g. in 40 mg s.c. o.d. enoxaparin

The most important component of management is to ensure adequate rehydration. This should be with normal saline (sodium chloride 0.9%; 150 mmol/L Na^+) with added potassium chloride sufficient to correct tachycardia, hypotension and ketonuria and return electrolyte levels to normal. This will usually entail 3 L of intravenous fluid per 24 h and at least 100 mmol of KCl. An alternative is Hartmann's solution (sodium chloride 0.6%; sodium lactate 0.25%; 131 mmol/L Na^+; potassium chloride 0.04%; 5 mmol/L K^+). Dextrose containing fluids are avoided except in women with diabetes as neither 5% dextrose nor dextrose saline contain sufficient sodium to correct the commonly associated hyponatremia. High concentrations of dextrose in particular may precipitate Wernicke's encephalopathy. Double-strength saline (2N saline) should also be avoided, even in cases of severe hyponatremia, as this results in too rapid a correction of serum sodium.

Wernicke's encephalopathy is prevented by routine administration of oral or intravenous thiamine. As requirements for thiamine increase during pregnancy (to 1.5 mg/day) women admitted with hyperemesis have a large potential deficit and should receive thiamine hydrochloride tablets 25-50 mg t.d.s. If intravenous treatment is required, this may be given as thiamine 100 mg diluted in 100 mL of normal saline and infused over 30-60 min once each week. Treatment (as opposed to prevention) of Wernicke's encephalopathy requires much higher doses of thiamine.

Antiemetics may be used liberally and safely in pregnancy. There are substantial data from systematic reviews and cohort studies to support the safety of conventional antiemetics in pregnancy including the first trimester. Antiemetics should be offered to women failing to respond to intravenous fluids and electrolytes alone.

The thalidomide disaster has resulted in an understandable reluctance on behalf of general practioners /primary care physicians to prescribe antiemetics for hyperemesis.

But women with nausea and vomiting in pregnancy, even if not requiring hospital admission, whose work and home life is disrupted, should be offered antiemetics.

Women with severe hyperemesis may require regular parenteral doses of more than one antiemetic to control their symptoms. There is no evidence of teratogenesis with antihistamines (H_1 receptor antagonists, e.g. promethazine, cyclizine), phenothiazines (chlorpromazine, prochlorperazine) and dopamine antagonists (metoclopramide, domperidone).

Drugs from each class can be used in combination. Powdered root ginger may also be used. A double-blind, randomized, cross-over trial demonstrated a reduced severity and greater relief of symptoms in the period in which ginger was given.

Side effects of antiemetics include drowsiness, particularly with the phenothiazines, and extrapyramidal effects and oculogyric crises, particularly with metoclopramide and the phenothiazines. Extrapyramidal effects usually abate after discontinuation of the drug and oculogyric crises may be treated with antimuscarinic drugs such as benzatropine 1-2 mg i.m. or i.v.

Ondansetron is a highly selective 5-HT_3 (serotonin) antagonist that has been used with success in intractable hyperemesis, but in a comparative study i.v. ondansetron 10 mg was no better than i.v. promethazine 50 mg. However in this study the hyperemesis was not very severe, which may explain the lack of difference in efficacy. Although there is no evidence of a teratogenic effect of ondansetron, there is insufficient information to be confident and it does cross the placenta.

In women with severe hyperemesis who do not improve with conventional antiemetic and intravenous therapy, a trial of corticosteroids may be considered. Corticosteroids have resulted in rapid improvement in small case series of women with severe refractory hyperemesis. A study of 25 women randomized to receive either 40 mg prednisolone or placebo daily demonstrated a trend towards improved nausea and vomiting and reduced dependence on intravenous fluids, but this did not reach statistical significance. However, women treated with corticosteroids reported an improved sense of wellbeing, improved appetite and weight gain. Steroids should be accompanied by histamine 2 receptor blockers, or proton pump inhibitors (e.g. omeprazole) to counteract gastric effects of the steroid. A suggested starting dose is hydrocortisone 100 mg i.v. twice daily followed by prednisolone 40-50 mg orally daily in divided doses once the woman is able to tolerate tablets. Response, if it occurs, is usually rapid such that the intravenous preparation is rarely needed for more than 48 hours. Steroids should be discontinued if there is no response after 2 days. If there is response, the dose of prednisolone should be reduced slowly to low doses and often cannot be discontinued until the gestation at which the hyperemesis would have resolved spontaneously (in some extreme cases this occurs at delivery).

In cases that fail to respond to all of the above therapies, the only remaining options are enteral or parenteral nutrition or termination of the pregnancy. The cost of enteral feeding is considerably less than that of total parenteral nutrition and it is safer. The successful use of enteral feeding via a nasogastric tube in hyperemesis unresponsive to antiemetics has been reported in women with meal-related nausea and vomiting only. However in pregnancy enteral hyperalimentation may be poorly tolerated because of nausea and vomiting and may even be contraindicated because of the risk of aspiration. Frequent tube displacement may also be a problem. Poor tolerance of a nasogastric tube may lead to consideration of a gastrostomy feeding tube. To minimize the risk of aspiration, a nasojejunal feeding tube may be placed beyond the pylorus, but this necessitates radiation exposure for correct positioning of the tube or insertion under endoscopic guidance.

Total parenteral nutrition (TPN) has been reported but is very rarely necessary. Because of its substantial metabolic, infectious, and thrombotic risks, it should be regarded as a measure of last resort. Because TPN involves the use of high concentrations of glucose, thiamine supplementation is mandatory.

GASTROESOPHAGEAL REFLUX

About two-thirds of women experience heartburn in pregnancy, commonly in the third trimester. This is partly because of reflux due to the decreased lower esophageal pressure, decreased gastric peristalsis and delayed gastric emptying, and partly due to the enlarging uterus. Reflux of acid or alkaline gastric contents into the esophagus causes inflammation of the esophageal mucosa, causing pain, waterbrash and dypepsia. Reflux may be asymptomatic or may present with heartburn, 'waterbrash', nausea and vomiting, cough or wheezing, or aspiration pneumonia. Recurrent or forceful vomiting may cause hematemesis from a Mallory–Weiss (esophageal mucosal) tear or abrasion.

Management

Postural changes, such as sleeping in a semi-recumbent position may help especially in late pregnancy. Avoiding food or fluid intake immediately before retiring may also prevent symptoms. Antacids are safe in pregnancy and may be used liberally. Liquid preparations are more effective and should be given to prevent and treat symptoms. Aluminum-containing antacids may cause constipation and magnesium-containing antacids may cause diarrhea. Metoclopramide increases lower esophageal pressure and speeds gastric emptying and may help relieve reflux. Sucralfate and histamine$_2$-receptor blockers, (e.g. ranitidine) are both safe throughout pregnancy. Proton-pump inhibitors (PPIs), such as omeprazole, are more powerful suppressors of gastric acid secretion, and, from limited data, appear safe. PPIs should be reserved for reflux esophagitis when histamine$_2$-receptor blockers have failed.

PEPTIC ULCER

Peptic ulceration is rare in pregnancy. This may be related to a postulated protective effect on the gastric mucosa of prostaglandins induced by pregnancy. Presentation is usually with epigastric pain rather than with complications such as hemorrhage or perforation. Gastrointestinal endoscopy is safe in pregnancy and should be used to investigate all but minor hematemesis as well as severe epigastric pain, particularly if accompanied by tenderness, in the absence of other causes of epigastric pain (Box 9.3) such as HELLP syndrome or pre-eclampsia.

Helicobacter pylori is found in the stomach of almost all patients with duodenal ulceration and is the dominant cause of peptic ulceration. There are serologic

Box 9.3 Causes of abdominal pain in pregnancy

Obstetric causes
- Ectopic pregnancy/miscarriage
- Labor
- Placental abruption
- Ovarian cysts
- Uterine fibroids
- Ligamentous pain
- Pre-eclampsia/HELLP syndrome
- Acute fatty liver pregnancy

Non-obstetric causes
- Constipation
- Infection (e.g. pyelonephritis, cholecystitis)
- Pneumonia
- Appendicitis
- Pancreatitis
- Peptic ulcer
- Renal colic
- Iliac vein thrombosis
- Metabolic (e.g. diabetic ketoacidosis, hypercalcemia, acute intermittent porphyria)
- Domestic violence

tests that reliably indicate infection in women with appropriate clinical symptoms. In these, endoscopy may be omitted. Eradication with antibiotic therapy increases ulcer healing and decreases relapse, and may be given in pregnancy, but is usually delayed in asymptomatic women. Smoking reduces mucosal resistance and therefore increases the risk of peptic ulceration.

Management

Antacids, sucralfate and histamine$_2$-receptor blockers are used for symptom control and are all safe in pregnancy. Definitive cure relies upon antihelicobacter therapy. Misoprostol, a prostaglandin analogue, protects the gastric mucosa, but is contraindicated during pregnancy because of the risk of miscarriage.

CONSTIPATION

This is another common symptom of normal pregnancy, affecting up to 40% of women. There are several contributory factors including a physiological reduction in colonic motility (with prolonged transit time) due to vasodilatory prostaglandins and vascular endothelial substances, poor dietary intake associated with nausea and vomiting, dehydration, and oral iron supplements. These commonly cause gastrointestinal upset and constipation. Pressure on the rectosigmoid colon by the gravid uterus may contribute to constipation in the third trimester. In the postpartum period, constipation may be particularly troublesome. This is related often to the use of opiate analgesic agents, but also to local perineal trauma and resultant reluctance to open the bowels for fear of pain.

Management includes reassurance and advice regarding increased intake of fluids and dietary fiber. Temporary cessation of oral iron supplements may help and laxatives should only be used if the above measures fail.

Bulk-forming drugs such as unprocessed bran, methyl cellulose, ispaghula husk or sterculia may be used in pregnancy. They should all be taken with adequate fluids to prevent intestinal obstruction. Stimulant laxatives such as glycerol suppositories and senna (Senokot®) tablets are safe for use in pregnancy but danthron should be avoided. Fecal softeners (liquid paraffin, castor oil and soap enemas) should be avoided in pregnancy. Docusate sodium (dioctyl sodium sulfosuccinate), which acts as a stimulant as well as a softening agent, is safe for use in pregnancy. Osmotic laxatives, such as lactulose and magnesium hydrochloride are safe.

INFLAMMATORY BOWEL DISEASE

Both Crohn's disease and ulcerative colitis (UC) tend to present in young adulthood. UC is more common in women and is encountered more commonly in pregnancy. The incidence of UC is about 5-10 per 100 000 and the prevalence is about 0.8 to 1 per 1000.

UC is confined to the colon and causes diarrhea, lower abdominal pain and passage of blood and mucus per rectum.

Crohn's disease affects both sexes equally. The incidence of Crohn's disease is about 5 per 100 000 and prevalence is about 0.5 in 1000. Crohn's disease may affect any part of the gastrointestinal tract from the mouth to the anus. It affects the terminal ileum alone in 30%, the ileum and colon in 50%, and the colon alone in 20% of cases. Women with involvement of the colon may present with any of the features mentioned above for UC, although bleeding is more common in UC than in Crohn's disease. Cases with ileitis present with cramping mid-abdominal pain, diarrhea or weight loss.

In addition inflammatory bowel disease (IBD) may be associated with extraintestinal manifestations including:

- arthritis (sacroiliitis, ankylosing spondylitis);
- aphthous ulcers (Crohn's disease);
- gallstones;
- ascending cholangitis;
- sclerosing cholangitis;
- conjunctivitis/irodocyclitis/episcleritis;
- erythema nodosum;
- increased risk of venous thrombosis.

Flexible sigmoidoscopy, colonoscopy and mucosal biopsy are usually diagnostic and allow histological examination to differentiate UC from Crohn's disease. These may all be safely performed in pregnancy.

Interaction of inflammatory bowel disease and pregnancy

Active IBD may affect fertility. In Crohn's disease inflammation and adhesions may affect the fallopian tubes and ovaries as may prior surgical intervention. Fertility is usually normal in quiescent IBD. The course of IBD is not usually affected by pregnancy. The risk of flare in pregnancy is reduced if colitis is quiescent at the time of conception. For Crohn's disease if conception occurs during disease remission, about one-third of women will experience an exacerbation , a risk equivalent to the non-pregnant patient. However if a pregnancy is conceived while the disease is active, two-thirds of women will have persistent disease activity and two-thirds of these will deteriorate. For UC, the risk of exacerbation is about 50% if disease is active at conception but falls to 30% if pregnancy is conceived during remission. Most exacerbations of IBD occur early in pregnancy and cause abdominal pain, diarrhea and passage of rectal mucous and blood. Women with Crohn's disease are at risk of postpartum flare. Pregnancy outcome is usually good in women with IBD although active disease at the time of conception is associated with an increased risk of miscarriage, and active disease later in pregnancy may adversely affect pregnancy outcome, with an increased rate of prematurity and low birthweight.

Prior surgery, including ileostomy, proctocolectomy and pouch surgery does not preclude successful pregnancy.

Management

Women with IBD planning pregnancy should be advised that pregnancy prognosis is best when they conceive during a period of disease remission. Maintaining adequate control of IBD is important for maternal and fetal health and necessitates multidisciplinary care between gastroenterologists and obstetricians. Management need not usually be altered because of pregnancy and patients on maintenance therapy have fewer relapses than those not on medication.

Nutritional deficiencies may be associated with inflammatory bowel disease related to malabsorption after extensive small bowel resection. Iron deficiency, hypoproteinemia, deficiencies in water- and fat-soluble vitamins and trace elements should be suspected and corrected using a combination of vitamins as indicated. Nutritional parameters should be assayed before pregnancy if possible and then at intervals during pregnancy.

Oral or rectal sulfasalazine (Salazopyrin), and the closely related aminosalicylate, mesalazine (Asacol®), and other 5-aminosalicyclic acid drugs may be safely used throughout pregnancy and breastfeeding. Since sulfasalazine is a dihydrofolate reductase inhibitor, 5 mg daily folic acid should be used before conception and in pregnancy to counter any possible increased risk of neural tube defects, cardiovascular defects, oral clefts, and folate deficiency. Oral and rectal preparations of corticosteroids may be required for acute treatment or maintenance and are safe in pregnancy. Azathioprine may be needed to maintain remission and this should continued in pregnancy (see Ch. 10). Follow up studies of more than 300 pregnancies in women with IBD treated with either azathioprine or 6 mercaptopurine suggest that these drugs although FDA category D (positive evidence of risk, see Ch. 6, Appendix A) are safe and well tolerated in pregnancy. Data from transplant patients are reassuring regarding the safety of ciclosporin A and tacrolimus. AntiT-NFα antibodies (infliximab) are also thought to be safe in pregnancy and breast feeding. Other teratogenic immunosuppressants such as methotrexate should obviousy be avoided in pregnancy. The common antibiotics used in Crohn's disease are metronidazole and ciprofloxacin and studies have failed to show any harmful effects of these in human pregnancy.

Indications for surgery in pregnant women with IBD remain the same as in the non-pregnant, i.e. obstruction, perforation, hemorrhage, abscess and toxic megacolon. A severely ill mother with active IBD provides a greater risk to the fetus than surgery. Most women with IBD may have vaginal deliveries. Cesarean section may be indicated in the presence of severe or active perianal Crohn's disease with a deformed, inelastic or scarred rectum and perineum. Active perianal Crohn's may prevent healing of an episiotomy. Recent recommendations also suggest Cesarean section in women with ileo pouch anal anastomosis because of the theoretical increased risk of damage to the anal sphincter with vaginal delivery. Women with a colostomy or ileostomy may deliver vaginally. If possible, the obstetrician should obtain information from the surgeon who performed previous surgery to better define the risk of vaginal delivery.

PANCREATITIS

This rarely complicates pregnancy, being no more common than in the non-pregnant patient with an incidence of about 1 in 10000. Most attacks occur in late pregnancy and clinical features and underlying causes are similar to the non-pregnant patient. The commonest causes are gallstones and alcohol. Rarer causes include hypertriglyceridemia and the hypercalcemia of primary hyperparathyroidism.

The serum amylase is invariably raised and levels > 1000 U/L suggest pancreatitis or common bile duct stones. Hyperlipidemia may mask the rise in amylase. Serum lipase is also raised in pancreatitis. Management is supportive with nasogastric drainage often required, particularly if there is evidence of paralytic ileus. Intravenous fluids and analgesia are given as required, and most cases resolve spontaneously. About 10% of patients may develop serious pulmonary, cardiac, renal or gastrointestinal complications with shock and an important feature of management is to identify this subgroup and ensure their rapid transfer to an intensive care unit.

Regular monitoring of cardiovascular status, hemoglobin, white cell count, amylase, renal function, oxygen saturation, liver function, prothrombin time, glucose and calcium are essential. Women with chronic pancreatitis or recurrent attacks require careful management in pregnancy as they often suffer from malabsorption, requiring enzyme replacement. In addition, gestational diabetes is frequent in these cases. In most there is a background of alcohol abuse, and their medical care needs to be supplemented by social work and psychological assistance. Fetal growth restriction is to be anticipated.

CONCLUSION

Gastrointestinal problems are common in pregnancy. Most of these relate to the pregnancy itself and symptoms of nausea, vomiting, constipation and reflux esophagitis are almost universal. Hyperemesis gravidarum has the potential to cause severe fetal and maternal morbidity and should be aggressively managed. Pre-existing gastrointestinal disease is usually well tolerated and active disease can be easily investigated and managed with the same armamentarium of drug therapies used in the non-pregnant patient.

Hepatic disorders
C. Williamson

INTRODUCTION

The hepatic disorders that present in pregnancy may be the consequence of diseases specific to pregnancy, e.g. obstetric cholestasis, hyperemesis gravidarum, acute fatty liver of pregnancy or hepatic manifestations of pre-eclampsia or may relate to usual hepatic disorders coincident with pregnancy. Alternatively women with pre-existing liver disease may present with specific symptoms or complications related to pregnancy. This chapter will cover the most common hepatic disorders of pregnancy with the exception of those related to pre-eclampsia which are covered in Chapter 3.

OBSTETRIC CHOLESTASIS

Obstetric cholestasis, that affects 0.5-1.5% of pregnancies in Europeans, is commoner in women of South Asian and South American origin. Most affected women are asymptomatic outside pregnancy, although up to 20% of cases have pruritus in the second half of the menstrual cycle or if they take estrogen-containing contraceptives.

Etiology

The etiology of obstetric cholestasis is complex. Most affected women have a genetic predisposition to the cholestatic effects of raised estrogens and/or progesterone. Evidence for genetic factors include sibling studies that report a 20-fold increase in risk for first-degree relatives, pedigree studies that demonstrate sex-limited autosomal dominant inheritance in a subgroup of cases and reports of heterozygous mutations in genes that encode biliary transporters. Raised serum levels of reproductive hormones are thought to play a role in the etiology of obstetric cholestasis because the condition is commoner in twin pregnancies where estrogen levels are higher, and because women with a history of cholestasis may develop pruritus and abnormal liver function when given exogenous oestrogens. The condition also occurs more commonly following the administration of progesterone to prevent preterm labor.

Maternal clinical features

Cholestasis characteristically presents with pruritus in the second half of pregnancy. This is most commonly a generalized itch, often first experienced on the palms and soles, and is not associated with a specific rash. The diagnosis is confirmed if abnormal liver function tests and/or raised serum bile acids are found and order causes (see below under 'Differential diagnosis') are excluded. The pruritus may precede the biochemical abnormalities by several weeks and therefore liver function tests and serum bile acids should be repeated after a week or two if initially normal in women where the diagnosis is suspected. Apart from pruritus, affected women may complain of dark urine and pale stools and approximately 10% have jaundice. There also is a reported association with postpartum hemorrhage. There is no consensus about whether the most reliable diagnostic test is the demonstration of raised transaminases or raised serum bile acids, and therefore many units use both. The normal ranges for serum transaminases in preg-

nancy should be used, and it is important to note that a minority of affected women have a raised bilirubin. Abdominal ultrasound may demonstrate gallstones. However, these may not be the cause of the cholestasis. Indeed, at least three genes that are thought to be mutated in obstetric cholestasis are also mutated in people with cholesterol gallstones. Hepatitis C infection is commoner in women with obstetric cholestasis than in the general obstetric population. It is therefore advisable to screen for hepatitis C and hepatitis B as affected women may be referred to a hepatologist for subsequent surveillance and treatment after delivery.

Fetal complications

Cholestasis is associated with spontaneous preterm labor, meconium stained amniotic fluid, cardiotocograph abnormalities and sudden intrauterine death. The perinatal mortality rate has reduced from 9-11% in older studies in the 1970s to < 3.5% in more recent studies where the fetus was delivered by 38 weeks gestation (Table 9.2). This is consistent with the results of a UK retrospective survey of pregnancies complicated by IUD that demonstrated that 90% of cholestasis-related fetal deaths occurred at 37 weeks of gestation or later. No fetal deaths were reported in two recent studies of < 100 cases. However, the authors are aware of several reports of pregnancies complicated by cholestasis-related IUD each year in the UK.

A recent Swedish study demonstrated that fetal complications of prematurity, asphyxial events and meconium stained liquor do not occur in their population in cases with serum total bile acids < 40 μmol/L. However, once the serum bile acids rise above this level, there is a 1-2% increase in these fetal complications with each rise of 1 μmol/L in the serum bile acid level.

Table 9.2 Summary of the major studies of fetal outcome in OC

	Number of cases	IUD[a] and/or NND (%)	Meconium staining (%)	Preterm labor (%)	Planned delivery < 37–38/40[b]
1964-1969	87	9	–	54	No
1965-1979	56	11	27	36	No
post-1969	91	3	–	–	Yes
1988	83	4	45	44	Yes
1994	320	2	25	12	Yes
1990-1996	91	0	15	14.3	Yes
1999-2001	70	0	14	6	Yes

[a]NND = neonatal death; IUD = intrauterine death rate as a percentage of all births.
[b]I.e. in the majority of cases in the study.

The etiology of fetal death in the rare cases in which it is observed is not fully understood. However, it is likely to be a sudden asphyxial event. Histological examination of placentas from OC pregnancies revealed non-specific changes, including reduced syncytial sprout formation, maturation defects, villous edema and trophoblastic swelling. In vitro studies using rodent cardiac cell cultures suggest that bile acids may have a toxic effect on the fetal heart.

The reason for the increased frequency of preterm labor is not clear, but it has been postulated that it may be a consequence of bile acid-induced release of prostaglandins, which in turn may initiate labor. Bile acids have also been shown to increase the incidence of preterm labor when given as an infusion to sheep. In the study in which bile acids were given as an infusion to sheep, all the bile acid-treated fetuses developed meconium stained amniotic fluid by the third day of infusion. This may be because the raised serum bile acids caused fetal distress and subsequent passage of meconium into amniotic fluid. Alternatively, it may be due to bile acids stimulating the smooth muscle of the fetal intestine resulting in increased bowel motility.

Pre-pregnancy advice and issues

If a woman has a previous history of obstetric cholestasis she has a high chance (90%) of recurrence in subsequent pregnancies. This is reduced if the previous affected pregnancy was a multiple pregnancy and subsequent pregnancies are not. It is advisable to ensure that baseline liver function tests and serum bile acids are normal, and to determine her hepatitis C status before she conceives. It is also sensible to establish whether she has asymptomatic gallstones and to enquire about gastrointestinal symptoms, drug reactions and a family history of cholestasis.

What to do at the first booking visit

Liver function tests should be checked at the first booking visit. There are no other specific management issues providing the woman is asymptomatic. If she had the condition previously she should attend for liver function tests and serum bile acids if she starts to itch.

Differential diagnosis

The diagnosis of OC is made by exclusion of other possible causes of pruritus and abnormal liver function. Therefore, once raised transaminases or bile acids are found, the following investigations should be carried out: viral serotoogy for hepatitis A, B, C,

EBV and CMW; liver autoantibodies (antismooth muscle antibody [suggesting chronic active hepatitis], antimitochondrial anitbody [suggesting primary biliary cirrhosis]).

Clinical pharmacology in pregnancy

Ursodeoxycholic acid (UDCA) is the most commonly used drug for treatment of obstetric cholestasis. In 2003 the Cochrane Database of Systematic reviews reported three trials comprising 56 cases in which UDCA is compared with placebo. In one trial, UDCA caused a greater reduction in liver function tests and serum bile acids than placebo. In the other trials there was no difference between UDCA and placebo in the relief of symptoms. A more recent study that randomized 130 women to either UDCA, dexamethasone or placebo demonstrated significant reductions in ALT and bilirubin in the UDCA group only. In a subgroup of cases with serum bile acids $\geq 40\ \mu mol/L$ UDCA also caused significant reductions in pruritus and serum bile acid levels. A review of the additional reports of UDCA treatment for obstetric cholestasis prior to 2001 reported that UDCA treatment resulted in a clinical and/or biochemical improvement in 74/85 (87%) of cases. Thus the available data suggest that UDCA should be used as a first-line agent for the treatment of obstetric cholestasis. UDCA is commonly started at a dose of 500 mg BD, but doses of up to 2000 g per day can be used for women who do not respond to lower doses. There have been no problems reported in the offspring of women with cholestasis that are attributable to UDCA treatment, although there has been no follow up of these babies. Aqueous cream with menthol can provide symptomatic relief, particularly for women who have difficulty sleeping as a consequence of pruritus, and can be a useful adjunct to UDCA treatment.

Dexamethasone has been used as a second-line treatment for women who have not responded to UDCA because one Finnish study reported a good clinical and biochemical response in all of 12 women who were treated. However, UK data do not replicate this response rate and dexamethasone did not result in significant reductions in liver function tests, serum bile acids or symptoms in the larger Swedish study in which it was compared with UDCA and placebo.

Other pharmacological agents that have been used to treat obstetric cholestasis include cholestyramine, guar gum and S-adenosyl methionine. None of these have been consistently shown to reduce serum bile acids or liver function tests although some studies report improved symptoms. It is thought that the increased prevalence of postpartum hemorrhage in obstetric cholestasis may be related to vitamin K deficiency. Therefore prophylaxis with oral vitamin K 10 mg OD or parenteral 5-10 mg once or twice before delivery is advisable.

Managing delivery

There is no form of antenatal surveillance that reliably predicts which pregnancies will be complicated by fetal distress, premature delivery or fetal death. However, the data shown in Table 9.1 and other population surveys indicate that the risk of fetal death increases if pregnancy continues past 37 weeks' gestation. Therefore delivery between 37 and 38 weeks' gestation is recommended. At this gestation the risks of respiratory distress drop considerably compared to those reported at 35 or 36 weeks' gestation. Many women with obstetric cholestasis have induction of labor, and this has raised concerns about increasing rates of Cesarean section in this group. There have been no studies that have addressed this issue specifically. However, an Italian study that reported a management protocol that included induction of labor at 37 weeks of gestation or earlier if there were unresponsive liver function tests or fetal distress also reported the rates of operative delivery in OC cases in whom labor was induced. For the 206 women managed using this protocol, the Cesarean section rate was similar to that of controls (15% vs. 16% respectively).

Post-pregnancy care, including advice on contraception

The maternal pruritus and abnormal liver function tests resolve within days or weeks of delivery in the majority of cases. If there are ongoing abnormalities in liver testing the woman should be referred to a hepatologist.

Estrogen-containing oral contraceptives may cause cholestasis in women with a history of obstetric cholestasis, so they should be avoided if possible. If a woman insists that she would like to take this form of contraception her liver function should be checked at regular intervals.

Box 9.4 summarizes the care that should be given to women with obstetric cholestasis.

GALLSTONES AND CHOLECYSTITIS

Cholesterol gallstones occur more commonly in pregnancy. There have been several prospective studies of the prevalence of gallstones or biliary sludge in pregnancy and the puerperium. In a Greek study of 669 pregnant women 6 (1%) had pre-existing gallstones

> ### Box 9.4 Management of women with obstetric cholestasis
>
> - Weekly LFT and serum bile acids
> - First-line treatment UDCA
> - Aqueous cream with menthol for itch
> - Vitamin K may protect against postpartum hemorrhage
> - Deliver between 37-38 weeks of gestation

identified on ultrasound and another 14 (2%) developed gallstones during pregnancy. An Italian study of 272 pregnant women demonstrated gallstones in 2% and sludge in 31%; after pregnancy sludge was found to have disappeared in 61% and stones resolved in 28%. A US study of 3254 women revealed either sludge or gallstones in 5% of women by the second trimester, 8% by the third trimester and in 10% by 4-6 weeks' postpartum. In this study body mass index was a strong predictor of gallstone disease. Gallstones are commoner in Chile, and a study of 980 women from this country revealed that 12% of women had gallstones in the early puerperium, compared with 1% of nulliparous healthy volunteers. The combination of gall bladder stasis and the lithogenic bile increases the formation of both sludge and stones during pregnancy. The reasons for this increased lithogenicity of bile in pregnancy are unclear but it is associated with increased concentrations of bile cholesterol, decreased concentrations of bile acids and increased ratio of cholic acid to chenodeoxycholic acid, all favoring the formation of stones. There are undoubtedly genetic factors as a family history of cholelithiasis is very common.

Acute cholecystitis is the second commonest cause of general surgical intervention in pregnancy after appendicitis, and complicates about 0.1% of pregnancies.

Maternal clinical features

Gallstones in pregnant women are commonly asymptomatic, although 28% of cases with stones in the Italian study complained of biliary pain. Gallstones may coexist with obstetric cholestasis, and this is likely to be because both conditions have shared genetic predisposing factors. Women with acute cholecystitis complain of right upper quadrant pain that commonly radiates to the back. This may be associated with nausea, vomiting, pyrexia and weight loss.

It should be considered in the presence of a raised white blood cell count, abnormal liver function tests, pericholecystic fluid, distension and thickening of the gall bladder wall, and ultrasound transducer-induced pain over the gall bladder.

A mildly (twofold) raised amylase is also consistent with a diagnosis of acute cholecystitis, although greater rises suggest pancreatitis or common bile duct stones.

The differential diagnosis of acute cholecystitis in pregnancy includes the causes of abdominal pain given in Box 9.3.

Management is the same as in the non-pregnant patient. Women should be given intravenous fluids, feeding should be stopped and they should receive antibiotic treatment and analgesia. Ultrasound examination will commonly confirm stones within the gall bladder but it is less useful at demonstrating gallstones in the common bile duct. If necessary a technetium-99 HIDA scan may be used as this exposes the fetus to minimal irradiation. Occasionally where there is suspicion of an impacted stone, endoscopic retrograde cholangiopancreatography (ERCP) is required.

Conservative management results in resolution of symptoms in over 75% of women. Laparoscopic cholecystectomy has been safely performed in pregnancy but is very difficult in later gestation. For this reason, assuming symptoms subside it is best deferred to the postpartum period. Endoscopic removal of common bile duct stones and stent drainage or sphincterotomy may be performed with minimal radiation.

A recent study that compared medical and surgical management of symptomatic cholelithiasis in 63 pregnant women demonstrated that surgical management was uncomplicated in 10 cases. In the 53 cases that were treated medically there was symptomatic relapse in 38% and 2 had premature delivery. With regard to surgical management, a retrospective review of the literature that compared the use of laparoscopic cholecystectomy with open cholecystectomy indicated that the former was associated with lower rates of spontaneous abortion in the first trimester and premature delivery in the third trimester. There is some debate about the best time to perform surgery. The second trimester is the optimal time to perform a cholecystectomy with regard to fetal outcome. Also in the third trimester uterine enlargement may result in mechanical problems. However, surgery must be performed if there is large duct obstruction as this will reduce the chance of pancreatitis and cholangitis.

ACUTE AND CHRONIC VIRAL HEPATITIS

Viral hepatitis is the commonest cause of jaundice in pregnancy worldwide. The course of most forms of viral hepatitis is not appreciably altered in pregnancy. The exceptions are hepatitis E and herpes simplex hepatitis, both of which are more likely to have adverse outcomes in pregnant women. Hepatitis A, B, C and E and herpes simplex hepatitis will be considered in turn.

Hepatitis A

Hepatitis A is spread by the fecal–oral route and occurs most commonly in areas of poor sanitation. In parts of Asia, Africa and South America there are extremely high rates of exposure in early childhood, and therefore acute infections are relatively rare in pregnancy. In Western countries hepatitis A infection should be suspected in women with acute hepatic dysfunction, particularly if they have a history of recent travel to an endemic area.

Maternal clinical features

Women with acute hepatitis A infection commonly present with anorexia, nausea, fever and jaundice. They may have considerably raised serum transaminases and bilirubin. The illness is usually self-limiting and there is no chronic carrier state. Fulminant liver failure is rare and the rates of this severe complication are no commoner in pregnancy than in the non-pregnant woman. Acute infection can be diagnosed by the demonstration of IgM anti-HAV antibodies in maternal serum.

Fetal complications

There are no studies to demonstrate an increased risk of congenital abnormality, fetal loss, intrauterine growth restriction or preterm delivery following hepatitis A infection in pregnancy. Vertical transmission at the time of delivery is rare, as the virus is only excreted in the maternal feces for a short time. If this does occur normal immune globulin (NIG), which contains anti-hepatitis A antibodies may be used. However, hepatitis A vaccine is not licensed for use in children < 2 years of age.

Post-pregnancy care, including advice on contraception

Breastfeeding is not contraindicated and the hepatitis A vaccine is safe for lactating mothers.

Hepatitis B

Hepatitis B affects approximately 280 million people worldwide, and is particularly prevalent in Asia and sub-Saharan Africa, with seropositivity in > 50% of the adult population in some countries. Its prevalence has fallen in Western countries with the introduction of the hepatitis B vaccination.

Maternal clinical features

Most women with acute hepatitis B infection will present with mild symptoms. Approximately 30% will have anorexia, nausea, vomiting, jaundice, abdominal pain or pyrexia. Approximately 1% will develop fulminant hepatic failure. Liver transaminase levels may rise to above 1000 IU/L (usual upper limit of normal is 40 IU/L). Chronic infection occurs more commonly in individuals who have had mild, anicteric illness, and is less common in those who had severe symptoms at the time of acute infection. Chronic infection with hepatitis B is associated with an increased risk of subsequent cirrhosis, chronic active hepatitis and primary liver cancer.

Fetal complications

The fetus may be infected following transplacental transfer of the virus or by direct inoculation at the time of delivery. In utero infection is rare except in cases where the mother has acute hepatitis B infection during pregnancy. In these cases the vertical transmission rate is 10% in the first trimester and approximately 90% if infection occurs in the third trimester. The rates of intrauterine death and preterm delivery are increased in pregnancies of women with acute hepatitis B infection.

In women with chronic infection, the subgroup of cases comprising women who are positive for hepatitis B e-antigen (i.e. consistent with high infectivity) also have vertical transmission rate of approximately 90%. The implications of vertical transmission to the fetus, or of horizontal transmission in the first years of life are considerable for the children of women with hepatitis B. Indeed, 40% of chronic carriers of hepatitis B contracted the virus by vertical transmission.

Pre-pregnancy advice and management

Women should be advised that hepatitis B is commonly spread by sexual contact and they should discuss the risk of transmission with their partner. They should minimize intake of alcohol and drugs that may be hepatotoxic and should have serological screening to establish whether they are hepatitis e-antigen positive. If acute infection is suspected they should also be screened for IgM anti-HBc as this is a marker of recent infection. It is also important to

ensure that they do not have HIV, or hepatitis C. Affected women should also have baseline checks of liver function. They should be advised of the risks of transmission to the offspring and the importance of immunoprophylaxis.

Clinical pharmacology in pregnancy

If a woman is at risk of acute hepatitis B infection, e.g. following needlestick injury, the current data do not indicate that treatment with hepatitis B immunoglobulin (HBIG) or hepatitis B vaccine is contraindicated. The woman should be screened to ensure that she is seronegative. There are no specific treatments used for affected women in pregnancy. However, it has been shown that high maternal HBV DNA levels are associated with failure of immunization in the infant of an affected pregnancy. In this group of highly viremic women, lamivudine has been used successfully to reduce the risk of vertical transmission.

Managing delivery

There is no evidence that mode of delivery has a significant influence on the rates of vertical transmission providing appropriate immunization is given to the neonate.

Post-pregnancy care, including advice on contraception

Breastfeeding should be encouraged as it does not alter the rates of transmission to the neonate providing the baby is receiving immunization. Hepatitis B vaccine is safe for breastfeeding mothers. HBIG and hepatitis B vaccine should be given to the neonate of hepatitis B-infected women at birth, and the vaccine should also be given at one month and six months of age (or a similar locally recommended regimen should be given). Combined immunoprophylaxis has been shown to have a protective efficiency rate of > 93%. There is no contraindication to other neonatal immunizations in babies given hepatitis B immunoprophylaxis.

There is no evidence that any specific form of contraception is contraindicated in hepatitis B. However, barrier methods should be used if the partner is not affected, to prevent sexual transmission.

Hepatitis C

Hepatitis C is common among intravenous drug users, people who have had multiple transfusions and those with HIV infection. However, it also occurs in women with no apparent risk factors. It is estimated to affect 0.5-1% of the antenatal population although its prevalence varies in different populations. Affected individuals develop chronic hepatitis after contracting the infection, but they are commonly asymptomatic for a considerable number of years. However, approximately 30% will develop cirrhosis after 10 years, and this group of patients are also at risk of hepatoma.

Maternal clinical features

Pregnant women with hepatitis C infection do not have an exacerbation of their disease during pregnancy. However, they do have an increased risk of obstetric cholestasis, and when this does occur the rate of premature delivery and the maternal symptoms are worse than in women with obstetric cholestasis who do not have hepatitis.

Fetal complications

The risk of vertical transmission is low providing the mother has a low circulating count of the virus. The level above which the risk of vertical transmission is believed to increase is 1×10^6 genome equivalents per milliliter. A meta-analysis of 77 studies performed between 1992-2000 indicated that another risk factor for vertical transmission is co-infection with HIV. The same study indicated that the mode of delivery does not influence the rate of infection in the offspring of women affected with hepatitis C. A recent multicenter study by the European Pediatric Hepatitis C Virus Network confirmed that mode of delivery and breast feeding do not influence the rate of mother-to-child transmission of hepatitis C, and also reported that female fetuses are more likely to be infected (adjusted odds ratio 2.1 [95% CI 1.2-2.5], $p = 0.006$).

Post-pregnancy care, including advice on contraception

Horizontal transmission of hepatitis C within a family is rare, but it can occur if the mother has high levels of viremia. Breastfeeding is not contraindicated as the current literature does not suggest that the rate of transmission to the newborn is increased in lactating women.

Women with hepatitis C should be referred to a hepatologist for long-term review and for consideration of antiviral treatment with interferon and ribavirin. Both drugs are contraindicated in pregnancy and when breastfeeding. Ribavirin is highly teratogenic and the manufacturers recommend that treatment is ceased at least 6 months before conception to allow 'washout' of body stores.

Hepatitis E

Hepatitis E is spread by the fecal–oral route and is endemic in many parts of Asia. It causes an acute self-limiting hepatitis in non-pregnant individuals.

Maternal clinical features

The course of hepatitis E is exacerbated by pregnancy, with a 12-fold increase in the fatality rate. Approximately 20% of pregnant women who have the infection develop acute liver failure, and the rates of hepatic failure and death increase with advancing gestation.

Fetal complications

A recent Indian study of the clinical features of hepatitis E infection in 28 pregnant women reported premature delivery in 67% of cases. Vertical transmission was observed in 6/18 cord blood samples and there was a high perinatal mortality rate in the 6 affected infants; two had hypoglycemia, hypothermia and died within 48 h and one had massive hepatic necrosis.

Herpes simplex hepatitis

Hepatitis secondary to herpes simplex is extremely rare, but it does appear to occur more commonly in pregnant women. Herpetic vesicles are not always present and the presenting features are non-specific. The commonest symptoms are fatigue and pyrexia, and liver function tests commonly reveal markedly high transaminases and mildly raised bilirubin. The condition carries a grave prognosis without antiviral therapy, and if suspected it should be treated with intravenous aciclovir.

WILSON'S DISEASE

Wilson's disease is an autosomal recessive disorder in which copper accumulates, resulting in hepatic impairment, neurological symptoms, particularly movement disorder, and behavior abnormalities. It is caused by mutations in the *ATP7B* gene that encodes a copper binding ATPase, resulting in abnormal hepatic excretion of copper that is destined for fecal excretion. Affected individuals usually have low serum levels of copper and ceruloplasmin, and raised urinary copper. Fertility is commonly reduced in women with suboptimally treated Wilson's disease, and they may have amenorrhea, irregular menses and increased miscarriage rates. However, maternal and fetal outcomes are generally good if the disease is adequately treated.

Clinical pharmacology in pregnancy

If a woman with Wilson's disease is stable on treatment she should be advised to continue her current medication. The three principal treatments used for Wilson's disease are D-penicillamine, trientine and zinc. D-penicillamine and trientine are chelating agents that combine with copper. Zinc acts on intestinal cells to prevent copper absorption. The use of D-penicillamine is associated with teratogenicity in animals and humans. The principal concerns for humans are a cutis laxa syndrome, micrognathia and low set ears. Trientine has been reported to cause teratogenicity in animal studies.

Despite these concerns there are encouraging data on pregnancy outcome following the use of these chelating agents as maintenance therapy for Wilson's disease. This may be because the dose used for maintenance therapy in Wilson's disease is lower than that used to treat cystinuria, and from which the data on teratogenicity were derived. There is more experience with the use of D-penicillamine in treating Wilson's disease in pregnancy and a recent summary of the current literature reported good outcomes in 144 of 153 pregnancies in 111 women. The adverse outcomes were 3 therapeutic abortions, 1 miscarriage, 1 premature delivery, 2 cases of cutix laxa, 1 of cleft lip and palate and 1 case of mannosidosis. The same author reported 19 good outcomes in 22 pregnancies in 17 women treated with trientine. The adverse outcomes were 1 therapeutic abortion, 1 miscarriage and 1 case of isochromosome X.

Zinc has also been continued as a maintenance therapy for pregnant women with Wilson's disease. A recent report of the outcome of 26 pregnancies in 19 women reported 2 congenital abnormalities (7.7%); one heart defect requiring surgery at 6 months and 1 baby with microcephaly who died soon after birth. All other babies were reported as normal.

Taken together these data indicate that maintenance therapy with D-penicillamine, trientine or zinc should be continued in pregnancy. This is particularly important as there are reports of hemolysis, hepatic deterioration and death in women who have stopped D-penicillamine treatment in an attempt to avoid teratogenicity. The congenital abnormalities associated with the chelating agents are thought to be related to fetal copper deficiency rather than a direct effect of the drugs. Therefore some authors have advocated aiming for relatively low doses of these agents providing the maternal disease is controlled. It should be remembered that the chelating agents also reduce serum levels of iron and zinc and therefore they should not be given together with iron supplements. Pyridoxine (vitamin B6) supplements should also be given as D-penicillamine also has anti-pyridine effects.

Newborn babies of women with Wilson's disease have normal copper and ceruloplasmin levels, even if the mother has not complied well with treatment.

Post-pregnancy care, including advice on contraception

Breastfeeding is not contraindicated in women with Wilson's disease. Concentrations of zinc and copper are reduced in the mothers' milk, but no adverse consequences have been reported in their babies.

HEPATIC FAILURE

Acute liver failure is defined as the development of hepatic encephalopathy secondary to severe liver dysfunction, and it can be classified as hyperacute, acute or subacute, depending upon whether the onset of encephalopathy takes < 7 days, 8-24 days or > 24 days. American demographic data from outside pregnancy show that acute liver failure affects women more commonly than men with a median age of onset of 38. It also occurs more commonly in Americans of Caucasian origin. In the USA and UK the commonest cause of acute liver failure is paracetamol toxicity, followed by viral hepatitis and idiosyncratic drug reactions. Other causes include autoimmune hepatitis, Wilson's disease and pregnancy-specific diseases. Table 9.3 lists the major causes of hepatic failure and the investigations that should be performed for each. All of these conditions may occur in pregnant women. However, the predominant cause of hepatic failure in pregnant women varies in different geographical locations. In Asian countries viral hepatitis is much commoner than in the USA and UK, and in particular hepatitis E is an important cause in South Asia. In contrast, paracetamol poisoning is commoner in women from the USA and UK.

Maternal clinical features

Once hepatic failure is suspected the woman must be managed by a multidisciplinary team that includes obstetricians, obstetric physicians, hepatologists, anesthetists and intensive care specialists. The main management priorities are, first, to establish the underlying diagnosis as this will influence the prognosis and specific management plans, and, second, to monitor the development of the associated complications of encephalopathy, hypoglycemia, renal impairment, aci-

Table 9.3 Causes of acute liver failure and relevant investigations

Diagnosis	Investigation/initial assessment
HELLP syndrome/severe pre-eclampsia	Hypertension, platelets, urinary protein, urate, transaminases
Acute fatty liver of pregnancy	As for HELLP syndrome, glucose, imaging may be performed
Hepatitis A, B, E	Viral serology
Herpes simplex hepatitis	Viral serology
Paracetamol poisoning	Drug levels in blood
Idiosyncratic drug reactions	Eosinophils
Wilson's disease	Copper, ceruloplasmin, urinary copper, slit lamp examination
Autoimmune hepatitis	Autoantibodies
Budd Chiari syndrome	MRI or ultrasound, if necessary venography
Malignancy	MRI or ultrasound, histology
Hemolytic uremic syndrome/thrombotic thrombocytopenic purpura	Blood film, platelet count, urea and electrolytes, creatinine, urate

Modified from O'Grady (2006).

dosis, electrolyte imbalance, prolonged prothrombin time, thromocytopenia and infection. Detailed management strategies for acute liver failure in non-pregnant patients are outlined in two recent reviews by Lee (2003) and O'Grady (2006). On the whole these will not differ in pregnant women, although decisions must also be made about early delivery, particularly when there is a pregnancy-specific diagnosis, e.g. acute fatty liver of pregnancy or severe pre-eclampsia. Also, hemostasis is a priority if delivery is contemplated and blood and blood products must be available.

A recent Chinese study of the clinical features of 55 women with acute liver failure demonstrated that hepatic encephalopathy occurred significantly more commonly in pregnant women (76% compared to 50% of non-pregnant women), as did hepatorenal syndrome (64% vs. 13%) and hemorrhage (56% vs. 3%). There were also significantly lower blood levels of glucose and higher levels of creatinine.

Fetal complications

There are limited data on the fetal outcome of maternal acute hepatic failure in pregnancy. The Chinese study reported high rates of fetal death (20%), preterm labor (33%) and fetal distress (28%). Maternal hypoglycemia is associated with fetal demise as well as maternal death, underlining the importance of regular measurement of blood glucose. Paracetamol metabolites can cross the placenta and may result in fetal liver damage, coagulation abnormalities and intraventricular hemorrhage.

Clinical pharmacology in pregnancy

N-acetylcysteine is a potent antioxidant that is used for the treatment of paracetamol overdose. It can also be used to treat other causes of acute hepatic failure and its use in pregnancy has been reported. Hypertension should be treated using standard protocols. However cerebral edema should also be considered in women with hypertension and tachycardia and this should be treated with mannitol. Women with renal failure should not be treated with mannitol as it is nephrotoxic. Vitamin K and folate should also be administered. Proton pump inhibitors or H_2 antagonists should be used to prevent gastrointestinal bleeding. Blood products, platelets, glucose and electrolytes should be replaced as required. All body fluids should be cultured regularly and prompt treatment given if infection is identified.

Managing delivery

For women with acute liver failure secondary to acute fatty liver of pregnancy or severe pre-eclampsia delivery is necessary to treat the condition. For other causes a decision about delivery will be made dependent upon the mother's condition and the gestational age of the fetus. If the mother has any coagulation defects they should be corrected prior to delivery.

Post–pregnancy care, including advice on contraception

Post-pregnancy care and advice will vary depending upon the condition that caused acute liver failure.

PREGNANCY AFTER LIVER TRANSPLANTATION

Most women find that their libido returns quickly after liver transplantation, as does regular menstruation, and therefore there have been a considerable number of pregnancies reported in women who have had successful liver transplants.

Pre-pregnancy advice and management

Women should be advised to avoid conception for 2 years after liver transplantation to allow stabilization of immunosuppression. Studies that include women who conceive less than 2 years after transplant have reported worse pregnancy outcomes in this group. Pregnancy after liver transplantation is rarely normal and most case series report increased rates of miscarriage, premature delivery, small for gestational age infants, hypertension and pre-eclampsia. Pre-eclampsia is particularly common in women with renal dysfunction or hypertension prior to conception. However, a recent case series in which all patients were treated with tacrolimus did not report a marked increase in the rates of hypertensive diseases in a center with considerable experience in the management of pregnant liver transplant patients. There is an increased risk of diabetes mellitus secondary to immunosuppression, and screening for diabetes should be performed prior to conception and in early pregnancy. Graft rejection occurs, but it is rare. It may be heralded by deterioration in liver function tests. However, it must be remembered that other relatively common pregnancy-specific disorders such as obstetric cholestasis or pre-eclampsia may also cause hepatic impairment.

There is an increased risk of cytomegalovirus infection in the period immediately after transplantation, and the risk is also higher during episodes of rejection where increased immunosuppression is required. This is important as cytomegalovirus infection may result in congenital abnormalities or fetal hepatic impairment if it occurs in early pregnancy.

Clinical pharmacology in pregnancy

The principal immunosuppressive drugs used in women who have had a liver transplant are ciclosporin, tacrolimus, azathioprine and corticosteroids. The clinical pharmacology of these agents is discussed in Chapters 4, 6 and 10.

Managing delivery

The presence of pregnancy complications may influence the timing and mode of delivery. Cesarean rates are high in the recent case series, but vaginal delivery is not contraindicated.

Post-pregnancy care, including advice on contraception

Women who have had liver transplants have increased rates of neoplasia, including cervical cancer. They should therefore be advised to have cervical smears regularly, and at least yearly.

Reliable, effective contraception is extremely important in life limiting states such as after hepatic transplantation. Women should be assisted by an expert in contraceptive aspects of medical disease as unplanned pregnancy adds one more potential disaster to a woman who has undoubtedly been through a series of life threatening events. Survival after transplantation is largely dependent on avoidance of major life stresses that destabilize the control of the medical disorder, and it is incumbent on physicians and obstetricians who deal with these patients to ensure that contraceptive advice is not relegated to inexperienced members of the team. Barrier methods, the Mirena® coil and implantation devices are the contraceptive agents of choice. Oral contraceptives are contraindicated in women who have had Budd-Chiari syndrome and they also can exacerbate the hepatotoxicity of ciclosporin.

CONCLUSION

Obstetric cholestasis affects approximately 1 in 200 pregnancies. It may be complicated by spontaneous preterm labor and rarely by IUD at relatively late gestation. UDCA is more effective than other drugs for control of symptoms.

Cholesterol gallstones occur more commonly in pregnancy. However most do not result in acute cholecystitis. If this occurs surgical management is more effective than medical management.

The principal maternal risks associated with hyperemesis gravidarum are hyponatremia, hypokalemia and Wernicke's encephalopathy secondary to thiamine deficiency. Conventional antiemetics are safe as first line treatment. If these are not effective there are data from small studies to support the use of corticosteroids or 5HT3 receptor antagonists. Most women with hyperemesis should be treated contemporaneously for gastroesophageal reflux.

The course of most forms of viral hepatitis is not altered by pregnancy. The exceptions are hepatitis E and herpes simplex hepatitis, both of which are associated with adverse outcomes.

Pregnancy in women with Wilson's disease is associated with good maternal and fetal outcomes providing the disease is adequately treated. Maintenance therapy with D-penicillamine, trientine and zinc should be continued.

Acute liver failure should be managed by a multi-disciplinary team. Specific management strategies will vary depending on the underlying diagnosis. Pregnant wome n with acute liver failure more commonly have hepatic encephalopathy, hepato-renal syndrome and hemorrhage than non-pregnant women.

Women who have had liver transplant should avoid pregnancy for 2 years. Most studies suggest that women with liver transplants have higher rates of miscarriage, preterm delivery, IUGR, hypertensive disease and diabetes. Graft rejection is rare.

Further reading

Alstead E A, Nelson-Piercy C 2002 Inflammatory bowel disease in pregnancy. Gut 52:159-161

American College of Obstetricians and Gynecologists Educational Bulletin 1998 Viral hepatitis in pregnancy. International Journal of Gynaecology and Obstetrics 63:195-202

Bacq Y et al 1997 Intrahepatic cholestasis of pregnancy: a French prospective study. Hepatology 26:358-364

Bailit J L 2005 Hyperemesis gravidarium: Epidemiologic findings from a large cohort. American Journal of Obstetrics and Gynecology 193:811-814

Beasley R P et al 1983 Prevention of perinatally transmitted hepatitis B virus infections with hepatitis B immune globulin and hepatitis B vaccine. Lancet ii:1099-1102

Brewee G J et al 2000 Treatment of Wilson's disease with zinc: XVII: treatment during pregnancy. Hepatology 31:364-370

Burrows R F, Clavisi O, Burrows E for the Cochrane Pregnancy and Childbirth Group 2003 Interventions for treating cholestasis in pregnancy. Cochrane Database of Systematic Reviews 3: CD000493

Campos G, Guerra F, Israel E 1986 Effects of cholic acid infusions in fetal lambs. Acta obstetricia et gynecologica Scandinavica 65:23-26

Caprilli R et al 2006 European Crohn's and Colitis Organisation European evidence based consensus on the diagnosis and management of Crohn's disease: special situations. Gut 55(suppl 1):i36-58

Costoya A et al 1980 Morphological study of placental terminal villi in intrahepatic cholestasis of pregnancy: histochemistry, light and electron microscopy. Placenta 1:361-368

Diav-Citrin O et al 2005 The safety of proton pump inhibitors in pregnancy: a multicentre prospective controlled study. Alimentary Pharmacology & Therapeutics 21:269-275

Dodds L et al 2006 Outcomes of pregnancies complicated by hyperemesis gravidarum. Obstetrics & Gynecology 107:285-292

Eloranta M L et al 2001 Risk of obstetric cholestasis in sisters of index patients. Clinical Genetics 60:42-45

Euler G et al 2003 Hepatitis B surface antigen prevalence among pregnant women in urban areas: implications for testing, reporting and preventing perinatal transmission. Pediatrics 111:1192-1197

European Paediatric Hepatitis C Virus Network 2005 A significant sex-but not elective cesarean section-effect on mother-to-child transmission of hepatitis C virus infection. Journal of Infectious Disease 192:1872-1879

Fagan E A 2002 Disorders of the liver. In: Medical disorders in obstetric practice, 4th edn. Blackwell Science, New York, p 282-345

Fell D B et al 2006 Risk factors for hyperemesis gravidarum requiring hospital admission during pregnancy. Obstetrics & Gynecology 107:277-284

Fisk N M, Storey G N 1988 Fetal outcome in obstetric cholestasis. British Journal of Obstetrics and Gynaecology 95:1137-1143

Gilat T, Konikoff F 2000 Pregnancy and the biliary tract. Canadian Journal of Gastroenterology 14(suppl D):55D-59D

Glantz A et al 2005 Intrahepatic cholestasis of pregnancy: a randomized controlled trial comparing dexamethasone and ursodeoxycholic acid. Hepatology 42:1399-1405

Glantz A, Marschall H U, Mattsson L A 2004 Intrahepatic cholestasis of pregnancy: relationships between bile acid levels and fetal complication rates. Hepatology 40:467-474

Gorelik J et al 2003 Dexamethasone and ursodeoxycholic acid protect against the arrhythmogenic effect of taurocholate in an in vitro study of rat cardiomyocytes. British Journal of Obstetrics and Gynaecology 110:467-474

Graham G, Baxi L, Tharakan T 1998 Laparoscopic cholecystectomy during pregnancy: a case series and review of the literature. Obstetrical and Gynecological Survey 53:566-574

Halfon P et al 1999 Mother-to-infant transmission of hepatitis C virus: molecular evidence of superinfection by homologous virus in children. Journal of Hepatology 30:970-978

Holzbach R, Sivak D A, Braun W E 1983 Familial recurrent intrahepatic cholestasis of pregnancy: a genetic study providing evidence for transmission of a sex-limited, dominant trait. Gastroenterology 85:175-179

Jain A B et al 2003 Pregnancy after liver transplantation with tacrolimus immunosuppression: a single centre's experience update at 13 years. Transplantation 76:827-832

Kenyon A et al 2001 Pruritus may precede abnormal liver function tests in women with obstetric cholestasis: a longitudinal analysis. British Journal of Obstetrics and Gynaecology 108:1190-1192

Ko C W et al 2005 Incidence, natural history, and risk factors for biliary sludge and stones during pregnancy. Hepatology 41:359-365

Kornfeld D, Crattingnuis S, Ekbom A 1997 Pregnancy outcomes in women with IBD – a population-based cohort study. American Journal of Obstetrics and Gynaecology 177:942-946

Kumar A et al 2004 Hepatitis E in pregnancy. International Journal of Gynecology and Obstetrics 85:240-244

Lee W M 2003 Acute liver failure in the United States. Seminars in Liver Disease 23:217-226

Li X M et al 2005 Clinical characteristics of fulminant hepatitis in pregnancy. World Journal of Gastroenterology 11:4600-4603

Locatelli A et al 1999 Hepatitis C virus infection is associated with a higher incidence of cholestasis of pregnancy. British Journal of Obstetrics and Gynaecology 106:498-500

Lu E J et al 2004 Medical versus surgical management of biliary tract disease in pregnancy. American Journal of Surgery 188:755-759

Madar J, Richmond S, Hey E 1999 Surfactant-deficient respiratory distress after elective delivery at 'term'. Acta Paediatrica 88(11):1244-1248

Maringhini A et al 1993 Biliary sludge and gallstones in pregnancy: incidence, risk factors, and natural history. Annals of Internal Medicine 119:116-120

Mazzotta P, Magee L A 2000 A risk-benefit assessment of pharmacological and non-pharmacological treatments for nausea and vomiting of pregnancy. Drugs 59:781-800

Müllenbach R et al 2003 ABCB4 gene sequence variation in women with intrahepatic cholestasis of pregnancy. Journal of Medical Genetics 40:E70

Nelson-Piercy C 1998 Treatment of nausea and vomiting in pregnancy: when should it be treated and with what? Drug Safety 19(2):155-164

Nelson-Piercy C, Fayers P, de Swiet M 2001 Randomised, double-blind, placebo-controlled trial of corticosteroids for the treatment of hyperemesis gravidarum. British Journal of Obstetrics and Gynaecology 108:9-15

Nesbitt T H et al 1996 Endoscopic management of biliary disease during pregnancy. Obstetrics & Gynecology 87:806-809

Oates-Whitehead R 2004 Nausea and vomiting in early pregnancy. Clinical Evidence 11:1840-52

O'Grady J G 2006 Acute liver failure. Postgraduate Medical Journal 81:148-154

Palmovic D 1986 Acute viral hepatitis in pregnancy. Results of a prospective study of 99 pregnant women. Lijecnicki Vjesnik 108:296-300

Reid R et al 1976 Fetal complications of obstetric cholestasis. British Medical Journal 1:870-872

Reyes H 1982 The enigma of intrahepatic cholestasis of pregnancy: lessons from Chile. Hepatology 2:87-96

Roncaglia N et al 2002 Obstetric cholestasis:outcome with active management. European Journal of Obstetrics, Gynecology and Reproductive Biology 100:167-170

Rosmorduc O, Hermelin B, Poupon R 2001 MDR3 gene defect in adults with symptomatic intrahepatic and gallbladder cholesterol cholelithiasis. Gastroenterology 120:1459-1467

Safari H R et al 1998 The efficacy of methylprednisolone in the treatment of hyperemesis gravidarum:a randomized, double-blind, controlled study. American Journal of Obstetrics and Gynecology 179:921-924

Selitsky T, Chandra P, Schiavello H J 2006 Wernicke's encephalopathy with hyperemesis and ketoacidosis. Obstetrics & Gynecology 107:486-490

Shimono N et al 1991 Fulminant hepatic failure during perinatal period in a pregnant women with Wilson's disease. Gastroenterology Japan 26:69-73

Sternlieb I 2000 Wilson's disease and pregnancy. Hepatology 31:531-532

Sullivan C A et al 1996 A pilot study of intravenous ondansetron for hyperemesis gravidarum. American Journal of Obstetrics and Gynecology 174:1565-1568

Trogstad L I et al 2005 Recurrence risk in hyperemesis gravidarum. BJOG 112:1641-1645

Tsimoyiannis E C et al 1994 Cholelithiasis during pregnancy and lactation. Prospective study. European Journal of Surgery 160:627-631

Valdivieso V et al 1993 Pregnancy and cholelithiasis: pathogenesis and natural course of gallstones diagnosed in early puerperium. Hepatology 17:1-4

van Zonneveld M et al 2003 Lamivudine treatment during pregnancy to prevent perinatal transmission of hepatitis virus infection. Journal of Viral Hepatitis 10:294-297

Wang J, Zhu Q, Zhang X 2002 Effect of delivery mode on maternal-infant transmission of hepatitis B virus by immunoprophylaxis. Chinese Medical Journal 115:1510-1512

Williamson C 2001 Gastrointestinal disease. Baillière's Best Practice & Research. Clinical Obstetrics & Gynaecology 15:937-952

Williamson C et al 2004 Clinical outcome in a series of cases of obstetric cholestasis identified via a patient support group. British Journal of Obstetrics and Gynaecology 111:676-681

Wong V C et al 1984 Prevention of the HBsAg carrier state in newborn infants of mothers who are chronic carriers of HBsAg and HBeAg by administration of hepatitis-B vaccine and hepatitis-B immunoglobulin. Lancet 1:921-926

Yeung L T, King S M, Roberts E A 2001 Mother-to-infant transmission of hepatitis C virus. Hepatology 34:223-229

Chapter 10

Connective tissue diseases

C.-S. Yee, C. Gordon, M. Khamashta, R. Foster, D. P. D'Cruz

Immunological diseases
C.-S. Yee, C. Gordon, M. Khamashta

IMMUNOLOGICAL CHANGES IN PREGNANCY

Following conception, a state of maternal tolerance to the fetus develops to prevent rejection of the fetus. However, the mechanisms involved in this change have not been fully understood. Briefly, this tolerance is a result of the properties of the fetoplacental unit and changes that occur in the maternal immune system.

The fetoplacental unit expresses special HLA antigens which protect it from maternal immune mediated cytotoxicity. At the maternal – fetal interface, trophoblasts inhibit fetal rejection by maternal lymphocytes and express regulatory proteins which protect against the action of maternal complements.

There is modulation of the maternal immune system in particular the development of T regulatory cells and a shift in the type of T cell response from T helper-1 to T-helper-2. This is mainly due to production of cytokines (especially IL-10, IL-4, IL-5, IL-6 and IL-13) by the uterus and fetoplacental unit. Hormonal changes during pregnancy with increase in progesterone, oestrogens, corticosteroids, human chorionic gonadotrophins and somatotropin probably contribute to these adaptations.

Complement and immunoglobulin levels are increased in pregnancy and this should be borne in mind when interpreting laboratory results.

SYSTEMIC LUPUS ERYTHEMATOSUS

Systemic lupus erythematosus (SLE) is a chronic multi-system autoimmune disease, which usually has a relapsing-remitting course. It predominantly affects women of childbearing age. With improvement in treatments resulting in better control of the disease, viable pregnancy is becoming more common. There is a tendency for the disease to flare during pregnancy with potentially catastrophic consequences to the mother and fetus. Hence pregnancy in lupus patients should be considered high risk.

Pre-pregnancy

Fertility is usually not affected by the disease as autoimmune ovarian failure is rare. Infertility in lupus is usually the result of drug treatment, especially with the use of cyclophosphamide. The risk of cyclophosphamide-induced ovarian failure is related to the total drug dose and the age of the patient when exposed (> 35 years is offered as a threshold). One has to be cautious when using hormonal manipulation in the treatment of infertility as there appears to be a risk of flare and thrombosis in patients with antiphospholipid syndrome.

The management of pregnancy in lupus should start before conception so as to optimize maternal health. The disease is not in itself a contraindication to pregnancy with the exception of organ-system complications such as pulmonary hypertension and renal failure. To minimize the risk of flare during pregnancy, the disease should be inactive for at least 6 months prior to conception.

At the pre-pregnancy assessment, the disease status of the patient and presence of organ-system complications need to be ascertained. It is particularly important to assess patients for the presence of cardiorespiratory (e.g. pulmonary hypertension, valvular heart disease and pulmonary fibrosis) and renal (e.g. proteinuria and renal failure) complications. In addition, the knowledge of the patient's status of anti-Ro and antiphospholipid autoantibodies (anticardiolipin antibodies and lupus anticoagulant) is essential. Patients with positive anti-Ro antibody are at increased risk of neonatal lupus syndrome affecting the baby while persistent strongly positive antiphospholipid antibodies are associated with antiphospholipid syndrome (with its associated risks to pregnancy).

Investigations that are commonly performed at the pre-pregnancy visit are:

- full blood count;
- urine dipstick;
- renal function tests;
- autoantibody profile;
- lung function test;
- echocardiography.

The medications taken by the patient to control the disease also need to be reviewed. Drugs that are considered safe in pregnancy include:

- prednisolone;
- hydroxychloroquine;
- azathioprine;
- ciclosporin A.

If the patient is on immunosuppressives that are contraindicated in pregnancy, it is preferable to change to the above drugs at least 3-6 months before conception. This is to allow the clearance of the medication from the system. More importantly, it allows the patient to be stabilized on the new medication to avoid the risk of a flare during this changeover period.

Traditional NSAIDs (e.g. ibuprofen and diclofenac) are generally safe during pregnancy but should be avoided in early pregnancy (due to risk of miscarriage) and after 34 weeks' gestation (due to the risk of premature closure of ductus arteriosus). NSAID preparations that contain misoprostol (e.g. Arthrotec) are contra-indicated in pregnancy. Newer NSAIDs especially COX-2 specific inhibitors should be avoided as there are inadequate data regarding safety in pregnancy. Paracetamol and codeine-based analgesia may be used and are preferred for pain relief.

Anti-hypertensives are commonly used in SLE to treat hypertension, for renoprotective effect or as a vasodilator for Raynaud's phenomenon. The most commonly used group of anti-hypertensives are angiotensin-converting enzyme (ACE) inhibitor and angiotensin-2 receptor antagonist. Unfortunately they are associated with congenital malformation and renal dysfunction in the fetus and hence should be avoided. Patients should have their anti-hypertensive medications switched to those that are safe in pregnancy (methyldopa, labetalol and nifedipine) before conception.

In summary, planning of a pregnancy in a patient with lupus is crucial to ensure the greatest likelihood of success while minimizing the risks (Box 10.1). Patient education is essential to ensure they fully understand all the issues at hand and the need for close monitoring during pregnancy.

Pregnancy

Many studies have shown that there is an increased risk of lupus flares in pregnancy. Fortunately with current management, most of these flares are usually not severe. The risk factors for flares appear to be the presence of an active disease during the 3 to 6 months prior to conception and a history of renal involvement. The majority of the flares occur towards the later part of pregnancy and during the puerperium.

Lupus has the potential to cause both maternal and fetal morbidities. There is increased likelihood of pre-eclampsia or pregnancy-induced hypertension. This is more so in those with previous lupus nephritis and those with associated antiphospholipid syndrome.

Lupus is associated with premature delivery, intrauterine growth restriction and fetal loss. Fetal loss which includes miscarriages and stillbirths occurs in about 20% of pregnancies in lupus. The risk factors for these adverse fetal outcomes are presence of antiphospholipid antibodies, history of renal involvement and severe active lupus activity. Patients who are anti-Ro positive are at risk of neonatal lupus syndrome.

In view of the above, all pregnancies in lupus patients should be considered to be high risk and ideally should be managed jointly by physicians and obstetricians (experienced in high-risk pregnancy) who have special interest in pregnancy in rheumatic diseases. As such, these pregnancies should be followed up closely to enable early detection of maternal and fetal morbidities.

During pregnancy, the patient should be carefully assessed for early signs of lupus flares and these flares (except for the mildest) should be actively managed to bring the flare under control promptly. In this respect, one should be aware that many pathophysiological changes of pregnancy may mimic features of lupus activity (Table 10.1).

One of the most difficult challenges is the differential diagnosis of pre-eclampsia and lupus nephritis as both of them result in significant proteinuria, and raised blood pressure may occur with nephritis. However, raised blood pressure is not a common feature in active lupus nephritis whereas it is the predominant feature of pre-eclampsia. One useful feature is the presence of urinary sediments (pyuria or hematuria or cellular casts) which would indicate the presence of lupus nephritis as they are not present in pre-eclampsia. However, it is essential to exclude other causes of hematuria or pyuria (e.g. infection, stones and vaginal bleeding) before attributing them to lupus, in the absence of cellular casts.

The well-being of the fetus should not be forgotten and fetal growth needs to be monitored closely. In pregnancies that are at risk of congenital heart block (anti-Ro positive), the fetal heart rate should be monitored closely. In specialized centers, fetal cardiac ultrasonographic assessments are performed at about 20 weeks gestation to look for complete heart block.

Anti-dsDNA and complements (C3 and C4) levels are helpful indicators of lupus activity. Rising anti-

---

Box 10.1 Lupus in pregnancy

- Planning for pregnancy essential.
- Patients with pulmonary hypertension and renal failure should avoid pregnancy.
- Disease should be inactive for 6 months before conception.
- Medications should be reviewed and changed to those that are considered safe in pregnancy.

Table 10.1 Pathophysiological pregnancy changes that may be confused with lupus activity

Features	Pregnancy-related	Lupus activity
Facial rash	Melasma/chloasma Facial blushing	Malar rash
Joint pain/swelling	Mechanical arthralgia Bland knee effusion	Inflammatory synovitis
Seizure	Eclampsia	Neuropsychiatric lupus
Stroke syndrome	Eclampsia	Neuropsychiatric lupus
Proteinuria	Pre-eclampsia	Nephritis
Anemia	Hemodilution	Anemia of chronic disease Hemolytic anemia
Thrombocytopenia	Pre-eclampsia HELLP syndrome	Immune thrombocytopenia

dsDNA titres above the normal range and decreasing complement levels suggest lupus activity. As absolute complement levels increase in pregnancy, a fall in the levels would be sufficient to indicate activity even if the levels are within normal range. It has been suggested that a fall of 25% should be considered significant.

Therefore the minimum investigations to be performed at every assessment are:

- urine dipstick;
- full blood count;
- renal function test;
- anti-double stranded DNA antibodies (anti-dsDNA);
- complement C3 and C4 levels;
- fetal ultrasonography;
- fetal heart rate (those at risk of congenital heart block).

The medications the patient is taking should be reviewed. If the patient is on any medication that is contraindicated in pregnancy, this should be discontinued immediately and the patient should be counseled on the risk of teratogenicity.

If the patient has lupus activity, this is usually treated with corticosteroids. In general, steroid doses should be kept to the minimum required to control the disease as they are associated with increased risk of pre-eclampsia/pregnancy induced hypertension, gestational diabetes and infection, particularly at doses above 10 mg daily of prednisolone or equivalent. Avoid using steroids that cross the placenta (e.g. dexamethasone and betamethasone) to minimize the effect on fetus that include impaired neuropsychiatric development even with short-term use. Prednisolone and prednisone are metabolized by the placenta, hence very little crosses the placenta at doses ≤ 20 mg daily. Intravenous pulses of methylprednisolone may be used to reduce disease activity rapidly, particularly in those with severe activity. This approach may reduce the risk of steriod-induced pre-eclampsia as it reduces the need for higher doses of oral steroids to control severe activity. Apart from steroids, hydroxy-chloroquine, azathioprine and ciclosporin A may additionally be used to control disease activity. Termination of pregnancy needs to be considered in patients with uncontrolled severe disease activity despite high dose steroids. There is no role for prophylactic use of corticosteroids in the prevention of disease activity.

Low-dose aspirin is commonly used in such high-risk pregnancies as there is an increased risk of pre-eclampsia. There is evidence from meta-analysis that

> **Box 10.2 Risks posed by lupus activity in pregnancy**
>
> - High-risk pregnancy with potential maternal and fetal morbidities.
> - Essential to differentiate lupus flare from pathophysiological changes of pregnancy.
> - Early detection and treatment of maternal lupus flare.
> - Close monitoring for fetal well-being.

asprin may reduce the risk of pre-eclampsia by up to 20%. It is also used along with subcutaneous low molecular weight heparin in patients with associated antiphospholipid syndrome. However, there is variation in the recommended optimal dose of low molecular weight heparin to be used. The need for low molecular heparin in obstetric antiphospholipid syndrome with no history of thrombosis is also debatable.

Delivery and postpartum care

The timing and method of delivery is dictated by obstetric indications and the presence of organ-system complication (especially pulmonary hypertension). Normal vaginal deliveries are usually achieved by at least 60% of pregnant lupus women.

In view of the increased risk of flare during this period, the patient should be monitored closely for any early indication of flare. In patients who are anti-Ro positive, the baby should be monitored for development of neonatal lupus syndrome. Assessment by a pediatric cardiologist is required if the baby has developed congenital heart block.

As with pregnancy, any evidence of lupus activity should be treated early and corticosteroids are usually used. All the drugs that are considered safe in pregnancy are also safe for lactation with the exception of ciclosporin A. Patients with antiphospholipid syndrome and a history of thrombosis, who were treated with heparin during pregnancy, should have their anticoagulation converted back to warfarin, which is safe for lactation. Those patients with antiphospholipid syndrome but without a history of thrombosis are at an increased risk of thrombosis during the postpartum period and should be treated with heparin throughout this period.

With regards to contraception, estrogen-containing preparations should be avoided as they may increase the risk of flare apart from the known increased risk of thrombosis. Progestogen-only preparations or intrauterine devices are preferred (Box 10.3).

Neonatal lupus syndrome

This is a syndrome of cutaneous lupus or congenital heart block (CHB) or both which appears in neonates born to mothers with anti-Ro autoantibodies. Occasionally there may be accompanying systemic involvement such as hemolytic anemia, thrombocytopenia, hepatitis, nephritis, aseptic meningitis and myelopathy. It may occur in infante of women with connective tissue disease or asymptomatic mothers. It is rare for both cutaneous lupus and CHB to occur together in the same infant.

The overall prevalence of CHB is around 0.005% but this increases to 2% in women with anti-Ro antibodies. This risk increases further to about 20% in women with anti-Ro autoantibodies and those who have had a previous child affected by CHB. CHB is not evident before 16 weeks' gestation and may be associated with pericarditis, myocarditis, endocarditis and cardiomyopathy in the fetus. Affected feterses may develop first and second degree heart block that becomes complete by the time of birth and may require a permanent pacemaker in the neonatal period. This condition has a high mortality of about 15 to 30% and the majority of deaths occur in the neonatal period. In view of this, mothers with anti-Ro autoantibodies should have the fetal heart rate assessed weekly from 16 weeks' gestation onwards as well as a detailed ultrasound scan to look for any cardiac abnormalities at around 20 weeks' gestation. An electrocardiogram (ECG) of the baby should be performed after delivery as babies with first- or second-degree heart block may progress to higher degrees of heart block after birth. A neonatologist should be present at the time of delivery of a baby with CHB.

The skin rash of neonatal lupus is typically a photosensitive annular erythematous lesion, which is similar to the rash of subacute cutaneous lupus. It usually appears shortly after birth as a result of exposure to ultraviolet light but may occur at any time during the first 6 months. Fortunately this is usually self-limiting and resolves without scarring. This is most likely due to transplacental transfer of pathogenic maternal IgG antibody as the rash does not persist beyond 6 months of age which is consistent with half-life of maternal IgG.

The cutaneous lupus rash usually does not require any treatment but in severe cases, topical steroids may be used. Systemic involvement may require systemic steroids. For CHB there is some evidence that fluorinated corticosteroids such as dexamethasone and betamethasone given to the mother may be helpful particularly with incomplete heart block. It is much less certain whether they are helpful in cases with complete heart block. These steroids are not rendered inactive by the placenta. Affected infants with CHB need to be assessed by a pediatric cardiologist and a pacemaker may be required in the neonatal period. Even if a pacemaker is not required immediately, the infant will need to be monitored as their condition may progress later in life and most children with CHB require a pacemaker by the age of 12 years.

SYSTEMIC SCLEROSIS

Systemic sclerosis is a multi-system autoimmune disease that is characterized by obliterative endarteritis and collagen proliferation in tissues. It is much less common than SLE and is classified according to the extent of skin involvement:

1. Limited cutaneous systemic sclerosis with acral distribution of skin involvement.
2. Diffuse cutaneous systemic sclerosis with more proximal and extensive skin involvement.
3. Systemic sclerosis sine scleroderma with systemic involvement but without skin involvement.

This condition usually affects women of post-menopausal age, hence pregnancy is not common with this disease. The main risks to pregnancy are pulmonary hypertension and development of renal crisis.

Pre-pregnancy

There is no evidence that fertility is affected by systemic sclerosis. However, it is essential that the condition is stable prior to conception. Prior history of renal crisis is not a contraindication to pregnancy but this is associated with an increased risk of pre-eclampsia or pregnancy-induced hypertension. During pre-pregnancy assessment, the patient should be assessed for the presence of organ complications that may pose risks during pregnancy. Patients with pulmonary hypertension and renal failure should avoid becoming pregnant in view of the high risk involved. Patients with extensive pulmonary fibrosis may also be unsuitable because of concern about hypoxia. The following investigations are commonly performed:

- renal function tests;
- autoantibody profile;
- echocardiography;
- lung function test.

Pregnancy

During pregnancy, Raynaud's phenomenon usually improves with the increased cardiac output in the second and third trimesters. However, gastro-esophageal reflux, which is common in systemic sclerosis, usually worsens especially in the third trimester. Renal crisis presents with acute-onset severe hypertension with deteriorating renal function. This may be confused with pre-eclampsia but the lack of proteinuria would support a diagnosis of renal crisis, rather than pre-eclampsia. The differentiation of the two is crucial as early delivery would have no effect on the renal crisis as opposed to pre-eclampsia. Therefore, blood pressure, the results of urine dipstick tests and renal function need to be monitored closely. If the patient has microstomia, assessment by an anesthetist is required as this may result in difficulty with intubation and pose an anesthetic risk.

Once pregnancy is confirmed, the patient's medications need to be reviewed. ACE inhibitors and angiotensin-2 receptor antagonists are commonly used in systemic sclerosis, and they need to be discontinued ideally before conception as they are associated with congenital malformation and renal

Box 10.5 Systemic sclerosis risks

- Avoid pregnancy if pulmonary hypertension, renal failure or extensive pulmonary fibrosis present.
- Previous renal crisis not considered to be a contra-indication to pregnancy.
- Gastroesophageal reflux usually worsens requiring treatment with ranitidine and a prokinetic agent.

dysfunction in the fetus. If renal crisis develops, it is essential to control the blood pressure aggressively. If required, ACE inhibitors may be used and this is one occasion when ACE inhibitors are indicated in pregnancy.

The majority of patients need treatment for gastro-esophageal reflux with ranitidine. It is not uncommon for a prokinetic agent such as metoclopramide to be used in addition due to the severity of the condition during pregnancy.

Delivery and postpartum

The timing and method of delivery is dictated by obstetric indications and the presence of organ-system complications (especially pulmonary hypertension). There is a high risk of the condition deteriorating after pregnancy, hence careful monitoring is required. Aside from these requirements, there are no special issues to be considered in this period.

OTHER CONNECTIVE TISSUE DISEASES

Apart from SLE and systemic sclerosis, the other connective tissue diseases of concern are:

- primary Sjogren's syndrome;
- dermatomyositis;
- polymyositis;
- overlap syndrome;
- undifferentiated connective tissue diseases.

Unfortunately there are very little clinical data on pregnancy in primary Sjogren's syndrome, dermatomyositis, polymyositis and undifferentiated connective tissue diseases. As these conditions usually occur in older age groups, pregnancy is much less common in patients with these conditions as compared to SLE. There is no evidence that fertility is affected by these conditions. From the authors' experience, patients with these conditions usually do well during pregnancy as long as the condition is stable at conception.

As with lupus, patients need to be assessed for the presence of organ-system complications (especially pulmonary hypertension and renal failure), anti-Ro antibodies and antiphospholipid antibodies. The management of patients will be along similar lines as with lupus depending on the presence of these risk factors. For disease flares, steroids may be used. Other medications should be reviewed before and in early pregnancy (as described in 'Systemic lupus erythematosus' above).

RHEUMATOID ARTHRITIS

Rheumatoid arthritis is a chronic autoimmune systemic disease that predominantly affects synovial tissue resulting in erosive inflammatory arthritis. Extra-articular involvement is not unusual but is becoming less common and less severe with modern management of this disease. Unlike SLE, inflammatory arthritis improves in at least 80% of pregnancies. The disease itself usually does not pose special problems during pregnancy and it is not commonly associated with anti-Ro antibodies or antiphospholipid antibodies.

Pre-pregnancy

The main issue during the pre-pregnancy visit is to review the medications that the patient is taking to control the disease. The following drugs are commonly used:

- disease modifying antirheumatic drugs (DMARDs);
- biological therapy (including anti-TNF);
- corticosteroids;
- NSAIDs;

Drugs that are considered to be safe during pregnancy are:

- prednisolone;
- hydroxychloroquine;
- sulfasalazine;
- gold;
- azathioprine;
- ciclosporin A;
- tacrolimus.

Patients on biological therapy and other DMARDs should discontinue or switch their drugs to those that are considered safe during pregnancy. Generally this should be done 3 to 6 months prior to conception.

However, leflunomide needs to be discontinued at least 2 years prior to conception and requires a washout with cholestyramine as it is stored in adipose tissue.

Traditional NSAIDs (such as ibuprofen and diclofenac) are generally safe during pregnancy but should be avoided in early pregnancy (due to risk of miscarriage), after 34 weeks' gestation (due to risk of premature closure of ductus arteriosus) and in patients who have hypertension. NSAID preparations that contain misoprostol (such as Arthrotec) are contraindicated in pregnancy. Newer NSAIDs especially COX-2 specific inhibitor should be avoided as there are inadequate data regarding their safety in pregnancy. Paracetamol and codeine-based analgesia may be used and are preferred.

Pregnancy

Rheumatoid arthritis usually improves during pregnancy; additional treatment to control the disease is usually not required (Box 10.6). Any disease activity usually responds to corticosteroids, which can be administered orally, intra-articularly, intramuscularly or intravenously. Occasionally a DMARD may be required especially if high doses of steroids are needed. However, it has to be borne in mind that DMARDs have a delayed onset of action and their full effect is usually evident only after 3 to 6 months.

The medications the patient is taking need to be reviewed if this has not been done pre-pregnancy. If the patient is on any medication that is contraindicated in pregnancy, this should be discontinued immediately and the patient should be counseled on the risk of teratogenicity.

NSAIDs, paracetamol and codeine-based analgesia may be used during pregnancy but NSAIDs should be avoided early in pregnancy and after 34 weeks' gestation. In practice, NSAIDs can often be discontinued in pregnancy as the arthritis usually improves significantly. Opiates such as pethidine and morphine

---

Box 10.6 Rheumatoid arthritis

- Condition usually improves with pregnancy.
- DMARDs should be reviewed and changed 3 to 6 months before conception.
- Flare of arthritis usually treated with steroids.
- Be aware of possibility of cervical spine involvement when intubation anticipated.

may be used for severe pain with caution as there is a risk of fetal cardiorespiratory depression.

Delivery and postpartum

For vaginal delivery, the delivery position of the patient needs to take into account the effects of inflammatory arthritis or deformities affecting the joints of the lower limbs. Patients with cervical spine involvement require special consideration by the anesthetist if intubation is anticipated. All patients with rheumatoid arthritis should be considered at risk of cervical subluxation if this has not been assessed before pregnancy.

Following delivery, the patient is at increased risk of flares during the postpartum period. As with pregnancy, disease activity can be treated with corticosteroids, which can be administered orally, intra-articularly, intramuscularly or intravenously. DMARDs that are safe for lactation include hydroxychloroquine, sulfasalazine, gold and azathioprine. If other DMARDs or biological therapy is required, patients should be advised to discontinue breastfeeding. Most of the traditional NSAIDs are safe during lactation but it is considered best to use short-acting drugs (such as ibuprofen) that are taken during or soon after breastfeeding in order to avoid accumulation of the drug in breast milk. There are inadequate data on the newer COX-2 specific inhibitors. There is no specific issue with any of the available contraception methods in rheumatoid arthritis.

Systemic vasculitides

R. Foster, D. P. D'Cruz

INTRODUCTION

Systemic vasculitides are rare in young women and knowledge of these disorders in pregnancy is limited to a relatively small group of patients. However, since it is known that pregnancy can have a disease-modifying effect on autoimmune connective tissue disease, and connective tissue diseases can have an adverse effect on pregnancy; these patients need to be actively managed in order to prevent negative outcomes for both mother and child.

This section focuses on primary systemic vasculitis, spondyloarthropathy and dermatomyositis. We will discuss how these conditions affect pregnancy outcome, and whether or not pregnancy affects the natural history of the disease. The available treatments will be discussed, and those treatments which are contraindicated in pregnancy will be highlighted. Issues pertinent to each disease before, during and after pregnancy will be discussed.

PRIMARY SYSTEMIC VASCULITIS AND PREGNANCY

The vasculitides are a heterogeneous group of uncommon diseases, characterized by inflammatory cell infiltration and necrosis of blood vessel walls. The evidence base for management of patients with vasculitis in pregnancy is mostly limited to small case series and case reports.

It is worth noting that patients with vasculitis have an increased risk of being antiphospholipid antibody positive. Untreated, antiphospholipid syndrome can predispose to pregnancy morbidity, and so it is important to screen all female patients with vasculitis for anticardiolipin antibodies and the lupus anticoagulant before they start trying for a family. Positivity would be an indication for low dose aspirin plus or minus low molecular weight heparin (see Ch. 8, p. 156) plus care under a rheumatologist and obstetrician.

In general, it is advisable to have the vasculitis in remission prior to pregnancy, where possible to use treatments with a good safety record during the pregnancy, and to manage the pregnancy in conjunction with a specialist rheumatologist. We will discuss further Wegener's granulomatosis, Takayasu's arteritis and Polyarteritis nodosa and will briefly mention microscopic polyangiitis.

Wegener's granulomatosis

Wegener's granulomatosis (WG) is a systemic vasculitis, predominantly affecting the blood vessels of the upper respiratory tract, lungs and kidneys. Antineutrophil cytoplasmic antibodies (ANCA) with a cytoplasmic staining pattern and specificity for proteinase 3 are characteristic. Pregnancy in patients with WG is not common for three main reasons. First, it is a rare disease which does not primarily occur in women of childbearing age; yearly incidence is around 5-12 per million, with peak incidence during the fourth and fifth decades Second, it is a potentially very severe disease, which in itself can discourage women from trying to conceive. Third, the major first-line agent in its treatment is cyclophosphamide which can cause ovarian failure, and which is usually prescribed in conjunction with contraception due to its potential for teratogenicity. As such, there have been relatively low numbers of women with WG who have undergone pregnancy. The only available literature consists of case reports and case series and there are no agreed guidelines on management.

Does pregnancy affect the disease course of Wegener's granulomatosis?

These case reports can be divided into three groups: women with WG who became pregnant while in remission, those who became pregnant during active disease and those who first developed WG while pregnant. Of those who became pregnant while in remission, roughly one-third relapsed, one-third remained in remission and one-third suffered complications (e.g. pre-eclampsia). Nearly one-third of all reported pregnancies in WG were diagnosed for the first time during pregnancy. This might suggest a tendency for pregnancy to have an adverse effect on WG, however it is important to consider potential publication bias, and the fact that relapses occur in more than 50% of non-pregnant women and male WG patients. There does not appear to be any beneficial effect of pregnancy on WG; of those patients reported who became pregnant whilst still in an active phase of disease, all experienced a flare or worsening of symptoms.

Does Wegener's granulomatosis affect pregnancy outcome?

WG appears to have an adverse effect on pregnancy. The outcome of patients in whom onset of disease was during pregnancy, or who had active disease when they became pregnant, seems to be worse than that of those in whom disease was controlled at conception; in the former groups there are higher rates of spontaneous and therapeutic abortions, and higher rates of maternal death. Prematurity and Cesarean sections are common in WG whether the disease is controlled at conception or not. As with lupus nephritis, patients with WG complicated by glomerulonephritis, even if inactive, may be at increased risk of pre-eclampsia, pregnancy induced hypertension, prematurity, intra-uterine growth restriction and late pregnancy losses. There is increasing evidence that WG patients are at increased risk of venous thrombotic events and given that pregnancy itself and the postpartum period increase the risk of venous thromboembolism, clinicians should have a low threshold for assessing women for thrombotic complications.

Treatment of Wegener's granulomatosis in pregnancy

Treatment of disease relapse
Any relapse of disease is potentially life threatening, as it is in the non-pregnant state, and therefore needs to be treated aggressively with appropriate medication. Where possible, drugs thought to be safe in pregnancy, e.g. azathioprine and prednisolone, should be used. If this is not sufficient treatment, then drugs with a potential or unquantified risk to the fetus will need to be considered. The risk of maternal death needs to be weighed up against the potential risk of such medication to the fetus. Such decisions should be discussed in a multidisciplinary setting and must take the patient's views into account. Clearly, if disease relapse occurs early in the pregnancy, consideration should be given to terminating the pregnancy in order to use cytotoxic agents such as cyclophosphamide. Later in the pregnancy, and depending on the major organs involved, patients may be stabilized with intravenous methylprednisolone or possible intravenous immunoglobulin after careful consideration of the risks.

Treatment for patients in remission
Most patients in remission continue immunosuppressive treatment during pregnancy. It is intuitive that those drugs with the best safety record in pregnancy should be used. A common therapeutic regime is azathioprine, often with low dose prednisolone.

Summary of drugs used in Wegener's granulomatosis
Azathioprine is thought to be relatively safe in pregnancy. A recent randomized, controlled trial suggests that, in non-pregnant patients, it is as effective as cyclophosphamide (the gold standard) in the remission phase of WG, and there are pilot data suggesting that high dose azathioprine is as effective at inducing remission in relapsed disease. This is probably the best first-line therapy for treatment of WG in pregnancy.

Cyclophosphamide is absolutely contraindicated in pregnancy – it is a known teratogen, with highest risk of fetal malformation during the first trimester. However, there are reports in which cyclophosphamide was used in a number of cases of severe WG relapse during pregnancy. This use was without short-term complication, although the long-term effects are not known.

Methotrexate is highly teratogenic during the first trimester and should be avoided where possible.

Prednisolone is relatively safe throughout pregnancy. Some patients have remained in remission on prednisolone alone during pregnancy, although the combination of prednisolone plus a cytotoxic seems to be a more effective treatment.

Co-trimoxazole is relatively contraindicated because of its antagonism of folic acid, although there is no proven teratogenic effect.

Intravenous immunologlobulin is safe in pregnancy, but of unknown efficacy in WG.

Mycophenolate mofetil is being increasingly used in the treatment of WG. It is probably teratogenic and it should be avoided in pregnancy.

Rituximab is used as a third-line treatment in WG, however there are not enough studies to draw conclusions about the safety of rituximab in pregnant women and should, at present, be avoided if possible.

Recommendations

Pre-pregnancy counseling is critical for women with WG. They need to be aware that WG is a serious disease in which relapses are not uncommon even on maintenance therapy. They need to know that any relapse during pregnancy needs to be treated aggressively to avoid the risk of maternal and fetal death, and this may involve the use of therapeutic agents with teratogenic potential. It should be explained that pregnancy probably has an adverse effect on WG and may increase the risk of disease relapse. They should be told that having WG gives them a probable increased risk of prematurity and spontaneous abortion, an increased risk of requiring therapeutic abortion and Cesarean section, and higher rates of maternal death than that of the general pregnant population. It is strongly advised that the woman be in remission prior to conception and that she continues maintenance therapy throughout pregnancy. Before a woman starts to try for a family, she needs to be switched from any potentially teratogenic medication to a safer alternative such as azathioprine, taking the half-life of the drug into consideration. Whilst on teratogenic medication such as cyclophosphamide, mycophenolate or methotrexate, she must take contraceptive measures which should be continued for 4 to 6 months after discontinuing these drugs prior to attempting conception.

Antenatal monitoring must involve members of a multidisciplinary team including a rheumatology or nephrology specialist early on. Close clinical monitoring during pregnancy, especially of renal function (U&Es, proteinuria, BP) and routine FBC, ANCA, ESR/CRP testing, is paramount. Relapses must be treated aggressively and effectively. Early induction is indicated in women who are experiencing a relapse or complications refractory to medical therapy.

Postnatal follow-up will vary in intensity from patient to patient. All patients will require continuing follow-up under a rheumatologist for their WG.

Takayasu's arteritis

Takayasu's arteritis (TA) is a rare chronic inflammatory arteritis predominantly affecting the aorta, its major branches and the pulmonary arteries. Vessel inflammation results in fibrosis, stenosis and thrombosis and can cause aneurysm formation. Complications of disease result from end-organ ischemia and include hypertension, cardiac valve disease, retinopathy and stroke. It predominantly affects women of childbearing age and so the issue of pregnancy is an important one. There exists only a small database of literature on pregnancy and TA, due to the disease itself being very rare, and our evidence is drawn from a case series of a total of 76 pregnancies.

Does pregnancy affect the disease course of Takayasu's arteritis?

TA disease activity as measured by serum CRP and ESR suggests that inflammation may actually be reduced during pregnancy. Other markers of disease activity, e.g. new bruits, fever or typical vascular imaging features, have not been assessed during pregnancy. Positron emission tomography (PET) scanning is increasingly being used to assess disease activity in patients with large vessel vasculitides: active aortitis is clearly demonstrated with increased FDG uptake in the aorta and its main branches. In this context, a negative PET scan may be useful when planning the optimum time for conception since patients with TA may have low-grade elevations of acute phase markers such as ESR and CRP without major disease acitivity. Hypertension is a common feature of TA and is frequently missed because the upper limb pulses may be absent or reduced. Thus, BP monitoring should be by femoral cuffs.

Does Takayasu's arteritis affect pregnancy outcome?

In general it appears that TA is compatible with favorable maternal and fetal outcome. Maternal complications include hypertension and pre-eclampsia, congestive heart failure, progressive renal failure, intracerebral hemorrhage during the second stage of labor and very rarely death. TA appears to be associated with an increased incidence of intrauterine growth retardation, there does not appear to be an increase in intrauterine mortality. Both maternal and fetal complications are more common in patients who have diffuse disease with abdominal aortic involvement, uncontrolled hypertension, and in those who present late. Fertility is not adversely affected.

Treatment of Takayasu's arteritis in pregnancy

Strict blood pressure control is paramount. Antihypertensive agents that have been used with success include alphamethyldopa, nifedipine, beta-blockers and hydralazine. Should anti-inflammatory medication be required, corticosteroids are first-line treatment as in non-pregnant disease. In non-pregnant cohorts, approximately one-half of all patients treated for TA respond to steroid therapy, about one-third of the non-responders achieve remission with subsequent cytotoxics. It follows that pregnant patients with active disease should trial a low-teratogenicity cytotoxic such as azathioprine if they do not respond to steroids. Prophylactic antibiotics should be administered at the time of delivery to prevent bacterial endocarditis and septicemia.

Recommendations

Pre-pregnancy counseling should stress the importance of disease-control prior to conception; women with active disease in pregnancy do worse in terms of both maternal and fetal outcome. A full medical assessment of the patient should be performed, including vascular imaging, ideally by MRI or PET scan, to assess disease activity and extent of vessel involvement. The patient should be aware that outcome is less favorable in extensive disease with abdominal aorta involvement. They must be aware of the importance of strict blood pressure control and intensive follow-up from a multidisciplinary team.

The patient needs to be monitored throughout pregnancy for hypertension and signs of heart and renal failure in particular. If these are controlled, outcome is generally good. Blood pressure monitoring during labor is particularly important because of the increased risk of intracerebral hemorrhage. Central arterial monitoring may be required, particularly if the subclavian arteries are diseased. Uncontrolled hypertension during the second stage of labor is an indication for low forceps delivery or vacuum extraction.

Postnatal follow-up will vary in intensity from patient to patient. All patients with TA will require lifelong follow-up under a rheumatologist and cardiologist.

Polyarteritis nodosa

Polyarteritis nodosa (PAN) is a necrotizing vasculitis of small and medium arteries, affecting all of the major organ systems. It causes weakening of the arterial wall and aneurysmal dilatation, resulting in characteristic nodules which can be demonstrated by radiology and which can rupture. Impaired perfusion can lead to ulceration, infarction, or ischemic atrophy in tissue supplied by the affected vessels. In general, severity and outcome of PAN is worse in the presence of proteinuria greater than $1\,g/24\,h$, creatinine $> 140\,mmol/L$, cardiomyopathy, gastrointinal (GI) or CNS involvement. There have been very few reports of pregnancy in women with PAN, with only small case series published.

Approximately 10% of patients with PAN are hepatitis B positive and this is highly relevant in terms of transmission of the virus to the fetus, and has implications for the patient's partner and carers. The management of the hepatitis B positive woman with PAN should include an attempt to eradicate viral carriage if possible prior to conception and Guillevin et al have published trials of low dose prednisolone in combination with plasma exchange and antiviral agents which have achieved seroconversion to negative in most patients.

Does pregnancy affect the disease course of polyarteritis nodosa?

Of the small numbers of patients reported, the majority of those who conceived while in remission did not suffer a relapse of disease, those who were diagnosed with PAN late in pregnancy had a poor outcome with high rates of maternal death from renal failure, gastrointestinal hemorrhage, respiratory failure and coma. There is inadequate evidence to reliably comment on whether or not pregnancy affects PAN disease activity.

Does polyarteritis nodosa affect pregnancy outcome?

Again, it is difficult to comment given the small numbers of patients studied. Of 14 pregnancies, 10 resulted in the delivery of healthy infants, 2 in spontaneous abortion and 2 in therapeutic abortion.

Treatment of polyarteritis nodosa in pregnancy

In the majority of cases, PAN should be controlled with steroid monotherapy in pregnancy. Life-threatening disease calls for stronger therapy such as cyclophosphamide, but not enough is known on this subject to comment further.

Recommendations

Pregnant patients do better when they are in disease remission, this must be stressed to the patient prior to conception. Careful monitoring of, in particular, renal function, GI signs and symptoms, CNS involvement and cardiac disease is mandatory. Patients require lifelong follow-up. Beyond this, it is not possible to make reliable recommendations.

Microscopic polyangiitis

Microscopic polyangiitis (MPA) is one of the ANCA associated vasculitides that is characterized by necrotizing crescentic glomerulonephritis and pulmonary hemorrhage. Serologically antibodies with a perinuclear staining pattern (pANCA) on neutrophils with specificity for myeloperoxidase are useful diagnostically. There have been five case reports of MPA in pregnancy one of which was fatal. Interestingly in two women, the babies developed neonatal pulmonary hemorrhage and renal impairment and cord blood showed the presence of anti-myeloperoxidase antibodies, suggesting neonatal transmission of the disease. Both babies responded to corticosteroids and exchange blood transfusion.

SPONDYLOARTHROPATHIES AND PREGNANCY

The spondyloarthropathies (or seronegative arthritidies) are a group of overlapping forms of inflammatory arthritis, which characteristically affect the spine and entheses, and which in contrast to rheumatoid arthritis are negative for serum rheumatoid factor. Disease may present at any age, although young adults are most commonly affected. We will discuss in detail ankylosing spondylitis and psoriatic arthri-

tis. Both diseases are more common than the vasculitides; prevalence is 1500 per million and 200-1000 per million, respectively. As would be expected, there is more of an evidence base relating to the course and recommended treatment of women with these diseases during pregnancy.

Ankylosing spondylitis

Ankylosing spondylitis affects predominantly men at a ratio of 2.5:1 with some older series suggesting that the ratio may be as high as 9:1. It causes arthritis of the spine and sacroiliac joints and can cause inflammation of the eyes, lungs and cardiac valves. Severe chronic inflammation can result in loss of mobility and deformity. In the non-pregnant patient, medical treatment consists of nonsteroidal anti-inflammatory and antimalarial agents, sulfasalazine is occasionally used, as is methotrexate for peripheral joint arthritis. More recently the anti-TNF agents, infliximab and etanercept, have had a dramatic effect on both the peripheral arthritis and spinal disease, and have revolutionized the outlook for these patients. Lifelong physiotherapy input is required to minimize disability. A number of retrospective and prospective studies have been published on pregnant patients with ankylosing spondylitis.

Does pregnancy affect the disease course of ankylosing spondylitis?

Small retrospective and prospective studies in the 1980s found ankylosing spondylitis activity not to be affected by pregnancy. A more recent prospective study of 10 pregnancies from before conception to 24 weeks' postpartum, used validated disease activity scores to assess disease in women with ankylosing spondylitis. The majority of these patients had disease activity at the time of conception, which remained throughout the first and second trimesters, and improved markedly during the third trimester. Disease became more active again, in most patients, a few weeks postpartum. Interestingly CRP levels in most of the patients were not elevated and did not fluctuate during the course of the study. This suggests that factors other than inflammation may be playing a role, for example the changes in posture and spinal mobility due to the relaxation of ligaments and presence of a gravid uterus during pregnancy, and the physical strain of caring for an infant postpartum.

Does ankylosing spondylitis affect pregnancy outcome?

Pregnancy outcome appears to be unaffected by anky-losing spondylitis, with no evidence of increased maternal mortality or fetal morbidity and mortality rates.

Treatment of ankylosing spondylitis in pregnancy

Drugs that have been used safely during pregnancy include antimalarials, NSAIDs, prednisolone and sul-fasalazine. Methotrexate should be avoided because of its teratogenic potential. At the moment the anti-TNF agents are also contraindicated in pregnancy but there may be a case for considering these agents to achieve remission in patients with severe disease prior to planning a pregnancy.

Recommendations

Patients should be advised that ankylosing spondyli-tis is unlikely to be significantly affected by preg-nancy, that symptoms can become a little worse in the first and second trimesters and that they are likely to improve during the third. It is safe for the patient to take most of the usual medications for symptom relief, but methotrexate should be avoided particularly during the first trimester. It is important to have regular physiotherapy input. The patient should be told that having ankylosing spondylitis has no known deleterious effect on pregnancy outcome. The patient may need extra help with childcare once the child is born, particularly if she has impaired mobility or fixed deformity. There is an argument for prescribing peripartum prophylactic antibiotics, especially in the presence of a known cardiac lesion.

Psoriatic arthritis

Psoriatic arthritis (PA) is an inflammatory arthritis associated with coincidental psoriasis. The arthritis can occur in five different patterns: asymmetrical oli-goarthritis; symmetrical small joint polyarthritis; distal interphalangeal joint arthropathy with nail changes; arthritis mutilans; and spondylitis. Extra-articular manifestations such as ocular and aortic root inflammation can occur. Treatment depends on site and severity of disease. In non-pregnant patients NSAIDs are first-line therapy for symptom control, intra-articular corticosteroids are also useful. Metho-trexate is probably the most widely prescribed second-line agent, sulfasalazine and ciclosporin are also used. New drugs such as leflunomide, an anti-lymphocyte drug, and anti-tumor necrosis factor alpha drugs are being evaluated and have recently been licensed for use in PA.

Does pregnancy affect the disease course of psoriatic arthritis?

Improvement of symptoms has been reported in patients with psoriatic arthritis who become preg-nant. No large studies have been performed to confirm these reports. Psoriatic arthritis often dis-plays a very variable and unpredictable clinical course, which can progress despite disease-modify-ing therapy, or enter remission spontaneously. This would make it difficult to assess whether or not any change in disease severity was due to pregnancy or other factors.

Does psoriatic arthritis affect pregnancy outcome?

Psoriatic arthritis is not known to have an adverse effect on pregnancy. The main risk would come from medication used to treat the disease, as such it is sen-sible to recommend the use of therapy thought to be safe in pregnancy.

Treatment of psoriatic arthritis in pregnancy

NSAIDs and local steroids alone may be sufficient to control symptoms during pregnancy. Intuitively, outcome will be better if the woman is in remission prior to conception, which may require disease-modifying drugs. Methotrexate should be avoided. Sulfasalazine and ciclosporin are probably safe. Leflu-nomide and the TNF-alpha antagonists have not been assessed for safety in pregnancy. In the presence of heart valve involvement peri-partum antibiotics should be prescribed.

Recommendations

The woman should be advised that it should be safe for her to become pregnant, and that provided she stops all unsafe drugs prior to conception there should be no adverse outcome to the fetus due to the ankylosing spondylitis. She could be told that her disease may improve symptomatically during pregnancy. She needs to be aware that childcare may be difficult if her disease is uncontrolled after delivery.

Polymyositis–dermatomyositis and pregnancy

Polymyositis and dermatomyositis are the most common forms of inflammatory myopathy. In dermatomyositis, the muscle inflammation is associated with characteristic skin changes. Yearly incidence is 1-9 cases per million, with peak incidences occurring during childhood and above the age of 45. In other words, it is a rare disease which does not typically affect women of childbearing age. As such there are only a small amount of data concerning these diseases and pregnancy, and this is confined to case reports and one retrospective series. Patients with the anti-synthetase syndrome comprising the association of an inflammatory myopathy, interstitial pneumonitis, skin lesions, naynaud; phenomenon, inflammatory polycarthritis and, at the biological level, antinuclear antibodies known as anti-synthetases, especially with anti-Jo-1 antibodies are at increased risk of interstitial lung disease which can occasionally be severe, leading to significant respiratory disability.

Does pregnancy affect the disease course of polymyositis-dermatomyositis?

There is no definite effect of pregnancy on polymyosi-tis-dermatomyositis disease activity. Some patients experience exacerbations and minor flares, some report improvement of symptoms, in many there is no change. A significant number of patients in these series were diagnosed for the first time whilst pregnant, which may suggest some pregnancy-related factor which predisposes to the development of disease.

Does polymyositis-dermatomyositis affect pregnancy outcome?

The majority of infants in these reported cases were delivered healthy and at term. However, for those mothers in whom disease was not well controlled, there was an increased rate of fetal loss and a greater number of premature births. There was a greatly increased risk of fetal loss if disease was diagnosed in the first trimester. If diagnosed in the second or third trimesters most pregnancies resulted in live, although premature, births. There have been two maternal deaths reported in patients with polymyositis-dermatomyositis.

Treatment of polymyositis-dermatomyositis in pregnancy

The majority of patients seem to be controlled with steroids alone during pregnancy. Azathioprine is the second-line agent of choice. It is important to treat disease-relapses and new onset of disease aggressively, as outcome appears to be worse in the presence of active disease.

Recommendations

In general, the patient should be advised that it should be safe for her to become pregnant, that there is no evidence that this will significantly worsen her disease, but that any disease relapse needs to be treated effectively in order to prevent fetal complications and death. However, this may not be true if the patient has significant interstitial lung disease which may lead to respiratory compromise during the pregnancy. In these patients very careful cardiac and respiratory assessments should be considered and the patient counseled accordingly on the advisability of a pregnancy in the presence of interstitial lung disease. Serum, creatinine kniase (CK) should be monitored throughout pregnancy, in conjunction with regular follow up from the obstetrics team and rheumatology expert.

Further reading

Andrews J et al 2004 Non-invasive imaging in the diagnosis and management of Takayasu's arteritis. Annals of the Rheumatic Diseases 63:995-1000

Benenson E et al 2005 High-dose azathioprine pulse therapy as a new treatment option in patients with active Wegener's granulomatosis and lupus nephritis refractory or intolerant to cyclophosphamide. Clinical Rheumatism 3:251-257

Doria A et al 2004 Pregnancy in rare autoimmune rheumatic diseases: UCTD, MCTD, myositis, systemic vasculitis and Bechet disease. Lupus 13:690-695

Guillevin L et al 1996 Prognostic factors in polyarteritis nodosa and Churg–Strauss syndrome. A prospective study in 342 patients. Medicine (Baltimore) 75:17-28

Guillevin L et al 2005 Hepatitis B virus-associated polyarteritis nodosa: clinical characteristics, outcome, and impact of treatment in 115 patients. Medicine 84:313-322

Harber M A et al 1999 Wegener's granulomatosis in pregnancy – the therapeutic dilemma. Nephrology, Dialysis, Transplantation 14:1789-1791

Jayne D et al 2003 A randomised trial of maintenance therapy for vasculitis associated with antineutrophil cytoplasmic antibodies 'CYCAZAREM'. New England Journal of Medicine 349:36-44

Langford C A, Kerr G S 2002 Pregnancy in vasculitis. Current Opinion in Rheumatology 14:36-41

Looper WO et al 2006 Congenital malformation after first-trimester exposure & ACE inhibitor. New England Journal of Medicine 354:2443-2451

Gordon C 2004 Pregnancy and autoimmune diseases. Best Practice and Research Clinical Rheumatology 18:359-379

Khamashta M, Ruiz-Irastorza G, Hughes G R V
1997 Systemic lupus erythematosus flares during
pregnancy. Rheumatic Disease Clinics of North
America 23:15-30
Kitridou R C 2005 Pregnancy in mixed connective tissue
disease. Rheumatic Disease Clinics of North America
31:497-508
Østensen M et al 2004 A prospective study of
pregnant patients with rheumatoid arthritis an
ankylosing spondylitis using validated clinical
instruments. Annals of the Rheumatic Diseases
63:1212-1217

Østensen M et al 2006 in press Anti-inflammatory and
immunosuppressive drugs and reproduction: Arthritis
Research and Therapy 8:209
Piccoli G B et al 2004 Vasculitis and kidney involvement in
pregnancy: evidence-based medicine and ethics bear
upon clinical choices. Nephrology, Dialysis,
Transplantation 19:2909-2913
Rees D et al 2006 Prevalence of the antiphospholipid
syndrome in primary systemic vasculitis. Annals of the
Rheumatic Diseases 65:109-111
Wallace D J, Hahn B H 2002 Dubois' lupus eryhtematosus,
6th edn. Lippincott Williams & Wilkins, London

Chapter **11**

Malignant disease in pregnancy

M. I. Shafi, S. A. Karim

INTRODUCTION

The combination of malignant disease and pregnancy presents a paradox whereby there is an association of controlled growth (pregnancy) and uncontrolled growth (malignancy). Generally the age at which malignancy arises does not correspond with the peak age of reproduction, but increasingly instances are encountered where these do occur together posing significant problems. For completeness, gestational trophoblastic neoplasia (GTN) is considered in this chapter.

Few individual clinicians will have significant experience of managing women with malignant disease and pregnancy. Management is not clear cut as there are various issues to consider. There is usually a conflict between optimal maternal therapy and fetal well-being. Consequently, either maternal or fetal well-being, or both, may be compromised. There is a paucity of literature relating to maternal outcomes after treatment for malignancy in pregnancy. Studies of published reviews and individual case reports may be useful to guide management.

Although cancer is the second most common cause of death during the reproductive years, it affects only approximately 1 in 1000 pregnancies. The most common malignancies associated with pregnancy involve the breast, cervix, leukemia, lymphoma, melanoma, thyroid, ovary and colon. Because of the current trend in women to delay pregnancy, these associations are likely to increase.

As optimization of both maternal and fetal outcomes is difficult to reconcile, compromise is often required. The main issues raised are:

- Does the presence of the malignancy require consideration of termination of the pregnancy?
- Is the prognosis for the malignancy affected by the pregnancy (and vice versa)?
- What effect will the malignancy, or any planned treatment, have on the fetus?
- Does the malignancy require deferment of treatment because of pregnancy?

The existence of pregnancy may have a direct (e.g. hormonal) or an indirect effect on the course and management of the disease. There is often a delay in diagnostic workup and treatment. The choice of treatment and psychological effects may be important. The decision making process can be difficult due to the various factors that input into making the decision. Maternal wishes are extremely important as is sharing what little information is available in relation to the specific tumor in pregnancy (Fig. 11.1).

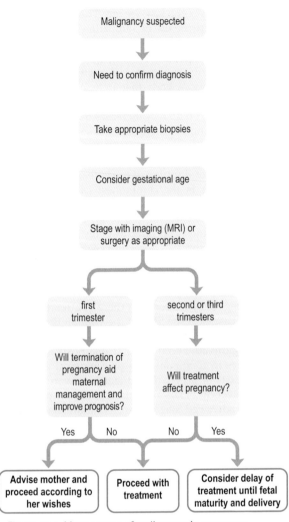

Figure 11.1 Management of malignancy in pregnancy.

EFFECTS OF CANCER THERAPY IN PREGNANCY

In general, malignant conditions during pregnancy are not associated with poor perinatal outcomes. The data relating to children's higher order brain functioning following in utero exposure to maternal cancer and its associated treatment are sparse. The literature that does exist has concentrated on structural observations of the fetus, made very close to the time of delivery. These observations suggest that exposure to antineoplastic drugs after the first trimester is not associated with increased teratogenicity. This is important as brain development continues throughout gestation, and exposure to antineoplastic drugs later in pregnancy may theoretically

have an effect on neurodevelopment. The potential undesirable effects on the developing fetus and its cognitive development in childhood relating to maternal cancer in pregnancy, remain largely unknown.

Surgery may be required to evaluate or treat malignancies in pregnancy. Surgery and anesthesia should be avoided in the first trimester if at all possible, because of the theoretical risk of teratogenesis and the potential to disturb the pregnancy and precipitate miscarriage. However, the clinical indication may be such that surgery cannot be deferred. As always the risks and benefits must be considered in the context of the particular clinical problem and the mother's wishes. Where surgery is required, attempts should be made to minimize any effect on the pregnancy. These include avoiding hypotension, hypoxia, coagulation and metabolic disturbance.

Almost all of the cytotoxic drugs used are able to cross the placenta and theoretically could be teratogenic or mutagenic. The common function of all chemotherapy is to affect cell division mechanisms. It is this property, with its antitumor function, that can have potentially detrimental effects on the developing embryo or fetus. Between 5-10 weeks' gestation is the period of maximal susceptibility for the fetus. With exposure at this time the estimated risk of major malformations from single agent chemotherapy is in the order of 10%, rising to 25% for combination chemotherapy (cf. 1-3% in general population). Fetal demise may also occur. After 13 weeks' gestation, organogenesis is completed, with the exception of the brain and gonads. Any effect after this period is likely to be manifest as intrauterine growth restriction rather than fetal anomaly. Chemotherapy will affect the fetal hemotopoietic system with about a third of babies at birth having pancytopenia if exposed to chemotherapy in utero.

When chemotherapy is used after the first trimester, the majority of cases have a normal pregnancy outcome. The central nervous system (CNS) develops throughout pregnancy and even after birth. Some chemical substances such as alcohol are known to have an adverse effect on CNS development in the second and third trimesters. With regard to chemotherapeutic agents, those studies that are available report no major impact on later neurodevelopment following in utero exposure. However, the database on which these conclusions are drawn remains small and lacks the power to detect small, but clinically significant, effects.

Radiation is used for diagnostic and therapeutic purposes in many malignancies. Exposure to less than 0.05 Gy does not increase the teratogenic risk. In most diagnostic procedures, the cumulative dose of

> **Box 11.1 Effects of cancer therapy in pregnancy**
>
> - In general, malignant conditions during pregnancy are not, per se, associated with poor perinatal outcomes.
> - Exposure to chemotherapy at 5-10 weeks' gestation, the period of maximal susceptibility for the embryo / fetus, has an estimated risk of major malformations from single agent chemotherapy of around 10%, rising to 25% for combination chemotherapy.
> - Chemotherapy use after the first trimester is associated with IUGR and pancytopenia.
> - Radiation treatment is associated with fetal damage, especially to the CNS where there are associations with microcephaly and developmental delay.

radiation does not reach this value, even if the abdomen is unshielded. However, imaging where malignancy is suspected will often push this exposure up considerably, and so increase the risk to the fetus. Radiation treatment will increase the exposure still further so that fetal damage may occur, especially to the CNS with cases of microcephaly and developmental delay. The developing embryo and fetus are extremely sensitive to ionizing radiation and the human brain seems to be the most sensitive organ. These effects are both time and dose dependent. Ionizing radiation is a known CNS teratogen and may be a more serious risk to the fetus than the cancer itself. Radiation is capable of producing cognitive and behavioral teratogenic effects, which are demonstrable at doses below those causing visible structural malformations.

Finally, cancer patients are more likely to experience febrile episodes either as a complication of the disease process or of treatment. Hyperthermia is associated with increased fetal abnormality rates in animal studies with the effect primarily limited to the period of organogenesis. The effect in humans is unclear (Box 11.1).

COMMON NEOPLASTIC DISEASES IN PREGNANCY

Breast cancer

Breast cancer is the commonest cancer in women, with a lifetime risk of 11% in the UK. While the overall incidence of breast cancer has increased, mortality has fallen by 30% over the last decade. The major factors in this decline are the use of Tamoxifen and the widespread application of breast cancer screening. Reproductive factors affect the subsequent risk for breast cancer. Nulliparity increases and parity reduces the risk of breast cancer. Early menarche and late age at first pregnancy are also associated with increased risk. Conversely, pregnancy increases the risk of breast cancer developing in carriers of BRCA1 and BRCA2 mutations. Breastfeeding confers a weak, but significant, protective effect for breast cancer especially in those with longer duration of breastfeeding.

Breast cancer is the commonest cancer in pregnancy and the puerperium, occurring in about 1 in 3000 women, representing 3% of all breast cancers. With many women choosing to delay childbearing, the incidence of breast cancer in pregnancy is likely to increase. Breast cancer pathology is similar in age-matched pregnant and non-pregnant women. However, the prognosis associated with breast cancer during pregnancy is worse as there is a tendency to late stage disease, especially if the woman is aged 30 years or less. This poorer prognosis is associated with both the more advanced stage at diagnosis and also with delays in treatment. The physiological changes in the breasts of pregnant and lactating women may hinder detection of discrete masses, thus explaining the more advanced stage at presentation than in an age matched non-pregnant control group. If breast cancer is suspected in pregnancy, ultrasound and mammography may be used for assessment. With proper shielding, mammography poses little risk of radiation exposure to the fetus. Mammograms are more difficult to assess during pregnancy, and the final arbiter is diagnostic biopsy. This may be achieved using fine needle aspiration, core biopsy or excisional biopsy. The pathologist should be made aware of the pregnancy to aid interpretation of the histological material.

Termination of the pregnancy has not been shown to have any beneficial effect on the outcome of breast cancer. However, it may need to be considered, if therapeutic options (chemotherapy and radiation therapy) are significantly limited by the pregnancy.

Treatment of the breast cancer is primarily surgical with deferred reconstruction. Chemotherapy is generally not advocated in the first trimester (because of organogenesis) but may be used later in pregnancy. Limited data suggests that chemotherapy may be associated with premature labor. Data on the immediate and long-term effects of chemotherapy on the fetus are limited. There is a general recommendation not to use Tamoxifen in pregnancy. Radiotherapy is not absolutely contraindicated but adequate shielding of the fetus should take place. Generally it is advised to wait until after delivery, as radiation may be harmful to the fetus at any stage of development.

Fertility may be influenced by treatment for breast cancer. Chemotherapy can cause premature ovarian failure. The likelihood depends on the regimens used and, particularly, the woman's age. Women over the age of 40 are more likely to develop amenorrhea and ovarian failure compared to those under age 40. For those women who do conceive following such treatment, there is no available evidence that any of these chemotherapeutic agents adversely affect subsequent fetal or neonatal development. Nor does there appear to be any adverse effect of subsequent pregnancy on maternal survival. Most authorities recommend a minimum delay of two years before contemplating pregnancy after breast cancer treatment to allow any early recurrences, which may influence the decision for any future pregnancy, to be detected. In younger women or those with more advanced disease, a longer interval may be preferred as these situations are associated with poorer outcomes.

Women may wish to preserve their fertility, prior to chemotherapy. Whilst egg freezing and ovarian tissue cryopreservation, are not well established, embryo freezing remains a viable alternative to those with a partner. The risk of ovarian stimulation on risk of recurrence of breast cancer is unknown.

Following completion of treatment for breast cancer, women may breastfeed from the unaffected breast. Suppression of lactation does not improve prognosis of breast cancer. During treatment with chemotherapy or radiation, women are advised not to breastfeed (Box 11.2).

Hodgkin's lymphoma

Hodgkin's lymphoma primarily affects young adults and is therefore a relatively common tumor associated with pregnancy. No set protocols exist for its management and an individualized program will need to be constructed. This will take into account the stage and severity of the Hodgkin's lymphoma, the gestation and the mother's wishes.

Magnetic resonance imaging (MRI) is the preferred imaging modality for assessment in order to avoid exposure to ionizing radiation. During the first trimester, continuation of pregnancy may pose risks to the long term outcome in respect of the Hodgkin's lymphoma. If the disease is supradiaphragmatic, then a more conservative approach may be adopted. Chemotherapy is not advised in the first trimester but radiation may be considered with proper shielding.

Box 11.2 Breast cancer and pregnancy

- Breast cancer is the commonest cancer in pregnancy and the puerperium.
- Nulliparity increases and parity reduces the risk of breast cancer.
- Pregnancy increases the risk of breast cancer developing in carriers of *BRCA1* and *BRCA2* mutations.
- Breastfeeding confers a weak, but significant, protective effect for breast cancer.
- Breast cancer pathology is similar in age-matched pregnant and non-pregnant women.
- The prognosis associated with breast cancer during pregnancy is worse as there is a tendency to late stage disease, associated with the more advanced stage at diagnosis and delays in treatment.
- Subsequent pregnancy does not appear to have any adverse effect on maternal survival.
- A minimum delay of 2 years before contemplating pregnancy after breast cancer treatment, to allow any early recurrence to be identified, is recommended.

In the second half of pregnancy, treatment can be delayed until delivery at 32-36 weeks. If chemotherapy is clinically warranted in late pregnancy, such as in women with symptomatic advanced stage disease, then vincristine alone may be used as it is not associated with fetal abnormalities in the second half of pregnancy. Corticosteroids may be employed for their antitumor effects, relief of specific symptoms, as well as hastening lung maturity in the fetus in preparation for preterm delivery. Many clinicians will favor combination chemotherapy over single agent chemotherapy or radiation therapy after the first trimester. Combination chemotherapy with ABVD (doxorubicin, bleomycin, vinblastine and dacarbazine) appears to be safe in the second half of pregnancy. Radiation therapy may also be considered for respiratory compromise secondary to a rapidly enlarging mediastinal lesion.

Survival of women with Hodgkin's lymphoma in pregnancy is similar to that of non-pregnant women when matched for stage of disease, age at diagnosis and calendar year of treatment. The long-term effect of chemotherapy on the progeny is uncertain, although the available evidence tends to be reassuring (Box 11.3).

Box 11.3 Hodgkin's lymphoma in pregnancy

- MRI is the preferred imaging modality for assessment in order to avoid exposure to ionizing radiation.
- Chemotherapy is not advised in the first trimester but radiation therapy may be considered with proper shielding.
- In the second half of pregnancy, treatment can be delayed until delivery at 32-36 weeks.
- Combination chemotherapy with ABVD (doxorubicin, bleomycin, vinblastine and dacarbazine) appears to be safe in the second half of pregnancy.
- Radiation therapy may also be considered for respiratory compromise secondary to a rapidly enlarging mediastinal lesion.
- Survival of women with Hodgkin's lymphoma in pregnancy is similar to that of non-pregnant women when matched for stage of disease, age at diagnosis and calendar year of treatment.

Non-Hodgkin's lymphoma

Non-Hodgkin's lymphoma (NHL) usually affects much older patients compared with Hodgkin's lymphoma. There are concomitantly fewer reports of NHL associated with pregnancy. MRI is the preferred investigation for staging purposes. Most NHLs are aggressive and a delay in treatment due to pregnancy may have an adverse outcome. Gestational age becomes very important in counseling the woman, with termination or preterm delivery having to be considered. The latter will minimize fetal exposure to chemotherapy or radiation therapy. Only in those with indolent NHL, may treatment be delayed.

Children exposed to high dose doxorubicin containing combination chemotherapy in utero, especially during the second and third trimesters, have been found to be normal on follow up ranging up to 11 years of age.

Leukemia

Pregnancy and the leukemias are rarely associated, possibly due to reduced fertility in these patients. There is no evidence that the course of either acute or chronic leukemia is altered by pregnancy, but the evidence on which this is based is limited. Leukemia affects fetal well-being. The earlier the diagnosis is made, the higher the perinatal mortality. This may be due to maternal anemia, disseminated intravascular coagulation, thrombosis or disruption of placental exchange. Acute leukemias are highly malignant but potentially curable. Without treatment, maternal death can occur within two months. The best chemotherapeutic regimen should be used irrespective of the gestation. Giving chemotherapy in the first trimester is associated with risk of fetal abnormality.

Thyroid tumors

Papillary adenocarcinoma is the commonest thyroid malignancy and has a peak incidence at age 30-35. Reviews have suggested a negligible effect on the malignancy of pregnancy. Usually, treatment consists of tumor ablation with radioactive iodine – this is contraindicated in pregnancy. In early disease, treatment may be deferred to the postpartum period. In more advanced disease, surgical excision followed by postpartum radioactive iodine is indicated.

Melanoma

About one-third of women diagnosed with malignant melanoma will be of reproductive age. There are conflicting reports, based on relatively small numbers of patients, in relation to prognosis when malignant melanoma is associated with pregnancy and also whether pregnancy may induce or exacerbate melanoma. However, there does not appear to be significant difference in survival between patients diagnosed during pregnancy and outwith pregnancy when controlled for tumor thickness (see Ch. 15).

Prognosis, as in all women with localized melanoma, depends primarily on tumor thickness and truncal anatomical site. As in the non-pregnant, the same rules apply for biopsy of worrying lesions. Moles which change in size, shape, or color, persistently itch, or are new and look different from other spots should be evaluated and biopsied if there is any concern.

Wide local excision around the melanoma site is conducted, irrespective of pregnancy status. Melanomas that have not spread beyond the site of at which they developed are highly curable. The treatment of localized melanoma is surgical excision with margins proportional to the microstage of the primary lesion. For most lesions < 2 mm thick, this means 1 cm radial re-excision margins. With increasing depth of invasion, the risk of lymph node and/or systemic disease increases. Local treatment remains surgical excision but with larger radial margins (2-3 cm). Sentinel lymph node biopsy if indicated (melanoma greater than 2 mm thick) can be performed safely in pregnancy as the dose of radioactive material used in this procedure carries negligible risk to the fetus. Sentinel lymph node biopsy should be performed prior to wide excision of the primary melanoma to ensure accurate lymphatic mapping. More advance cases (> 4 mm depth) should be considered for adjuvant therapy with high dose interferon.

There is no evidence to suggest that pregnancy following a diagnosis of melanoma alters prognosis. Recurrences can occur in lymph nodes or internal organs. If this happens during pregnancy, management is undoubtedly more complex and carries a potential, albeit small, risk of spread to the fetus. In those women with advanced melanoma (stage III or IV), the placenta should be examined for the presence of melanoma metastases. If these are present, there is a 20% risk of death of the baby from transplacental spread of the melanoma. The decision as to how long to wait before conceiving following a diagnosis of melanoma depends on the risk of recurrence weighed against the desire for pregnancy and age of the patient. The wait should typically be up to 5 years depending on these factors although it is not possible to provide evidence based recommendations. For example, a woman with localized disease greater than 1 mm thickness who wishes to become pregnant after surgery for stage I or II melanoma should be advised to delay pregnancy for 2 years postsurgery, as the likelihood of recurrence is highest during this period.

Colon cancer

Colon cancer in pregnancy is uncommon but not rare. This is associated with poor prognosis attributable to delays in diagnosis and advanced disease at diagnosis. The diagnosis is frequently delayed by attributing symptoms to pregnancy rather than colonic cancer, such as rectal bleeding, nausea, vomiting or constipation. Pregnancy will affect the diagnostic evaluation and treatment of colon cancer. Appropriate evaluation of significant lower gastrointestinal symptoms during pregnancy can lead to an earlier diagnosis and improved prognosis.

Standard treatment for colon cancer is open surgical resection of the primary lesion and regional lymph nodes for localized disease. When resection can be achieved with clear margins, the survival rate does not differ depending on whether the tumor extends through the bowel wall as compared to similarly staged patients without such invasion. Preoperative imaging allows better selection of patients for resection. Surgery may also be curative in 25-40% of patients with resectable metastases to the liver. Chemotherapy may be contemplated in those with stage III cancer of the colon. Adjuvant radiation appears to have no current standard role in the management of

patients with colon cancer following curative surgery.

Gynecological malignancies

Malignancies of the genital tract during pregnancy are relatively uncommon. The tendency to delay childbearing may result in an increased association in the future. In most instances, management should be as if the woman was not pregnant. Surgical approach is preferred for the various site-specific tumors.

Vulval cancer

This mainly affects postmenopausal women. There does appear to be a younger cohort that are at risk of vulval cancer and these are usually related to oncogenic human papilloma virus infections. If such tumors occur during pregnancy, surgery should be undertaken as in the non-pregnant woman. After 36 weeks' gestation, delay in treatment to the puerperium is advocated. Pregnancy has no effect on long-term outcome of vulval cancer. If a woman has been successfully treated for vulval cancer, then pregnancy is not contraindicated. Vaginal delivery is possible in this situation but is influenced by the postsurgical vulval functionality.

Cervical cancer

This is the commonest gynecological malignancy associated with pregnancy. Cervical cytology is not recommended during pregnancy as part of routine screening. Despite this, if preinvasive disease is detected, it may be managed conservatively in the absence of cytological and colposcopic features of invasive disease. Biopsy of the cervix may be associated with significant risk for hemorrhage and suitable precautions should be taken. Only if there is a significant suspicion of invasive disease, should a suitable biopsy be contemplated to confirm the diagnosis. This may be in the form of a wedge or cone biopsy.

Women with cervical cancer during pregnancy will often present with vaginal bleeding. Whilst the bleeding is usually pregnancy associated, this can not be assumed. The cervix and vagina should therefore be visualized to identify any pathology if present.

Early stage cervical cancers, may be cured using local treatment in the form of a suitably tailored cone biopsy. For more advanced tumors, radical surgery or chemo-radiation will need to be considered. This will depend on the stage of disease and gestation. Institutional expertise may also be a relevant factor. The wishes of the woman and the stage in the pregnancy are obviously very important in the discussions (Fig. 11.2).

The major dilemma occurs during the 20-32 week gestation period. Delays to treatment to allow fetal maturity may impact on prognosis. If possible, delay until after 32 weeks and confirmation of fetal lung maturity will allow a surgical approach to be utilized and Cesarean-radical hysterectomy may be conducted. A classical Cesarean section should be performed to minimize risk of tumour disruption. At surgery, the ovaries may be conserved. Vaginal delivery while feasible may be associated with a risk of significant hemorrhage from the cervical tumor.

In those women with more advanced disease (Ib2-IV), chemo-radiation is the preferred treatment. In early pregnancy, external beam radiation results in miscarriage but in later pregnancy, surgical evacuation of the pregnancy or delivery may be required.

Endometrial cancer

This is a rare association with pregnancy. The age profile of women with endometrial cancer is postmenopausal. The high circulating progesterone levels during pregnancy may have a beneficial effect in preventing endometrial cancer. The abnormal endometrium is unfavorable for successful implantation and most of the reported cases are associated with first trimester miscarriage. There are a few case reports of live births in association with endometrial cancer. Some contend that these are cases of misdiagnosis. Usually diagnosis occurs in the postpartum period and standard treatment protocols may be applied.

Ovarian cancer

This is rarely diagnosed during pregnancy. Management is based on experience of treatment in the non-pregnant woman. Any ovarian mass greater than 5 cm in diameter should be viewed with caution. Recent case reports have described the laparoscopic approach to adnexal masses in pregnancy. The aim is to undertake the surgery prior to 16 weeks gestation if possible. In the latter half of pregnancy, ovarian tumors are particularly difficult to diagnose due to the gravid uterus.

If ovarian cancer is diagnosed during pregnancy, treatment is essentially similar to that in the non-pregnant woman. Staging laparotomy may be followed by adjuvant chemotherapy if indicated.

GESTATIONAL TROPHOBLASTIC NEOPLASIA

Gestational trophoblastic neoplasms (GTN) are rare but highly curable tumors arising from the products of conception in the uterus. The prognosis for cure is good even when the disease has spread to distant organs. There is ethnic variation in the incidence of GTN in the UK, with women from Asia having a higher incidence compared with non-Asian women (approximately a doubling of risk). Persistent GTN may develop after a molar pregnancy, a non-molar pregnancy or a live birth. The incidence after a live birth is low and is estimated to be in the order of 1:50 000. The importance of GTN is that it is almost always curable, with preservation of fertility, if treated appropriately and in a timely manner.

There is no universally accepted staging system for GTN. Recent attempt at unifying a staging system was developed by the Federation Internationale De Gynecologie et d'Obstetrique (FIGO) and published in 2002. It was recommended that 'GTN' should preferentially be used instead of gestational trophoblastic disease (GTD). This staging combines the classical anatomical staging with other prognostic indicators that have been identified as clinically important in managing

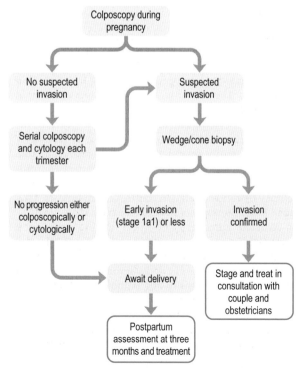

Figure 11.2 Cervical cytological abnormality or suspected malignancy during pregnancy.

Table 11.1 FIGO anatomical staging and scoring system

FIGO scoring	0	1	2	4
Age	<40	≥40	–	–
Antecedent pregnancy	Mole	Abortion	Term	–
Interval months from index pregnancy	<4	4-<7	7-<13	≥13
Pre-treatment serum HCG (IU/L)	$<10^3$	10^3-$<10^4$	10^4-$<10^5$	$≥10^5$
Largest tumor size (including uterus) cm	<3	3-<5	≥5	–
Site of metastases	Lung	Spleen, kidney	Gastrointestinal	Liver, brain
Number of metastases	–	1-4	5-8	>8
Previous failed chemotherapy	–	–	Single drug	2 or more drugs

Stage I: Disease confined to the uterus.
Stage II: GTN extends outside of the uterus, but is limited to the genital structures (Adnexa, vagina, broad ligament).
Stage III: GTN extends to the lungs, with or without known genital tract involvement.
Stage IV: All other metastatic sites.

Table 11.2 Premalignant and malignant disorders

Premalignant disorders	Malignant disorders
Complete hydatidiform mole (CHM)	Invasive mole
Partial hydatidiform mole (PHM)	Gestational choriocarcinoma
	Placental site trophoblastic tumor (PSTT)

women with GTN (Table 11.1). A patient is allocated to a stage as represented by Roman numeral I, II, III, and IV. This is then separated by a colon from the sum of all the actual risk factor scores expressed in Arabic numerals e.g. stage II:4, stage IV:8.

Both CHM and PHM can develop into invasive moles and choriocarcinoma, however only CHM has been shown to develop into PSTTs (Table 11.2).

The commonest form of GTN is the hydatidiform mole, which occurs in approximately 1:1000 pregnancies in the UK. It is defined as products of conception that lack an intact fetus and show gross cyst-like swellings of the chorionic villi due to accumulation of fluid. There is disintegration and loss of blood vessels in the villous core. It is subdivided into complete and partial mole based on genetic and histopathological features. CHM arises when an ovum devoid of maternal nuclear DNA is fertilized either by two sperm or by a single sperm which duplicates its chromosomes to give a diploid complement of DNA. PHM are triploid in origin with two sets of paternal haploid genes and one set of maternal haploid genes. This is invariably as a result of dispermic fertilization of an ovum. These proliferate into abnormal trophoblast with variable amounts of fetal tissue.

The widespread use of ultrasound has led to earlier diagnoses of molar pregnancies. They usually present as threatened or missed miscarriage. Other associated features are rare with hyperemesis, early severe pre-eclampsia or hyperthyroidism occurring.

CHM is more common in women who become pregnant at either extreme of childbearing age (< 16 or > 40 years) although PHM appears not to be age assoicated. Hydatidiform moles are also more common in women who have had previous molar pregnancies; the incidence rises to 1:76 with one previous mole, and to 1:6.5 with two previous moles.

The trophoblast forms hydropic villi which are most obvious in complete moles and macroscopically resemble a bunch of grapes. In PHMs these changes are milder and focal, such that macroscopically in spontaneous abortions the diagnosis may not be apparent. The ability to synthesize human chorionic gonadotrophin (HCG), is preserved in molar tissue, enabling it to be used as an extremely sensitive tumor marker.

Patients with a suspected molar pregnancy should undergo pelvic ultrasound scan (USS), HCG estimation in serum and/or urine, and chest radiography (CXR) to look for possible metastatic disease. In CHM, the classical USS appearance is described as a snow storm, although this is not often seen until the second trimester of pregnancy. In PHM, occasionally fetal parts may be identified on USS, in association with a grossly abnormal placenta.

The primary treatment for these patients is prompt suction evacuation of the uterine contents. Medical termination of CHM including prostanoids to ripen a nulliparous cervix is not recommended as this may induce uterine contractions and trigger trophoblastic embolization. The latter may be fatal and is probably also the explanation for a higher risk of needing subsequent chemotherapy if medical or other surgical methods are used to evacuate the uterus. Similarly, use of potent oxytocic agents have the potential to cause the same effect. It is recommended, that where possible, oxytocic infusions are only commenced once evacuation has been completed.

In the UK, all patients with GTN are registered centrally in one of three centers which coordinate the national follow-up service. Central pathology review can be undertaken. All patients send two weekly blood and urine samples to the center for serial HCG estimations. In the majority of cases the mole regresses and the HCG levels return to normal ($\leq 4\,IU/L$). To enable early detection of disease relapse using HCG, patients are advised to avoid a further pregnancy for 6 months. The hormones in the oral contraceptive pill are probably growth factors for trophoblastic tumors and for this reason patients are advised not to use the pill until the HCG levels have returned to normal.

The rate of fall of HCG after uterine evacuation can predict the likelihood of subsequently developing a trophoblastic tumor. If the HCG has fallen to normal within 8 weeks of evacuation then marker follow-up can be safely reduced to 6 months. However in patients whose HCG levels are still elevated beyond 8 weeks from the date of evacuation, follow-up is continued for 2 years. As patients who have had a previous mole or GTN are at an increased risk of having a second molar pregnancy, HCG levels are measured at 6 and 10 weeks following the completion of each subsequent pregnancy.

The indications for chemotherapy in patients with a CHM or PHM are shown in Box 11.4. HCG values > 20 000 IU/L four weeks after evacuation of a mole or rising values in this range at an earlier stage, indicate that the patient is at increased risk of uterine perforation or severe hemorrhage. These complications can be life threatening and the risk can be reduced by starting chemotherapy. About 15-20% of CHMs and 0.5% of PHMs ultimately require chemotherapy.

Staging investigations are performed and information used in the scoring system to determine the risk of developing drug resistance to methotrexate. Women who are low risk receive single agent chemotherapy with methotrexate, which is given intramuscularly, alternating daily with oral folinic acid for 1 week followed by a week of rest prior to recommencing treatment. Chemotherapy shrinks the disease very rapidly, and this predisposes the patient to an increased risk of tumor hemorrhage. The other side effects are

Box 11.4 Indications for chemotherapy

- Evidence of metastases in brain, liver or gastrointestinal tract, or radiological opacities > 2 cm on chest X-ray.
- Histological evidence of choriocarcinoma.
- Heavy vaginal bleeding or evidence of gastrointestinal or intraperitoneal hemorrhage.
- Pulmonary, vulval or vaginal metastases unless HCG falling.
- Rising HCG after evacuation.
- Serum HCG > 20 000 IU/L more than 4 weeks after evacuation, because of the risk of uterine perforation.
- Raised HCG 6 months after evacuation even if still falling.

mucosal ulceration, conjunctivitis and occasionally serositis.

Women scoring as high risk receive combination chemotherapy. One such regimen comprises etoposide, methotrexate and actinomycin D (EMA) alternating weekly with cyclophosphamide and vincristine (CO). Acute side effects include myelosuppression, alopecia, peripheral neuropathy and those associated with single agent methotrexate therapy.

Treatment with either regimen is continued until the HCG has been normal for 6 weeks. During this time the serum HCG is measured twice a week, so that the tumor response can be closely monitored and appropriate treatment changes made promptly.

CHORIOCARCINOMA

Choriocarcinoma most commonly follows a molar pregnancy but can follow a normal pregnancy, ectopic pregnancy or abortion. The incidence of choriocarcinoma following term delivery is approximately 1:50 000. Although choriocarcinoma can arise following any type of pregnancy, CHM is probably the most common antecedent with an estimated 3% of CHMs developing into choriocarcinomas. It should be considered when a patient has continued vaginal bleeding in the postdelivery period. Other common signs include unusual neurologic symptoms or signs in a female within the reproductive age group and asymptomatic lesions on routine chest X-ray.

Choriocarcinoma is a highly malignant tumor, which appears as a soft purple largely hemorrhagic mass. Microscopically it mimics the appearances of an early implanting blastocyst with central cores of mononuclear cytotrophoblast surrounded by a rim of multinucleated syncytiotrophoblast and a distinct absence of chorionic villi. The surrounding areas are usually necrotic and hemorrhagic and tumor is frequently seen within venous sinuses. Genetic analysis frequently demonstrates multiple karyotype anomalies, but none as yet are specific for choriocarcinoma.

Choriocarcinoma following an apparently normal pregnancy or non-molar abortion usually presents within a year of delivery. The presenting features may be similar to hydatidiform moles with vaginal bleeding, abdominal pain, pelvic mass and symptoms due to a high serum HCG. However, one-third of all patients with choriocarcinomas present without gynecological features, and instead manifest symptoms and signs associated with metastases. Pulmonary, cerebral and hepatic deposits are most frequent but any site may be involved.

Although these tumors are highly vascular, excision biopsy of a metastasis should be considered where it can be safely achieved. This not only enables histological confirmation of the diagnosis but also permits genetic analysis to prove the gestational nature of the tumour. Thus, if there are only maternal genes and no paternal genes present then the patient has a non-gestational tumor e.g. an ovarian choriocarcinoma or more rarely an epithelial tumor which has differentiated into choriocarcinoma. Frequently, however, biopsy is not possible and the diagnosis is made on the clinical history and other investigation findings. The patients are then scored and treated as described for molar disease.

PLACENTAL SITE TROPHOBLASTIC TUMOR

Placental site trophoblastic tumor (PSTT) can develop following a term delivery, non-molar abortion, or CHM. PSTT is thought to constitute about 1% of all trophoblastic tumors. They are slow growing malignant tumors composed mainly of cytotrophoblast with very little syncytiotrophoblast and so produce little HCG. However, they often stain strongly for human placental lactogen (HPL), which helps to distinguish this tumor from, carcinomas, sarcomas, exaggerated placental-site reaction and placental nodule. The raised HPL may cause hyperprolactinemia which can result in amenorrhea and/or galactorrhea. PSTT usually spreads by local infiltra-

tion with distant metastasis occurring late via the lymphatics and blood. The behavior of PSTT is thus quite different from other forms of GTN and it is often relatively chemoresistant. Consequently, the mainstay of treatment is hysterectomy when the disease is localized to the uterus. When metastatic disease is present, individual patients can respond and be apparently cured by multi-agent chemotherapy either alone or in combination with surgery.

Follow-up

On completion of their chemotherapy, patients are advised to:

- Avoid conceiving for one year.
- To use adequate sun-block to minimize the effect of therapy induced skin photosensitivity.
- To remain on HCG follow-up for life to confirm that their disease is in remission.

About 2% of low-risk and 4% of high-risk patients relapse. All low- to middle-risk patients can be salvaged with further chemotherapy (EMA/CO or alternative regimens) and thus this group has a close to 100% cure rate. High-risk patients have an overall 86% 5-year survival rate. Deaths in this group usually occur due to delays in making the diagnosis. Drug resistance is the other main cause of death in high risk patients, but salvage rates for relapse following EMA/CO therapy can be in excess of 70%.

In the long term, EMA/CO therapy increases the risk of second tumors by 1.6-fold compared to the general population, and may expedite the menopause by an average of 3 years. Low risk chemotherapy with methotrexate, however, is not associated with any long-term toxicity. Importantly neither treatment affects fertility or rates of fetal abnormality in subsequent pregnancies.

Women who become pregnant after a molar pregnancy have a 98% chance of this being normal.

The combined oral contraceptive pill may increase the need for treatment if taken while the HCG levels are still raised. Other forms of hormonal contraception do not appear to have the same effect. Once HCG levels return to normal, it is then safe to use the combined oral contraceptive pill.

CONCLUSION

Malignant disease in pregnancy represents a complex situation with differing medical and ethical issues. Delays in diagnosis can occur when symptoms of malignancy are attributed to pregnancy. Once malignancy is diagnosed, then gestational age becomes an important factor in further management. MRI is safe in pregnancy and can be used for staging purposes. Maternal counseling is of paramount importance in the decision making process.

The general concept of treating malignancy in pregnancy is to proceed as in the non-pregnant. There are obviously variations to this as detailed in this chapter. If possible chemotherapy should be avoided in the first trimester due to an associated teratogenic risk.

With GTN, correct diagnosis and appropriate management is important. In the UK, there is a centralized GTN service allowing considerable expertise to be developed in managing this condition.

Further reading

Altman J F et al 2003 Placental metastasis of maternal melanoma. Journal of American Academic Dermatology 49:1150-1154

Barthelmes L et al 2005 Pregnancy and breast cancer. British Medical Journal 330:1375-1378

Gwyn K, Theriault R 2001 Breast cancer during pregnancy. Oncology 15(1):39-46; discussion 46, 49-51

Koren G, Lishner M, Farine D (eds) 1996 Cancer in Pregnancy: Maternal and Fetal Risks. Cambridge University Press, Cambridge

Mackie R M et al 1991 Lack of effect of pregnancy on outcome of melanoma. Lancet 337:653-655

Royal College of Obstetricians and Gynaecologists 2004 The management of gestational trophoblastic neoplasia. Guideline no. 20

Chapter 12

Infections in pregnancy

M. M. Khare, M. D. Khare

INTRODUCTION

Infections in pregnancy are common and contribute significantly to maternal and neonatal mortality and morbidity mainly in the developing countries. About one-quarter of maternal deaths in the developing nations are related to infections in pregnancy with puerperal sepsis and septic abortions as predominant contributors. Maternal infections are also one of the commonest preventable causes for preterm birth in these settings. Maternal deaths due to infections in the UK have dramatically reduced in the last two decades although not completely disappeared. There were 13 direct deaths from genital tract sepsis in the last triennium (2000-2002) in the Confidential Enquiry into Maternal Deaths in the UK. There were 14 other deaths due to infection not related to genital tract sepsis. Three of these deaths were from meningitis. Although the patterns of infectious disease in pregnancy are different across the globe, increasing foreign travel and immigrant population in developed countries makes it essential for health professionals caring for these women to have increased awareness of unusual infections that may present. Also the increase in sexually transmitted disease worldwide is a major public health issue. Some maternal infections may pose increased risks of infection to the fetus in utero or intrapartum with variable consequences in the short and long term. The involvement of multidisciplinary teams involving the obstetricians, neonatologists, maternal-fetal medicine specialists, microbiologists, genitourinary specialists, midwives, pharmacologists, intensivists, general practitioners and community health workers is vital in providing good quality of care in the preconception, antenatal and postnatal periods.

This chapter will discuss the common infections in pregnancy that may have consequences for the health of the mother, fetus or newborn baby. Some rare infections have also been briefly discussed.

EFFECTS OF PREGNANCY ON THE IMMUNE SYSTEM IN RELATION TO BACTERIAL AND VIRAL INFECTIONS

Fetal–maternal interaction is a complex phenomenon. It involves some element of maternal immune suppression to minimize the risk of rejection of the fetus, while maintaining enough immunity to fight infection. The immune system has two arms viz. innate or non-specific immunity and adaptive or specific immunity. Adaptive immunity is needed to eliminate infections. This adaptive immunity is coordinated by activated helper type of T lymphocytes called Th cells. These Th cells have the capacity to differentiate into Th1 and Th2 cells. Th1 cells secrete chemical substances called cytokines such as gamma-interferon, tumor necrosis factor (TNF)-beta, interleukin (IL)-2 and TNF-alpha. These stimulate cytotoxic T-cells and macrophage phagocytic activity, both responsible for cell-mediated immunity. Th2 cells secrete cytokines like IL-1, IL-4, IL-5, IL-6, and IL-13 and stimulate B-cells and eosinophils that are responsible for antibody-mediated immunity. Diminished Th-1 response during pregnancy can lead to an increase in incidence of infections such as listeria monocytogenes, group B streptococcus, malaria, tuberculosis, leprosy, viral infections such as infectious hepatitis, varicella zoster and coccidioiodomycosis. Diminished Th-1 response coupled with over-stimulation of innate immunity and non-specific tissue damage can compound the effect of persistent infection.

EFFECTS OF BACTERIAL AND VIRAL INFECTIONS ON THE FETUS

Infection of the fetus may occur transplacentally via hematogenous route or directly from the genital tract to amniotic fluid, during pregnancy or just before delivery. Varying characteristics of micro-organisms and maternal–fetal factors are responsible for the variability of manifestations in the fetus. For example, the virulence of microbes, the size of the inoculum, the status of the immune response of the fetus at different gestational ages and passively derived maternal antibody are all factors in determining the effects of infections on the fetus.

Bacteria, viruses or parasites may cause cell death, abnormalities of cell growth by mitotic inhibition or direct cytotoxic effects such as chromosomal injury or cell necrosis and may lead to inflammatory responses. Some organisms have a propensity to affect certain stages of organogenesis. Rubella virus inhibits cell growth and thus causes structural damage if primary infection occurs in the first trimester. Toxoplasmosis has a higher risk of fetal infection in the third trimester (60%). Toxoplasma, cytomegalovirus (CMV) and herpes simplex virus (HSV) may be associated with intrauterine growth restriction. There is a receptor for parvovirus B19 on the red blood cell called p antigen which affects the fetus at the time of the rapid increase in erythrocyte numbers during the second trimester and causes hemolytic anemia and hydrops fetalis. Infection in pregnancy may lead to miscarriage, stillbirth, premature delivery, structural defects and intrauterine growth restriction. Neonatal persistence of infection and further damage may occur with some infections, including rubella, CMV, HSV and varicella-zoster virus (VZV) infections.

There is increasing interest in research related to perinatal infections and brain injury in preterm and term infants and emerging epidemiological data supports the key role of inflammatory processes in the pathogenesis of perinatal brain injury with increased risk of cerebral palsy.

PRINCIPLES OF BACTERIAL AND VIRAL DIAGNOSIS

Isolation, detection and identification of bacteria

Conventional culture methods use solid or liquid media for isolation of bacteria from clinical specimens. For blood cultures automated continuous monitoring blood culture systems are now available in most laboratories. Identification may use conventional procedures, which include observation of physical characteristics and biochemical reactions, or more recently, miniaturized biochemical reactions which are compared with established profiles for identification of bacteria.

Newer rapid systems use novel substrates that may react with bacterial enzymes to elicit responses detectable in as early as 2-4 h compared to 24-48 h required by standard methods. They are more expensive at present and hence not widely used.

Susceptibility testing utilizes methods such as disc diffusion, broth microdilution, antibiotic gradient or short-incubation automated methods. Disc diffusion is the most popular and widely used method.

Diagnosis of viral infections – isolation and identification of the virus in cell culture

The growth of viruses requires cell culture as viruses only replicate in living cells. Because viruses are inactivated at room temperature, it is important to transport and inoculate them as soon as possible after collection. Further identification is done by observing the characteristic cytopathic effect (CPE) on cell culture e.g. CMV. If a virus does not produce CPE then further techniques (e.g. hemadsorption) may be helpful. Definitive identification employs techniques including complement fixation, hemagglutination inhibition, neutralization, fluorescent-antibody assay, or enzyme immunoassay (EIA).

Microscopic identification directly in the specimen

Electron microscopy may be used to detect viral particles by their morphology and size e.g. identification of HSV in vesicular fluid.

Serology

Serological methods detecting the presence of IgM antibodies (e.g. IgM antibody to parvovirus-B19) suggest acute infection, as does a fourfold or greater rise in titer of IgG antibodies in samples taken 10-14 days apart (e.g. herpes simplex infection). Low IgG avidity is useful for diagnosis of primary infection, based on the fact that antibody binds less avidly to antigens during early phases than in the later or chronic phase of infection. This has been demonstrated for primary viral infection with CMV, HSV, rubella and Epstein-Barr virus (EBV).

Detection of viral antigen in blood or body fluids

This is most often done by ELISA, e.g. surface antigen of hepatitis B, CMV antigenemia assay.

Detection of viral nucleic acids in blood or the patient's cells

If only a small amount of DNA is present in the specimen, the polymerase chain reaction (PCR) may be used to amplify the viral nucleic acids. Qualitative assays on amniotic fluid are used for prenatal diagnosis of congenital infection such as CMV after 21 weeks of gestation. Quantitative assays of viral load include RNA of HIV and hepatitis C virus (HCV), and DNA of CMV; these are used to monitor the course of the disease.

BACTEREMIA, SEPTICEMIA AND SEPTIC SHOCK

The presence of bacteria in the blood with or without symptoms is defined as bacteremia. Septicemia is defined as the presence of bacteremia or their toxins in the blood accompanied by systemic symptoms. Septic shock is defined as septicemia complicated by decreased cardiac output, systemic hypotension, decreased tissue perfusion and cellular dysfunction leading to multi-organ failure. Women with septicemia may present with vomiting, diarrhea, abdominal pain, tachypnea, tachycardia and high fever. *Escherichia coli* is the most common cause of Gram-negative bacteremia. Other organisms such as *Klebsiella pneumoniae* and *Proteus* are less frequent. Septic shock occurs in 30-40% of patients with Gram-negative bacteremia. The high frequency of septic shock in bacteremia caused by *Enterobacteriaceae* is due to the toxic effect of the endotoxin, lipopolysaccharide (LPS) on the circulatory system.

The reported incidence of bacteremia after vaginal delivery is 0.1-0.4% while after Cesarean section it is 3-4%. After Cesarean, it is more commonly associated with endometritis. With early recognition and appropriate treatment, mortality in obstetric bacteremia is very low (< 1%). Bacteremia is reported in 8-10% of women with chorioamnionitis and in up to 7% of patients with pyelonephritis. Bacteremia may rarely be associated with infective endocarditis complicating pregnancy and in this instance is associated with very high maternal and fetal mortality rates of around 22% and 15%, respectively.

The immunocompetence of the host and virulence of organisms determine prognosis in cases of septic shock. Early recognition and diagnosis of septic shock with prompt treatment are essential. Treatment involves correction of hemodynamic derangement, treatment of infection with broad spectrum antibiotics followed (after bacteriologic identification) by specific antibiotics, ventilation and other intensive care interventions. Mortality in septic shock has been reported as 15-20%.

Group A streptococcal (GAS) toxic shock syndrome (TSS) is an uncommon, but life-threatening infection during pregnancy and should be considered in cases where there is a rapid onset of shock, accompanied by deep tissue necrosis in limbs, Cesarean scar or other tissues (necrotizing fasciitis). Sometimes the initial presentation is with limb pain that may mimic deep vein thrombosis, or myalgia. Such women may not always be tachycardic and febrile.

Staphylococci may cause septic shock and *Listeria monocytogenes* may cause septicemia. Listeriosis may cause preterm labor in around 70% of infected mothers and the risk of stillbirth and miscarriage is 40-50%. Early recognition and treatment improves the prognosis.

UTERINE INFECTIONS INCLUDING CHORIOAMNIONITIS AND POSTPARTUM ENDOMETRITIS

Chorioamnionitis

Chorioamnionitis refers to inflammation or infection of the placenta and or the chorion and amnion. It may be a clinical or histological diagnosis. Clinical chorioamnionitis is present in up to 5% of term and 10-25% of preterm deliveries with higher risk in those with preterm premature rupture of membranes (PPROM). Histologic chorioamnionitis is observed more commonly than clinical chorioamnionitis. The majority of cases occur secondary to ascending infection from the vagina and cervix, however, some may be caused by hematogenous spread or invasive prenatal procedures. The infection is polymicrobial in etiology and organisms commonly seen include mycoplasma, coliforms, group B streptococci and anaerobes. Table 12.1 summarizes features of chorioamnionitis.

Several studies have shown an association between intrauterine infection and cerebral white matter lesions or cerebral palsy in preterm neonates. Chorioamnionitis and neonatal sepsis are more common following preterm delivery than term. In a meta-analysis, preterm deliveries with clinical chorioamnionitis were found to be significantly associated with periventricular leukomalacia (RR 3.0; 95% CI 2.2-4.0), and cerebral palsy (RR 1.9; 95% CI 1.4-2.5) while in term infants there was increased relative risk of 4.7 (95% CI 1.3-16.2) for cerebral palsy.

Management of clinical chorioamnionitis includes expediting delivery and treatment with broad spectrum antibiotics such as gentamicin and ampicillin intravenously. In case of operative delivery by Cesarean section appropriate anaerobic cover may be added by using clindamycin or metronidazole. Intrapartum maternal pyrexia should be treated promptly as it is associated with neonatal seizures and encephalopathy in the immediate postnatal period. Prompt treatment is likely to reduce adverse maternal and neonatal outcomes.

Postpartum endometritis

Puerperal infection of the uterus is a common cause of fever postnatally. There is an increased risk of endometritis following emergency Cesarean section with prolonged rupture of membranes. Other risk factors for post Cesarean endometritis include all the risk factors for chorioamnionitis as discussed previously. Endometritis is a polymicrobial infection caused by a variety of organisms found in the vagina including group B streptococci, *E. coli, Gardnerella vaginalis, Bacteroides* species, peptostreptococci, *Mycoplasma hominis* and *Ureaplasma urealyticum*. It is important to collect appropriate specimens from the upper genital tract without contamination from the vagina and to send blood cultures as approximately 20% cases have bacteremia.

Postpartum endometritis should be suspected when there are symptoms of lower abdominal pain with high grade temperature, uterine tenderness and leukocytosis. An antibiotic regimen containing gentamicin and clindamycin is recommended.

Routine use of prophylactic antibiotics for elective and emergency Cesarean sections is recommended by national guidelines in the UK. Prophylactic antibiotics, such as a single dose of first-generation cephalosporin or ampicillin should be given to reduce the risk of postoperative infections such as endometritis, urinary tract and wound infections which other wise occur in up to 8% of women who have had a Cesarean section.

SEXUALLY TRANSMITTED DISEASES IN PREGNANCY

Sexually transmitted diseases (STD) in pregnancy are a major public health problem that may affect women's health during pregnancy and may have immediate and long-term postpartum consequences. Also some of the infections may be transmitted to the fetus transplacentally and others may cause neonatal infections due to intrapartum transmission. The risk of co-infection with more than one STD and re-infection after treatment is high due to exposure to infected partners. The pregnancy related problems caused by STDs include risk of preterm delivery, premature rupture of membranes, puerperal sepsis and post-

Table 12.1 Risk factors and clinical features of chorioamnionitis

Risk factors	Clinical features
Nulliparity	Maternal fever
Prolonged labor	Maternal tachycardia
Prolonged rupture of membranes	Fetal tachycardia
Repeated vaginal examination	Flat cardiotocograph
Internal fetal monitoring	Uterine tenderness
Bacterial vaginosis	Malodorous liquor
Group B streptococcal colonization	Preterm labor
Meconium stained liquor	

partum infection. The risks to the fetus include stillbirth, low birthweight, congenital abnormalities and specific symptoms in the neonate as outlined in Table 12.2.

Herpes simplex virus

Herpes simplex virus (HSV) is a DNA virus of the *herpesviridae* family. The two types of HSV that infect humans are HSV-1 and HSV-2. Both types cause genital herpes and the clinical manifestations are identical, however HSV-2 is more common and is the cause of most HSV-related perinatal mortality and morbidity. Genital herpes is the most common ulcerative sexually transmitted infection in the UK. The risk of devastating congenital herpes is reported as 1 in 5000 neonates in the USA and 1 in 33000 in the UK.

HSV-1 is transmitted through direct contact with skin or mucous membranes. HSV-2 is spread sexually and to the infant by contact of infected secretions in the genital tract during passage through the birth canal. Most primary infections are asymptomatic and hence not recognized clinically. Following the primary infection the virus remains latent in the local sensory ganglia until it is reactivated when there may be symptomatic lesions or asymptomatic shedding of the virus. Most patients have 4-6 recurrences annually. Immunocompromised pregnant women are at increased risk for reactivation. Co-infection with HIV increases the risk of perinatal transmission of both HSV and HIV. Recurrence rates are higher in pregnancy with increased risk at term. Symptomatic patients may present with malaise, fever, myalgia, dysuria, urinary retention, enlarged tender nodes in the groin, or cutaneous lesions with tingling, burning, itching and pain at the site of eruption.

Booking

Women should be asked for a history of genital herpes in self or partner. Women should be advised regarding the increased rate of recurrence in pregnancy and information about the risks of neonatal infection and preventive strategies should be given. Advice to avoid sexual intercourse when partner has HSV recurrence should be given. In areas of high

Table 12.2 Sexually transmitted diseases in pregnancy, risk of fetal/neonatal infection, features of congenital/neonatal infection and treatment of mother during pregnancy

STD	Risk of transmission to fetus/neonate with untreated maternal infection	Congenital infection/neonatal infection	Treatment of mother during pregnancy
Genital herpes simplex	Intrapartum 40% (primary herpes at time of delivery) Recurrent herpes <1%	Fever, vesicular rash, irritability, convulsions, jaundice, breathing difficulties, thrombocytopenia	Aciclovir
Hepatitis B	90% in chronic carriers. 60% if infection at term or delivery	70-90% of babies will remain chronically infected and have risk of developing cirrhosis or hepatocellular carcinoma	Supportive
Hepatitis C	Up to 6%, increased to 15% if co-infected with HIV	In adult life – cirrhosis and hepatocellular carcinoma	Supportive
Syphilis	Almost 100% in untreated primary or secondary infection <5% with late latent infection	Early-anemia, petechiae, purpura, osteochondritis/periostitis, jaundice, hepatosplenomegaly, lymphadenopathy, ascites and hydrops Late-interstitial keratitis	Benzathine penicillin/ procaine penicillin
Chlamydia	Intrapartum 30-50%	Conjunctivitis (3-40%), pneumonia (10-20%)	erythromycin/ amoxycillin
Gonorrhea	Intrapartum 30-50%	Conjunctivitis, disseminated neonatal infection	ceftriaxone/ spectinomycin

prevalence of neonatal herpes women should be tested for susceptibility.

Primary infection

Antenatal

Women should be referred for evaluation by a specialist and for screening for other sexually transmitted infections. Treatment is with oral aciclovir or valaciclovir for 5 days. Daily suppressive aciclovir in the last 4 weeks of pregnancy may prevent genital herpes recurrence at term.

Intrapartum

Cesarean is recommended for women who have a first episode of genital herpes at delivery or within six weeks of the expected due date of delivery.

The risk of neonatal transmission is higher in these cases as there may be inadequate maternal antibodies for transfer across the placenta to yield a protective effect. In women who opt for vaginal delivery, fetal scalp electrode monitoring should be avoided, as should fetal blood sampling, if possible.

Recurrent herpes simplex during pregnancy

Antenatal

There is insufficient evidence to support use of preventative aciclovir in the last 4 weeks of pregnancy or the use of viral cultures to detect viral shedding in the third trimester.

Intrapartum

For women presenting with recurrent genital herpes lesions at the onset of labor, the risks to the baby of neonatal herpes are small but should be considered in the discussion of risks and benefits of Cesarean section. A recurrent episode of genital herpes occurring at any other time during pregnancy is not an indication for delivery by Cesarean section.

Hepatitis B

Hepatitis B (HB) is a DNA virus that may be transmitted sexually, from an infected mother to the fetus (vertical transmission) or through transfusion of blood products. Hepatitis in pregnancy is not associated with increased miscarriage, stillbirth or congenital malformation. However, prematurity seems to be increased if hepatitis is acquired in the last trimester.

Pre-pregnancy

In high-risk women HB vaccine could be considered. If there is evidence of cirrhosis or chronic active hepatitis, consultation with a specialist in liver diseases should be sought.

Booking

All women are offered screening for hepatitis B at the booking visit in most Western nations. In high risk women it is important to ask about unprotected intercourse during pregnancy with infected partners as there is the potential for infection during pregnancy; seronegative women may need to be tested again later in the pregnancy. Partners and children of infected women should be offered screening and follow-up, with hepatitis B immunization as appropriate.

Antenatal

During the acute phase of infection, hepatitis B surface antigen (HBsAg) and e antigen (HBeAg) will be detected on serology. Perinatal transmission of HB virus occurs if the mother has had acute HB infection during late pregnancy or in the first months postpartum, or if the mother is a chronic HB antigen carrier (Table 12.2). Since the administration of hepatitis B vaccine is safe during any stage of pregnancy, nonimmune, seronegative pregnant women with risk factors may be immunized.

Postnatal

Neonatal infection may be prevented by administering HB vaccine in newborns of mothers who are HBsAg positive and in addition they should be given hepatitis B immune globulin at another site within 12 h of birth if the mother is HBeAg positive. This has an efficacy of more than 95%. There is no contraindication to breastfeeding. Hepatitis B vaccination of the newborn is standard in Australia and various other nations because the prevalence in the general population is considered sufficient to justify prophylactic measures.

Hepatitis C

The antenatal prevalence of hepatits C virus (HCV) infection in the UK is estimated to be below 1%. Hepatitis C is transmitted by transfusion of unscreened blood, through injecting drugs, from mother-to-child and uncommonly by the sexual route. For risk of transmission to the neonate and effects see Table 12.2.

Booking

Hepatitis C antibody screening should be offered to high risk women, i.e. those who are HIV positive, have multiple sexual partners, are injecting drug users and women exposed to blood or blood products. These women may need to be tested again later in the pregnancy if they continue to be exposed to the risk factors.

Intrapartum and postnatal

Current evidence does not suggest a benefit of elective Cesarean section for HCV-infected women in terms of prevention of neonatal infection nor a need to refrain from breastfeeding, with the exception of HIV/HCV co-infected women.

Syphilis

The seroprevalence rate has been low for many years in the developed countries although there has been a resurgence of syphilis in the UK in the last 5 years. Syphilis is caused by a spirochete, *Treponema pallidum*, and its sexual mode of transmission has been recognized for many years, although it may also be acquired congenitally, through blood transfusion. Vertical transmission results in more than 1 million infants born with congenital syphilis annually worldwide.

The chronology of infection with this organism is prolonged over decades. The various stages in evolution of the infection have been termed primary, secondary, latent and tertiary syphilis. The incubation period averages 3 months but may lie between 3 and 90 days depending on the size of the inoculum at infection. Primary infection is characterized by a lesion at the site of entry of the infection that is usually painless, the chancre. This appears as a small red papule or crusted erosion that breaks down and exudes serous fluid, with non-tender regional lymphadenopathy (bubo). Multiple chancres may be seen in immunocompromised individuals. In untreated individuals, the secondary stage follows in 6-8 weeks with widespread macular lesions appearing on the mucous membranes, trunk, extremities, palms and soles. After 4-8 weeks these lesions disappear and the patient enters the latent stage. Relapses may occur in the next 3-4 years. If untreated, reactivation may occur between 5-50 years after the primary infection. The typical lesion of tertiary syphilis, the gumma, is a chronic area of inflammatory destruction presenting as an indolent lesion with a necrotic center. Gumma are single or multiple, they vary in size from microscopic to large and tumor-like and predominantly affect the skin, liver, bones and spleen.

Transmission to the fetus can occur at any stage of pregnancy by the hematogenous route if there is maternal spirochetemia. If pregnancy occurs in the early stages of syphilis and is untreated, the risk of transmission is almost 100%. The probability of fetal transmission is up to 70% even 4 years after primary infection although the risk is low after 2 years, and is low for babies born to mothers with latent syphilis.

Spirochetes cannot be grown in artificial media. Also there are no current methods to distinguish between *T. Pallidum* infection from the other three forms of human treponemal infection, namely yaws, pinta and non-venereal syphilis. Serological tests remain the method of choice for diagnosis. The Venereal Diseases Reseach Laboratory (VDRL) test and the rapid plasma reagin (RPR) tests are used as screening tests as they are simple and inexpensive with high sensitivity during early infection. Specific tests that are used to confirm positive screening tests include *T. pallidum* hemagglutination assay (TPHA), the *T. pallidum* particle agglutination test (TPPA) and the fluorescent treponemal antibody absorption test (FTA-ABS).

Pre-pregnancy

If syphilitic infection is diagnosed, it is important to advise the woman to take strict contraceptive precautions, because of the risk of fetal transmission, until an effective course of treatment has been administered.

Booking

Screening for syphilis is an integral part of the booking visit in the UK. If positive for VDRL, further specific tests from a reference laboratory should be arranged along with referral to a specialist in sexually transmitted disease for treatment if required, investigation for other STDs, contact tracing and treatment of partners.

Antenatal

The suspicion of infection during pregnancy requires VDRL testing to seek increasing titres from the booking sample. If there has been clearly documented evidence of treatment with a decline in titres, further treatment is not necessary.

Treatment

The Centers for Disease Control and Prevention (CDC) and WHO recommend treating early syphilis (primary, secondary or early latent) with a single dose of 2.4

million units of benzathine penicillin G (2.4 million units weekly for 3 weeks if the suspected duration of syphilis is at least a year). In the UK, the recommendation is for daily injections of procaine penicillin (0.6-0.9 million units) for 10-14 days. There are limited data from randomized clinical trials that compare the various therapeutic regimen. Serial scans should be performed for signs of fetal infection (Table 12.2) and to monitor fetal growth.

Postnatal

Neonatologists should be alerted before delivery so that appropriate examination, management and follow up may be arranged for the neonate.

Chlamydia

Chlamydiae are obligate intracellular bacteria. This has become the commonest sexually transmitted bacterial infection reported in the genitourinary medicine (GUM) clinics in the UK and elsewhere in the Western world. It is a significant public health issue with 10-30% infected women at risk of developing pelvic inflammatory disease. Subfertility can occur in 20% untreated women and there is increased risk of ectopic pregnancy following infection.

Chlamydial infections in the mother may cause miscarriage, stillbirth, intrauterine infection, preterm rupture of membranes, preterm delivery and postpartum endometritis. Approximately 20% of postpartum upper genital tract infections are caused by chlamydia. In untreated chlamydial infection in pregnancy there is risk of transmission to the fetus or neonate (Table 12.2).

Acute *C. trachomatis* infections are diagnosed by cell culture, direct immunofluorescence, EIA, direct DNA hybridization and recently by nucleic acid amplification tests (NAATs). In chronic or persistent chlamydial infections, the level of standard chlamydia serology may not be diagnostic, with detection requiring the NAAT. Erythromycin is the drug of choice, however amoxicillin should be considered if the woman cannot tolerate erythromycin due to its gastrointestinal side effects. The recommended dose of erythromycin is 500 mg 4 times daily for 7 days. There are a number of reports confirming the efficacy of a single oral dose of 1 g of azithromycin, and this may be preferred where compliance is doubted.

Gonorrhea

Neisseria gonorrhoeae, the causative organism for gonorrhea is the second most common bacterial STD in the UK with 22 320 infections diagnosed in GUM clinics in 2004. *N. gonorrhoeae* may infect the genitourinary tract, rectum, pharynx or eye. Gonococcal infection in women is frequently asymptomatic. When symptomatic, women may present with dysuria or a mucopurulent discharge. Disseminated forms of the disease may be seen in untreated cases, characterized by bacteremia, pustular dermatitis, low-grade fever, myalgia and migratory polyarthritis.

The perinatal implications include an increased risk of preterm birth, chorioamnionitis with preterm rupture of the membranes, postpartum endometritis and risk of transmission to the neonate causing conjunctivitis (Table 12.2).

Booking

If there is a history of gonorrhea in the partner, the woman should be tested for gonorrhea and chlamydia. For women at high risk of acquiring STDs during pregnancy, these tests along with testing for syphilis should be repeated in the third trimester.

Antenatal

In cases of uncomplicated gonorrhea, ceftriaxone 250 mg IM in a single dose or spectinomycin 2 g IM in a single dose are recommended. It is good practice to treat empirically for chlamydia even if this has not been tested as concurrent infection is frequent. In disseminated disease the woman should be hospitalized and parenteral therapy with ceftriaxone or cefotaxime for 24-48 h followed by oral therapy for a total duration of a week.

Postnatal

The possibility of neonatal infection should be considered if gonorrhea has complicated late pregnancy.

Bacterial vaginosis

Bacterial vaginosis (BV) is a common condition with poorly understood etiology and natural history. It is the commonest cause of vaginal discharge in women of childbearing age. It seems to result from an imbalance of the normal vaginal flora, with an overgrowth of anaerobic bacteria and a reduction in lactobacillary flora. The implicated microorganisms include *Gardnerella vaginalis, Ureaplasma urealyticum, Mycoplasma hominis, Mobiluncus* species, *Prevotella* species and other anaerobes, although no single bacterial agent consistently predominates. It may be asymptomatic, or associated with the production of a vaginal discharge with a fishy odor and occasionally vaginal burning or itching. It has been implicated as a cause of preterm birth, premature rupture of membranes, low birth weight and postpartum sepsis.

BV is diagnosed if three of the following four criteria are present:

1. Vaginal pH higher than 4.5.
2. The presence of clue (vaginal epithelial) cells in the vaginal fluid.
3. Thin, gray or white homogenous discharge.
4. Positive KOH 'whiff' test.

Currently it is advisable to test and treat all women who are symptomatic or have a vaginal discharge on physical examination, or those with a previous history of preterm birth. In general, routine treatment of partners is not recommended. The recommended treatment includes oral metronidazole 400 mg or clindamycin 300 mg, each taken twice daily for 7 days.

Trichomoniasis

Although the incidence of *Trichomonas vaginalis* (TV) infection has fallen in the developed countries up to 30% pregnant women in the developing countries carry this infection. It is usually sexually transmitted and women may remain asymptomatic for many months. It has been associated with preterm birth and low birthweight but treatment of asymptomatic TV did not reduce the risk of preterm birth in a randomized, controlled trial. Symptomatic women may be treated with metronidazole.

FUNGAL INFECTIONS IN PREGNANCY

Vaginal candidiasis (moniliasis or thrush) is a common and frequently distressing infection for many women. About 30-40% of women are colonized with candida and around 75% of all women develop symptomatic infection at some time in their lives. Vulvo-vaginal itching or irritation, and vaginal discharge are common symptoms. Thrush is more common in pregnancy. The possible reasons are increased levels of estrogen enhancing action of mannose-containing receptors that increase adherence of candida to mucosal cells. There is an increase in mucosal glycogen content that increases the growth of candida. The reduced cell-mediated immunity during pregnancy may contribute to candidal infection. Of candidial infections 80-85% are caused by *Candida albicans* and remaining infections by other species including *C. glabrata, C. tropicalis, C. krusei*.

There is no evidence that thrush in pregnancy is harmful to the developing fetus. A Cochrane database systematic review has shown that topical imidazoles such as clotrimazole and miconazole are more effective than nystatin for treating symptomatic vaginal candidiasis in pregnancy. Treatment for seven days may be necessary in pregnancy rather than the shorter courses more commonly used in non-pregnant women. The use of topical azoles for the treatment of superficial fungal infections is safe and efficacious. However, there are some data suggesting a dose-related increase in the risk of teratogenicity associated with the use of systemic azoles.

Systemic candidiasis is extremely rare in healthy women of childbearing age. It may occur in women with underlying immunodeficiency due to chemotherapy for malignancy, acquired immunodeficiency syndrome (AIDS), prolonged use of steroids, antibiotics or total parenteral nutrition. It may also be seen as a complication of intravenous drug use. Amphotericin B is the drug of choice for the treatment of systemic fungal infections in pregnancy. There are serious risks of fetal malformations associated with the use of griseofulvin, ketoconazole, flucytosine and the newer azole voriconazole and hence these are contraindicated in pregnancy. At present, there are insufficient data regarding the use of the newer antifungal agent caspofungin in pregnancy.

PARASITIC PROBLEMS IN PREGNANCY

Parasitic infections are more prevalent in tropical countries. But with the increasing mobility of most populations, economy of airline travel and immigration from these countries parasitic infections during pregnancy must now be considered even in temperate climates. Women on immunosuppressant regimes and those with AIDS are also at increased risk of parasitic infections. Most of the infections discussed below are acquired by the fecal–oral route

Schistosomiasis

Schistosomiasis is a systemic infection caused by *Schistosoma hematobium, S. japonicum and S. mansoni*. Most cases are seen in Africa, the Middle East and South America, but the diagnosis may be found in immigrant populations worldwide. Schistosomiasis does not cause any direct effect on the fetus, but chronic infection may cause miscarriage or preterm delivery secondary to maternal debilitation. Diagnosis requires demonstration of eggs in urine, feces or vaginal secretions. If treatment is needed during pregnancy praziquantel as a single dose is the agent of choice.

Giardiasis

This common enteric infection is caused by *Giardia intestinalis or G. lamblia* and may present with bulky watery diarrhea and abdominal pain. Usually there are no effects on pregnancy or the fetus. Diagnosis is by demonstation of trophozoites in feces in early stage or cysts in later stage. Treatment of choice during pregnancy is paromomycin 500 mg 4 times daily for 7 days. Metronidazole may be used in the second or third trimester.

Enterobiasis

Enterobius vermicularis or pinworm infection may present as perianal itching, that can be intense. There is no effect on pregnancy or the fetus. The diagnosis may be confirmed by demonstrating pinworms on adhesive tape, which is applied to perianal region, first thing in the morning. Treatment is with a single dose of pyrantel palmoate and may be used after the first trimester.

Hookworm infection

This intestinal helminthic infestation is caused by *Ankylostoma duodenale* or *Necator Americanus*. It is a major cause of maternal anemia in the developing world and the WHO has estimated that up to 40 million pregnant women are infected each year. In fact anemia is a major contributor to maternal mortality in the developing world and up to 60% of cases of anemia are due to helminthic infestation. It has no direct effect on the fetus, but maternal ill health is always of concern for fetal well-being. Diagnosis is made by demonstration of eggs in the feces. Treatment of the anemia requires iron supplements. Studies from Nepal and from Sri Lanka have shown less anemia, slightly higher birthweight and considerably lower infant mortality in the first six months when routine treatment with mebendazole or albendazole is given in the second and third trimester, even without laboratory diagnosis. This seems a sensible course of action, particularly when there is anemia. This would not be appropriate in the developed world where other causes of anemia predominate. But the diagnosis of helminth infction must be considered carefully in women at risk anywhere in the world. For severe infection pyrantel palmoate may be given for three days.

Amebiasis

This results from infection with *Entamoeba histolytica*. Infection is acquired by ingestion of cysts. Infection may result in severe colitis with or without fecal blood and mucus, and also in amebic abscess. This is suggested by a high swinging fever with right lower chest and upper quadrant pain, and a mass usually detectable by ultrasound. There is no direct effect on the fetus, but severe maternal illness and debilitation impair fetal growth. Diagnosis is made by demonstration of trophozoite forms in fresh fecal samples. Treatment of choice during pregnancy is paromomycin for seven days.

MALARIA

Although not common in the developed nations, malaria is seen commonly in women from the developing countries and in immigrant populations of women who have traveled from endemic areas. Almost 40% of pregnant women are exposed to malarial infections worldwide. Pregnant women are more severely affected than non-pregnant women. Drug resistance is increasingly becoming a problem. It is associated with high maternal mortality mainly in the developing countries where anemia in the mother further increases the morbidity. HIV in sub-Saharan Africa and south Asian countries is increasingly seen as a co-infection with malaria in pregnancy, making both an issue of high priority for public health services. In Africa an estimated 200 000 newborn babies die of malaria annually.

Malaria is caused by four species of *Plasmodium* (*P. falciparum, P. vivax, P. ovale* and *P. malariae*). The worst prognosis for mother and baby is seen in cases with falciparum malaria. The mode of transmission is through the bite of an infected anopheline mosquito, transfusion of blood products and sharing of infected syringes and needles.

The severity of disease in pregnancy is dependent on the previous immunity of the mother derived from exposure to malarial infection. The main complications for the mother are severe hemolytic anemia, hypoglycemia, hyperpyrexia, acute renal failure, pulmonary edema, hemorrhagic or endotoxic shock, and cerebral malaria. Primigravide are at higher risk in endemic areas and develop immunity with repeated exposure in subsequent pregnancies, even when they are asymptomatic. Thus, a low threshold of suspicion is required in these cases to detect malaria especially among immigrant populations from these areas. Diagnosis is by demonstration of parasites in a thick blood film.

Affected pregnancies are at higher risk of miscarriage, premature delivery and neonatal death. The possible mechanisms for preterm labor include anemia in the mother, placental malaria and hyperpyrexia. Congenital infection is seen in 1-4% of non-immune infected mothers and may present as hepatosplenomegaly.

In placental malaria, parasites may be found sequestrated in the placenta even when peripheral blood films are negative. This problem may be overcome in the future by the use of new antigen-based rapid diagnostic tests. This has practical considerations for women who may be potentially semi-immune during pregnancy. The mechanisms for low birth weight may be explained by this process of parasitic sequestration in the placenta affecting placental function and this thesis has been supported by finding abnormal uterine artery Doppler studies in association with malaria during pregnancy. This also has implications for women co-infected with HIV as there may be risks of increased vertical transmission of both infections.

Prompt symptomatic and supportive treatment with appropriate antimalarial therapy remains the mainstay of treatment. In symptomatic cases intensive care unit admission and management is appropriate. Severity of the disease, patterns of resistance to the drugs based upon the country in which malaria was acquired, previous immunity to malaria and safety of the drugs in pregnancy should be considered in deciding the optimal antimalarial drug. In uncomplicated falciparum malaria, chloroquine is the drug of choice. In chloroquine resistant cases, quinine is used in the first trimester and for the second and third trimester, quinine, sulfadoxine-pyremethamine or amodiaquine may be used. In cases with severe malaria, artemisinin drugs may be used as they achieve a more rapid clearance of parasites. In non-falciparum malaria cases, chloroquine should be used for the initial treatment until delivery and primaquine should be used for radical cure postpartum.

Preventive strategies include regular chemoprophylaxis, intermittent preventive treatment (IPT) with antimalarials and insecticide-treated bednets. The only drug that has been extensively used for IPT during pregnancy in the last decade is sulfadoxine-pyremethamine. Women from non-endemic areas should avoid travel in pregnancy to endemic areas. The American Center for Disease Control recommends mefloquine for prophylaxis although it should be avoided in the first trimester if possible due to theoretical concerns of teratogenicity. There is no current evidence of adverse consequences following prophylactic dosages. Proper prophylactic measures should be taken if travel cannot be avoided and early medical advice should be sought if there is suspicion of infection. Advice about prophylaxis should be obtained from a specialist in travel medicine as recommendations vary from year to year and for different destinations.

FUNGAL DISEASE

Fungal disease or systemic mycoses are very rare in healthy pregnant women. Some cases of systemic mycosis caused by either opportunistic pathogens like *Aspergillus* or by pathogens like *Coccidioides immitis* and *Blastomyces dermititidis* have been reported. They are associated with high mortality in pregnancy and hence a high index of suspicion is needed to hasten diagnosis and prompt treatment.

Pulmonary aspergillosis with possible cerebral involvement in a previously healthy pregnant woman has been reported. Coccidioidomycosis should be considered in the differential diagnosis of febrile illness with pneumonia in pregnant women from endemic areas such as south-western USA and northern Mexico or those that have traveled to these areas during pregnancy. It is especially important to consider the diagnosis if fever is accompanied by bilateral nodular infiltrates in the lung, with or without erythema nodosum or meningitis.

Blastomycosis is an exceedingly uncommon complication of pregnancy but should be considered in an immunosuppressed gravida with multisystem infectious disease, frequently with central nervous involvement. Recognizing its presence during pregnancy and initiating appropriate therapy is of critical importance to the mother and fetus as transplacental disease has been reported, with high mortality. In one paper there were 20 babies born from mothers with blastomycosis, two (10%) of whom had transplacental transmission and both succumbed to blastomycosis. Localized disease is treated with itraconazole, but generalized disease may require amphotericin B to reduce the likelihood of mortality.

TOXOPLASMOSIS, RUBELLA, CYTOMEGALOVIRUS, VARICELLA, PARVOVIRUS AND EPSTEIN-BARR VIRUS INFECTION

Toxoplasmosis

The prevalence of maternal toxoplasma infection in the UK is 1-2 per 1000. It is caused by the protozoan *Toxoplasma gondii*. About 85% of women of childbearing age are susceptible to infection at booking in UK. It is acquired by pregnant women through ingestion of sporocysts. This may be secondary to inadequately washed vegetables or salads contaminated with cat litter or from inadequate hand washing following gardening or eating inadequately cooked meat containing viable parasitic tissue cysts. Usually acute maternal toxoplasmosis is asymptomatic. The clinical features occur in 5-15% infected women and present with flu-like symptoms and lymphadenopathy.

The risk of transmission to the fetus is significant if the mother is infected in the immediate preconception period or early in pregnancy with vertical transmission complicating 30-40% of maternal infections leading to congenital toxoplasmosis. The risk of transmission is 10-15% in the first trimester and the consequences are severe disease or fetal loss. In the second trimester, there is 25-40% transmission, with usually non-fatal sequelae. In the third trimester, over 60% of fetuses are infected, with typically mild or asymptomatic manifestations.

Although there is limited information regarding the risks of congenital infection in infants of mothers with infection of longstanding duration before pregnancy, it seems the risk of transmission is low. However, there are exceptions in mothers who are immunocompromised or may have acquired the infection very late in the third trimester and may remain seronegative until after delivery of baby.

Pre-pregnancy and antenatal

Women should avoid eating unwashed fruits, vegetables and inadequately cooked meat. Wearing gloves for gardening and good handwashing techniques after gardening and handling cats should be emphasized.

Serological methods are commonly used for diagnosis. Absence of IgG antibodies in early pregnancy identifies susceptible women. Presence of IgG antibodies suggests previous infection. These are detected 1-2 weeks after infection and the individual remains positive for these antibodies for life. Low IgG avidity suggests recent infection. Absence of IgM rules out recent infection. Also, IgM may be present for years after initial infection, hence limiting its value in testing for recent infection. It is important to remember that although positive IgM may be a true-positive result it does not establish acute infection. Definitive diagnosis should be made following confirmation of a rise in IgG titers in serial samples. Direct techniques using PCR amplification can be used for prenatal diagnosis of congenital toxoplasmosis.

Spiramycin 1 g orally 8 hourly is recommended as first line treatment when the mother is diagnosed. This also reduces the risk of vertical transmission to the fetus. However, if fetal infection is suspected on ultrasound findings (Table 12.4) or amniotic fluid infection confirmed by amniocentesis, pyrimethamine and sulfonamides are more effective than spiramycin. This regimen should be supplemented with folinic acid 5 mg daily. The treatment needs to be continued until delivery.

Neonatal toxoplasmosis may present with hydrocephalus, intracranial calcifications, microcephaly, chorioretinitis, blindness, strabismus, epilepsy, psychomotor or mental retardation, petechie and anemia.

Rubella

Rubella is a RNA virus of *togaviride* family. The incidence of rubella in females has fallen considerably since the introduction of the rubella vaccine program in most nations of the developed world. Even so, about 40 infants with congenital rubella syndrome have been reported since 1991 in the UK. In adults, rubella causes a febrile illness, often mild, with transient red rash, post-auricular and sub-occipital lymphadenopathy and occasionally, arthritis.

Pre-pregnancy

Rubella vaccine is available as a single vaccine or combined with measles and mumps vaccine (MMR). It is offered to previously non-immunized and seronegative women before pregnancy. About 5% of the population do not respond to rubella vaccine and therefore remain susceptible to the infection. Women presenting before pregnancy for any reason, and in fact all women of reproductive age, should be checked for rubella immunity, and vaccinated if demonstrated susceptible to the infection.

Booking

Pregnant women are routinely screened for rubella IgG. If they are not immune they should avoid contact with rubella during pregnancy. A history of exposure to or possible recent infection with rubella in early pregnancy is sought, particularly in recent immigrants, and the laboratory is informed of a suspicious history so that the appropriate tests for primary rubella infection (IgM and IgG avidity) are performed.

Antenatal

If recent infection is suspected rubella IgM and rubella specific IgG avidity will help in confirming primary infection. Table 12.3 summarizes risk from

Table 12.3 Risk from rubella infection in pregnancy

Gestation	Defects	Risk
Before 11 weeks	Heart, central nervous system, eyes, ears	Over 90%
11–16 weeks	Fetal defects	20%
16–20 weeks	Deafness	15%
After 20 weeks		Normal background risk

infection in pregnancy. In maternal reinfection, the risk to the fetus is speculated to be less than 5%. Amniotic fluid PCR or fetal blood IgM and PCR may confirm fetal infection (Table 12.4). If fetal infection is confirmed at an early gestation, therapeutic termination of pregnancy should be discussed as an option, with a frank and detailed appraisal of the risks to the fetus. No specific treatment for rubella is currently available.

Postnatal

Vaccination should be offered to non-immune women post delivery and they should be advised to avoid pregnancy for three months after vaccination.

Table 12.4 Prenatal diagnosis of fetal infections with characteristic ultrasound findings, invasive diagnostic tests and interventions during pregnancy

Infection	Ultrasound findings	Diagnostic tests	Interventions if infection confirmed
Toxoplasmosis	Intracranial calcifications, venticulomegaly, hepatic enlargement, ascites and increased placental thickness.	PCR[a] on amniotic fluid or cordocentesis to detect fetal IgM[b]	Pyrimethamine and sulfadiazine
Rubella	Fetal growth restriction, hydrops, congenital heart defects (pulmonary valvular stenosis, ventricular septal defect), microcephaly, cataracts.	Chorion villous sampling in the first trimester, RT-PCR[c] on amniotic fluid and fetal blood for IgM and RNA[d]	Offer termination of pregnancy
Cytomegalovirus	Ventriculomegaly, periventricular calcification, microcephaly, echogenic bowel and intra-abdominal calcification.	Culture or PCR on amniotic fluid	Offer termination of pregnancy if significant viral load
Varicella-zoster	Fetal growth restriction, limb hypoplasia and microcalcification of the liver or spleen.	Culture or PCR on amniotic fluid	
Parvovirus B19	Hydrops.	PCR on amniotic fluid, cordocentesis to detect fetal anemia	Intrauterine fetal transfusion
Syphilis	Hepatosplenomegaly, Hydrops in severe cases, polyhydramnios and placentomegaly in later stages of the disease.		

[a]polymerase chain reaction
[b]Immunoglobulin M
[c]reverse transcriptase polymerase chain reaction
[d]ribonucleic acid

Cytomegalovirus

CMV is a double-stranded DNA virus of *herpesviridae* family. Whilst most primary CMV infections in adults are asymptomatic, some present with flu-like illness or glandular fever. Following primary infection, CMV like other herpes viruses remains latent but may cause infection due to reactivation during pregnancy. Sometimes recurrent infection with CMV occurs with a different strain of virus. The virus is excreted in body fluids including saliva, semen, blood, breast milk, cervical secretions, urine and tears. Women of child-bearing age acquire infection from sexual contacts or from children.

Antenatal

The diagnosis of primary CMV infection is made by demonstration of seroconversion of CMV-specific IgG antibodies from negative to positive, but not by rise in titre, as this also occurs with recurrent infection. CMV specific IgM is not a reliable marker for diagnosis of primary infection. It may remain positive after pre-conceptional CMV infection or may be falsely positive due to cross-reactivity with tests for other herpes viruses. Low IgG avidity of serum indicates primary CMV infection. EIA which detects IgG response to glycoprotein B of CMV is useful in the diagnosis of primary infection. It becomes positive 50-120 days after the primary infection.

Transplacental infection of the fetus occurs in 40% of mothers with primary CMV infection during pregnancy but only 1% transmission is reported with reactivation of infection. It is important to note that infection of the fetus does not imply that defects or disease will result. Fetal CMV infection may be suspected by ultrasonographic findings (Fig. 12.1 and Table 12.4). Fetuses infected with CMV are likely to have positive amniotic fluid cultures after 21 weeks of gestation because fetal kidney infection is common. Higher viral load (> 10^5/mL) is associated with a higher risk of an affected fetus. At present, no specific therapy is available for in utero treatment of primary infection.

Postnatal

The incidence of congenital CMV is 0.3-4% worldwide and 0.35% in the UK. Overall, only 7-10% of congenital CMV infected fetuses born to mothers with primary CMV infection are affected. They may present with jaundice, hepatosplenomegaly, rash, chorioretinitis, microcephaly and developmental delay. Of those that are asymptomatic at birth around

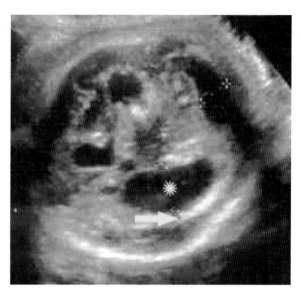

Figure 12.1 Ultrasonographic image demonstrating ventriculomegaly (asterix) and periventricular calcification (arrow) in a case of fetal CMV infection.

10-15% develop sensorineural deafness by five years of age.

Varicella

Chickenpox is an acute, infectious disease caused by the *varicella zoster* virus (VZV) of *herpesviridae* family. This virus is also the cause of shingles (herpes zoster) following reactivation. Chickenpox is highly contagious, infecting up to 90% of people who come into contact with the disease. Transmission is through significant contact with an infected person, airborne droplet infection or contact with infected articles. The incubation period is from 10 to 21 days. The most infectious period is from 1-2 days before the rash appears but infectivity continues until all lesions have crusted over. Chickenpox presents with an intensely itchy, vesiculo-pustular rash (Fig. 12.2) mostly over the trunk, associated with fever. Varicella infection in non-immune pregnant women may cause severe chickenpox with risk of varicella pneumonia in up to 10% and is more likely in smokers. The severity of pneumonia may worsen with increasing gestation.

Pre-pregnancy

In the USA and some European countries, varicella seronegative women undergoing infertility treatment or those presenting for preconception counseling are offered vaccination. Currently, vaccine is not licensed for this indication in the UK.

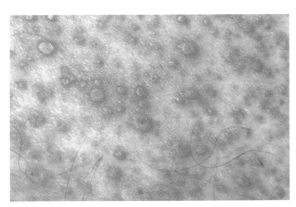

Figure 12.2 Typical skin rash in chickenpox (courtesy Dr Mike Sladden, Specialist Registrar in Dermatology, University Hospitals of Leicester NHS Trust, Leicester, UK).

Booking

If there is no history of previous chickenpox, women must (see below) be advised to avoid contact with chickenpox during pregnancy and to contact healthcare workers following a potential exposure. There is some justification for checking varicella immunity before pregnancy, to expedite administration of immune globulin after exposure to varicella during pregnancy. The woman with antibodies needs no such treatment and may be reassured.

Antenatal

In the event of contact with chickenpox during pregnancy, an assessment should be made of the likelihood that varicella is the diagnosis to assess infectiousness and the degree of exposure (household, face-to-face contact for 5 min or indoors contact for more than 15 min). In cases of uncertainty, serum should be checked for VZV IgG. If the woman is not immune to VZV, she should be given Varicella zoster immunoglobulin (VZIG) up to a maximum of ten days after significant contact. Women should be asked to notify their doctor early if a rash develops.

Chickenpox during pregnancy

The infected woman should be advised to avoid contact with other pregnant women and babies until at least 5 days after the rash appears or all blisters have crusted over. If the pregnant woman develops chickenpox in the first 20 weeks of pregnancy, there is 1-2% risk of fetal varicella syndrome (FVS) characterized by shortened limbs, skin scarring, cataracts and growth restriction. A detailed ultrasound examination at 16-20 weeks or approximately 5-6 weeks after the infection should be performed (Table 12.4). VZV DNA is detectable by PCR in amniotic fluid. It is important to note that the presence of VZV DNA only indicates fetal infection and not FVS. Maternal infection at 21-36 weeks is usually not associated with adverse fetal effects but may present as shingles in the first few years of life. Infection with varicella after 36 weeks of pregnancy may cause neonatal chickenpox. This is particularly serious if the mother becomes infected within 7 days before delivery. The UK Advisory Group on Chickenpox recommends that oral aciclovir be prescribed for pregnant women with chickenpox if they present within 24 h of the onset of the rash after 20 weeks of gestation. The newborn infant is very vulnerable to varicella if the mother sustains the illness from 5 days before delivery to 2 days postpartum. The fatality rate is up to 30% without prophylaxis or treatment. Although no adverse fetal or neonatal effects have been reported with the use of aciclovir in pregnancy, there is slight theoretical risk of teratogenesis in the first trimester and treatment, as with the use of many drugs in pregnancy, requires a discussion with the mother of relative risks and benefits in the context of informed consent.

All women with chickenpox should be referred to hospital if chest symptoms, neurological symptoms, hemorrhagic rash or bleeding develop, or if there is underlying significant immunosuppression. Delivery during the viremic period should be avoided if possible. The mother is at risk of bleeding due to thrombocytopenia and disseminated intravascular coagulation. There is also a high risk of varicella of the newborn, which is associated with high morbidity and mortality. Intravenous aciclovir and symptomatic treatment with paracetamol, chlorpheniramine and topical soothing agents can be used. (See also Ch. 6, p. 130.)

Postnatal

If the mother has had chickenpox 5 days before delivery or within 2 days of giving birth, the newborn should be given VZIG. Breastfeeding should be avoided until the new mother has passed the infectious period, and isolation is necessary if she is an inpatient in a maternity unit.

Parvovirus B19

Booking

Pregnant women should be given information about parvovirus B19. Screening for parvovirus IgG may be done on booking blood to find susceptible women (both parvovirus IgG and IgM absent) although currently routine screening is not justifiable as no prophylaxis or vaccine is available. Screening may be considered in women in risk occupations, including childcare, junior primary school teaching and pediatric healthcare, as lack of immunity to parvovirus may be of sufficient concern to recommend removal from the workplace, particularly at times of a known outbreak of the disease.

Antenatal

Parvovirus B19 is a DNA virus of the *parvoviridae* family and is commonly spread by respiratory secretions. The virus usually replicates in rapidly dividing erythroid progenitor cells. A flu-like illness is followed by a characteristic facial rash, which spreads to the trunk and limbs. and is known as 'erythema infectiosum', 'fifth disease' or 'slapped cheek syndrome'. Mothers, nursery teachers and health workers who come in contact with school-aged children are at highest risk of contracting the infection, although 30-60% of adults are immune.

Gestational parvovirus B19 infection is usually a minor illness for the mother, but it has been associated with serious fetal consequences including miscarriage (about 6% overall, 10% before and 2% after 20 weeks) and occasionally hydrops fetalis as a result of hemolytic anemia and congestive cardiac failure. Spontaneous recovery of hydropic fetuses may occur with subsequent delivery of a normal infant. There is no evidence of teratogenicity or congenital anomalies in the newborn.

If primary parvovirus infection during pregnancy is confirmed (parvovirus IgM positive or DNA detection by PCR) serial fetal ultrasound starting from about three weeks after infection or seroconversion is used for the detection of hydrops fetalis (Table 12.4) that occurs in 3-4% of cases. Hydrops is of great concern and may lead to fetal cardiac failure from severe anemia. For this reason, fetal anemia should be sought by cordocentesis and intrauterine transfusion performed if severe anemia confirmed. This lowers the fetal mortality rate. Careful follow-up is necessary. There is no indication for therapeutic termination of pregnancy. Specific antiviral treatment is not available for parvovirus B19 infection.

Epstein–Barr virus infection

Epstein–Barr virus (EBV) is a member of *herpesviridae* family. Most infections are asymptomatic. It usually present as infectious mononucleosis with fever, sore throat, and swollen lymph nodes. There are no known adverse effects for the fetus of EBV infection in pregnancy. There is a probable association of reactivation of maternal EBV infection with childhood acute lymphocytic leukemia. Primary EBV infection is diagnosed if IgM antibody to the viral capsid antigen (VCA) is present and antibody to EBV nuclear antigen (EBNA) is absent. Vaccine is currently not available.

MEASLES, MUMPS, INFLUENZA AND OTHER VIRAL INFECTIONS

Measles

Measles is an acute highly infectious viral illness caused by measles virus and is transmitted via droplet infection. A prodromal phase of 2 to 4 days is followed by fever, conjunctivitis, coryza and Koplik spots on the oral mucosa. The characteristic widespread red macular rash appears on the body between the third and seventh days, spreads over 4 days and lasts for a week. Encephalitis is a severe complication of measles although rare in pregnant women. Serum testing for measles specific IgG and IgM is available for the diagnosis of acute infection.

Pre-pregnancy

In non-immune women of childbearing age two doses of MMR vaccine can be given separated by a 3-month interval.

Antenatal

Measles during pregnancy is associated with increased maternal mortality secondary to pneumonia. Hence women with suspected pneumonia should be referred to a tertiary center. Measles infection increases risk of prematurity and growth restriction.

Contact with measles infection during pregnancy

In susceptible exposed women, passive immunization with pooled immunoglobulins may be offered within 72 h of exposure.

There is no specific treatment for measles.

Mumps

Mumps is characterized by parotoditis, which may be unilateral or bilateral. Complications of mumps include oophoritis, aseptic meningitis and deafness. Maternal illness in pregnancy is generally benign, although it may cause fetal loss within 2 weeks of infection in the first trimester. There is a possible association between mumps infection and endocardial fibroelastosis. There is no reported association with congenital anomalies. There is no specific treatment for mumps.

Influenza

Influenza is a respiratory illness associated with infection by the influenza virus. Symptoms include headache, fever, cough, sore throat, myalgia and arthralgia. There is a wide spectrum of illness ranging from minor symptoms to pneumonia and death. There are two main types that cause infection, influenza A and influenza B. Influenza pneumonia in pregnant women is associated with higher morbidity and mortality than in non-pregnant women. Neuraminidase-inhibitors such as oseltamivir or zanamivir may be used if potential benefits outweigh risks. There is no increased risk of congenital malformation from influenza infection. (See Ch. 6, p. 129.)

Hepatitis A

Hepatitis A virus is transmitted by the feco–oral route and is endemic in Mexico, South America, Africa, Eastern Europe and Asia, although cases occur in all populations. Although there is no risk to the fetus or neonate from vertical transmission, there is increased risk of systemic infection, miscarriage and premature delivery. (See Ch. 9.)

Hepatitis E

Hepatitis E virus (HEV) is RNA virus that causes outbreaks of acute viral hepatitis in the developing countries and sporadic hepatitis in non-endemic areas. It may lead to fulminant hepatic failure in pregnancy. Mortality rate of HEV infection has been reported to be 20-50% during pregnancy. It can lead to preterm delivery and vertical transmission. Vaccine is currently not available and treatment is supportive.

Enteroviruses

Enteroviruses such as coxsackie virus, and echovirus may cause intrauterine infection. Coxsackie virus B3 has been associated with non-immune hydrops fetalis, myocarditis and varicella-like congenital skin lesions in neonate. Human echovirus 11 infection has been reported with Bornholm disease (costochondritis) in late pregnancy and infection of the neonate.

IMMUNIZATION IN PREGNANT WOMEN

In active immunization, an immunizing antigen is administered to induce a timely, long-lasting or permanent protective immune response in the patient.

The antigen may be a whole organism (killed or live), a purified subcellular fraction of the organism, a recombinant protein, or an inactivated exotoxin (toxoid). In passive immunization, there is transfer of protective antibodies pooled from immune individuals or transfer of immunoglobulin G (IgG) transplacentally from mother to fetus. Such immunity is short lasting due to the short half-life of the antibodies.

Indications for immunization during pregnancy include:

- pregnant women traveling to endemic areas;
- occupational exposure to the pathogen;
- accidental exposure or contact with a person suffering from the disease;
- immunodeficiency states.

Live vaccines are avoided in pregnancy due to the theoretical concerns of teratogenicity. If immunization is to be given in anticipation of later risks, it is preferable for administration during the second and third trimester. However, in situations where the risk of acquiring the disease or the risk associated with the disease exceeds the risk of immunization, it should be given even during the first trimester. This would apply when there is serious concern about infection with serious infections such as rabies, yellow fever, hepatitis B, tetanus, diphtheria, hepatitis A and meningococcal disease. Breastfeeding should not be withheld by mothers who receive immunization during pregnancy or post delivery.

Research for development of CMV and malarial vaccines is ongoing and of high priority. With advances in molecular technology, newer vaccines for influenza, hepatitis A and B, *H. influenze* type b, poliomyelitis, pneumococcus, cholera and pertussis that are more immunogenic or have fewer side effects may become available.

Immunization for some common infections in pregnancy is discussed below.

Rubella

Pregnant women found susceptible to rubella should be immunized after delivery. Nevertheless, termination of pregnancy following inadvertent immunization should not be recommended as there is no evidence that the vaccine is teratogenic from surveillance of women who received rubella vaccine during pregnancy.

Influenza

There is no evidence that influenza vaccine prepared from inactivated virus causes damage to the fetus. Pregnant women with medical conditions such as chronic respiratory diseases, cardiac disease, renal failure, previous splenectomy or immunodeficiency related illness, all of which increase the risk of complications from influenza, should be vaccinated before the influenza season, regardless of the stage of pregnancy.

Hepatitis A

Post exposure prophylaxis can be given using immunoglobulin and hepatitis A vaccine to the pregnant woman. A second dose of vaccine is recommended 6 months later.

Hepatitis B

Vaccine may be given for high risk cases. In some countries (e.g. Australia), vaccination of every newborn against hepatitis B is routine (see Chs 9 and 19).

Bacteria

It is important to ensure that pregnant women are immune to tetanus, as an important means of preventing neonatal tetanus. Pregnant women may safely be given tetanus toxoid or combined diphtheria-tetanus toxoids.

SUMMARY OF PRACTICE POINTS

Infections in pregnancy may lead to miscarriage, stillbirth, premature delivery, congenital anomalies and intrauterine growth restriction. There is a causal link between maternal infection, fetal inflammation and brain injury in both term and preterm infants. Intrauterine infections may be associated with adverse neonatal outcomes such as periventricular leukomalacia, intraventricular hemorrhage, cerebral palsy, bronchopulmonary dysplasia and neonatal death.

Molecular methods are increasingly used for rapid diagnosis of maternal, fetal and congenital infections.

Women with septicemia may present with vomiting, diarrhea, abdominal pain, tachypnea, tachycardia and temperature over 38 °C. The onset of sepsis may be insidious but may rapidly worsen.

In cases of suspected sepsis, active management with parenteral broad spectrum antibiotics, intravenous fluids and oxygen are important measures.

Amniotic fluid infection and or fetal infection do not imply that the fetus is affected.

Rash in pregnancy or significant contact with a person with a suspected viral illness should be investigated and managed appropriately. Infections in pregnancy associated with rash include varicella, rubella, parvovirus B19, measles, infectious mononucleosis, streptococcus, meningococcus, enterovirus and syphilis.

Women suspected or diagnosed to have STD during pregnancy should be tested for other common STDs that may potentially have impact on maternal and fetal health.

Chickenpox in pregnancy may be complicated by life threatening pneumonia. Falciparum malaria and hepatitis E in pregnancy are associated with high maternal mortality mainly in the developing nations.

Pregnant women should avoid travel to areas with endemic infections if possible. If traveling is mandatory appropriate advice regarding immunization, prophylactic treatment and preventive measures should be available to these women.

Further reading

Adam I, Elwasila el T, Homeida M 2004 Is praziquantel therapy safe during pregnancy? Transactions of the Royal Society of Tropical Medicine and Hygiene 98(9):540-543

Christian P, Khatry S K, West K P, Jr 2004 Antenatal anthelmintic treatment, birthweight, and infant survival in rural Nepal. Lancet 364(9438):981-983

Enders M et al 2004 Fetal morbidity and mortality after acute human parvovirus B19 infection in pregnancy: prospective evaluation of 1018 cases. Prenatal Diagnosis 24:513-518

Confidential Enquiries into Maternal Deaths in the United Kingdom. Why mothers die: the sixth report of Confidential Enquiries into Maternal Deaths in the United Kingdom. CEMACH, 2000-2002. London: RCOG, 2004

Department of Health 2003 Screening for infectious diseases in pregnancy DoH standards to support the UK Antenatal Screening Programme. The Stationery Office, London

French L M, Smaill F 2004 Antibiotic regimens for endometritis after delivery. The Cochrane Database of Systematic Reviews 4:CD001067

Gulmezoglu A M 2002 Interventions for trichomoniasis in pregnancy. The Cochrane Database of Systematic Reviews 3:CD000220

McDonald H, Brocklehurst P, Parsons J 2005 Antibiotics for treating bacterial vaginosis in pregnancy. Cochrane Database of systematic Reviews. 1:CD000262

MacLean A, Regan L Carrington D (eds). 2001 Infection in pregnancy. RCOG, London

Morgan-Capner P, Crowcraft N S 2002 Guidelines on the management of, and exposure to, rash illness in pregnancy (including consideration of relevant antibody screening programmes in pregnancy). Communicable Disease and Public Health 5:59-71

WHO. Maternal and congenital syphilis. Bulletin of the World Health Organization 2004;82. Online. Available at: http://www.who.int/bulletin/volumes/82/6/en/index.html

Wu Y W, Colford J M Jr 2000 Chorioamnionitis as a risk factor for cerebral palsy: a meta-analysis. Journal of the American Medical Association 284:1417-1424

Young G L, Jewell D 2001 Topical treatment for vaginal candidiasis (thrush) in pregnancy. Cochrane Database of Systematic Reviews 3:CD000225

Chapter **13**

HIV and pregnancy

D. A. Hawkins, S. E. Barton

INTRODUCTION

The global HIV pandemic continues to evolve from its initial epicenter in sub-Saharan Africa. Current particular areas of increasing prevalence include Eastern Europe and Asia. Women of childbearing age are disproportionately affected and it is estimated by the World Health Organization (WHO) that some 750 000 children are infected by vertical transmission annually. This is not surprising as the risk of transmission in a breastfeeding population is 25-45% and the majority of HIV infected women have no access to effective interventions to reduce transmission. However, in countries where comprehensive interventions including formula feeding are available, the risk of mother to child transmission may be well below 2% as is the case in many parts of Western Europe and North America.

Epidemiology in the UK

The prevalence of HIV among women giving birth is highest in metropolitan areas, reaching 1:179 (0.56%) in Inner London and 1:278 (0.36%) in Outer London in 2004. Figures for the rest of England were just over 1:1000 (0.1%), while Scotland was around half that level at 1:2000 (0.05%). The highest seroprevalence was found in those women who were born outside the UK from countries where HIV prevalence is substantial. Thus, in 2004 1:45 (2.2%) of antenatal women born in sub-Saharan Africa were HIV infected. Another group with a relatively high prevalence is women born in Central America and the Caribbean giving birth in the UK of whom 1:164 (0.61%) women were positive. Meanwhile, the HIV prevalence in women born in the UK, having remained low and stable in recent years at around 0.03%, has increased significantly in 2004 to 0.07%. While still low, this may be an indicator of increasing infection rates in the UK-born population.

Screening in pregnancy

In the UK as a whole there are now estimated to be over 800 births per year to HIV infected women (2004 data from the unlinked anonymous dried blood spot survey). In the past, the majority of women were unaware of their infection and most women who were known to be positive in pregnancy were diagnosed prior to becoming pregnant. In view of this, a multi-collegiate working party report in 1998 agreed a national policy to offer and recommend HIV testing, along with other screening tests to all pregnant women as an integral part of antenatal care. The aim of 90% uptake of antenatal testing by the end of 2002 was more than achieved and the ascertainment has been reversed with more women now diagnosed in the antenatal period than prior to pregnancy.

With the increasing prevalence of HIV, cost-effectiveness analysis even in lower prevalence areas justifies the policy of universal screening compared to selective screening. Furthermore, in the areas of higher prevalence it is being proposed that an expanded screening program be adopted, including an HIV test in the third trimester to detect those women who might have become infected during pregnancy. This is timely as in London there have recently, in 2005, been a number of positive children identified whose mothers were HIV negative at first trimester booking and who must have acquired the infection at a later stage of pregnancy. This expanded screening program might also include testing of potentially discordant partners. If a woman's HIV status is unknown – again in areas of higher prevalence – it may also be appropriate to consider HIV testing in labor, as has been mandated in some urban areas in the USA. This would allow instigation of HIV post exposure prophylaxis (PEP) to the neonate, with the chance that it may still be effective at that stage.

Risk of transmission

Without intervention, the risk of mother to child transmission of HIV in Europe is around 15-25% in non-breastfeeding women. Most of this transmission is thought to occur intrapartum, although both early and late in utero infection has been documented. Transmission early in pregnancy may be related to factors such as a high viral load associated with seroconversion during pregnancy or placental damage associated with substance misuse. Fortunately, the institution of antiretroviral therapy by the third trimester or earlier, appears to be effective in preventing almost all late maternal–fetal transmission.

Risks of vertical transmission

In untreated women, a number of risk factors for vertical transmission have been described. They are related to maternal health, prematurity and obstetric factors and are listed in Box 13.1. The single most important variable however, shown in a number of studies, is the association of transmission with high maternal plasma viral load. All of the other listed factors are much less important in terms of HIV transmission risk.

Box 13.1 Factors associated with risk of vertical transmission

- HIV infection acquired during gestation
- maternal health
- maternal CD4 lymphocyte count
- maternal viral load
- maternal nutrition
- chorioamnionitis
- preterm labor
- low birthweight
- duration of rupture of membranes
- order of birth if twin
- genetic, e.g. neonatal CCR-5 genotype
- breastfeeding.

The above factors can be viewed variously as surrogates for viral load, length of exposure to HIV, or susceptibility to HIV. The level of viral load in blood and genital fluids is however of overriding importance and will significantly affect the risk seen with all the other factors

---

Several studies have related mother-to-child transmission rates to maternal viral load. Two large studies showed that no transmission occurred where the maternal plasma viral load was < 1000 copies per mL (0/57) and < 500 copies per mL (0/84). However, a recent meta-analysis of seven prospective studies in the USA and Europe revealed 44 transmissions in 1020 women (4%) with plasma viral load of < 1000 HIV copies/mL at around the time of delivery. The rates were lower for mothers on antiretroviral therapy. Multivariate analysis showed that transmission was lower with antiretroviral therapy, Cesarean section, greater birthweight and higher CD4 count. However, it should be noted that these data were collected when HIV RNA PCR assays were less sensitive than currently used. Thus, the additional protective effects of Cesarean section shown in these studies may not remain significant in the presence of combination antiretroviral therapy and undetectable plasma viremia at < 50 copies per mL (see Section 13.8).

PRE-PREGNANCY ISSUES AND SUBSEQUENT PRE-CONCEPTION ADVICE

Pregnancy does not seem to have a major effect on HIV prognosis, although there may be some effect in women who are already significantly immunosuppressed. Conversely, late stage HIV disease in particular may have an adverse effect on pregnancy and lead to an increased risk of complications such as miscarriage, stillbirth, fetal abnormality, perinatal morbidity, intrauterine growth restriction, low birth-weight and preterm delivery. Therefore, as well as the standard advice for any pregnancy, an HIV positive woman considering pregnancy should be strongly advised to commence antiretroviral therapy should her immunity be waning and near or at the levels for initiation of antiretroviral treatment recommended by the adult British HIV Association (BHIVA) and other guidelines.

The fact that a woman is of childbearing age should be taken into consideration when deciding which antiretroviral drugs to prescribe. Most would recommend avoiding efavirenz. It has been classified as a Food and Drugs Administration (FDA) Group D drug in pregnancy due to neural tube defects (in cynomolgus monkeys), and similar CNS malformations described retrospectively in humans taking the drug in the first trimester. However, there have been no reports of neural tube defects in a prospective registry or, indeed, any excess of congenital malformations above expected background levels. The nucleoside backbone combination of stavudine (D4T) and didanosine (DDI) should also be avoided due to increased risk of lactic acidosis (there have been three deaths reported), although this combination is now uncommonly prescribed out of pregnancy.

Management of discordant couples

In a relationship where the male partner is infected by HIV but his female partner is not, assisted conception with either sperm washing or donor insemination is considered significantly safer than timed, unprotected intercourse and should be advised in all cases. In such relationships, assuming they are monogamous, HIV transmission risk per act of unprotected intercourse is between 0.3 and 1%. This risk can be reduced, but not to zero, by limiting exposure to the fertile period of the female's reproductive cycle. In a prospective study of couples trying to conceive through this method, 4% of women sero converted which is considered an unacceptably high rate. However, a retrospective study in Spain of 77 discordant couples conceiving, in which the infected partner had fully suppressed HIV replication on therapy for at least 6 months, reported no transmission. The couples were taught how to limit unprotected intercourse to the fertile period of each cycle. However, no data were presented on seroconversion risk in discordant couples who did not conceive. The numbers are too small to comment on transmission

rates but the study does reflect common advice given to patients.

Donor insemination removes the possibility of genetic parenthood from the HIV infected male partner, but does eliminate any risk of HIV transmission during conception.

Sperm washing has an advantage of allowing genetic parenting: sperm, from the HIV infected partner, are separated from HIV contaminated semen by centrifugation before being used in insemination or an IVF procedure. The efficacy of the wash is verified with a post wash HIV assay by PCR or NASBA before being used in treatment. This treatment is relatively simple and significantly safer than timed, unprotected intercourse with no reported cases of seroconversion in either female partners or children born to women who have conceived in over 3000 cycles of sperm washing, combined with intra-uterine insemination, IVF or intra-cytoplasmic sperm injections.

It is recommended that couples should have natural cycle insemination unless fertility factors are identified, when fertility drugs for supra-ovulation or IVF can be considered. The disadvantage of sperm washing is that the treatment is at present only provided in a limited number of fertility centers in the UK, Europe and North America. The majority of patients who receive treatment are required to fund themselves for this procedure. However, in the UK the National Institute of Clinical Excellence (NICE) guidelines published in 2004 on fertility, recommend sperm washing to be considered in discordant couples. This has led to a significant increase in the number of patients funded by the NHS to allow three cycles of sperm washing on the basis that this is a risk-reduction rather than a fertility treatment.

Before sperm washing, couples should be provided with adequate information and counseling on the technique, and also the options for donor insemination including advice on how to access such treatment to allow them to make an informed choice.

In a situation where the discordant couple have a female partner who is infected by HIV, whilst the male remains seronegative, unprotected intercourse should be avoided and instead the couple be provided with quills, syringes and sterile containers and advised on the use of self-insemination during the most fertile time of the woman's reproductive cycle. If conception has not been achieved within 6-12 months of regular self-insemination, then fertility investigation may be initiated. This may be considered sooner in women who are over 35 or who have irregular menstrual cycles or a history suggestive of tubal disease. In women above 35 years without HIV, the success rate of assisted reproduction therapy is low, falling from 15% per cycle at 36 years in most units to under 2% after 40 years. It may be even lower in HIV positive women.

Concordant couples should also avoid unprotected intercourse and be advised to consider sperm washing to minimize the risk of transmitting a resistant viral variant between partners, and potentially to the child by vertical transmission.

Guidelines for the fertility management of HIV discordant couples have recently been published by the British Fertility Society. It should be remembered that depression is extremely prevalent, perhaps even universal, in this population and a response to depression is often an unrealistic desire for pregnancy. Pregnancy never cures depression and attention should always be paid to this aspect of healthcare in these patients. It is usually omitted in guidelines produced by those who concentrate on the technology of fertility enhancement.

OTHER SEXUALLY TRANSMITTED DISEASES AND GENITAL INFECTIONS IN PREGNANCY

Asymptomatic pregnant women in the UK are not routinely offered screening for genital infections apart for serological tests for HIV, hepatitis B and syphilis. However, worldwide the prevalence of sexually transmitted infections and other genital infections is relatively high in HIV positive women, and this appears also to be true to some extent in Europe and the United States. The authors found a 50% prevalence of genital infections in mainly sub-Saharan African women. These, together with the Afro-Caribbean population, make up a high proportion of the antenatal HIV positive cohort in the UK. Bacterial vaginosis was particularly common (50%) with 10% having STIs (Chlamydia, HPV and HSV). Bacterial vaginosis may lead to chorioamniomitis which, in turn, may lead to prolonged ruptured membranes, premature birth and higher risk of mother-to-child transmission of HIV. For these reasons, despite the lack of clear evidence supporting routine screening, it is prudent to recommended screening and treatment of BV in this high-risk group (see Ch. 12).

In addition, other genital infections such as ulcerative STIs and gonococcal and chlamydial cervicitis may be associated with increased local HIV production with higher viral load in genital secretions. Genital tract viral loads may be discordant with blood viral loads particularly in those not on fully suppressive antiretroviral therapy. This may thus increase the risk of HIV transmission and be an additional reason for prompt diagnosis and treatment. The recommendations are therefore to screen HIV positive pregnant women for genital infections, soon after booking and repeat this at around 28 weeks. Syphilis serology should also be repeated on the latter occasion. As always partner notification should take place, where possible, to reduce the risk of re-infection.

Finally there is an association between CIN, cervical cancer and HIV related immunosuppression. However with highly active antiretroviral therapy (HAART), CIN tended to regress with a rising CD4 count and falling viral load. In terms of management, cytology should be undertaken in pregnancy as for HIV seronegative women and referral for colposcopy should be undertaken if an abnormality is detected. Invasive cancer management would be as in the HIV seronegative.

ANTENATAL CARE

Early detection of the mother's HIV status via routine screening as discussed above is essential to allow early implementation of measures to reduce mother to child transmission. All who provide antenatal care should thus be appropriately trained to include HIV tests in the routine screening offered and should have the knowledge to explain the measures required to reduce mother to child transmission. Protocols should be in place for prompt communication of any positive result and organization of confirmatory tests.

Psychosocial issues

HIV positive women are best looked after by a multidisciplinary team, including an HIV physician, obstetrician, midwife, health advisor, pediatrician and a pediatric nurse. At times the team will need to be augmented with others such as a psychiatric team, social worker, legal advocates and interpreters. Substance misusers will require referral to, and liaison with, the drug dependency team. Early assessment of the social circumstances of newly diagnosed HIV positive pregnant women is important. They may need help with housing or immigration problems. In both cases it is important to identify the issues as early as possible, so that women can be referred for appropriate special advice and support. The policy of dispersal applied in the UK, for example, is a particularly important issue and will affect continuity of care. Thus it must be made clear that adverse medical consequences may follow dispersal late in pregnancy or in those who have recently delivered.

Disclosure

It should be explained to the woman that it is necessary for members of the healthcare team to know of her HIV status to allow appropriate clinical management. However, it should also be made clear that every care will be taken to respect confidentiality. For example the woman herself can be involved in explicit instructions to all staff about the level of exposure to visitors. One important issue relates to disclosure to a sexual partner whom a woman may not wish to inform for fear of violence or other reasons. A significant number of male partners will be HIV negative at the time of their partner's initial diagnosis. Clearly women should be encouraged to disclose their HIV status to reduce the likelihood of onward transmission. If the woman declines, it should be recognized that breaking of confidentiality to inform a sexual partner of her HIV positive status is sanctioned 'in the last resort' by a variety of bodies including the World Health Organization (WHO) the General Medical Council (GMC) in the UK and the British Medical Association (BMA). Clearly such a decision would not be taken lightly and it may be helpful to discuss difficult disclosure cases in the multidisciplinary team and consider approaches that might be taken. Of particular importance is understanding the reasons why disclosure is feared in a particular case and to discuss and support the patient through these various difficulties. This may take some time and it is important that the patient is encouraged to protect their partner from infection while disclosure is being considered.

In particular ethnic groups there may be issues of cultural diversity which need to be recognized and responded to empathetically. Different health beliefs may impact on the acceptance of various interventions including antiretroviral therapy.

Antenatal visits

The principles of intervention to reduce mother-to-child transmission should be discussed at an early stage, reassuring the mother that the likelihood of transmission to the neonate is very low with the interventions suggested. In addition to the routine aspects of antenatal care, HIV monitoring tests such as plasma viral load and CD4 positive lymphocyte measurements should be reviewed in conjunction with the HIV physician. A baseline viral resistance assay should also be requested. Antiretroviral toxicity monitoring including liver function tests will also be necessary and abnormalities distinguished from pregnancy related conditions.

The choice and timing of antiretroviral therapy will need to be considered and discussed at the multidisciplinary team meeting with attention to management during delivery, mode of delivery and prophylaxis for the neonate. A written treatment plan should be finalized at an early stage and placed in the medical file to be readily available in the delivery suite or theater.

There may be a need for prophylaxis against opportunist infections such as *Pneumocystis carinii* pneumonia (PCP) and toxoplasmosis if the CD4 count is below 200/mL.

A detailed ultrasound scan for anomalies should be performed at around 21 weeks, particularly if the woman has been on antiretroviral therapy during the first trimester or has taken folate antagonists such as Septrin during this time. This will also provide valuable data for the prospective antiretroviral registry as to the safety of these drugs at critical stages in development.

Invasive procedures such as chorionic villus biopsy or amniocentesis should however be avoided. If considered absolutely essential then attempts should be made to reduce viral load to a minimum with antiretroviral therapy.

VIRAL LOAD AND RESISTANCE

Given its central importance to the risk of transmission, the level of viral load should be assessed every 1-2 months and at approximately 36 weeks' gestation, (provided a prompt result is made available) in order to be able to make informed decisions regarding mode of delivery and appropriate post exposure prophylaxis (PEP) regimen for the infant(s).

In many countries, including the UK, many HIV positive pregnant women are infected with subtypes that are prevalent in Africa. At times there may be concern that the viral load level reported does not appear to fit with CD4 cell number or clinical status and in this situation it may be prudent to re-test with another assay as, on occasion, technical factors may contribute to falsely low results.

It is good practice to assay for antiretroviral drug resistance as soon as a woman presents to inform decisions about treatment. Resistance is usually due to acquisition of resistant virus at initial infection but at times there are other reasons. For example a single dose of nevirapine to prevent mother to child transmission in a previous pregnancy may cause significant resistance.

It is appropriate to determine HIV genotype (or phenotype) if a woman having had suppressed virus, becomes viremic on therapy to assess if this is due to resistance or some other cause. The latter may include insufficient drug levels associated with non-compliance or altered pharmacokinetics in pregnancy that may be assessed by therapeutic drug monitoring. Finally a resistance assay 2-3 weeks after stopping suppressive therapy is recommended, particularly if a non-nucleoside combination has been prescribed (see later).

ANTIRETROVIRAL THERAPY IN PREGNANCY

When deciding on antiretroviral therapies it is important to balance the decrease in risk of HIV transmission that might be achieved versus possible adverse effects of treatment. Such unwanted effects might be evidence of mitochondrial toxicity in HIV negative children – as was first described by a French group – of mothers who had received AZT and/or 3TC in pregnancy.

Pre-eclampsia has been reported to be less common in HIV positive pregnant women not on fully suppressive antiretroviral therapy but HAART appears to restore or even increase the risk of pre-eclampsia and premature delivery. It may also of course lead to maternal toxicity.

Finally it is important to consider that the treatment given must not compromise future maternal options for therapy.

One of the benefits of combination antiretroviral therapy, given sufficiently early (at the latest, the beginning of the third trimester), is that by the time of delivery the viral load may be fully suppressed below the current sensitive detection level of 50 HIV copies per ml. If this is the case, by the time of confinement, it allows the mother the option of a vaginal delivery. The risk of transmission in this situation appears to be exceedingly low (< 1%). Moreover, should any untoward obstetric problems occur, the decisions about management may be based on obstetric grounds rather than modified by concern about a significant added risk of transmission of HIV to the neonate. There have, however, been concerns raised in the publications of the European Collaborative Study (although interestingly not by various US studies) that combination antiretroviral therapy significantly increases the risk of premature labor. Furthermore a recent paper from Spain suggests that the duration of HAART both prior and during pregnancy increases the risk of both pre-eclampsia and premature delivery and that incidence of these adverse events has continued to increase over the last few years. Despite these reports we feel that the balance of risks for both

mother and baby remains in favor of continuing to treat the mothers with fully suppressive combination therapy.

Nucleoside analogues

AZT (zidovudine) monotherapy

An early randomized, placebo controlled trial of antiretroviral therapy in pregnancy from USA and France published in 1994 was the AIDS Clinical Trial Group (ACTG) 076 Study. This showed that use of zidovudine commencing from 14-28 weeks antenatally, IV AZT during delivery and for 6 weeks as post exposure prophylaxis to the neonate, reduced the risk of HIV transmission by about two-thirds (24% down to 8%). The viral load reduction was modest and averaged only 0.24 log 10 by the time of delivery due to viral load rebound following incomplete suppression. Thus a major part of the beneficial effect was attributed to pre and post exposure prophylaxis. A similar study from Thailand used AZT from week 36 without the neonatal component. Here despite a greater viral load reduction at term (0.5 log 10) there was only a 50% reduction in transmission. Planned Cesarean section was shown to have a similar efficacy to AZT monotherapy and a combination of both approaches lead to overall transmission rates of less than 1-2%.

A Cochrane analysis of these randomized studies along with randomized studies of nevirapine to mother and baby (see below) confirmed the benefit of the above interventions. However these regimens allow unacceptable transmission rates particularly in women with higher viral loads, do not address the mothers' need for treatment, and are not the current standard of care.

The consequence of this early experience has led many authors and guidelines to recommend that AZT should be part of the antiretroviral regimen, even when used as part of combination therapy (see below), and that other aspects of this regimen, including IV AZT during delivery, should be continued even if a fully suppressive combination therapy is being used and there is likely to be very low levels of virus in the mother's blood and genital tract. This recommendation that AZT is a required component in any maternal regimen should probably be questioned in the future as other drugs may be just as effective, and possibly less likely to cause adverse effects, such as mitochondrial toxicity or anaemia. Notwithstanding this, AZT, usually in combination with 3TC (lamivudine), has been used extensively in pregnancy and therefore we have confidence in its reasonable safety and tolerability. Maternal adverse effects of combination therapies including AZT are similar to those in the non-pregnant population such as nausea, headache and anemia.

The risk of mitochondrial toxicity varies according to the affinity of the nucleoside analogues for the gamma polymerase. Mitochondrial toxicity was reported in a French study in exposed but uninfected children, whose mothers have received AZT and/or 3TC in pregnancy, with occasional significant neurological morbidity or death. A review of over 20 000 children in the USA did not support a significant effect, but mitochondrial toxicity remains a concern both in pregnant and other populations receiving antiretroviral therapy. Several new backbone combinations are under investigation in non-pregnant populations but further experience of these drugs is required particularly in pregnancy.

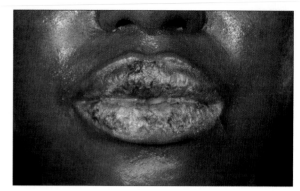

Figure 13.1 Stevens–Johnson syndrome affecting the oral mucosa.

Non–nucleoside reverse transcriptase inhibitors

Nevirapine has been the most widely used non-nucleoside reverse transcriptase inhibitors (NNRTI) in pregnancy and has generally been well tolerated. However, concerns have been raised because of liver toxicity which may develop in the first few weeks of treatment and warrant discontinuation of therapy. Occasionally this may lead to fulminant hepatitis and deaths have occurred. The risk has been shown to be greater in women, than in men, and with better immunity, and the drug should not be prescribed in women with CD4 counts above 250/mL or men with CD4 counts above 400/mL. Thus, this excludes its use as short-term antiretroviral therapy to prevent mother-to-child transmission in pregnancy in women who do not need treatment in their own right. Nevirapine may also cause a generalized rash which may or may not be associated with liver function abnormalities. The risk is less clearly associated with CD4 level. Again, the rash may be severe enough to warrant discontinuation of treatment, and 0.3% may develop Stevens-Johnson syndrome (see Fig. 13.1).

Nevirapine is also being used in the developing world solely to prevent mother-to-child transmission (MTCT) as mentioned above. The HIVNET012 study evaluated a stat dose of nevirapine given to the mother in labor with an additional dose to the neonate within 48-72 h of birth, and this approach became the basis of the extensive use of nevirapine to reduce vertical transmission of HIV. This, along with other suboptimal therapies; short course of AZT and/or 3TC, has led to significant reductions of mother-to-child transmission, and where no other intervention was

possible or practicable may have been an ethical approach. However, most would agree that it would be preferable to give antiviral treatment to the mother for her own health where this was indicated, and this will also be more effective in preventing vertical transmission. These single dose nevirapine regimens have been closely evaluated and have raised concern in that given the long pharmacokinetic half-life of nevirapine of 2-3 weeks and the fact that only a single mutation may cause significant resistance, this may prejudice the mother's future therapeutic response to combination antiretroviral therapy should it become available to her. Resistance rates appear to be high, particularly when investigated with more sensitive assays and reduced therapeutic response has been shown with subsequent nevirapine based regimens. Recent reports however suggest that similar efficacy may be achieved by omitting the maternal dose thus preventing the emergence of maternal resistance.

These considerations are particularly important because fixed dose combinations including nevirapine are the generic antiretrovirals which are most commonly available in the developing world at the present time and alternative options may not be available or be much more expensive.

Finally it should be noted that there is also a risk of nevirapine resistance developing on stopping combination therapy including nevirapine because of the long half life of this drug (~60 h) and significant drug levels may persist for a 14-21 days. This period of essential functional monotherapy may allow resistance to develop.

There is little experience with efavirenz in pregnancy, although it remains first line treatment in combination in the general non-pregnant population (see discussion in scenarios and Table 13.1).

Table 13.1 HIV drugs

Drug	Points of note	Maternal side effects	Neonatal side effects
Nucleoside/tide analogues		*Nausea, vomiting, fatigue, headache	
Lamivudine (3TC)	3TC has activity against hepatitis B	Abdominal pain, insomnia, rash, tiredness	Mitochondrial toxicity
Zidovudine (AZT)	Only licensed drug for HIV in pregnancy IV peripartum if on AZT monotherapy or VL > 50/mL on HAART including AZT	dizziness, weakness, muscle pain, anemia	Mitochondrial toxicity Anemia
Combivir (AZT + 3TC	Commonest backbone in pregnancy	See AZT and 3TC	see AZT and 3TC
Kivexa (lamivudine + abacavir)	Further experience awaited	Hypersensitivity to abacavir	
Truvada (tenofovir + emicitricabine)	Both drugs active against hepatitis B Further experience awaited	Renal toxicity-monitor monthly Low blood phosphate levels	
Stavudine (D4T)	Avoid combination of DDI + D4T	Lactic acidosis + death	
Didanosine (DDI)	From the prospective registry, increased congenital malformations with first trimester use	Diarrhea, peripheral neuropathy, rash	? excess congenital malformations
NNRTIs		[a]Rash, nausea, headache	
Nevirapine	Use only when CD4 < 250/mL Rapid placental transfer Monotherapy – Used in developing countries to decrease MTCT but long t1/2 + high resistance potential	Liver toxicity Stevens-Johnson syndrome (rare)	
Efavirenz	Avoid if possible: neural tube abnormalities reported in animal studies + from retrospective reporting in humans	Dizziness, tiredness, sleep disturbance Impaired concentration Vivid dreams	
Protease inhibitors		[a]Diarrhea, nausea, vomiting, abdominal pain, headache, rash, raised LFTs	
Kaletra (Ritonavir + lopinavir)	Limited experience but appears well tolerated		
Ritonavir + saquinavir	" "		
Ritonavir + atazanavir	Further experience awaited	Mild hyperbilirubinemia	Mildly elevated bilirubin
Ritonavir + fosamprenavir			

[a]class effects.

Protease inhibitors

Because of the problems associated with non-nucleoside drugs, it may be preferable to use protease inhibitors in pregnancy. They are not without their complications however, and the development of hyperglycemia or exacerbation of diabetes has been described with one study showing a two- to threefold increase in risk of the latter complication.

Most experience of protease inhibitors in pregnancy is with Nelfinavir, but this is no longer first choice in adult treatment guidelines and pharmacokinetic studies also show reduced drug exposure in pregnancy.

The use of low dose ritonavir to pharmacokinetically boost the levels of a number of protease inhibitors is now standard practice. These boosted combinations such as ritonavir/lopinavir and ritonavir/saquinavir in various formulations seem to achieve generally therapeutic levels in pregnancy, be clinically effective and are reasonably well tolerated. However drug levels achieved are quite variable and further studies including therapeutic drug monitoring (TDM) are underway. Thus at present where available TDM for PIs in pregnancy is recommended.

Treatment for pulmonary tuberculosis is discussed in Chapter 6. There are important pharmacokinetic interactions requiring possible close adjustment of both antituberculous and antiretroviral medication. Expert advice and TDM is required to manage this complex situation.

Finally, there are a few patients who have been treated in pregnancy with another protease inhibitor called Atazanavir. So far the concerns over raised bilirubin levels (the drug inhibits UDP-glucuronyl transferase causing elevations of unconjugated bilirubin) have not led to significant problems in the neonates but further experience is awaited.

OTHER DRUG TREATMENTS IN PREGNANCY

There may be a number of circumstances where HIV positive women need to be on other therapies in pregnancy. These include folate antagonists such as Cotrimoxazole as prophylaxis against *Pneumocystis jiroveci* pneumonia (PCP) and other opportunistic infections. A multicenter retrospective study of 148 infants exposed to ART in utero showed that the risk of congenital malformations was significantly raised in those additionally exposed. However a subsequent study suggested that administration of small doses of folic acid appears to negate this risk.

In any event the need for continuing any treatment into pregnancy needs to be critically reviewed not least because prophylactic therapies may be safely discontinued with the improving immunity associated with antiretroviral therapy.

OBSTETRIC MANAGEMENT AND MODE OF DELIVERY

The aim is to minimize the risk of mother-to-child transmission while at the same time not increasing maternal or other neonatal morbidity. Discussion on the mode of delivery as part of the risk assessment should be commenced from the first booking visit, and a provisional delivery plan discussed with a multidisciplinary team, including the HIV physician. The wishes of the mother must be determined and the possibility of a vaginal delivery considered, depending on obstetric factors and whether or not the mother is likely to have an undetectable viral load at the time of delivery.

Pre-labor Cesarean section

There are many studies supporting use of pre-labor Cesarean section in the presence of intact membranes as an effective method of reducing the risk of vertical transmission. These include a number of prospective cohort studies from either side of the Atlantic and a randomized, controlled study of mode of delivery in Europe. The benefits were shown to persist in the presence of the then available antiretroviral therapy. However, Cesarean section was less effective in reducing transmission when performed in labor or after membrane rupture. In the latter case the risk increased in proportion to the duration of ruptured membranes. However, these studies were done before the era of highly suppressive combination antiretroviral therapy and whether such risks persist at very low viral load levels (< 50/mL) is unknown.

The level of viral load in the blood correlates well with that in the genital tract in women on suppressive therapy, and a variety of studies have shown less than 1% transmission from women with blood HIV levels below 1000 copies/mL. However, transmission has been reported on occasion when maternal viremia was not detected, although some of the centers in these studies were not using the more stringent copy number of < 50/mL.

Early reports suggested that the complication rates for Cesarean section are higher in HIV positive women, particularly those undergoing emergency caesarean sections. Postpartum fever was the main complication and noted more commonly in women with low CD4 counts. However, this appears to be almost completely averted by the routine use of prophylactic antibiotics and is, thus, the current recommendation for all HIV positive women undergoing Cesarean section. Indeed, in a recent case controlled study from the UK where all HIV positive women were treated with antiretroviral therapy in pregnancy and all received prophylactic antibiotics, there was no difference in the incidence of post operative morbidity. Data from Central and South America following both vaginal and prelabor pre-ruptured membranes elective Cesarean section, showed low complication rates in both cases of just over 3%.

The timing of the Cesarean section should probably be a little earlier than in an HIV negative woman, partly because there does appear to be a tendency to earlier labor associated with the antiretroviral therapy. Thus possible increased transmission risks associated with premature labor or ruptured membranes needed to be balanced against the increased risks of respiratory distress in the neonate.

Intrapartum considerations include the avoidance of traumatic procedures such as invasive monitoring, or scalp lacerations which might occur with the use of the ventouse. Thus, forceps are the preferred mode of delivery if assistance should be required. However, if there is any likelihood of obstetric complications there must be a low threshold for making a decision in favour of Cesarean section.

It is important to ensure that antiretroviral therapy is continued up to delivery. However intravenous zidovudine during labor, used in the original study, was shown not to be necessary in a French study of women with undetectable viral load at the time of delivery, whether vaginally or by Cesarean section. In view of this and other data from the USA suggesting that omitting i.v. zidovudine in labor does not increase the risk of HIV transmission it has been dropped from the UK guidelines. It remains a recommendation in the current American guidelines.

The umbilical cord should be clamped as quickly as possible after birth. Following delivery the neonate should be bathed to remove any maternal blood and body fluids.

MANAGEMENT OF HIV 2 IN PREGNANCY

HIV 2 is endemic in West Africa. Other areas of high prevalence include Portugal and its former colonies in Africa, Brazil and India. Co-infection with HIV I and HIV 2 may occur. HIV 2 is less pathogenic than HIV I and is less easily transmitted both vertically and horizontally. This is probably because HIV 2 specific viral loads are often very low and indeed they are usually undetectable where the CD4 count is greater than 300/mL. Where disease progression occurs and with lower CD4 counts, HIV 2 specific viral loads become detectable and the risk of disease progression and transmission will increase. Overall however rates of vertical transmission are said to be between 0 and 5.4% in breastfeeding populations with no specific interventions.

Less than 100 cases of HIV 2 infection have been reported within the UK with only a handful of cases in pregnant women. However, migration from areas of higher prevalence is not uncommon and it is likely that we will see more cases in the future. There will also be cases of HIV2/HIV1 co-infection.

As there is limited experience with the management of HIV 2 positive women in pregnancy interventions are based on expert opinion. Clearly where the patient is significantly immunosuppressed with a low CD4 count and detectable HIV 2 viral load, she should receive combination antiretroviral therapy. In this regard, it should be noted that HIV 2 is naturally resistant to non nucleoside drugs and decreased susceptibility has also been shown in vitro to zidovudine and also to the protease inhibitor amprenavir. Other boosted protease inhibitors plus alternative nucleoside backbones such as abacavir/3TC or tenofovir/3TC might be considered. Monitoring should include HIV 2 specific viral loads where these can be accessed from reference laboratories. Delivery can either be by caesarean section or vaginal delivery when the viral load is undetectable with or without antiretroviral treatment.

Where the CD4 count is above 300/mL, it is known that the HIV 2 specific viral load is almost always undetectable. As the risk of transmission in this situation is very low, we have refrained from antiretroviral therapy. To date no transmissions have occurred with such an approach. Although the risk of breastfeeding is probably also very low, where formula feed is easily available, this should probably be recommended.

MANAGEMENT OF CO-INFECTION IN HEPATITIS B AND HEPATITIS C

Co-infection of hepatitis B and C

The management of hepatitis viruses in pregnancy is discussed in Chapter 12. However a few comments should be made here concerning co-infection with HIV.

Hepatitis C co-infection

There is evidence that the level of HCV viremia is greater in patients co-infected with HIV and this may account for the threefold increased risk of HCV transmission in mothers co-infected with HIV. There is also evidence that antiretroviral treatment is associated with a reduced HCV transmission although the mechanism for this is unclear. In view of this increased risk of transmission and evidence from one study that delivery by Cesarean section may reduce the rate of transmission, we usually recommend pre-labor Cesarean section in all HIV/ hepatitis C co-infected mothers.

Hepatitis B co-infection

Immunosuppression with HIV may increase the levels of HBV DNA but there is no clear evidence of increased risk of maternal fetal transmission. There are however raised levels of HBV viremia and it should be remembered that some antiretroviral agents such as lamivudine Emicitriabine and Tenofovir are active against both HBV and HIV. It is thus recommended that antiretroviral therapy for pregnant women with HIV/HBV co-infection should include drugs with activity against HBV.

Guidelines on the management of co-infection of HIV/HBV and HIV/HCV are on the BHIVA website (http://www.bhiva.org).

NEONATAL MANAGEMENT

Post-exposure prophylaxis

Some form of post-exposure prophylaxis (PEP) is recommended for all infants born to HIV positive mothers. There is no evidence that this needs to be given longer than 4 weeks although some guidelines recommend up to 6 weeks of therapy following the arbitrary example of the ACTG O76 study. When the mother has an undetectable viral load at the time of delivery – whether by vaginal delivery or Cesarean section – it is recommended to give the neonate AZT monotherapy unless there is evidence that the mother has a virus that might be resistant to this drug. In this situation an alternative agent from the mothers regimen should be used. It is possible that PEP adds no additional benefit in this situation because of the very low risk of transmission when the mother has an undetectable viral load but this has not been tested. Thus it is generally recommended to give AZT although this does of course increase the child's exposure to antiretroviral drugs.

Conversely, where there is a detectable maternal viral load, there will be an increased risk of transmission correlating with the level of the viral load. Triple PEP therapy should be considered in this situation with infants born to untreated mothers or mothers with detectable viremia despite combination therapy. The regimen used would depend on pharmacokinetic data, experience of use of the drug in neonates, drug formulation available and evidence of resistance.

It is beyond the scope of this chapter to discuss antiretroviral therapy in children. However a brief mention should be made of neonates in relation to post-exposure prophylaxis regimens. Dosing regimens have been developed for the nucleoside analogues such as AZT and 3TC and for the non nucleoside drug nevirapine. Experience for protease inhibitors is increasing. Should intravenous therapy be required, as with sick and/or premature neonates zidovudine is the only antiretroviral therapy available for intravenous use. One practical way of providing additional antiretroviral treatment is to give nevirapine to the mother at least 2 hours prior to delivery. This drug readily crosses the placenta and in view of its long half-life, provides therapeutic levels for 7–10 days. Should the mother have had nevirapine for more than 3 days, the neonatal metabolism of nevirapine will have been induced from the antenatal in utero exposure and full dose therapy based on body weight may be started at birth rather than the usual induction dose.

Laboratory diagnosis of HIV infection in non-breastfed infants

Maternal antibodies may persist until 18–24 months of age, accounting for a positive HIV antibody test. While this test should be performed, HIV infection can confidently be excluded in neonates only by HIV DNA PCR on peripheral blood lymphocytes. It is recommended to test infants at day 1, at 6 weeks and at 12 weeks of age. If all are negative and the infant is not being breastfed, mothers/parents can be reliably informed that the infant is not HIV infected. It is possible that the test at day 1 could be negative in an infant subsequently proven infected as HIV DNA levels are very low and may fail to amplify following a very recent (intrapartum) infection. Indeed, positive tests at this stage may suggest earlier intrauterine transmission. Combination post-exposure prophylaxis in neonates has also been shown in one study to delay the detection of HIV DNA and RNA. However, should only 4 weeks of combination PEP be given as is recommended, PEP will have been discontinued for a sufficient length of time to allow a reliable result on the 6 weeks DNA PCR test.

As the likelihood of HIV infection in neonates following appropriate intervention is so low, it is no longer felt necessary to provide routine prophylaxis against *Pneumocystis carinii* pneumonia (PCP) with co-trimoxazole. However, PCP prophylaxis should still be given to high-risk infants at increased risk of HIV transmission. Other infant immunizations are indicated although it is recommended not to give BCG vaccine until the infant is confirmed uninfected with two negative HIV DNA PCRs after one month of age. Other live vaccines are contraindicated (none are currently given in the UK).

Child protection

On occasion pregnant mothers refuse antiretroviral treatment or other interventions to reduce the risk of transmission to their unborn child. Attempts will be made by the multidisciplinary team to influence the mother's decision but when unsuccessful a prebirth planning meeting should be arranged with social services. The mother should then be informed that court permission will be sought at birth to treat the infant for 4 weeks with combination PEP. Furthermore breastfeeding will strongly be discouraged.

INFANT FEEDING

Formula feeding is recommended for all infants born to HIV infected mothers. There is evidence that breast-feeding provides an ongoing risk of HIV transmission and clearly where there are appropriate facilities and clean water supplies, formula feeding is safer. Of course worldwide breastfeeding has been promoted for good reason for its beneficial effects in the developing child. Thus the results of studies that evaluate the efficacy of antiretroviral treatment (given to the mother as part of her antiretroviral regimen and/or to the neonate as pre- and post-exposure prophylaxis) in allowing breastfeeding with minimal risk of HIV transmission are eagerly awaited. The costs versus benefits of such strategies will need to be carefully evaluated.

Most mothers from the developing world want to breastfeed and failure to do so may lead to concerns about unwilling disclosure of HIV status. Unfortunately there are no reliable data on the effects of maternal antiretroviral therapy on concordance of HIV in plasma with free or cell associated virus in breast milk. It is likely of course that such levels will be significantly reduced. Additional concerns about this approach also relate to further antiretroviral drug exposure and its possible associated toxicity for the child.

CLINICAL SCENARIOS

The UK guidelines recommend pre-labor Cesarean section at 38 weeks where the most recent viral load is detectable at greater than 50 /mL or where the viral load is unknown. However the risk of transmission is very low (< 1%) with women on stable therapy and undetectable viral load (< 50/mL) and it is now felt reasonable to offer a vaginal delivery in this situation. Indeed it is unclear from currently available data whether Cesarean section reduces transmission of HIV further and of course there are recognized morbidities with this procedure. Notwithstanding this, there needs to be a low threshold for proceeding to Cesarean section where there is a likelihood of obstetric complications. These issues and uncertainties need to be discussed with the patient and the medical and obstetric team in deciding on the individual birth plan.

Women who conceive on antiretroviral therapy

Where women conceive on combination antiretroviral therapy they should generally be advised to continue their current treatment. Evidence from the antiretroviral databases shows no additional fetal risk with this approach. There is also concern at possible viral rebound on cessation of therapy with a significant decline in immunity associated with the CD4 lymphocyte loss. The mother's health might thus be compromised and there is a theoretical risk of reactivation of infections associated with congenital abnormalities such as cytomegalovirus. Furthermore, many women will not realize or report their pregnant status until well into the period of organogenesis. Efavirenz should not be used in a woman who is considering pregnancy. In a woman taking it who finds herself pregnant, it should be continued only when there is no alternative. At present perhaps the only truly contraindicated drugs are ddI and D4T because of their association with lactic acidosis, and possibly ddI itself, the only drug in the prospective registry which has shown an increased risk of malformation at 6% compared to baseline of 2-3%.

Women who become pregnant while treatment naïve and who require treatment for their own health according to guidelines for established HIV infection

These women should start antiretroviral therapy at the end of the first trimester (12-13 weeks). Consideration should be given to the current safety and efficacy data of drugs that have been used in pregnancy. As most experience is with zidovudine and lamivudine as a nucleoside backbone, these are usually recommended in combination with a boosted protease inhibitor. The regimen may be subsequently modified post delivery depending on patient criteria for non-pregnant adults.

Antiretroviral treatment in mothers who do not yet require treatment for their HIV disease

It is reasonable to use combination antiretroviral therapy at all levels of viral load commencing in the second trimester with the intention to achieve undetectable levels of viral load prior to delivery. Boosted protease inhibitor based combinations are preferred for their resilience to the development of resistance compared with NNRTI combinations and because they may be stopped post delivery at the same time as the nucleoside backbone. There are also other contraindications and difficulties with NNRTIs as discussed earlier.

Although AZT monotherapy plus pre-labor Cesaman section is still recommended as an option in the BHIVA guidelines for women who have low levels of viral load < 6-10000/mL, a short-term course of combination antiretroviral therapy has a low toxicity for the fetus and has advantages. In particular, it allows the mother the option of vaginal delivery.

Women who present very late in gestation or in labor

Here it is sensible to include compounds that rapidly cross the placenta and have reliable pharmacokinetics in neonate. The preferred antiretroviral regimen would then include a non-nucleoside drug and there is most experience with nevirapine (PIs would be eschewed because they have limited transplacental transfer). Combination therapy (usually with AZT and 3TC) should be utilized to reduce the likelihood of resistance development in mother and child as has been shown with single dose nevirapine monotherapy. In addition zidovudine should be used intravenously and all treatments continued after delivery until details of the mother's clinical, immunological and virological status have been determined.

Threatened premature delivery

Here, management depends on optimum obstetric management (e.g. the use of antibiotics and steroids where indicated) along with appropriate antiretroviral therapy to the mother and infant.

Presentation after delivery or mother of unknown status in labor

If a woman presents in labor, attempts should be made to discuss an HIV test and where agreed a rapid test undertaken to assess status. Should HIV be thought likely on risk assessment then triple PEP should not be postponed if the results of the test are delayed. Similarly where it is ascertained after delivery that the infant's mother is HIV positive, or where maternal interventions have been declined or were only commenced after labor had begun, PEP to the neonate should be commenced as soon as possible. Standard risk assessment procedures should be followed as per post exposure prophylaxis following sexual exposure (see clinical effectiveness guidelines http://www.bashh.org). PEP is only likely to be effective if given within a few days. However, if the mother continues to breastfeed subsequently these is still a case for giving it later on.

REPORTING AND LONG-TERM FOLLOW-UP

International antiretroviral pregnancy registry

As mentioned there is a prospective international registry of the use of antiretroviral therapy in pregnancy. It is of great importance that this is supported to inform the safety of the increasing number of drugs in use. Forms and details are given in the references below.

National

Many countries will have their own reporting requirements. In the UK it is the responsibility of clinicians caring for women with HIV and their children to report women prospectively to the UK National Study of HIV in Pregnancy (NSHPC), and infants to the British Pediatric Surveillance Unit (BPSU) after birth (see Boxes 13.2 and 13.3 for details). There is now an anonymous flagging system from the NSHPC in the Office of National Statistics dealing with death and cancer registration.

Box 13.2 National Study of HIV in Pregnancy and Childhood (NSHPC)

This is the UK surveillance system for obstetric and pediatric HIV, based at the Institute of Child Health, London. Diagnosed pregnant women are mainly reported through a parallel reporting scheme run under the auspices of the Royal College of Obstetricians and Gynaecologists. HIV infected children and children born to HIV infected women are mainly reported through the British Paediatric Surveillance Unit of the Royal College of Paediatrics and Child Health.

Box 13.3 Antiretroviral Pregnancy Registry

Greenford Rd, Greenford, UB6 0HE
   Tel: 020 8966 4500; Fax 0208 966 2338; URL:
http://www.apregistry.com

Further reading

Brocklehurst P 2002 Interventions for reducing the risk of mother-to-child transmission of HIV infection. Cochrane Database System Review CD000102.

Connor E M et al 1994 Reduction of maternal-infant transmission of human immunodeficiency virus type 1 with zidovudine treatment. Pediatric AIDS Clinical Trials Group Protocol 076 Study Group. New England Journal of Medicine 331:1173-1180

Cooper E R et al 2002 Combination antiretroviral strategies for the treatment of pregnant HIV-1-infected women and prevention of perinatal HIV-1 transmission. Journal of Acquired Immune Deficiency Syndrome 29:484-494

European Collaborative Study 1999 Maternal viral load and vertical transmission of HIV-1: an important factor but not the only one. AIDS 13:1377-1385

European Mode of Delivery Collaboration 1999 Elective caesarean-section versus vaginal delivery in prevention of vertical HIV-1 transmission: a randomised clinical trial. Lancet 353:1035-1039

Garcia P M et al 1999 Maternal levels of plasma human immunodeficiency virus type 1 RNA and the risk of perinatal transmission. Women and Infants Transmission Study Group. New England Journal of Medicine 341:394-402

Gilling-Smith C HIV prevention. Assisted reproduction in HIV-discordant couples Guidelines ref A randomised trial of two post exposure prophylaxis regimens to reduce mother -to-child HIV – I transmission in infants of untreated mothers.

Gray G E et al 2005 Guidelines for the management of HIV infection in pregnant women and the prevention of mother-to-child transmission of HIV. AIDS 19: 1289-1297

Hawkins D et al 2005 on behalf of the BHIVA Guidelines Writing Committee. Management of HIV in pregnancy. HIV Medicine 6(suppl.2):107-148

International Perinatal HIV Group 2001 Duration of ruptured membranes and vertical transmission of HIV-1: a meta-analysis from 15 prospective cohort studies. AIDS 15:357-368

International Perinatal HIV Group 1999 The mode of delivery and the risk of vertical transmission of human immunodeficiency virus type 1: a meta-analysis of 15 prospective cohort studies. New England Journal of Medicine 340:977-987

Ioannidis J P et al 2001 Perinatal transmission of human immunodeficiency virus type 1 by pregnant women with RNA virus loads <1000 copies/mL. Journal of Infectious Disease 183:539-545

Jungmann E M et al 2001 Is first trimester exposure to the combination of antiretroviral therapy and folate antagonists a risk factor for congenital abnormalities? Sexually Transmitted Infections 77:441-443

Kourtis A P et al 2001 Understanding the timing of HIV transmission from mother to infant. Journal of the American Medical Association 285:709-712

Lawn S D et al 2000 Correlation between human immunodeficiency virus type 1 RNA levels in the female genital tract and immune activation associated with ulceration of the cervix. Journal of Infectious Disease 181:1950-1956

Mofenson L M et al 1999 Risk factors for perinatal transmission of human immunodeficiency virus type 1 in women treated with zidovudine. Pediatric AIDS Clinical Trials Group Study 185 Team. New England Journal of Medicine 341:385-393

National Institute for Clinical Excellence. Antenatal care: routine care for the healthy pregnant woman. RCOG, London, 2003

Wimalasundera R C et al 2002 Pre-eclampsia, antiretroviral therapy, and immune reconstitution. Lancet 360:1152-1154

Chapter 14

Neurological disease in pregnancy

S. A. Lowe

SYNOPSIS

Headache
Epilepsy
Disorders of the peripheral nervous system
Multiple sclerosis
Myasthenia gravis
Cerebrovascular diseases
Cerebral tumors
Summary

HEADACHE

Headache is a very common experience in pregnancy and only a small proportion of cases warrant detailed assessment and management, although a careful history and appropriate physical examination are always necessary. Primary headache syndromes consist of a spectrum of conditions ranging from tension-type headache to migraine as well as rarer forms such as cluster headache and benign exertional headache. Secondary headaches are associated with a broad range of conditions including head and neck trauma, vascular events, e.g. stroke or subarachnoid hemorrhage, increased cerebrospinal fluid pressure, substance withdrawal, infection or space occupying lesions. The association of headache with pre-eclampsia is not as strong as many suppose, but the condition must always be considered in the differential diagnosis when a woman presents with headache in late pregnancy.

Tension headache is more commonly bilateral than unilateral and is often described as squeezing or pres-sure-like and not associated with nausea. These generally improve with rest or with simple analgesics although excessive use of medication (particularly containing codeine) may lead to chronic daily headache.

Migraine

Migraine is a common problem in pregnancy. Women with migraine are equally likely to experience worsening, improvement or no change in pregnancy. Pre-existing migraine is associated with an increased incidence of early onset pre-eclampsia. In contrast with tension headache, migraine is usually unilateral, throbbing and severe and may or may not be preceeded by aura, most commonly visual. Typical visual aura symptoms develop over greater than 5 min and last no more than 60 min. They are generally homonymous, often hemianopic in distribution and expanding in the shape of a crescent with a bright ragged edge which scintillates. Scotoma, photopsia or phosphenes may occur. Other symptoms of aura may include numbness or paresthesiae most commonly on the face and hand. Less commonly motor weakness, symptoms of brainstem dysfunction or altered level of consciousness may occur indicating particular subtypes of migraine, e.g. hemiplegic or basilar-type.

Migraine is often accompanied by more general symptoms, e.g. nausea (80%), vomiting and light or noise sensitivity. More prolonged focal neurological symptoms, e.g. sensory or speech disturbance may occur and will arouse anxiety in the patient and her medical attendants, but are entirely consistent with the diagnosis. These cases mimic transient ischemic attacks, presumably on the basis of migrainous vaso-spasm, and are particularly concerning when there is little or no accompanying headache (typical aura without headache). Although there are no specific clinical signs or investigations to diagnose migraine definitively, the clinical picture is sufficiently distinctive to allow reassurance of the patient, and defer consideration of neuroimaging until postpartum. The majority of epidemiological studies indicate that primary headache generally improves in pregnancy, particularly after the 16th week when the lethargy of pregnancy resolves. Those with menstrual migraine show the greatest improvement. New onset migraine is uncommon in pregnancy and often occurs in women with a family history of migraine. These women do require appropriate clinical assessment but it is very rare to discover underlying structural pathology and investigation may be deferred until after delivery in most cases. The differential diagnosis of new onset headache in pregnancy and the puerperium includes all causes of secondary headache as well as conditions unique or more common in pregnancy such as pre-eclampsia, idiopathic (previously called benign) intracranial hypertension and cerebral venous sinus thrombosis.

Management of headache in pregnancy

There are three aspects to the management of migraine:

1. avoidance of triggers;
2. treatment of the acute attack; and
3. prophylaxis against recurrent migraine.

If migraine occurs infrequently, acute therapy and avoidance of triggers (such as cheese, chocolate, wine, oranges, bright sunlight, overwork) may be all that is required. Simple analgesics, e.g. paracetamol (sometimes with codeine) or aspirin, may be adequate with or without an antiemetic, e.g. metoclopramide. Non-steroidal anti-inflammatory drugs, e.g. naproxen or ibuprofen, are often useful analgesics in this condition but in the second and third trimester they should be avoided as they may cause premature closure of the ductus arteriosus and oligohydramnios. Ergot agents, with or without caffeine, are commonly used outside pregnancy for the acute treatment of migraine and are particularly effective during the aura phase. Theoretically, these drugs may vasoconstrict the placental bed vessels and they are therefore contraindicated during pregnancy. If they are used inadvertently, the woman should be reassured as there is no evidence of adverse effects. Five hydroxytryptamine receptor antagonists, e.g. sumatriptan, naratriptan and zolmitriptan, are highly effective for treating acute migraine. They are also vasoconstrictors, but the limited data available about their use in pregnancy do not suggest any increase in adverse events.

Migraine attacks that are severe, prolonged or unresponsive to the above may require treatment with narcotic analgesics given parenterally. Intravenous metoclopramide 20-30 mg has been shown to be superior to placebo in the treatment of acute migraine outside pregnancy. These agents are safe although narcotics may cause neonatal respiratory depression when given close to the time of delivery. In general parenteral opiates should not be the first choice for treatment of migraine, and are subject to abuse, and dependency considerations.

Prophylactic treatment may be necessary if migraine is frequent or uncontrolled. During pregnancy, the most appropriate agents for this purpose are propranolol (20-80 mg nocte), low dose aspirin (75-100 mg per day), cyproheptadine (2-4 mg nocte), amitryptyline (10-25 mg nocte) or verapamil (40-80 mg nocte). Antiepileptic drugs, serotonin antagonists, e.g. pizotifen and methysergide and selective serotonin reuptake inhibitors (SSRI) are also used for prophylaxis outside of pregnancy but may be associated with adverse fetal outcomes and should be avoided.

Headache in the postpartum period

Acute headache in the postpartum period is often a concerning symptom. The differential diagnosis includes primary headache but a number of specific causes need to be excluded. If the patient has received an epidural or spinal anesthetic, a dural puncture is often blamed. It has been estimated that 39% of parturients report symptoms of headache unrelated to dural puncture following delivery. The symptoms of post-dural puncture headache (PDPH) are a fronto-occipital, throbbing or dull headache appearing within seconds of arising from the bed, relieved promptly by lying down, with onset usually within 3 days. Dizziness, nausea and vomiting, visual disturbances, interscapular pain, neck stiffness, photophobia or auditory symptoms may accompany the headache. This headache is related to loss of cerebrospinal fluid and lowering of the cerebrospinal fluid pressure. The differential diagnosis of PDPH includes migraine, meningitis, pre-eclampsia, epidural abscess, cerebral tumor, cerebral venous sinus thrombosis and intracranial hemorrhage. Careful clinical assessment and the judicious use of cerebral imaging are required to differentiate these conditions. If PDPH is likely, a request for review by the anesthetist is necessary as application of an epidural blood patch is promptly and remarkably effective at terminating the headache.

Cerebral venous sinus thrombosis

Cerebral venous sinus thrombosis (CVST) is a rare condition with an estimated incidence of 1 per 100 000 deliveries in developed countries, although in developing countries the incidence may be as high as 200-500 per 100 000 deliveries. Thrombophilias, pre-eclampsia, dehydration and puerperal infection may be significant risk factors. CVST can present at any stage of pregnancy, however most present in the second to third week postpartum. Presentation is extremely varied, from isolated slowly developing headache, focal neurological signs and symptoms, seizures, papilledema and behavioral changes to impaired consciousness, ranging from slight confusion to deep coma. The typical description is of a woman with a severe and persistent headache for some days who proceeds to a focal or generalized seizure. Diagnosis is often delayed owing to the rarity of the condition and the lack of specificity of the presenting symptoms. Early diagnosis and treatment may reduce the risk of fatal outcome or permanent disability. Imaging is essential for the diagnosis. Plain CT scan may be negative but should be performed to exclude hemorrhage or space occupying lesion. The gold standard for diagnosis is magnetic resonance imaging and angiography (MRI/MRA) or intra-arterial four-vessel angiography. Digital subtraction angiography or helical CT venography are alternatives. CSF examination is necessary if infection is suspected.

Therapeutic anticoagulation, even in the presence of hemorrhage, is the mainstay of treatment, although rarely surgery or thrombolysis may be life saving. Within a few days of delivery, systemic thrombolysis is contraindicated. Even so, cerebral venous thrombosis is such a serious condition that catheter directed thrombolysis to minimize systemic effects and maximize local efficacy may be considered. Antiepileptic drugs should be given as treatment or prophylaxis for seizures. The prognosis for CVST is better than previously thought, however mortality ranges from 6-20% despite anticoagulation. The presence of severely altered state of consciousness and intracranial hemorrhage are strongly indicative of a poor prognosis. Anticoagulation is usually continued for 3-6 months until MRI demonstrates sinus patency. Recanalization occurs in the majority of cases. The risk of recurrence is low, even in future pregnancies and most recurrence is within one year. A thrombophilic etiology should always be sought in investigating CVST but such investigation is best deferred until the patient is no longer taking anticoagulants.

Idiopathic intracranial hypertension

Idiopathic intracranial hypertension (previously called benign intracranial hypertension or pseudotumor cerebri) is a rare but serious disorder that occurs more commonly in the first half of pregnancy, particularly in those who are obese. There is a tendency for pre-existing idiopathic intracranial hypertension to worsen during pregnancy, possibly due to weight gain and hormonal changes. Most patients (95%) present with retro-orbital headaches and 15% have diplopia. The headache in this condition is usually constant, throbbing, bifrontotemporal, and often associated with nausea and vomiting. In keeping with its origin in raised intracranial pressure, the headache is usually present on arising in the morning and is somewhat lessened in the erect posture, although by the time of diagnosis, the headache has often lost such variability. The diagnosis is confirmed by the finding of papilledema with or without visual loss or cranial VI nerve palsies. Neuroimaging is required to exclude alternative causes of raised intracranial pressure prior to lumbar puncture and to exclude conditions such as cerebral sinus and venous thrombosis.

Women with idiopathic intracranial hypertension should be encouraged to lose weight prior to pregnancy. Treatment, with therapeutic lumbar puncture, thiazide diuretics, acetazolamide (a carbonic anhydrase inhibitor), analgesics and or corticosteroids, is directed towards controlling symptoms and preventing visual loss. Surgical options include optic nerve sheath fenestration and lumbo-peritoneal shunting. Pregnancy outcome appears to be unaffected by the disorder and apart from close supervision of the visual acuity and fields, obstetric management should be unaffected. There is a 10% risk of recurrence in subsequent pregnancy, sometimes more than once, and a risk of permanent visual impairment of 10%.

Pre-eclampsia

The majority of women with pre-eclampsia do not have headache. There are no specific features of headache in pre-eclampsia although there may be associated neurological symptoms of visual scintillations, visual loss or jitteriness. Headache in this condition is thought to be secondary to vasoconstriction, cerebral edema and/or side effects of anti-hypertensive medications, particularly the vasodilators hydralazine and nifedipine. Rarely, focal neurological signs such as cortical blindness, altered mental state, or transient lateralizing features may be present. A peculiar and easily demonstrable hyperreflexia of unknown genesis often accompanies severe pre-eclampsia and may lead to concern at the likelihood of eclamptic seizures. It has not been demonstrated as a risk factor for eclampsia. Severe headache in a woman with pre-eclampsia should lead to consideration of the possibility of intracerebral hemorrhage, a feared but rare complication of severe pre-eclampsia.

EPILEPSY

The epilepsies comprise a group of disorders characterized by recurrent seizures and classified according to clinical or specific electroencephalographic EEG features. Most types of epilepsy are characterized by more than one type of seizure. Patients with focal or partial epilepsy syndromes may have simple partial, complex partial and secondarily generalized tonic-clonic seizures. Patients with generalized epilepsy may have one or more of the following seizure types: absence, myoclonic, tonic, clonic, tonic-clonic and atonic. Although epilepsy is the most commonly encountered neurological disease in pregnancy, it is still relatively rare with a prevalence of 0.6-1.0%. Medical therapy utilizing anticonvulsant drugs is the most common form of treatment (Table 14.1) although surgery – or no treatment – may have a role in specific cases.

Table 14.1 Anticonvulsant drugs

Drug	Indications
Carbamazepine	Focal and secondary GTC
Clonazepam	Generalized focal and secondary GTC
Ethosuximide	Absence
Felbamate	Focal and secondary GTC
Gabapentin	Focal and secondary GTC
Lamotrigine	Focal and secondary GTC, tonic atonic, primary GTC, myoclonic
Levetiracetam	Focal and secondary GTC
Oxcarbazepine	Focal and secondary GTC
Phenobarbital/ Primidone	Focal and secondary GTC, primary GTC
Phenytoin	Focal and secondary GTC, primary GTC
Tiagabine	Partial, focal and secondary GTC, tonic atonic, myoclonic
Topiramate	Focal and secondary GTC, absence, tonic atonic, myoclonic
Valproate	Focal and generalized
Vigabatrin	Focal and secondary GTC
Zonisamide	Focal and secondary GTC, primary GTC

GTC: generalized tonic-clonic.

Preconception care

Ideally, all women with epilepsy should undergo counseling prior to pregnancy. The principles of drug review at this time are:

1. Withdraw any unnecessary medication where possible.
2. Use the smallest effective dose of medication.
3. Withdraw drugs with fetal effects and replace with safer drugs if possible.

In the case of epilepsy, tampering with stable and effective medication does carry hazards for the patient. Anticonvulsant therapy is usually chosen with great care by the patient's neurologist, and often after the failure of other drugs. For these reasons, it is advisable to consult with the neurologist before making any substantive change.

Preconception counseling may identify women who have been seizure free for a number of years on minimal medication, particularly those with a normal electroencephalogram (EEG) and normal cerebral imaging. In these cases, careful weaning of therapy over 6 months prior to pregnancy may be entirely appropriate, accepting a small risk of recurrence of seizures. All women with epilepsy taking anticonvulsant drugs (ACDs) should receive folate supplementation with higher doses (5 mg) reserved for those women taking valproate or carbamazepine. During pregnancy, antenatal screening for neural tube defects with maternal serum alpha-fetoprotein and ultrasound should be performed at or near 12 weeks of amenorrhea. A careful 18-20 week morphology scan should be performed, ensuring the sonographer is aware of the patient's additional risks. Most clinicians agree that for both the mother and her fetus, the benefits of controlling seizures outweigh the potential risks associated with the ACDs. The genetics of epilepsy are complex and advice regarding heritability should be guarded.

Pregnancy

A minority of women with epilepsy experience an increase in seizure frequency during pregnancy, particularly those with poorly controlled epilepsy prior to pregnancy. This may be explained by changes in anticonvulsant drug pharmacokinetics as well as vagaries of patient compliance. In practice tiredness, nausea, vomiting, sleep disturbance and emotional stress may be important factors affecting seizure frequency during pregnancy. These factors may be magnified around the time of delivery and immediate puerperium. Whether seizure disorders themselves may cause an increase in congenital malformations or adverse pregnancy outcomes remains controversial. Seizures have been reported to cause significant fetal heart rate decelerations, presumably secondary to maternal hypoxemia and acidosis. Single seizures are unlikely to be a significant problem while status epilepticus is associated with significant maternal (33%) and fetal mortality (50%). Trauma during seizures can result in placental abruption or uterine injury, as well as the usual maternal hazards of self-injury and aspiration pneumonitis. Some older studies suggested that epilepsy was associated with adverse pregnancy outcomes such as pre-eclampsia, lower birth weight and stillbirth although other studies failed to confirm this.

Anticonvulsant drugs

A large number of drugs with differing mechanisms of action are used in the treatment of epilepsy, either individually or in combination. During pregnancy, a number of factors influence drug levels including altered absorption, protein binding, metabolism, renal clearance and non-compliance. Overall, there is a tendency to require an increase in ACD dose during pregnancy. ACD levels should be monitored by observation of the clinical response and regular (3-monthly) plasma unbound drug levels where these are available. As the adverse effects of ACDs are believed to relate to peak levels, a change to smaller doses at more frequent intervals or sustained release preparations should be considered. Treatment should be maintained around the time of delivery and dosage reassessed postnatally as toxicity may occur if the gestational higher dose is continued in the puerperium.

For most ACDs, transplacental drug transfer results in significant fetal exposure. This is true for both the older ACDs and newer agents. The use of ACDs during pregnancy has been associated with an increased incidence of congenital malformations (see Table 14.2), both major and minor, impairment of intrauterine and postnatal growth, neonatal toxicity syndromes, hemorrhagic complications in the neonate and neuro-developmental delay. Determining the magnitude of these risks is extremely difficult as epidemiological data are highly variable and large, randomized prospective studies are neither available nor feasible. Observational data from a number of national prospective drug registers is gradually becoming available and will contribute significantly to our knowledge in this area.

Although the ACDs are all considered major teratogens, the majority of babies exposed to ACDs, particularly in monotherapy (> 95%) have a normal outcome. Evidence exists for teratogenicity with all commonly

Table 14.2 Incidence of major congenital malformations following monotherapy with ACDs: based on the prospective data from the UK Epilepsy and Pregnancy Register, 2005

Anticonvulsant drug	Number of malformations/total	Major malformation rate % (95% CI)
Valproate	44/715	6.2 (4.6-8.2)
Carbamazepine	20/900	2.2 (1.4-3.4)
Lamotrigine	21/647	3.2 (2.1-4.9)
Phenytoin	3/82	3.7 (1.3-10.2)
Gabapentin	1/31	3.2 (0.6-16.2)
Topiramate	2/28	7.1 (2.0-22.6)
Levetiracetam	0/22	0.0 (0.0-14.9)

used older ACDs. Of the newer anticonvulsant drugs, prospective studies have indicated that monotherapy with lamotrigine and oxcarbazepine is associated with a low rate of malformations. Virtually no data are available about other new agents such as levetiracetam, zonisamide and felbamate. The incidence of major malformations in women with epilepsy is also related to a previous pregnancy with a major malformation, polytherapy with ACDs, higher dosages of valproate (> 1000 mg/day), low folate levels and low education levels. Strong epidemiological data exist implicating valproate (1-2%) and carbamazepine (0.2-1%) as particular risk factors for neural tube defect, specifically spina bifida. Even high dose folate supplementation has not been shown to alter the incidence of neural tube defects in women with epilepsy, although current recommendations suggest folate 4-5 mg/day be commenced before conception. The predominant malformations seen in women with epilepsy are cleft lip or combined cleft lip and palate (valproate 1.5%, phenytoin 1.2%, carbamazepine 0.4%, lamotrigine 0.2%) and cardiovascular malformations (phenytoin 1.2%, valproate 0.7%, carbamazepine 0.7%). Hypospadias and gastrointestinal defects are also overrepresented. The relative risk of facial clefting has been estimated at 2.7 for untreated epileptics and 4.7 for woman taking anticonvulsants. Although the relative risk of congenital malformation with valproate is higher than with alternative agents, overall the risk of monotherapy is low. This should be taken into account when changes in therapy are contemplated.

Almost all of the older ACDS (benzodiazepines, carbamezepine, phenobarbitone/primidone, phenytoin, trimethadione, valproate) have been associated with the fetal anticonvulsant drug syndrome consisting of minor malformations and dysmorphism, e.g. hypertelorism, lowset abnormal ears, short neck with low posterior hairline, bilateral single transverse palmar creases and distal digital hypoplasia. The incidence of this syndrome has varied with the population studied but in general the risk appears to be about 10% in exposed fetuses. Aspects of this syndrome also appear to occur more commonly in children of women with epilepsy, even when untreated. Many of these features improve with age. A number of ACDs appear to exert their teratogenic effect through the toxicity of their metabolites. During pregnancy, the metabolism of carbamazepine is increased leading to increased levels of the 10,11 epoxide metabolite which accumulates in amniotic fluid and may be fetotoxic. Fetal epoxide hydrolase levels are genetically determined and an association has been demonstrated between low levels and an increased incidence of fetal anticonvulsant drug syndrome. The same pathway metabolizes phenytoin, phenobarbital and tiagabine. This might explain the similarity of teratogenic effects with various ACDs. Newer agents such as lamotrigine, topiramate, gabapentin and oxcarbazepine are not metabolized through this pathway. Nevertheless, as the mechanism of most adverse fetal effects is unknown, reassurance about safety in pregnancy depends almost entirely on observed clinical experience, and this is accruing with increased use of the newer drugs.

The use of ACDs, particularly valproate but also carbamazepine and phenytoin, has also been associated with neuropsychological abnormalities in the offspring of women with epilepsy. A recent Cochrane review concluded that there is little evidence about which drugs carry more risk than others and further prospective studies are required. Assessment at 18 months of age revealed that exposure to intrapartum seizures, high dose of ACDs and small head circumference at birth were also associated with neuropsychological abnormalities. Again these studies remain imperfect and the results are variable. A number of ACDs induce vitamin K deficiency which is reflected in elevated production of neonatal PIVKA (protein induced by vitamin K absence). Vitamin K deficiency bleeding, previously called hemorrhagic disease of the newborn, is said to occur in 6-12% of babies of women exposed to these drugs. The deficiency is easily corrected with oral vitamin K during the last month of pregnancy or maternal (10 mg) and neonatal (1 mg) parenteral vitamin K at delivery.

Delivery and postpartum

In practice stress, sleep deprivation, pain, hyperventilation and erratic absorption of ACDs contribute to an increased risk of seizures during the emotional turmoil of labor and the immediate postpartum period. The route of delivery should be selected on obstetric grounds although precautions should be taken whatever the mode of delivery. All women with epilepsy should have a cannula inserted on admission to the delivery suite. Vitamin K, 10 mg parenteral may be administered to the mother prior to delivery as an alternative to weeks of oral vitamin K. Anticonvulsant drugs should be continued at pregnancy doses during and immediately after delivery, but reduced stepwise over the first 2 or 3 postnatal days as the increased requirements of pregnancy abate quickly. Where oral therapy is not possible, intravenous preparations of phenytoin may be given. Intravenous valproate and fosphenytoin are available in some countries.

If seizures do occur, appropriate supportive treatment with protection of the airway, oxygen and monitoring of the fetal heart rate should be commenced. Most seizures are self-limiting, however if seizures are prolonged, treatment with intravenous clonazepam (1-2 mg over 2-5 min), lorazepam or diazepam (2 mg/min to max 10 mg) will usually terminate the seizure. Treatment with these drugs may cause maternal respiratory depression and fetal and neonatal sedation. Careful clinical assessment is required to exclude other causes of seizure in labor such as eclampsia (see Box 14.1).

The days following delivery are a time of particular risk for recurrent seizures. Adequate pain relief, assistance with mothercrafting, and measures to allow the new mother as much rest as possible will reduce the risk of postpartum seizures. The patient can return to pre-pregnancy ACD dosages within the first week following delivery. Most ACDs are considered compatible with breastfeeding although the newborn should be observed for sedation.

Box 14.1 Differential diagnosis of seizures in pregnancy

- Eclampsia.
- Vagal episode/faint.
- Subarachnoid hemorrhage.
- Thrombotic thrombocytopenic purpura.
- Amniotic fluid embolus.
- Cerebral venous sinus thrombosis.
- Water intoxication/hyponatremia.
- Toxicity of local anesthetics.
- Hypoglycemia.
- Cerebral vasculitis angiopathy.

Oral contraceptive and levonorgestrel implant failures are more common in women taking phenytoin, carbamazepine, oxcarbazepine, felbamate, topiramate and phenobarbitone. Higher dose estrogen agents (at least 50 µg ethinylestradiol) or medroxprogesterone injections given every 10 weeks are alternatives. Preconception counseling is important for any chronic medical disorder, including epilepsy. It is useful to encourage the woman to return for this purpose when she is considering another pregnancy, to review the state of her general health, her epilepsy and its treatment.

DISORDERS OF THE PERIPHERAL NERVOUS SYSTEM

Certain peripheral entrapment neuropathies occur more commonly in pregnancy and may lead to troublesome symptoms. Lower limb neurological defect may develop during or immediately following delivery due to stretch or compression of branches of the lumbosacral plexus or peripheral nerves. These need to be distinguished from neurological complications secondary to spinal/epidural anesthesia or pre-existing lesions such as nerve root compression. Unusual causes of peripheral nerve disease such as inflammation in Guillain–Barre syndrome may also be seen in the pregnant woman. A careful neurological examination is imperative and further investigation with electrophysiologic testing and or imaging may be required. Generally, treatment is supportive and involves input from physiotherapists and rehabilitationists.

Bell's palsy

Acute mononeuritis of the facial nerve is now thought to be almost always secondary to herpes simplex infection although inflammation or compression cannot be excluded as a cause. If typical vesicular lesions are visualized in the external auditory meatus or soft palate, a diagnosis of Ramsay–Hunt syndrome (acute herpes zoster of the geniculate ganglion) can be made which is clinically indistinguishable from acute Bell's palsy. The incidence of Bell's palsy is increased in pregnancy particularly in late pregnancy and early in the puerperium. In these cases, the generally noted association with the herpes virus is almost always absent, thereby suggesting that peripartum Bell's palsy has a different etiology, quite feasibly related to swelling of the nerve in an anatomically narrow canal. The patient usually describes the onset over hours of weakness of one side of the face with or without pain in the ear, loss of taste on that side of the tongue and/or hyperacusis. On examination there are signs of a unilateral lower motor neurone weakness of the VIIth cranial nerve. If the patient is seen within 72 h of onset of symptoms, high dose corticosteroids e.g. prednisolone 40 mg/day tapering over 2 weeks may speed recovery but probably does not influence the long-term prognosis which is generally very good. If there is a complete facial palsy, about 85% of women recover full function, whereas 95% of those with partial palsy recover. If a herpes infection is considered likely, steroids should be avoided or combined with antiviral therapy such as aciclovir, which has been shown to be effective in the non-pregnant patient. Physiotherapy and eye care may also prevent morbidity and improve long-term outcome. Bell's palsy is not an indication for delivery per se but has been associated with an increased incidence of pre-eclampsia.

Carpal tunnel syndrome

Compression of the median nerve during pregnancy usually occurs due to edema in the carpal tunnel, where a number of structures compete for space in a canal bounded by the carpal bones and the flexor retinaculum at the wrist. It leads to symptoms of parasthesiae in the median three and one half digits and pain in the hand or forearm. It occurs in 2-3% of women, mostly beginning in the third trimester. Symptoms are frequently worse at night and may be bilateral in more than half, although the dominant hand may be more symptomatic. Tinel's sign may be present (parasthesiae in the median three digits with percussion over the carpal tunnel at the wrist) with or without motor and/or sensory loss in the median nerve distribution. Weakness of the thenar eminence is a sign of severe compression and if prolonged may cause wasting of the affected muscles. Definitive diagnosis can be made by nerve conduction studies if the symptoms or signs are atypical. Women with mild carpal tunnel syndrome may be reassured that the symptoms usually abate within weeks of delivery, although cases that present early in pregnancy may persist longer. More severe cases may be treated with wrist splints worn at night that maintain the wrist in a neutral position. Occasionally local injection of steroid or a combination of steroid and local anesthetic may be required. Surgical decompression may be required, particularly if motor signs are prominent or symptoms fail to resolve after delivery. Not all cases of hand symptoms are due to carpal tunnel syndrome and thought must be given to the differential diagnoses that include cervical radiculopathy and de Quervain's tenosynovitis.

Meralgia paresthetica

Compression or stretch of the anterior branch of the lateral cutaneous nerve of the thigh at the groin during pregnancy leads to dysesthesia, numbness or pain on the anterolateral aspect of the thigh, usually unilaterally. The condition is aggravated by obesity and generally occurs in late pregnancy. Objective sensory loss may be detected but is not always present. Again, like carpal tunnel syndrome, symptoms generally abate within weeks of delivery. No specific treatment is required.

Traumatic mononeuropathies and plexopathies

Injuries to the femoral nerve, sciatic nerve, common peroneal nerve, obturator nerve and lumbosacral plexus have all been described following delivery (Table 14.3). Pressure from the fetal head on the L4, L5 and S1 nerve roots as they course over the pelvic brim, unusual stretch during prolonged lithotomy position, particularly in patients with epidural anesthetics, account for the majority of these injuries. Women most at risk are nulliparas with a prolonged second stage of labor. Sensory, motor and even autonomic neural loss may occur but most are neurapraxias and resolve within 2 months. Foot drop is one of the most common obstetric neurapraxias and may be caused by injury at the level of the lumbosacral root or plexus, sciatic nerve or common peroneal nerve. It is associated with fetal macrosomia or malposition, or, more commonly from compression in lithotomy or while squatting.

Neurological complications of spinal/epidural anesthesia in obstetrics

Regional analgesia has become the method of choice for pain relief in labor and Cesarean section, and both the epidural and spinal techniques are very safe with an extremely low incidence of adverse effects. Even so, meningitis, epidural abscess, epidural hematoma and direct needle trauma to nerve roots or the spinal cord have all been described following spinal or epidural anesthesia. Meningitis or epidural abscess generally have a delayed onset with an incubation period of up to 1 week. Epidural abscess is characterized by lower back pain, usually very severe, and fever with or without radiating segmental pain. If the diagnosis is suspected, urgent imaging with MRI or CT is required. Conservative management consists of analgesia and appropriate intravenous antibiotics. If neurological deficit develops, operative decompression may be required. In contrast, epidural hematoma

Table 14.3 Neurological features of obstetric traumatic neuropathies

Site of injury	Neurological signs
Lumbosacral trunk (L4-5)	Weakness ankle dorsiflexion and eversion. Sensory loss over lateral aspect of the thigh, lower leg and dorsum of foot.
Sciatic nerve (L4-S3)	Weakness of knee flexion, ankle dorsiflexion, plantar flexion, inversion, eversion, weakness of the toes. Sensory loss posterior thigh, lateral and posterior calf, foot. Absent ankle jerk and plantar response.
Common peroneal nerve (L4-5)	Weakness of ankle dorsiflexion and eversion, weakness of extension of toes. Sensory loss minimal, lateral lower leg and dorsum of foot. Reflexes intact.
Obturator nerve (L2-4)	Weakness of hip adduction to a lesser extent, internal and external rotation. Sensory loss medial lower thigh. Reflexes intact (except adductor reflex).
Femoral nerve (L2-4)	Weakness of knee extension, hip flexion. Sensory loss anterior and anteromedial thigh, medial lower leg. Loss of knee jerk.

usually develops within 12 h of the spinal or epidural anesthetic. The persistence or recurrence of neurological block may be the first sign and again urgent neuroimaging is required if the diagnosis is suspected. The risk of epidural hematoma increases with the use of indwelling epidural catheters or the concomitant use of agents that affect hemostasis such as low molecular weight heparin particularly in the presence of non-steroidal anti-inflammatory drugs. Low dose aspirin is not considered a risk factor for epidural hematoma.

Guillain–Barre syndrome

Guillain–Barre syndrome is a rare condition of acute inflammatory demyelinating polyneuropathy.

Although the incidence is not increased in pregnancy, it is more common in the first 2-4 weeks postpartum. In the majority of cases an infection, most commonly campylobacter, cytomegalovirus or Epstein–Barr virus precedes the symptoms and signs. The disease is thought to be immune mediated, but its pathogenesis is unclear. The pathological finding is stripping of myelin from axons throughout the peripheral nervous system secondary to immune activation of macrophages. Symptoms and signs include rapidly progressive symmetrical weakness, loss of tendon reflexes, facial diplegia, oropharyngeal and respiratory paralysis, and impaired sensation in the hands and feet. The symptoms evolve rapidly over days to weeks, followed by a period of stability and then gradual improvement, often back to normal. Of cases described in pregnancy, about one-third required ventilatory support and the maternal mortality rate was 13%. Intravenous immunoglobulin and plasmapheresis are used in many cases and have been employed in pregnancy. Any case of a paralytic illness in pregnancy leading to reduced mobility should be given thromboprophylaxis for the period of impairment, as the incidence of thrombosis is high.

MULTIPLE SCLEROSIS

Multiple sclerosis (MS) is a demyelinating disorder characterized by recurrent or chronically progressive neurological dysfunction. Lesions may be found in the brain, optic nerves or spinal cord. Women are more commonly affected and the onset of disease is commonly in the child bearing years. The progress of MS may be highly variable with some patients remaining normal for years between attacks while others develop cumulative neurological disability. The most recent study of the natural course of MS during pregnancy found that the risk of relapse was lowest in late pregnancy but increased in the 3 months following delivery. This was unaffected by epidural anesthesia or breastfeeding. The net result from the year surrounding pregnancy, i.e. including the three postnatal months, seems to be that there is no greater likelihood of disease activity than in any other 1-year period. Women with MS should be counseled before pregnancy regarding the maternal and fetal risks of the disease and its treatment. The tendency for a natural improvement during pregnancy may allow the suspension of disease suppressing therapy prior to or early in pregnancy. Treatment of acute relapses and supportive measures, both pharmacological and rehabilitation, may be used as an alternative approach during pregnancy.

The management of relapses depends on their clinical severity. Mild relapses may need supportive treatment only whilst more severe relapses are usually treated with high dose corticosteroids. Prophylactic treatment is reserved for patients with relapsing-remitting MS to reduce the frequency of attacks, the rate of MS lesion appearances on MRI and the accumulation of disability. Beta-interferons are the standard therapy used for prophylaxis. Glatiramer is a synthetic amino acid polymer administered intramuscularly which is also useful for the prevention of progress in relapsing MS. Best results are seen when the drugs are initiated early in the course of the disease.

Supportive drug treatment is directed towards symptom management, e.g. imipramine for urinary urgency or bethanecol for urinary retention. Spasticity may be a significant symptom in more severe cases and drugs such as baclofen may be required. Paroxysmal pain and dysesthesia are disabling symptoms that may require treatment with drugs such as carbamazepine or gabapentin. Even prior to pregnancy, fatigue and depression can be prominent symptoms and these may be exacerbated by pregnancy. Treatment with amantadine or antidepressants may be appropriate. Probably just as important as pharmacologic treatment is support from a caring family for the woman with multiple sclerosis after delivery. If she is left to deal alone with the difficulties and challenges of a new child, lactation, sleeplessness and the emotional turmoil of new motherhood, a relapse is all the more predictable.

MYASTHENIA GRAVIS

Myasthenia gravis is an autoimmune condition characterized by muscle fatiguability and weakness. Specific antibodies to acetylcholine receptors can be measured in many affected patients and transplacental passage of these immunoglobulins during pregnancy may rarely lead to arthrogryposis multiplex congenita, a syndrome of nonprogressive congenital contractures resulting from lack of fetal movement in utero. More commonly, transient signs of myasthenia are seen in the neonate (10-30%). Although myasthenia gravis is an uncommon disorder, it primarily affects young women in the second and third decades of life, overlapping with the childbearing years. Pregnancy generally leads to an improvement in symptoms with a tendency to deteriorate postpartum.

The treatment of myasthenia gravis may include drug therapy and/or thymectomy. Drugs may be used for acute management or disease suppression. In mild cases, anticholinesterase drugs alone may be adequate. During early pregnancy, vomiting may impair absorption of these agents and occasionally parenteral administration will be required. Symptoms may result from both inadequate treatment and overdosage (cholinergic crisis) and careful supervision and dose/dose interval modification may be needed. A number of commonly used drugs including aminoglycosides, local anesthetics, beta-blockers and neuromuscular blockers, as well as infections may cause exacerbations in women with myasthenia gravis. Women with myasthenia gravis should *not* be given magnesium sulfate as this may precipitate acute weakness.

Immunosuppressive agents including prednisolone, cyclosporine and azathioprine are used for long-term disease control. On balance, the benefits of these therapies in this condition outweigh the associated risks. Intravenous immunoglobulin and plasmapheresis have also been used for myasthenic crisis or in severe cases. These modalities are considered safe for use in pregnancy. Thymectomy is utilized as a primary disease controlling modality and is generally performed prior to pregnancy. Studies indicate that thymectomized patients have fewer clinical exacerbations during pregnancy and a lower incidence of neonatal myasthenia.

CEREBROVASCULAR DISEASES

Although rare, cerebrovascular disease remains a significant cause of maternal morbidity and mortality. Stroke is an acute neurological injury due to ischemia or infarction caused by embolization, occlusion or rupture of a vessel. Amongst the causes of stroke (see Table 14.4), arterial infarction is the most common in pregnancy. The incidence of stroke is slightly increased during pregnancy, particularly in the third trimester, although the majority of pregnancy related stroke occurs in the 6 weeks postpartum. Epidemiological studies suggest an attributable risk (i.e. the excess caused by the pregnancy) of 8.1 strokes per 100 000 pregnancies [CI 6.4,9.7]. In the acute period, management is directed towards localizing the site of the lesion and determining the cause. This will involve careful history taking, clinical examination and appropriate neuroimaging. Cerebral CT scanning with appropriate shielding of the fetus and MRI/MRA are both considered safe in pregnancy. Lumbar puncture may also be required if infection or inflammatory vasculitis is considered a possibility.

Table 14.4 Causes of stroke in pregnancy

Cause	
Ischemic	Pre-eclampsia/eclampsia
	Arterial thrombosis
	Venous thrombosis
	Arterial embolism: direct and paradoxical
	Amniotic fluid embolism
	Vasculitis, e.g. systemic lupus erythematosus
	Thrombotic thrombocytopenic purpura
	Carotid artery dissection
Hemorrhagic	Severe pre-eclampsia
	Disseminated intravascular coagulation
	Cerebral venous thrombosis
	Arteriovenous malformation
	Cerebral aneurysm
	Hypertension
	Cocaine, anticoagulants

Ischemic stroke

In the older pregnant woman, atherosclerosis may be a cause of stroke, particularly in association with risk factors such as hypertension and smoking. In younger patients, underlying thrombophilias including the antiphospholipid antibody syndrome, or vasculitis should be considered. In this age group, carotid artery dissection should be excluded and its presence is suggested by a history of trauma or neck pain. Arteritis is a rare cause of stroke in pregnancy and may be associated with underlying immune or infectious diseases. Postpartum cerebral angiopathy is a poorly understood condition in which the patient develops stenosis and ectasia of the cerebral vessels with associated areas of hemorrhage or ischemia. It presents with headache, seizure and focal neurological deficit and may represent a form of eclampsia. Disorders of coagulation including thrombophilias, platelet abnormalities and hemoglobinopathies such as sickle cell disease may be associated with stroke in pregnancy. The hypercoagulability of pregnancy may exacerbate a pre-existing thrombophilia, particularly around the time of delivery. Thrombotic thrombocytopenic purpura is three times more common in pregnancy. In this condition, endothelial damage leads to increased platelet fibrin thrombi deposition within cerebral arterioles causing cerebral ischemia and subsequent headache, disorientation, seizures and stroke. The condition is diagnosed by the associated findings of microangiopathic hemolytic anemia, high lactic dehydrogenase, fever and renal impairment.

Arterial emboli from the heart cause approximately 30% of strokes observed in patients under the age of 40. They may be secondary to structural heart disease such as septal or valvular abnormalities, endocarditis or arrhythmias. Peripartum cardiomyopathy or myocardial infarction may cause stroke by hypoperfusion or from cerebral emboli secondary to mural thrombi. Paradoxical emboli associated with venous thrombosis and septal defects although rare may be an important cause of stroke in pregnancy as increased right heart pressure during labor and delivery may increase the risk of right-left shunting. The cause of stroke is not always apparent and a subgroup is designated 'cryptogenic stroke'. In this group the prognosis in terms of recurrence risk is relatively low. Cerebral venous sinus thrombosis is discussed above.

The treatment of ischemic stroke in pregnancy or the puerperium includes supportive care, antiplatelet agents and anticoagulants. Thrombolytic therapy may be indicated but the potential benefits of its use in pregnancy must be considered in the context of its recognized risk of bleeding. Percutaneous or surgical management of structural heart disease, such as the closure of a septal defect or valve replacement is usually delayed until after delivery.

Hemorrhagic stroke

Intracranial hemorrhage accounts for between 38 and 51% of all strokes associated with pregnancy. Subarachnoid hemorrhage (SAH) is the leading cause, most commonly from rupture of a pre-existing cerebral aneurysm. The remainder of SAH cases are due to bleeding from arteriovenous malformations (AVMs). Hypertension, family history, previous SAH, smoking and 'crack' cocaine are known risk factors. Patients with SAH present with sudden severe headache and rapid onset of photophobia, neck stiffness, impaired consciousness and stroke. Management consists of localizing the aneurysm or AVM with cerebral angiography and securing it to prevent further bleeding. Additional measures to control raised intracranial pressure may be required. In view of the high mortality rate in this condition, the decision to clip or embolize the lesion during pregnancy should be based on neurosurgical criteria. Delivery will have no benefit for the mother and should only be considered on compelling obstetric grounds. However, in terminal and irretrievable cases where there is evidence of maternal progression towards death, it may be necessary to consider perimortem Cesarean delivery to secure at least one survivor of the catastrophe.

Intracerebral hemorrhage during pregnancy or the postpartum period may be associated with hypertension, coagulopathies, the use of anticoagulants, or vascular malformations. Hemorrhage may occur in the context of pre-eclampsia/eclampsia (particularly systolic hypertension), placental abruption, massive postpartum hemorrhage or amniotic fluid embolism. Cerebral hemorrhage was for many years the chief cause of death in pre-eclampsia and eclampsia, justifying aggressive management of severe hypertension. Correction of any coagulopathy associated with the above conditions is also necessary.

The presentation of hemorrhage may be indistinguishable from ischemic stroke and urgent cerebral imaging with non-contrast CT will identify most hemorrhages. MRI may be required for the identification of petechial hemorrhages. Management is directed to correcting any coagulopathy, controlling hypertension and general supportive measures. Surgical management of an underlying AVM may be considered as the risk of rebleeding in the same pregnancy has been estimated at 27%.

Pre-conception counseling

Women with a previous stroke or transient ischemic episode may be at increased risk of stroke in pregnancy depending on the etiology of their previous event. Women with a recognized thrombophilia, history of cerebral emboli or pre-existing vasculitis, e.g. SLE may require prophylaxis with antiplatelet agents or anticoagulants in pregnancy. Most of these events are arterial and it is difficult to estimate the additional risk associated with pregnancy, although studies have shown a very low risk of recurrence. Large randomized studies have demonstrated the safety of low dose aspirin in pregnancy. Less information is available about clopidogrel and dipyridamole although animal studies suggest no evidence of adverse effect in pregnancy. If anticoagulation is required, low molecular weight heparin is preferred although warfarin may be have to be considered in certain situations. It may be appropriate to consider surgery or percutaneous management of a structural cardiac lesion prior to pregnancy to reduce the risk of complications. The postpartum period is probably the time of greatest risk and consideration should be given to the administration of prophylactic anticoagulation for 6 weeks postpartum, analogous to the recommendations for thromboprophylaxis after previous venous thrombosis.

Some women may present for pre-conception counseling because of a known risk factor for stroke such as a family history of cerebral aneurysm. Unruptured aneurysms are detected in 4% of such patients. Consideration should be given to neuroimaging to further assess the risk although prospective figures are not available to specifically estimate the risk of rupture during pregnancy or labor. A small study of the prognosis of women in subsequent pregnancies following a pregnancy with stroke has indicated a zero risk of recurrence. Some of these women were treated with prophylactic anticoagulation or antiplatelet agents. Larger studies indicate a recurrence rush up to 2%.

Labor and delivery

Vaginal delivery is associated with a potential increase in intracranial and intrathoracic pressure. There are therefore concerns regarding labor in women with stroke secondary to paradoxical emboli or septal defects. It is impossible to calculate the risk but it would seem adequate to continue aspirin and allow normal delivery, taking precautions to minimize the period of Valsalva or breath holding, and providing assistance to shorten the second stage and minimize its exhaustive effects on the mother. Intracranial pressure rises of 53-70 cm of water have been described with bearing down during labor. For this reason and others, the mode of delivery in women with previous hemorrhagic stroke or known unrepaired cerebral anomaly is controversial. It would seem prudent to avoid vaginal delivery in women with an unrepaired cerebral aneurysm or arteriovenous malformation whilst the decision for Cesarean or vaginal delivery should be on obstetric grounds alone if the risk of recurrent hemorrhage is very low.

CEREBRAL TUMORS

Although very rare, cerebral tumors or metastases are the fifth most common cause of cancer death in young women and may present during pregnancy. They may present with symptoms of headache, which is most often gradual in onset, progressive and unremitting. The headache is generally exacerbated by maneuvers that raise ICP such as coughing or exercise. Other symptoms depend on the site and size of the tumor and may include altered mentation, focal neurological deficits, seizures or nausea and vomiting. The latter must be distinguished from hyperemesis gravidarum by careful examination of the retinal fundi for papilledema. Any suspicion of raised ICP should prompt consideration of neuroimaging. The expansion of intravascular fluid volume and hormonal changes that accompany pregnancy may exacerbate a pre-existing tumor. In addition, metastases from choriocarcinoma must also be considered if cerebral tumor is suspected during pregnancy. MRI is the preferred method of imaging when cerebral tumor is suspected although CT scanning before and after IV contrast (with appropriate fetal shielding) is a more convenient and available modality for initial assessment.

Primary cerebral tumors

The hormonal effects of pregnancy may alter primary tumor growth while the dramatic shifts in intravascular volume around the time of delivery may lead to a rapid increase in tumor mass in the postpartum period. These changes have been seen with a number of malignant and benign tumors in pregnancy including gliomas, meningiomas and acoustic neuromas. The timing of surgery and or radiotherapy must be guided by neurosurgical indications but close to term, delivery may be indicated to expedite maternal treatment, with close observation in the postpartum period. Following delivery, excess tumor growth is said to regress.

Low-grade malignant gliomas are generally observed during pregnancy and treatment deferred until after delivery. Higher grade tumors, e.g. anaplastic astrocytomas and glioblastoma multiforme, although very rare, have a poor prognosis, even with treatment. Surgical intervention is often required urgently and craniotomy during pregnancy may be required. Radiotherapy (60 Gy to the tumor) is often commenced 2-3 weeks after surgery but may be delayed if delivery is possible in a short time. Adjunctive chemotherapy may also be necessary and the development of implantable chemotherapy, placed at the surgical site at the time of craniotomy, allows the delivery of high dose chemotherapy with minimal systemic exposure. If systemic chemotherapy is required, it may be delayed until completion of the pregnancy with little effect on overall prognosis. Meningiomas and acoustic neuromas, although benign, may cause significant morbidity by their space occupying effects. Evidence suggests that the majority of menigiomas contain estrogen and progesterone receptors. During pregnancy, meningiomas may increase in size and decrease following delivery. The patient should be closely observed during pregnancy and the immediate postpartum period and surgery is generally deferred until after delivery.

Pituitary tumors

These are generally classified on the basis of their size with microadenomas measuring < 1 cm and larger tumors being macroadenomas. They may exert their effects by means of their hormonal secretions (functional) or by their mass effect. The latter may produce neurological symptoms such as headache or visual deficit or endocrine effects of pituitary insufficiency. Diagnosis is generally made by MRI/CT or analysis of serum hormone levels. The latter may be difficult to interpret during pregnancy. Prolactinomas are a recognized cause of infertility often presenting with oligo/amenorrhea and anovulation. Treatment with dopamine antagonists, e.g. bromocriptine or carbergoline, can restore fertility. Once pregnant, women with pituitary tumors should be monitored closely for signs of increasing tumor size with visual field testing each trimester. Monitoring of prolactin levels is of no value in pregnancy. MRI is utilized for those with known macroadenomas or evidence of neurological deterioration. Prolactin secreting microadenomas rarely grow significantly in size and in these women, dopamine antagonists do not need to be continued during pregnancy or while breast feeding. Pituitary hormone deficiency must be managed in the standard manner during pregnancy. Treatment with surgery or radiation therapy should be based on neurosurgical indications.

Choriocarcinoma

Brain metastases commonly occur in women with choriocarcinoma and may be the presenting symptom in up to 20% of women with this rare tumor. The symptoms may have a gradual onset or there may be sudden onset of headache or neurological deterioration, particularly if there is sudden hemorrhage into the tumor. Concurrent pulmonary metastases are often detected along with the characteristic elevation of betaHCG. These tumors are very sensitive to chemotherapy and radiotherapy and craniotomy is rarely required. As there is no viable fetus, prompt treatment is the norm and the prognosis is very good.

Labor and delivery

The same concerns regarding changes in ICP in women with stroke apply to the woman with cerebral tumor. Epidural anesthesia is contraindicated if there is any risk of 'coning'. In patients with larger lesions and raised intracranial pressure, prolonged bearing down should be avoided. If there is disturbed mentation or focal neurological deficit, elective Cesarean delivery may be more appropriate. In all cases of macroadenoma, the risk of postpartum deterioration should be considered and the woman closely observed.

SUMMARY

- The diagnosis and management of neurological disorders in pregnancy requires a careful history and examination as well as appropriate investigations to anatomically localize the abnormality and determine the likely pathophysiology.
- Pre-existing neurological conditions should be carefully assessed prior to pregnancy. Appropriate advice needs to be given to the woman and her family regarding the prognosis and effects of her condition during and after pregnancy as well as the potential effects of therapy during pregnancy.
- Detailed information should be sought regarding the potential adverse effects of medications used for the treatment of neurological diseases particularly anticonvulsant drugs. Modifications to anticonvulsant therapy, e.g. monotherapy at the lowest possible dose, should be made to reduce these risks.
- The development of new neurological symptoms and signs in pregnancy requires careful assessment and prompt management.
- Appropriate plans should be made for the management of labor and delivery in those conditions that may be adversely affected by rises in intracranial pressure or the stresses of labor.

Further reading

Adab N et al 2005 Common antiepileptic drugs in pregnancy in women with epilepsy. Cochrane Database of Systematic Reviews 3:CD004848

Bleeker C P et al 2004 Postpartum post-dural puncture headache: is your differential diagnosis complete? British Journal of Anaesthesia 93:461-464

Cheng Q et al 1998 Increased incidence of Guillain-Barre syndrome postpartum. Epidemiology 9:601-604

Djelmis J et al 2002 Myasthenia gravis in pregnancy: report on 69 cases. European Journal of Obstetrics Gynecology Reproduction and Biology 104(1):21-25

Jaigobin C, Silver F L 2000 Stroke and pregnancy. Stroke. 31:2948-2951

Lowe S A 2001 Drugs in pregnancy. Anticonvulsants and drugs for neurological disease. Best Practia Research in Clinical Obstetrics Gynaecology 15(6): 863-876

Mabie W C 2005 Peripheral neuropathies during pregnancy. Clinical Obstetrics Gynecology 48:57-66

Martin J N Jr et al 2005 Stroke and severe preeclampsia and eclampsia: a paradigm shift focusing on systolic blood pressure. Obstetrics & Gynecology 105(2): 246-254

Morrow J I et al 2006 Malformation risks of anti-epileptic drugs in pregnancy: a prospective study from the UK Epilepsy and Pregnancy Register. Journal of Neurology, Neurosurgery, and Psychiatry 77(2):193-198. Epub 2005 Sep 12

Stevenson C B, Thompson R C 2005 The clinical management of intracranial neoplasms in pregnancy. Clinical Obstetrics and Gynecology 48(1):24-37

Turan T N, Stern B J 2004 Stroke in pregnancy. Neurologic Clinics 22:821-840

Vukusic S et al 2004 Pregnancy and multiple sclerosis (the PRIMS study): clinical predictors of post-partum relapse. Brain 127(Pt 6):1353-1360

Wong C A et al 2003 Incidence of postpartum lumbosacral spine and lower extremity nerve injuries. Obstetrics & Gynecology 101(2):279-288

Zahn C A et al 1998 Management issues for women with epilepsy: a review of the literature. Neurology 51(4):949-956

Chapter **15**

Dermatological disease in pregnancy

S. A. Vaughan Jones

SYNOPSIS

Physiological skin changes
Specific dermatoses of pregnancy
Dermatoses exacerbated by pregnancy

PHYSIOLOGICAL SKIN CHANGES

During pregnancy a number of physiological skin changes occur which are believed to result from the hormonal changes induced by pregnancy. It is important that these should be recognized as normal findings, distinct from the pregnancy dermatoses. Some of these changes may be of cosmetic significance to the woman and of importance to the dermatologist or obstetrician (see Table 15.1).

Hyperpigmentation

Hyperpigmentation of varying degrees is common during pregnancy and occurs in up to 90% of pregnant women. This is often localized to the areolae, genitalia, neck, axillae and periumbilical skin. It is often more pronounced in women with darker hair and skin color. The linea alba darkens to become the linea nigra, a hyperpigmented vertical streak on the midline of the abdomen. Pre-existing freckles, scars and naevi may also darken, although these pigmentary changes tend to regress postpartum. This phenomenon is thought to be due to increased levels of alpha and beta-melanocyte stimulating hormone (MSH), beta-endorphin, estrogen and progesterone all of which can stimulate melanogenesis, although this is still disputed.

Previous reports have suggested that pigmented lesions may darken in color due to increased pigmentation in pregnancy. A recent study of 22 patients found that pregnancy is not associated with any significant change in melanocytic naevi. There is also no convincing evidence in the literature that pregnancy induces malignant change within melanocytic naevi. However moles with a history of change in color should be examined closely to exclude malignant melanoma (see later).

A related phenomenon is melasma (formally called chloasma) which is seen both in pregnancy and with oral contraceptive therapy. This is a symmetrical brown hyperpigmentation commonly involving the cheeks, forehead, upper lip, nose and chin. It can occur in three patterns – centrofacial, malar or mandibular depending on the distribution of pigmentation. Histologically, excessive melanin deposition is seen either in the epidermis or dermal macrophages. This condition is exacerbated by excessive sun exposure and treatment should therefore include potent sunscreens, avoidance of ultraviolet radiation and irritating cosmetics. Fortunately, unlike the melasma associated with oral contraceptives, the melasma of pregnancy usually regresses postpartum, with only 10% of cases persisting.

Striae distensae (gravidarum)

Striae distensae develop in both puberty and pregnancy and are often preceded by stretching of the skin or rapid weight gain. They are seen in up to 90% of pregnant women and are uncommon in black and Asian women. These irregular, linear, pink or viola-

Table 15.1 Physiological changes in skin, nails and hair

Hyperpigmentation	Vascular changes
Melasma	Decreased apocrine gland activity
Striae distensae	Increased sebaceous gland activity
Pruritus gravidarum	Increased eccrine gland activity
Hair changes	
Nail changes	

ceous atrophic bands of tissue develop on the abdomen initially and then on the thighs, breasts, upper back, buttocks and inguinal areas later in pregnancy. The etiology of striae is still unclear. Stress-induced rupture of the connective tissue was proposed as a possible explanation although other studies have shown dense elastic tissue deposition compatible with scar formation. Liu (1974) proposed that pregnancy produces an increase in relaxin, estrogen and corticosteroid production. These hormones relax the adhesiveness between collagen fibers and promote the formation of polysaccharide ground substance, causing separation and striae formation at sites of distension. Striae may form due to structural changes which include realignment and reduced elastin and fibrillin fibres in the dermis. There also appears to be a significant association between the occurrence of striae and heavier babies as well as heavier or obese women. A recent report showed that family history and race were significantly predictive of striae distensae development. The role of massage in prevention of striae is still debated. One report showed a good response to topical tretinoin although this would not be recommended during pregnancy. A second report showed no beneficial effect of topical tretinoin 0.025% cream. Postpartum the discolouration of striae fades to leave persistent pale atrophic lines.

Pruritus gravidarum

Pruritus is one of the commonest physiological skin changes, affecting between 3-14% of all pregnancies. The etiology is probably multifactorial. It is thought that estrogen impairs transport of bile to the bile canaliculi, leading to an increase in circulating bile salts, while prostaglandins reduce the threshold for pruritus. Many women report an increase in skin dryness during pregnancy which may also contribute to pruritus. However a detailed history and physical examination is essential to exclude a systemic cause such as diabetes, thyroid, liver or renal disease. Obstetric cholestasis (OC) should be excluded by analysis of serum liver function tests and bile acids as

this is the most important differential diagnosis (see Ch. 9). Physiological pruritus is generalized or localized to the abdomen whereas the itch in OC is often nocturnal and localized especially to the palms and soles. A positive family history may help point towards the diagnosis of OC as this appears to have a genetic component. The treatment of pruritus gravidarum is antihistamine therapy (e.g. chlorpheniramine). Soothing emollients such as aqueous cream (with 1-2% added menthol) can also be helpful.

Hair changes

On the scalp the proportion of hairs in the anagen (growing phase) increases during pregnancy as the conversion from anagen to telogen (resting phase) hairs is slowed, thus creating thicker hair growth. However, this process is altered postpartum with a greater number of hairs entering the telogen phase and consequent shedding. Normally about 15% of scalp hairs are in the telogen phase and in pregnancy this falls to 5%, rising within a few months of delivery to 25%. This marked increase in telogen hair shedding is seen frequently in the postpartum period and can be a source of concern to the patient. This phenomenon is known as telogen effluvium and is also seen 3 months after stress or severe illness. This hair loss is generally diffuse but there can be a tendency to fronto-parietal hair loss, with so-called male pattern alopecia. Hair growth generally returns to normal up to 6-12 months after delivery although it may take as long as 15 months.

Mild hirsutism may appear in pregnancy to a varying degree most commonly involving the face, arms, legs and back. It generally reverses and disappears following delivery. It is thought to be due to increased ovarian production of androgens during pregnancy. Other causes such as polycystic ovary syndrome and androgen-secreting ovarian tumors should be excluded if marked hirsutism persists postpartum. Treatment is with reassurance and if necessary cosmetic removal (depilatory creams, electrolysis or ruby laser).

Nail changes

Nail changes during pregnancy include transverse and longitudinal grooving, brittleness and distal onycholysis. The pathogenesis of these nail changes is unknown. An attempt should be made to eliminate external sensitizers (nail polish, nail removers) and infections. The nails should be kept short if they are brittle or prone to onycholysis. Longitudinal melanonychia has also been reported to develop during pregnancy.

Vacular changes

The vascular system of a pregnant woman undergoes profound changes to accommodate the fetus and its growth. There is a substantial increase in blood volume, vascular distention, capillary permeability and new blood vessel formation. These changes are probably mediated by increased pituitary, adrenal and placental hormone secretion.

Vascular proliferation can result in the development of spider naevi particularly on the face and upper chest. Palmar erythema appears as diffuse mottled erythema localized to the thenar or hypothenar eminences. It often appears in the first trimester and resolves rapidly following delivery. Unilateral naevoid telangiectasia syndrome is a collection of spider naevi in a dermatomal distribution, often on face, neck and chest. This can occur in pregnancy where estrogen levels are high, and also in alcoholic liver disease and with oral contraceptive therapy.

Other vascular changes during pregnancy include flushing due to vasomotor instability and an increase in venous varicosities resulting from increased venous pressure in femoral and pelvic vessels. Non pitting edema is also very common in the third trimester affecting the face, hands, ankles and feet, occurring in between 50% and 70% of women. Edema generally subsides soon after delivery. Other causes such as preeclampsia, thyroid and cardiac abnormalities should be excluded. Management of varicosities, peripheral edema and flushing is generally conservative. Small hemangiomas can arise in pregnancy usually on the trunk and frequently regress following delivery.

Eccrine/apocrine gland activity

Eccrine gland activity is increased in pregnancy leading to an increase in hyperhidrosis and dyshidrotic eczema, while apocrine gland activity is reduced so that Fox–Fordyce disease and hidradenitis suppurativa tend to improve. Sebaceous gland activity tends to increase particularly in the third trimester so that acne vulgaris may either be exacerbated or develop for the first time. The rate of excretion of sebum tends to increase in pregnancy and returns to normal after delivery. In 30 to 50% of pregnant women brown papules appear on the areolae in early pregnancy. These are called Montgomery's tubercles and result from hypertrophy of the sebaceous glands but do not persist postpartum.

Immune system changes

There are key changes in the immune system during pregnancy and this may help to explain the effects of pregnancy on the skin and the increased susceptibility to certain skin diseases. During pregnancy the immune response is biased towards antibody production and away from cell mediated immunity to enable the fetus (allograft) to survive and to prevent fetal rejection. This may explain the apparent increase in autoimmune skin disease and increased incidence of skin infections (see later). It may also explain why there is often an improvement in psoriasis (Th1-mediated) while there is a deterioration in atopic eczema (Th2-mediated).

The Th2 (subset of CD4 + cells) cytokine pattern is associated with antibody responses suggesting that Th2-type cytokines predominate in the regulation of the maternal immune response. IL-3, IL-4, IL-5, IL-10 and IL-13 are all Th2 cytokines. Animal studies have shown that these cytokines can be detected in the placenta in all three trimesters of pregnancy. IL-10 suppresses Th1-mediated cellular immunity. The switch from Th1 to Th2 cytokine profile within the placenta thus allows fetal tolerance despite the presence of paternal MHC antigens.

Box 15.1 lists the key points in management of skin conditions in pregnancy.

SPECIFIC DERMATOSES OF PREGNANCY

The specific dermatoses of pregnancy have led to much confusion in the past due to the clinical overlap between the various conditions and lack of agreed terminology. A rationalized clinical classification is now widely recognized (see Table 15.2). Apart from pemphigoid gestationis (PG) no reliable diagnostic criteria exist to differentiate between these conditions. It was hoped that this classification would facilitate clinical investigation and thereby improve our understanding of the etiology of these dermatoses. Papular dermatitis of pregnancy is not included in this classification and is now thought to overlap with prurigo and PEP and not to be a separate clinical entity.

So far in published data there have been two prospective studies which have examined the prevalence of these disorders in pregnant populations.

Pemphigoid gestationis

Pemphigoid gestationis (PG) is a rare autoimmune bullous disease of pregnancy and the puerperium first described by Milton (1872) as 'herpes gestationis' because of the morphological similarity of individual lesions to herpetic vesicles. This term has now been abandoned as it caused confusion with the herpes virus-mediated skin infection. PG has a consistent relationship to pregnancy, the puerperium and rarely,

Box 15.1 Management: key points

- It is important to recognize the key physiological skin changes in pregnancy.
- Melasma is commonly seen in pregnancy or with oral contraceptive therapy.
- Pre-existing moles/naevi may darken during pregnancy but should be examined closely to exclude malignant melanoma.
- Striae gravidarum are common and may respond to local massage with emollients. The role of topical retinoids postpartum is debatable.
- Physiological pruritus is common but obstetric cholestasis (OC) should be excluded in cases of late and persistent pruritus.
- Emollients and systemic antihistamines are useful in the management of all cases of pruritus gravidarum.
- Telogen effluvium often presents as diffuse hair loss post partum but hair growth generally starts to improve within 6-12 months after delivery.
- Common vascular changes in pregnancy include spider naevi, palmar erythema, varicosities and peripheral edema.
- Maternal androgens may cause hirsutism and increase sebaceous gland activity thus causing acne vulgaris.
- Immune changes in pregnancy may partly explain the exacerbation of certain skin diseases, e.g. atopic eczema.

Table 15.2 Specific Dermatoses of pregnancy

New classification	Previous terminology
Pemphigoid gestationis	Herpes gestationis
Polymorphic eruption of pregnancy (PEP)	Toxemic rash of pregnancy
	Late-onset prurigo of pregnancy
	Pruritic urticarial papules and plaques of pregnancy (PUPPP)
	Toxic erythema of pregnancy
	Erythema multiforme of pregnancy
Prurigo of pregnancy	Prurigo gestationis of Besnier
	Early onset prurigo of pregnancy
Pruritic folliculitis	Unknown

Box 15.2 Pemphigoid gestationis

- Neonatal PG occurs in 5-10% cases causing transient rash for 3-4 weeks.
- Direct IMF is the diagnostic test (skin biopsy) with positive staining for Complement 3 +/− IgG.
- Rx – usually oral prednisolone 30-40 mg daily.
- Alternative Rx – plasmapheresis, ciclosporin, intravenous immunoglobulins for severe cases.
- Women should be counseled to avoid oral contraceptives, which can exacerbate the disease.
- Recurrence in subsequent pregnancies is common.

hydatidiform mole and choriocarcinoma. It is closely related to the pemphigoid group of autoimmune bullous diseases and its incidence has been reported in the literature as between 1 in 10 000 and 1 in 60 000 pregnancies. In a study the incidence of PG was 1 in 7000 pregnancies (Box 15.2).

The onset of a rash varies from between 9 weeks' gestation and 1 week postpartum, but it presents most frequently in the second and third trimesters. In approximately 14% of women PG presents in the postpartum period. If PG presents in the second trimester there is often a period of relative remission in the final few weeks of pregnancy followed by an abrupt postpartum flare of disease activity. Characteristically it recurs with increased severity and at an earlier gestation in subsequent pregnancies, although 'skipped' pregnancies can occur in approximately 8% of cases. A 'skipped' pregnancy refers to the situation when a patient presents with classical PG in one pregnancy, but in a subsequent pregnancy does not develop a cutaneous eruption. One hypothesis for this is when mother and fetus share HLA-DR antigens. The proposed mechanism may be via the induction of an exaggerated suppressor T-cell response in the presence of common HLA-DR antigen subtypes. Change of partner may also influence disease activity or expression. Recurrences of pruritus and blistering in PG are also seen when some women take oral contraceptives with estrogens or progestogens and around the menstrual cycle. For this reason counseling regarding family planning and further pregnancies is extremely important for women with PG.

In PG, early lesions are pruritic erythematous urticated plaques which may become annular or polycyclic. Gradually vesicles or bullae predominate so that lesions can closely resemble bullous pemphigoid. Lesions are often most marked in the periumbilical skin in 87% of cases before spreading over the abdomen, thighs, palms and soles. Blisters can occur de novo on otherwise clinically uninvolved skin and are usually intact blisters containing serous fluid. The face and oral mucosae are generally spared.

The histopathological features include marked edema with subepidermal separation and eosinophilic spongiosis. Basal cell necrosis may be a prominent feature. However, the diagnosis is confirmed by direct immunofluorescence (IMF) which demonstrates linear C3 basement membrane zone deposition in all cases, and in addition IgG in 27% cases. Circulating antibodies are detectable by indirect IMF and are usually of the complement-binding IgG1 subclass. These antibodies classically bind to the epidermal side of saline-split normal human skin and are directed against a component of hemidesmosomes of the basement membrane zone. Epitope mapping has shown that PG and bullous pemphigoid antibodies bind a common antigenic site within the non-collagenous domain (NC16A) of the transmembrane 180 kDa PG antigen. However there appears to be no good correlation between disease antibody titres and disease activity (see Fig. 15.1).

Neonatal pemphigoid gestationis

Transplacental transfer of these IgG anti-basement membrane zone antibodies can occur and may result in a neonatal blistering eruption which is milder and more transient than the maternal eruption – neonatal PG. This is seen in approximately 5-10% of women with PG. Skin lesions in cases of neonatal PG generally resolve within a few weeks as the maternal antibodies are catabolized so require no specific treatment other than simple wound care and prevention of secondary infection.

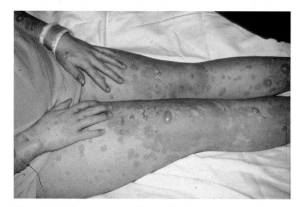

Figure 15.1 A severe case of pemphigoid gestationis with blistering on the arms and legs on a background of urticated erythema.

The fetal prognosis in PG has been a controversial issue, with only results from a few studies available. One study compared fetal outcome in pregnancies from 74 women with PG with normal pregnancies from the same women. The results clearly indicated a significant increase in premature deliveries in the PG pregnancies, as well as a tendency for small-for-dates babies. They concluded that these findings were compatible with low-grade placental dysfunction in PG.

We previously reported two cases, both of whom initially presented with a bullous disorder of pregnancy typical of PG, but who later progressed into bullous pemphigoid over a long period of time. This indicates that the two conditions are part of the same continuum of disease but with differing clinical patterns. One of these cases responded initially to treatment with a luteinizing hormone releasing hormone analogue, inducing a reversible 'chemical oophorectomy', but then relapsed and continued to have active disease despite hysterectomy and bilateral oophorectomy. The other case developed ulcerative colitis and thyrotoxicosis due to underlying Graves' disease, again highlighting the strong association with other autoimmune disease. A higher incidence of antithyroid autoantibodies in patients with a history of PG has already been established.

The aim of treatment in PG is to suppress bullae formation, relieve pruritus and prevent erosions, secondary infection and scarring. In mild cases of PG potent topical corticosteroids combined with emollients and systemic antihistamines may be sufficient to suppress disease activity. However, once bullae are established systemic corticosteroids are usually necessary, generally starting at a dose of 30-40 mg of prednisolone daily. More severe cases may need doses of 40-80 mg prednisolone daily. Gradual reduction of the dose should then be possible over the following weeks. However, a postpartum flare often occurs so the dose may need to be increased following delivery in anticipation of this. Systemic corticosteroids do not appear to affect fetal prognosis directly. However, maternal gestational diabetes and hypertension are important side effects that can be encountered with high dose steroid administration over a prolonged period. These side effects should be screened for and managed appropriately. High doses of steroids can also be associated with premature rupture of the membranes and preterm delivery. Close liaison between the obstetrician and dermatologist are required to ensure that close maternal and fetal monitoring is maintained. Parental steroid supplements will be required in labor. Infants of women with PG treated with significant doses of systemic corticosteroids during pregnancy require assessment at birth by a neonatologist. Evidence of adrenal insufficiency should be sought by estimation of serum sodium, potassium and cortisol levels.

For those cases in whom systemic corticosteroids do not appear to be effective, other possible treatment modalities include ciclosporin, plasmapheresis and intravenous immunoglobulins. Postpartum, minocycline and nicotinamide have been reported to be effective in a few cases.

Polymorphic eruption of pregnancy

Polymorphic eruption of pregnancy (PEP) (previously named pruritic urticarial papules and plaques of pregnancy or PUPPP) was first described in 1979. Although the latter term is still used to describe this condition particularly in the USA, it is generally agreed that PEP and PUPPP are identical dermatoses. PEP more accurately describes the variable morphology of individual lesions which can be papular, plaque-like urticated wheals, vesicular and bullous. PEP is the commonest gestational dermatosis with an incidence of approximately 1:160 pregnancies and is now regarded as a distinct clinical entity although the clinical features can resemble other specific dermatoses of pregnancy. Three-quarters of patients are primigravida and the rash usually develops in the third trimester or postpartum period. In contrast to PG, PEP is predominantly a disease of primigravida women and when it recurs the second eruption is less severe than the first (Fig. 15.2, Box 15.3).

Pathogenesis

In contrast to PG, in PEP there is no association with autoimmune disease or HLA type and fetal prognosis is normal.

The common clinical presentation of PEP in abdominal striae led to the suggestion that abdominal distension may be an important factor in the etiology. Indeed, there is a significant association with excess maternal weight gain, increased fetal weight and multiple pregnancy. One group have postulated that increased maternal weight gain and abdominal girth due to rapid abdominal expansion may cause trauma to the overlying skin so triggering the inflammatory response of PEP. An earlier study described 25 patients with PEP and found four cases with twins (16%). The association with maternal or fetal weight gain has however been debated.

One study of sex hormones (serum beta-hCG, estradiol and cortisol) in women with PEP found no significant differences in these hormone levels in women with PEP. However a more recent prospective study of 44 cases of PEP found low serum cortisol levels compared with controls. The relevance of this finding is unclear, and requires further investigation.

The same study of 44 women with PEP found a male: female fetal sex ratio of 2:1 suggesting that PEP was commoner in women carrying a male fetus. Further data from a later study showed the presence of male DNA in the skin of women with PEP carrying male fetuses, suggesting a phenomenon of microchimerism whereby fetal cells migrate to maternal skin

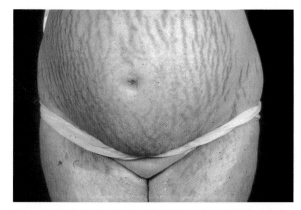

Figure 15.2 Polymorphic eruption of pregnancy (PEP) showing papules and plaques within striae on the anterior abdomen in a woman in her third trimester. Periumbilical sparing as seen here is typical of PEP.

Box 15.3 Polymorphic eruption of pregnancy (PEP)

- Commonest specific dermatosis – incidence 1:160.
- Usually affects primigravida women and recurrence is unusual.
- Fetal prognosis normal.
- Increased prevalence in multiple pregnancy – twins and triplet pregnancies.
- No diagnostic tests – direct IMF negative in most cases.
- Skin biopsy may be necessary to differentiate from PG in severe cases.
- Treatment usually involves use of topical steroids, emollients, antihistamines for pruritus.
- Early delivery should be considered if severe and resistant to treatment.
- Possible link with male fetus and microchimerism.
- True pathogenesis unknown.

during pregnancy. Whether this initiates the inflammatory response in PEP remains speculative. Thus although PEP is now a well-recognized entity the true pathogenesis of this condition has not been fully established.

Clinical features

The eruption tends to be short-lived with an average duration of 6 weeks. Lesions begin on the lower abdomen within striae, but sparing the umbilicus. Urticarial papules develop that coalesce to produce plaques, vesicles, target lesions and polycyclic wheals, and subsequently spread on to distal sites. Pruritus is a prominent symptom and as the lesions resolve fine scale and crusting appear, reminiscent of eczema. Clinically the lesions can occasionally appear similar to PG and can also be confused with scabies, erythema multiforme and drug eruptions. In PEP the umbilicus is frequently spared in marked contrast to PG, and this can be a helpful distinguishing feature between the two conditions. In a recent paper the authors categorized the clinical features into three types:

Type I   Mainly urticarial papules and plaques.
Type II   Non-urticarial erythema, papules or vesicles.
Type III Combinations of the two forms.

Histopathology of PEP varies with the clinical stage of the eruption, but often demonstrates variable features including upper dermal edema, scanty eosinophils and a perivascular lymphohistiocytic infiltrate. Some of these histopathological features are also seen in the other specific dermatoses of pregnancy.

Direct and indirect immunofluorescence and immunoelectron microscopy are characteristically negative and are important investigations to distinguish this condition from PG, which can appear clinically similar. Immunohistochemical studies in PEP have been limited but have so far suggested a predominantly T-helper lymphocytic response.

As PEP is self-limiting and often resolves after delivery without sequelae, symptomatic treatment alone is required. Moderately potent topical corticosteroids are usually more effective in relieving pruritus than antihistamines. The eruption can be severe for 1-2 weeks when a short reducing course of oral prednisolone may be indicated. A severe case of PEP unresponsive to therapy dramatically improved within 2 h of delivery by Cesarean section.

Maternal morbidity is a significant consideration in this group of patients, as the eruption classically occurs late in pregnancy when intense pruritus can cause loss of sleep with severe depression in some cases. For some patients induction of labor is an option if pruritus is severe and intractable.

In the remaining cases the most effective treatments used are antihistamines (chlorpheniramine), emollients (aqueous cream with 1-2% menthol) and topical corticosteroids (clobetasone butyrate 0.05% or betamethasone valerate 0.1%). Although the use of systemic corticosteroids has been reported in this condition this is generally reserved for severe cases.

Prurigo of pregnancy

Prurigo of pregnancy remains perhaps the least studied and least understood of all the pregnancy dermatoses. The incidence of prurigo varies from 1:300 to 1:450 pregnancies. It presents predominantly in the second or third trimester of pregnancy with grouped excoriated or crusted papules over the extensor aspects of the limbs and occasionally on the abdomen. Some lesions may appear eczematous and differential diagnosis from eczema can be difficult. The disease runs a protracted course and usually resolves shortly after delivery but can persist for up to three months. Recurrence in subsequent pregnancies is common. Serological tests are normal, histopathology non specific and immunofluorescence is negative. The hormonal abnormalities (elevated beta-hCG and reduced serum cortisol and estrogen concentrations) previously reported have not been confirmed in any other studies. There are no maternal risks, and the outcome of pregnancy is normal. Treatment is symptomatic only (Fig. 15.3, Box 15.4).

Since the original description there have been two further studies of patients with similar eruptions. One group discussed five patients with what they described as 'prurigo of late pregnancy' and noted some additional features to the original cases. Histopathological examination in four cases demonstrated a perivascular lympho-histiocytic infiltrate with occasional eosinophils, with both upper dermal edema and focal epidermal edema causing areas of vesicular spongiosis. Immunofluorescence studies in all cases were negative.

A later study of eight patients with prurigo found that each patient had features of an underlying atopic diathesis although none had typical eczematous lesions. Two studies showed elevation of serum IgE levels. The authors therefore postulated that prurigo of pregnancy may arise as a result of pruritus gravidarum occurring in atopic women. They based this argument on the finding that 18% of pregnancies are complicated by pruritus and that 10% of the population demonstrate atopy. It would therefore be predicted that both conditions would coexist in approximately 2% pregnancies.

Papular dermatitis of pregnancy previously described is now thought to be a variant of prurigo in pregnancy.

Pruritic folliculitis of pregnancy

The first description of pruritic folliculitis of pregnancy (PFP) was of six patients with pruritic erythematous follicular papules, and urticarial lesions in addition in two cases. In one case the eruption was confined to the limbs and abdomen, but in all others it was widespread. Onset during pregnancy was variable with the majority between the fourth and ninth months of pregnancy with resolution within 2-3 weeks of delivery. One patient experienced pre-menstrual recurrence of the rash, while two other patients gave a history of a similar eruption during a previous pregnancy. There were no other systemic features associated with this eruption, and both maternal and fetal prognoses were normal. Histopathological features of the papular lesions showed acute folliculitis in five of the six cases, with intra-follicular pustules comprising mixed inflammatory cells and some eosinophils. Direct immunofluorescence in four cases was negative, and bacteriological examination of the lesions with Gram staining revealed no significant organisms (Fig. 15.4, Box 15.5).

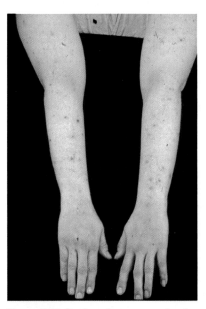

Figure 15.3 Prurigo of pregnancy showing excoriated papules on the arms.

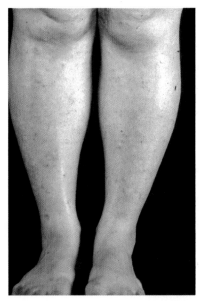

Figure 15.4 Pruritic folliculitis showing follicular papules on the extensor aspect of the lower legs.

Box 15.4 Prurigo of pregnancy

- Incidence 1:300 pregnancies.
- Pruritic papules on extensor aspects of the limbs or abdomen.
- Possible link with atopy – elevated serum IgE in some cases.
- Differential diagnosis from eczema may be difficult.
- Responds to emollients and antihistamines.
- Fetal prognosis normal.

Box 15.5 Pruritic folliculitis of pregnancy

- Pruritic eruption on acne sites – chest, back and rarely limbs.
- Generally improves during late pregnancy.
- No apparent increase in maternal serum androgen concentrations.
- Responds to topical acne treatments such as benzoyl peroxide 10% with 1% hydrocortisone.
- One case of good response to narrow band ultraviolet B therapy.
- Fetal prognosis normal.

The exact incidence of this eruption is not known but it is thought to be a hormonally induced acne. The clinical appearances are of a papulo-pustular folliculitis similar to the monomorphic acne seen in patients taking corticosteroids or progestogenic steroids. PFP classically occurs on acneiform sites i.e. on the upper chest and upper back but is also frequently seen on the lower limbs. There are no specific immunopathological features, and the histopathology is that of an inflammatory folliculitis.

PFP may respond to anti-acneiform treatments such as topical benzoyl peroxide 10% and 1% hydrocortisone. A recent study demonstrated the benefit of treatment with narrow band UVB (TL-01) in a patient who had failed to respond to other treatment.

DERMATOSES EXACERBATED BY PREGNANCY

The dermatoses exacerbated by pregnancy can largely be subdivided into inflammatory, infective, autoimmune, metabolic, miscellaneous skin disorders and skin tumors (Table 15.3). Of the inflammatory disorders such as eczema, psoriasis and acne vulgaris these appear to behave unpredictably in pregnancy. In those cases with pre-existing skin disease there may be relative remission during pregnancy but in the majority of cases there is exacerbation of disease or indeed these disorders may appear for the first time during pregnancy in individuals not previously affected.

Psoriasis

Psoriasis affects 1.5-2% of the normal population and is characterized by inflammatory scaly plaques on the skin surface, accompanied by a seronegative arthropathy in up to 7% of cases. Trauma or injury to the skin often results in localized psoriasis at the injury site (the Koebner phenomenon). Psoriasis has several distinct clinical types. The commonest of these is plaque-type with characteristic silvery scaly plaques on the extensor aspects of the limbs, sacrum and scalp. The guttate form consists of small scattered pink papules occurring in crops mainly on the trunk. It often follows an upper respiratory tract infection, particularly with streptococci. In erythrodermic psoriasis there is widespread erythema and a fine scale present often over the entire skin surface. Finally in pustular psoriasis there are small sterile pustules occurring either in pre-existing plaques or de novo on the skin surface.

The effect of pregnancy on psoriasis is unpredictable, although for most women there is usually an

Table 15.3 Dermatoses exacerbated by pregnancy

Inflammatory
  Psoriasis
  Atopic dermatitis
  Acne vulgaris/acne rosacea
  Urticaria
  Lichen planus
  Erythema nodosum
  Pityriasis Rosea
  Erythema multiforme
Infective
  Viral (herpes simplex, zoster)
  Bacterial (impetigo, TB, leprosy)
  Fungal (candida, pityrosporum sp.)
Autoimmune
  Lupus erythematosus (LE)
  Systemic sclerosis
  Polymyositis/dermatomyositis
  Pemphigus vulgaris/foliaceus
Metabolic
  Porphyria cutanea tarda
  Acrodermatitis enteropathica
  Connective tissue
  Ehlers-Danlos syndrome
  Pseudoxanthoma elasticum
Miscellaneous
  Erythrokeratoderma variabilis
  Mycosis fungoides
  Neurofibromatosis
  Acquired immune deficiency syndrome
Skin tumors
  Naevoid
    Melanoma
  Vascular
    Pyogenic granuloma
    Hemangioma
  Others
    Dermatofibroma
    Keloid
    Leiomyoma

Source: Winton (1989).

improvement during pregnancy while up to 15% of patients may deteriorate. The disease may flare in the postpartum period, usually within 4 months of birth. In psoriasis proinflammatory Th1 cytokines are up-regulated and play a key role in the mechanisms of chronic inflammation. In pregnancy the Th1 to Th2 switch that occurs may help to down-regulate the immune response in psoriasis and have anti-inflammatory effects.

Management is particularly difficult as systemic agents such as methotrexate, etretinate and acetretin are specifically contraindicated. The use of ultraviolet B therapy, topical corticosteroids, topical calcipotriol and dithranol, however, appear to be safe. Ciclosporin is safe in pregnancy but should be used with caution and during breastfeeding. The use of PUVA may carry a risk of mutagenesis and teratogenesis and should therefore not be used as first line therapy in pregnancy. However, a large study assessing pregnancy outcome in women treated with PUVA found no increased risk of spontaneous miscarriage or therapeutic termination or congenital malformations in pregnancies occurring after or during PUVA treatment. As always in pregnancy the risk benefit ratio must be considered and there may be a place for such treatment in severe psoriasis.

Impetigo herpetiformis

Impetigo herpetiformis is a rare acute form of pustular psoriasis precipitated by pregnancy. It can occur without a prior history of psoriasis and generally presents in women in their third trimester, with symptoms often persisting until delivery and in some cases postpartum. Occasionally it presents in the postpartum period. It is reminiscent of pustular psoriasis and classically presents with erythematous patches and pustulation at the margins. These typically begin in flexural areas and then spread centrifugally on to trunk and around the umbilicus but usually spare the hands, feet and face. Mucosal sites such as the tongue, buccal mucosa and esophagus can also become affected. Lesions tend to heal with post-inflammatory hyperpigmentation. There is often accompanying constitutional upset with fever, delirium, diarrhoea and vomiting and tetany due to hypocalcemia.

Histopathology of a skin biopsy is identical to pustular psoriasis with spongiform pustules of Kogoj and large collections of neutrophils within foci of spongiotic epidermis.

Laboratory investigations often reveal hypocalcemia (in some cases associated with hypoparathyroidism), and an elevated leucocyte count. Outside pregnancy the erythrocyte sedimentation rate (ESR) will be high, however this is not useful to assess disease in pregnancy due to the physiological increase in the ESR that occurs.

Management is usually systemic corticosteroids with doses of prednisolone up to 30-40 mg daily. However, stillbirth and placental insufficiency are still seen frequently even when disease activity appears to be controlled. Remisssion postpartum is common, but recurrence in successive pregnancies is typical, often with increased severity and at an earlier gestation, thus careful counseling is essential. Recurrence with the oral contraceptive pill has also been described.

Atopic eczema

Atopic eczema is a chronic relapsing pruritic dermatosis affecting 1-5% of the general population, and in many cases accompanied by other atopic features. It often deteriorates in pregnancy due to excessive excoriation from pruritus gravidarum. In some cases it may present for the first time during pregnancy. One prospective study of pregnancy dermatoses showed that atopic eczema was the commonest skin condition presenting in pregnancy. A past history or family history of atopy significantly increases the risk of developing eczema during pregnancy.

The immune system and hormonal changes that occur during pregnancy may help to explain the increase in incidence of atopic eczema.

The cytokine profile within the placenta switches from Th1 to Th2 cytokine profile during pregnancy to prevent fetal rejection. The T lymphocytes with a Th2 cytokine profile increase IL-4 and IL-13 synthesis which may stimulate B lymphocytes to increase production of IgE. In contrast, T lymphocytes with a Th1 profile increase interferon-gamma cytokine synthesis which inhibits IgE production. This may be one of the mechanisms to explain the increase in atopic eczema during pregnancy. Increased circulating levels of the pregnancy hormones estrogen and progesterone may also influence skin dryness, blood flow and pruritus.

It has been suggested that several factors are important in determining the infant's risk of developing atopic eczema, including fetal sex, maternal or paternal atopy, breastfeeding, maternal diet and smoking. The prevalence of infantile atopic eczema appears to be the same regardless of whether the disease was inherited from father or mother. Recent research has demonstrated that probiotics (Lactobacillus and Bifidobacterium species) in the maternal diet during pregnancy and breastfeeding may reduce the risk of infantile atopy in up to 50% of cases. This can be explained by the hygiene hypothesis which suggests that lack of exposure to infections early in life predisposes individuals to atopic disease. Probiotics (orally administered micro-organisms) might therefore help to prevent atopic eczema by altering intestinal microflora.

Management of atopic eczema in pregnancy should include liberal emollients and mild to moderately potent topical corticosteroids (clobetasone butyrate 0.05% or betamethasone valerate 0.1%). Topical corticosteroid ointments should be applied to all affected areas once to twice daily, preferably with emollients used beforehand. Soap and detergents should be avoided and a soap substitute such as aqueous cream or emulsifying ointment used instead. Antihistamines such as chlorpheniramine are safe in pregnancy and can be effective in reducing pruritus and assisting sleep but the newer non-sedating antihistamines (cetirizine and loratadine) are not recommended in the first trimester of pregnancy. The newer topical immunosuppressants tacrolimus and pimecrolimus have been avoided in pregnancy. However experience with systemic Tacrolimus in pregnancy in growing in patients with problems such as liver transplant and the current data on fetal outcome are reassuring. Thus, topical tacrolimus may be used if required after weighing up the risk–benefit ratio and the alternative therapies. Occasionally systemic corticosteroids such as prednisolone are required for a short time. Prednisolone is usually the drug of choice in pregnancy because of the extensive experience of its use. However, attention should be placed on screening for glucose intolerance and hypertension if the woman is on significant doses for a prolonged period. In this situation steroid supplements will be required in labor. Breastfeeding is considered safe during systemic steroid administration (Fig 15.5).

Nipple dermatitis can be provoked by breastfeeding with dry cracked skin and fissures which become secondarily infected with *Staphylococcus aureus*. This can be treated with frequent moisturisers and a mild topical corticosteroid such as hydrocortisone, combined with a topical antibiotic fucidin if infected.

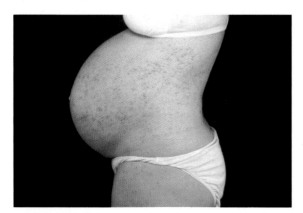

Figure 15.5 Acute exacerbation of eczema during pregnancy with excoriated papules on the trunk and limbs in a patient with pre-existing atopic eczema.

Hand dermatitis is often exacerbated in the puerperium because of the constant exposure to irritants used in the care of the young infant. Prophylactic measures such as the protection of hands using gloves and liberal emollients can be effective. As there is a higher incidence of contact dermatitis during pregnancy, rubber gloves should be avoided and should be replaced with vinyl gloves instead. Moderately potent or potent topical corticosteroids (betamethasone valerate 0.1%) can also be used and again these should be used in conjunction with liberal emollients and soap substitutes such as aqueous cream or emulsifying ointment.

Acne vulgaris

Acne vulgaris can improve during pregnancy but is occasionally exacerbated. As most of the systemic anti-acne drugs are teratogenic treatment should be with topical therapy such as benzoyl peroxide (2.5-10% cream, lotion or gel) or topical antibiotics such as clindamycin or erythromycin. Oral tetracyclines should be avoided in treatment as they may lead to yellow discoloration of developing teeth and impaired bone growth. Oral erythromycin is safe during pregnancy and can be used systemically as a treatment for acne. Treatments for severe acne (isotretinoin and cyproterone acetate) are specifically contraindicated in pregnancy at any stage. Isotretinoin is teratogenic while the anti-androgen, cyproterone acetate, can produce feminization of a male fetus. Topical retinoids should also be avoided as they too carry a risk of teratogenesis through systemic absorption.

Acne rosacea often flares in pregnancy and may also require treatment with topical or oral antibiotics (as above). There is a rare severe variant of acne rosacea called rosacea fulminans (also known as pyoderma faciale) which can flare in pregnancy and is characterized by the abrupt onset of a severe facial eruption with papules, nodules, pustules and erythema on the face. During pregnancy this requires treatment with oral erythromycin and oral corticosteroids. There has been a recent report of rosacea fulminans complicated by stillbirth (Fig. 15.6).

Erythema nodosum

This is an inflammatory process involving the subcutaneous fat which can be precipitated by a number of systemic conditions (streptococcal infection, tuberculosis, leprosy, sarcoidosis, inflammatory bowel disease) or drugs (sulfonamides and oral contraceptives). However, it can also present in pregnancy for the first time with tender symmetrical erythematous nodules or plaques classically on the anterior shins,

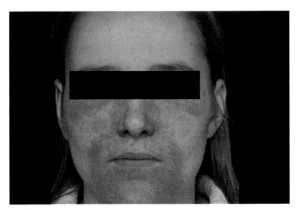

Figure 15.6 Acute rosacea presenting in pregnancy with marked facial erythema and a pustular eruption. Involvement of the cheeks and perioral area is typical of rosacea.

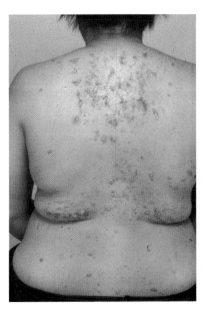

Figure 15.7 Pemphigus vulgaris in the second trimester with crusted superficial erosions on the upper and mid back with no intact blisters.

but lesions can also occur on the calves, arms, trunk and face. It can be associated with fever and arthralgia and usually resolves over a period of 6 to 8 weeks. Treatment in pregnancy should consist of bed rest and mild analgesics such as paracetamol. Non-steroidal anti-inflammatory agents should be avoided in pregnancy, especially the third trimester as they may cause premature closure of the ductus arteriosus in utero. They are also associated with oligohydramnios through the effects on the fetal kidney. Thus if these agents are used for any length of time, it is important to monitor amniotic fluid volume by ultrasound.

Erythema multiforme

Erythema multiforme is characterized by acute, self-limiting but often recurrent episodes of erythematous urticarial or maculopapular lesions which coalesce to form the classic 'target' lesions. These generally occur on the extremities and extensor aspects of the forearms and legs and on the palms and soles. Mucosal involvement is common, affecting eyes, mouth and vulva. Severe cases (Stevens-Johnson syndrome) may develop visual impairment due to scarring of the conjunctivae and can be indistinguishable from toxic epidermal necrolysis (TEN). Erythema multiforme can flare in pregnancy and this has been linked to herpes simplex virus which is implicated in the etiology. There is evidence of increased shedding of HSV during pregnancy and a prophylactic 6-month course of aciclovir has been shown to be effective in the prevention of recurrent erythema multiforme in non-pregnant individuals.

Pemphigus

Pemphigus vulgaris and foliaceus are both characterized by autoantibodies directed against desmosomal antigens desmoglein 3 (130 kDa) and desmoglein 1 (160 kDa), respectively, both transmembrane glycoproteins of desmosomes belonging to the cadherin supergene family of cell adhesion molecules. Pemphigus vulgaris reported during pregnancy is extremely rare and usually requires treatment with systemic corticosteroids or other immunosuppressive agents. Exacerbation of pre-existing disease can also occur during pregnancy, generally in the first or second trimesters. It often improves in the third trimester and this may be due to increased serum cortisol levels and consequent immunosuppression. Close fetal monitoring is required for severe maternal pemphigus (Fig. 15.7).

As in the non-pregnant individual pemphigus presents with non healing erosions on the trunk and limbs and associated mucosal lesions. Differential diagnosis from pemphigoid gestationis is important and direct and indirect immunofluorescence confirm the diagnosis, with an intercellular pattern of IgG deposition between the keratinocytes of the epidermis. There is a reported increase in fetal morbidity and mortality although several authors have reported cases with normal outcome. During pregnancy immunosuppressants (cyclophosphamide, methotrexate and gold) should all be avoided to minimize possible teratogenicity. Antibody titers (indirect immunofluorescence) may be helpful as a guide to disease activity and response to treatment. Control of disease with corticosteroids only is preferable and, as noted above, this can be continued while breastfeeding. The use of plasmapheresis has also been reported in the treatment of severe cases.

The trauma of vaginal delivery can result in worsening of vulval erosions and Cesarean section provides an alternative if there is already severe vulval involvement. However, Cesarean section routinely is of no benefit as blisters and increased rates of infection may occur in the surgical wound.

Neonatal pemphigus can occur due to transplacental transfer of maternal anti-epidermal IgG autoantibodies. Twenty-three cases of neonatal pemphigus worldwide have been confirmed. In these cases the majority of mothers had pemphigus vulgaris with a few cases of pemphigus foliaceus and one case of pemphigus vegetans. Stillbirths have been reported in four cases, and these were associated with high levels of maternal pemphigus antibodies. In addition the affected mothers had disease which was difficult to control requiring high doses of corticosteroid (100-300 mg) with or without dapsone or azathioprine. There have been cases of neonatal pemphigus vulgaris associated with mild oral pemphigus vulgaris in the mother during pregnancy, and also with more severe oral disease. This may be explained by the fact that neonatal skin has a similar desmoglein distribution pattern to adult mucosal epithelia. Hence, the antibody titers or clinical presentation of the mother do not predict the severity of the disease in the neonate. Most neonates who have neonatal pemphigus vulgaris usually improve spontaneously within two to three weeks, thus requiring only careful handling and topical antibiotics if clinically indicated. Breastfeeding is not contraindicated although local blister formation may occur and passive transfer of antibodies to the infant via breast milk is a potential risk.

Malignant melanoma

There has been considerable interest in the relationship between pregnancy and malignant melanoma. Since 1951 a number of case reports have suggested that pregnancy may induce or exacerbate melanoma. There are now five well-controlled studies that evaluate the effect of pregnancy on the prognosis of melanoma, when the melanoma was diagnosed during pregnancy. In all five studies there was no statistically significant difference in survival between patients diagnosed during pregnancy (study group) and controls. However in two studies the study group had tumors of greater thickness. One hypothesis for this is that diagnosis of melanoma may have been delayed because it is often stated that naevi may darken and

enlarge during pregnancy due to hormonal influence. However a recent prospective study of changes in melanocytic naevi during pregnancy showed no significant increase in lesion size based on sequential photography during pregnancy.

As in non-pregnant individuals it appears that prognosis of melanoma should be based on tumor thickness. MacKie et al's study of 388 women with stage 1 primary cutaneous disease during childbearing years showed the two most important prognostic factors to be tumor thickness and truncal anatomical site. When controlled for tumor thickness, however, pregnancy did not alter the prognosis of melanoma, as might be expected. The authors conclude that women with melanoma should be advised about pregnancy on the basis of thickness and site of tumor rather than hormonal status. In 1998 Grin et al reviewed the literature which examined the effect of pregnancy on prognosis of melanoma and the effect on future pregnancies after diagnosis. Their review concluded that pregnancy after or at the time of diagnosis of stage 1 melanoma did not appear to alter 5-year survival. However, there is little information about the prognosis of stage 111 and IV pregnancy-associated melanomas as statistical trials for such cases do not exist.

Transplacental transmission of melanoma to the fetus is extremely rare although placental metastases have been reported. Histological examination of the placenta is recommended to look for metastatic disease in women presenting with melanomas during pregnancy. Metastases to the placenta are generally blood-borne and occur only in women with widely disseminated malignant disease. It has been reported that there is about a 25% risk of stage IV malignant melanoma spreading from mother to fetus (Fig. 15.8).

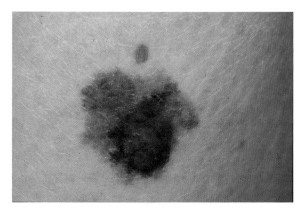

Figure 15.8 A superficial spreading melanoma with an asymmetrical outline and irregular dark pigmentation.

Box 15.6 Management of melanoma

- Malignant melanoma can present in pregnancy.
- Close examination of any changing mole in pregnancy is important to exclude early melanoma.
- Prognosis depends on tumor thickness.
- Placental metastases have been reported.
- Transplacental transmission to the fetus has been reported but is rare.
- Recognized 25% risk of stage IV melanoma spreading from mother to fetus.

Congenital malignant melanoma is an uncommon condition that is defined as malignant melanoma recognized at birth (Box 15.6). Congenital malignant melanoma in utero can develop in one of three ways:

1. Transmission by metastasis through the placenta from a mother with melanoma.
2. Primary melanoma arising within a giant congenital melanocytic nevus
3. Primary de novo cutaneous congenital malignant melanoma arising in utero.

Further reading

Aractingi S et al 1998 Fetal DNA in skin of polymorphic eruptions of pregnancy. Lancet 352:1898-1901

Aronson I K et al 1998 Pruritic urticarial papules and plaques of pregnancy: clinical and immunopathological observations in 57 patients. Journal of the American Academy of Dermatology 39:933-939

Boyd A S et al 1996 Psoriasis and pregnancy: hormone and immune system interaction. International Journal of Dermatology 35(3):169-172

Chanco Turner M L 1999 The skin in pregnancy in medical complications during pregnancy, G Burrow, N Duffy, P Thomas (eds). W.B. Saunders, Philadelphia

Driscoll M S, Grin-Jorgensen C M, Grant-Kels J M 1993 Does pregnancy influence the prognosis of malignant melanoma? Journal of the American Academy of Dermatology 29:619-630

Garcia Gonzales E et al 1999 Immunology of the cutaneous disorders of pregnancy. International Journal of Dermatology 38(10):721-729

Goldberg N S, DeFeo C, Krishenbaum N 1993 Pemphigus vulgaris and pregnancy: risk factors and recommendations. Journal of the American Academy of Dermatology 28:877-879

Grin C M, Driscoll M S, Grant-Kels J M 1998 The relationship of pregnancy, hormones and melanoma. Seminars in Cutaneous Medicine and Surgery 17:161-171

Grin C M, Driscoll M S, Grant-Kels J M 1998 The relationship of pregnancy, hormones and melanoma. Seminars in Cutaneous Medicine and Surgery 17(3):167-171

Holmes R C, Black M M 1983 The specific dermatoses of pregnancy. Journal of the American Academy of Dermatology 8:405-412

Jenkins R E et al 1999 Clinical features and management of 87 patients with pemphigoid gestationis. Clinical and Experimental Dermatology 24(4):255-259

Kalayciyan A et al 2002 A retrospective analysis of patients with pemphigus vulgaris associated with pregnancy. British Journal of Dermatology 147:385-410

Kalliomaki M et al 2003 Probiotics in primary prevention of atopic disease: a randomised placebo-controlled trial. Lancet 361:1869-1871

Kemmet D, Tidman M J 1991 The influence of the menstrual cycle and pregnancy on atopic dermatitis. British Journal of Dermatology 125:59-61

Liu D T Y 1974 Striae gravidarum (letter) Lancet 1:625

Mackie R M, Bufalino R, Morabito A et al 1991 Lack of effect of pregnancy on outcome of melanoma. Lancet 337:653-655

Milton J L 1872 The Pathology and Treatment of Diseases of the Skin; page 205 published Robert Hardwick, London

Pennoyer J W et al 1997 Changes in size of melanocytic naevi during pregnancy. Journal of the American Academy of Dermatology 36:378-382

Vaughan Jones S A et al 1999 A prospective study of 200 women with dermatoses of pregnancy correlating the clinical findings with hormonal and immunopathological profiles. British Journal of Dermatology 141:71-81

Wilkinson S M et al 1995 Androgen levels in pruritic folliculitis of pregnancy. The Journal of Investigative Dermatology 20:234-236

Winton G B 1989 Skin diseases aggravated by pregnancy. Journal of the American Academy of Dermatology 20:1-13

Zurn A et al 1992 A propsective immunofluorescence study of 111 cases of pruritic dermatoses of pregnancy: IgM anti-basement membrane zone antibodies as a novel finding. British Journal of Dermatology 126:474-478

Chapter 16

Drug misuse in pregnancy

M. Hepburn

BACKGROUND AND PREVALENCE

Problem drug use has been on the increase nationally and internationally for the past 20 years. An initial sharp increase in prevalence in the mid to late 1980s, particularly among women of childbearing age, led to a marked increase in drug misuse in pregnancy. Heightened awareness and consequently better identification contributed to rising numbers. The rate of increase slowed during the mid 1990s then rose again so that the number of pregnant drug using women has risen considerably during the past few years demonstrated by the fact that the number of pregnant drug using women attending a specialist service in Glasgow has doubled in the 5 years from 2000-2004.

While drug use occurs throughout the social spectrum, problem drug use associated with significant medical and social problems closely correlates with socioeconomic deprivation. Poverty increases mortality and morbidity among mothers and their babies.

Maternal mortality is increased 20-30-fold while the rates of prematurity, low birthweight and sudden infant deaths, are much higher among babies of socially disadvantaged women. Smoking is more common among these mothers further increasing the risk of low birthweight and cot death. These adverse effects on pregnancy outcome are exacerbated by superimposed problem drug use. Moreover, since the original increase in drug use occurred 20 years ago, the average age of pregnant drug users has increased and the combination of increased maternal age and increased duration of drug use is reflected in even greater increases in maternal and perinatal mortality and morbidity. There have also been changes in patterns of drug use with most notably an increase in use of cocaine and crack cocaine and with polydrug use now the norm including combined use of drugs and alcohol. These changes have also adversely affected outcomes. However on a positive note there has also been increased recognition by health services of the need to provide appropriate care for socially disadvantaged pregnant women whose problems have been highlighted by the inclusion of social information in the last two maternal mortality reports; similarly there has been increased recognition by addiction services of the particular needs of pregnant women who use drugs. Consequently there has been increased and improved health and social service provision for pregnant drug using women with production of national multidisciplinary management guidelines. Nevertheless there is still considerable room for improvement.

It has been widely stated that pregnant women who use drugs attend late or not at all for antenatal care. However drug using women do not differ from other women in their motivation to have children and to behave responsibly towards their children both before and after birth. As a consequence of improved, specialist service provision there is now considerable evidence that if provided with services that are appropriate in design and delivery, drug using women will attend early and regularly for antenatal care.

SERVICE DESIGN AND DELIVERY

Poverty and associated social problems affect pregnancy outcome so should be addressed by health, including maternity, services in a comparable manner to health problems that affect pregnancy outcome. Pregnant drug using women therefore need multidisciplinary care that addresses all their problems both medical and social in an integrated way within a single setting. Moreover, women who use drugs during pregnancy should be regarded as pregnant women who have a drug problem and not as drug users who are pregnant. Therefore, as in the case of women with health problems that can affect pregnancy outcome, their care should not only be provided by integrated teams but should be embedded in maternity services. Social and addiction workers should therefore provide input in antenatal care settings and pregnant drug using women should not have their maternity care provided by a midwife visiting addiction services.

EFFECTS OF DRUG USE ON REPRODUCTIVE HEALTH

Any problem or chaotic drug use can decrease fertility indirectly by impairing general health and nutrition. Heroin also affects fertility directly. Drug use, especially heroin use can therefore cause amenorrhea and anovulation but not necessarily simultaneously. Consequently, while many drug using women and service providers assume that conception cannot occur in the absence of menstruation, this is incorrect and drug using women who do not want to become pregnant should use effective contraception. Prescription of methadone to opiate users will increase fertility with resumption of menstruation. However since the effects of heroin on menstruation and fertility are exacerbated by the associated chaotic lifestyle and poor nutrition, any treatment that improves these factors will also increase fertility and this can happen before resumption of menstruation. Consequently information about and provision of appropriate effective contraception should be the responsibility of any service providing treatment for addiction problems. Such action should help to ensure that drug using women have pregnancies only if and when they choose and this helps to optimize outcomes. Conversely drug using women may complain of infertility and interventions aimed at cessation or stabilization of drug use and/or lifestyle may be sufficient to restore fertility. Treatment for such women is often viewed as inappropriate. However, they may conceive without intervention and their presentation provides an ideal opportunity to address their drug use and associated medical and social problems and consequently to improve the likelihood of good medical and social outcomes.

The alleged failure of drug using women to attend early for antenatal care is sometimes attributed to lack of awareness of pregnancy. In practice however it appears that women, if confused about diagnosis of pregnancy, are more likely to overdiagnose than underdiagnose pregnancy. The offer of free pregnancy testing in multiple sites including those providing addiction care will increase early detection of pregnancy and will have other benefits as well including earlier referral for termination if the pregnancy is unwanted, provision of effective contraception if the woman is not pregnant and does not want to conceive and provision of pre-pregnancy care including prescription of folic acid if she is planning pregnancy.

EFFECTS OF DRUG USE ON PREGNANCY

In problem drug use the drugs used are usually illegal, of unknown purity and taken in an uncontrolled way. Consequently it is difficult to carry out controlled studies of effects of drug use in pregnancy and there is a paucity of scientifically reliable data to inform recommendations on management of drug use in pregnancy. Nevertheless such management has traditionally been quite directive, based on observational data of unknown significance. With the increasing prevalence of problem drug use in pregnancy, practical experience has shown many of these older recommendations to be unfounded.

Of the common drugs currently in use, few have direct effects on pregnancy and most of the observed adverse effects are indirect. A major concern of most drug using women is the possibility of fetal anomalies caused by their drug use but this is in fact very uncommon. There has been conflicting evidence on the effects of benzodiazepine use on the risk of cleft palate; current evidence indicates an increased relative risk but the absolute risk remains low. High levels of alcohol consumption in early pregnancy may cause fetal alcohol syndrome which includes craniofacial abnormalities and microcephaly. The main effect of excessive maternal alcohol consumption during pregnancy is low birthweight, and there is evidence of subsequent neurodevelopmental delay. Cocaine is a powerful vasoconstrictor and vasoconstriction with consequent ischemia is presumably the etiology for the effects on brain development and the underdevelopment of organs including limbs and gut occasionally described in association with heavy chaotic cocaine use. An association between the use of amphetamines (and other vasoconstrictors) and gastroschisis has been reported with the hypothesis that vascular disruption early in development is culpable but a causal link remains unproven.

Other effects are limited. In the case of short-acting heroin the adverse effects actually result from the smooth muscle spasm caused by repeated minor degrees of withdrawal. In early pregnancy this could theoretically cause spontaneous abortion. Later in pregnancy it would cause preterm delivery but while this outcome is observed in association with chaotic heroin use it is difficult to determine whether the adverse outcomes result from the contribution of associated socio-economic deprivation and chaotic lifestyle or the drugs themselves. Placental insufficiency of similar etiology is presumably the cause of the low birthweight associated with heroin use but again it is difficult to separate the effects of heroin use and chaotic lifestyle. Prescription of substitute medication for problem opiate use is beneficial by stabilizing lifestyle and promoting access to services. Prescription in pregnancy of a long acting opiate such as methadone will protect against the increased risk of miscarriage or preterm labor associated with heroin use in pregnancy. However even though the rate of preterm delivery is not increased with the use of methadone in pregnancy, it is not clear to what extent this results from its duration of action compared to the social stabilization with general improvement in health that accompanies prescribed substitute medication.

Many adverse pregnancy outcomes have been associated with cocaine use. Cocaine is a powerful vasoconstrictor and this action may affect fetal development through ischemia of developing organs, and may cause placental abruption and intrauterine death. Cocaine use is also associated with preterm rupture of membranes and consequently with increased preterm delivery but use of cocaine does not cause withdrawal symptoms in the baby. However while neonatal withdrawal symptoms do not occur, the effects of cocaine use on the mother and therefore indirectly on the pregnancy may result in neonatal morbidity with some features such as irritability in common with withdrawal symptoms. Again adverse outcomes are more likely with heavy use of cocaine

that is itself associated with chaotic lifestyles and poor general health, certainly major contributory factors.

Birthweight is reduced among babies of women using substantial quantities of many types of drugs but it is difficult to separate the drug effects from lifestyle effects. Low birthweight is the most common effect seen in babies of women drinking alcohol heavily and those using heroin. With cocaine, vascular spasm is presumably the etiology. Smoking tobacco also causes low birthweight but there is conflicting evidence about the effects of marijuana on birthweight and other fetal parameters. Evidence of chromosomal effects is difficult to interpret in that the long-term significance of these is unknown. Nevertheless it is wise to advise women to reduce all illicit drug use as well as use of tobacco and alcohol during pregnancy as much as possible.

The other main concern of pregnant drug using women is that their babies will develop neonatal withdrawal symptoms. Withdrawal symptoms can be caused by a number of drugs as well as tobacco, alcohol and antidepressants. Among the drugs commonly misused in pregnancy opiates and benzodiazepines commonly cause neonatal withdrawal that requires treatment. Babies born to women using other drugs including stimulants such as cocaine or amphetamines can be unwell as a consequence of the effects of the drugs on the mother (see Ch. 19). Maternal opiate and/or benzodiazepine use is also associated with increased rates of sudden infant death, which is also increased in association with socio-economic deprivation.

SOCIAL EFFECTS OF DRUG MISUSE

The social effects of drug use in pregnancy are as important as the medical effects. Drug misuse is often associated with a chaotic lifestyle that can cause or exacerbate the effects of socio-economic deprivation on health and service use. Similarly medical factors can affect social outcomes of pregnancy. While parenting is compromised directly by drug intoxication the lifestyle associated with drug use is often the more important factor. However caring for a sick baby is particularly demanding for any mother and will be especially stressful for women having to address additional problems such as drug use. This relationship between medical and social factors demonstrates why pregnant women who use drugs need multidisciplinary care with input from health and social services. Moreover, regardless of the mechanism, drug using women overall have poorer outcomes of pregnancy. They therefore have high-risk pregnancies so their maternity care must be obstetrically led although much of their care can be delivered by midwives in the community.

IDENTIFICATION OF DRUG USE IN PREGNANCY

The primary care team, in their referral to maternity services, should provide all available relevant medical and social information. This should include information about problem drug and/or alcohol use. However the midwife or obstetrician who sees the woman for booking should also routinely enquire about such use. A positive response should prompt further detailed enquiry to assess the severity of the problem and the consequent type and level of input required from mainstream and/or specialist services. It is important to document the type of drugs used, the route, level and pattern of use, the source, cost and method of financing of use. With the exception of occasional recreational use of non-addictive drugs such as cannabis or ecstasy any history of illicit drug use or consequent use of prescribed substitutes should be regarded as an indication for assessment by addiction services. Regular prescription of benzodiazepines is likely to indicate an addiction problem that may benefit from addiction service assessment while prescription of antidepressants, which can cause neonatal withdrawal would not.

A full social history should be taken in the usual way. However there is considerable overlap between information required by maternity and social/addiction services and collection, documentation and sharing of this information will be determined by local collaborative arrangements. As for any pregnant woman information is required about the partner, the state of the relationship, any history of violence by the partner or other person, whether the partner is the father of the baby and/or existing children and whether he or she and/or other family members have a drug and/or alcohol problem. Domestic circumstances should be documented including care arrangements for previous children, current housing, tenancy arrangements and with whom the patient shares the accommodation. For any pregnant woman with problem drug and/or alcohol use any history of involvement with the criminal justice system should be ascertained and details recorded. Previous involvement with social, including addiction services should also be identified and the woman's permission sought to collaborate and share relevant information with social services. Drug use is a relapsing condition and

it is essential to recognize that even if abstinent in early pregnancy, a woman with a history of drug use is at risk of relapse during pregnancy or after delivery although the level of risk declines the longer the period of abstinence. A history of abstinence of a year or more at the time of conception is a reasonable cut off for involvement of specialized maternity and/or addiction services but even with such a history it is often worthwhile offering input from a professional experienced in dealing with addiction to provide support and information about sources of help if relapse should occur. It is also worth remembering that women may exaggerate the duration of abstinence to avoid involvement with social or addiction services so if there is any doubt about her current status or level of risk specialized assessment should be provided. Even if a woman is stable on substitute medication at booking the physiological, psychological and social changes of pregnancy can jeopardize stability. Such a woman will be in contact with addiction services and should have at least some input from specialized maternity services even if only to provide her with relevant information about possible effects on pregnancy and management of the baby and to establish management pathways should stability be lost.

Social and/or addiction services should be involved as early in the pregnancy as possible to provide specialized support to prevent crises. Drug use in pregnancy is not necessarily a child protection issue. However, if a woman has a drug and/or alcohol problem, is not in contact with social and/or addiction services and refuses to agree to information sharing or referral maternity staff will ultimately have a duty under child protection legislation to notify social services of their concerns. However, it is always preferable to obtain the woman's consent, if possible, before involving other agencies. Women refuse referral because they fear they will lose custody of their children. With sympathetic but honest discussion most will come to realize that acceptance of support offers the best chance of a good social outcome.

ANTENATAL MANAGEMENT

Addiction management

Substitution therapy

As already discussed there is ample evidence of the medical and social benefits of substitution therapy for opiate users and during pregnancy the increased risk of early delivery is further indication for such therapy. Methadone is the commonest substitute drug prescribed and there is considerable evidence of its safety during pregnancy while its long half-life also makes it particularly suitable in this situation. However like heroin it may cause withdrawal symptoms in the neonate although its protective effect against early delivery is of much greater importance for long term health of the baby. Buprenorphine is increasingly used as a substitute for opiate users so increasingly women will become pregnant while using it. Since buprenorphine was the opiate drug of choice in Scotland during the 1980s there is considerable experience of its illicit use by pregnant women although at levels lower than current therapeutic doses. While it is difficult to obtain sound data comparing use of prescribed methadone and buprenorphine during pregnancy experience of illicit use suggests it is equally safe but without advantages over methadone and it also causes neonatal withdrawal symptoms comparable to those caused by methadone. There is as yet no evidence to support prescription of other substitute opiates during pregnancy and there is some anecdotal evidence that use of codeine during pregnancy is associated with poorer outcomes. Consequently women using any opiate when they become pregnant should be offered substitution therapy and methadone remains the opiate substitute of choice in pregnancy. However, if women become pregnant while taking prescribed substitute buprenorphine there is no indication to transfer them to methadone. Naltrexone is another possible option. An opioid antagonist that blocks opiate receptors, it blocks the euphoric effect of opiates and is therefore sometimes used to prevent relapse in opiate users who have undergone detoxification. It may also be used in pregnancy but attempts to overcome the block may lead to acute opiate intoxication that is potentially harmful for the fetus. Selection of appropriately stable patients is therefore essential and women should be warned about risks of misuse during pregnancy. However, since there is no single ideal drug treatment, choice of management during pregnancy should be dictated by individual circumstances and preference.

There is no evidence to support maintenance substitute prescribing for any other type of drug.

Antenatal detoxification

Opiates

It has been claimed that antenatal opiate detoxification carries a significant risk of fetal death. It has been further claimed that reduction carries a risk of miscarriage in the first trimester and premature delivery in the third trimester and should therefore be carried out only very slowly and only during the mid trimester. The traditional recommendation is therefore that women using opiates during pregnancy should be maintained on substitute medication throughout pregnancy. The evidence supporting this recommendation however is weak. There is no evidence indicating a risk of fetal death and while an increase in amniotic fluid catecholamine levels following abrupt maternal opiate withdrawal has been interpreted as indicating fetal stress there is no evidence that this is of clinical significance. On the contrary, clinical experience in Glasgow has shown no evidence of adverse fetal effects from maternal opiate detoxification at any speed or at any stage of pregnancy. Pregnant women should therefore be allowed to reduce or withdraw substitute opiate medication. Conversely they should not be put under pressure to do so unless it is their choice and likely to be successful.

Reduced serum methadone levels in the third trimester have been reported, leading to the advice that methadone doses should be increased at this time. However practical experience does not support this recommendation. In fact, faced with imminent delivery and fear of neonatal withdrawal, many women manage significant reductions in methadone dose in the third trimester. Many factors including stress may necessitate an increase in methadone dose while reduction in stress may facilitate a reduction. Women may use illicit drugs in addition to prescribed methadone because their dose of methadone is inadequate while some will 'top up' even if this is not the case. Increasing the dose of methadone will eradicate illicit drug use in the former but not the latter situation. Total abstinence from illicit drugs during pregnancy is difficult to achieve for many women. While significant illicit drug use must be addressed, occasional use of small amounts of illicit drugs may be less harmful to the fetus than continuing to increase the dose of methadone to ever higher levels in the futile pursuit of total abstinence from illicit drugs. During pregnancy it is therefore necessary to titrate the dose of methadone against external factors that affect the woman's ability to cope with the aim of maintenance at the lowest dose compatible with reasonable stability of drug use. It is also essential to involve the woman in planning realistic therapeutic goals, whilst accepting responsibility for her management and any consequences for her baby.

Benzodiazepines

Benzodiazepines cause severe and prolonged neonatal withdrawal so the aim should be to limit fetal exposure. Immediate withdrawal from benzodiazepines however carries the risk of maternal convulsions so a short course of a longer acting benzodiazepine such as diazepam should be prescribed.

Clinical experience indicates that a seven day course is adequate for any level of maternal use. While rapid detoxification may fail or may result in only short-term abstinence, it has advantages and may be repeated if necessary. Pregnant women using opiates and benzodiazepines often view benzodiazepine use as less damaging to the fetus, less important and consequently less shameful than opiate use. They may express the view that detoxification from methadone is their primary objective. This is not the case. Not only should benzodiazepine detoxification precede any reduction in methadone dose but it may also be necessary to increase the methadone dose to facilitate withdrawal from benzodiazepines.

Other drugs

For all other types of drug there are no appropriate substitutes for either short- or long-term use and in all cases the aim should therefore be detoxification as quickly as possible. Many drug using women also smoke tobacco heavily. This may be more physically harmful to the baby than drug use but is less socially damaging so addressing their drug use takes priority. While trying to reduce or control their use of illicit drugs most women will not be able to reduce or stop smoking and in fact may increase their use of nicotine at this time. The use of nicotine patches is safe in pregnancy and, in theory beneficial for the fetus by reducing transplacental passage of carbon monoxide and other toxic substances derived from the combustion of tobacco. Nicotine, of course, remains, but oxygenation and placental blood flow are probably increased with the use of nicotine replacement therapy compared with smoking.

Obstetric management

Although drug using women have potentially high risk pregnancies there is no evidence to support variations from standard obstetric management unless there are specific grounds for doing so.

Cervical cytology and genital tract infections

Many pregnant drug using women will have had at best erratic contact with reproductive health services; for many women their cervical smear will be overdue while many have had previous abnormal smears. Those who have funded their drug use by prostitution will be at increased risk of sexually transmitted infections while some will have partners at increased risk. There is no contraindication to cervical cytology during pregnancy and the contact with services during pregnancy provides a useful opportunity for taking a smear. If a cervical smear is taken swabs to screen for genital tract infection should be taken at the same time. At any time, pelvic examination and screening for infection should be undertaken if indicated by the history.

Blood-borne virus infection

Pregnant drug using women should be offered the routine antenatal screening tests including screening for blood-borne virus infection. However in addition to screening for human immunodeficiency virus (HIV) infection and for hepatitis B (HBV) surface antigen to detect carrier status they should also be offered screening for HBV core antibody to detect immunity resulting from prior infection with HBV. Women with a history of current or past injecting drug use should be given information about hepatitis C infection and advised to consider being tested. However, since no interventions have been identified that reduce the risk of vertical transmission, since knowledge of HCV PCR positive status should influence maternity management and since a positive diagnosis may destabilise during use, testing during pregnancy is not necessary and may be counter productive. For these reasons a review of the past 10 years' experience of routine offering of antenatal testing in Glasgow led to its discontinuation. In many countries it is the policy to offer drug users immunization against HBV and, especially in the case of those with persistent HCV infection, immunization against hepatitis A (HAV). Given the frequent difficulties in maintaining sufficient contact to complete the course, pregnancy may be a good time to vaccinate susceptible women using an accelerated regimen such as 0, 1 and 2 months or even 0, 7 and 21 days. While each regimen requires a booster dose at 12 months, even in the absence of a booster they are better than an incomplete course using standard regimes. HBV vaccine is beneficial for all babies, especially those of drug using women. Those born to women shown to be infectious carriers should also have immunoglobulin at birth. Maternal prior infection may indicate that others in the family have also been infected and consequently be a marker for a high-risk home environment so babies born to women immune but not infectious should receive active immunization but do not require immunoglobulin. Provided the baby of an infection carrier is immunized and receives immunoglobulin at birth breast feeding is not contraindicated.

Women who test positive for HIV infection should receive multidisciplinary management according to national guidelines with the offer of interventions to reduce the risk of vertical transmission from mother to baby. These include selective use of delivery by Cesarean section, antenatal and intrapartum antiretroviral treatment for mother, antiretroviral treatment for the neonate and avoidance of breast feeding. Women with persistent HCV viremia should be offered referral for specialist assessment but provided they are well and their liver function is within normal limits there is no indication for urgent referral during pregnancy when in any case drug treatment would be contraindicated. There are as yet no interventions shown to reduce the overall low risk of vertical transmission estimated to be around 5% in the absence of co-infection with HIV. The management of women who are HCV PCR+ve should therefore not be modified because of their infection. Procedures carrying a risk of fetal inoculation including use of scalp electrodes and fetal blood sampling should, as in the care of all women, be used only when clinically indicated. Screening babies for HCV antibody at 18 months to 2 years of age with subsequent PCR testing for the few who are antibody positive will identify the small number of babies with ongoing infection who could benefit from follow up. Breast feeding is not contraindicated in the presence of persistent maternal HCV viremia.

Other health problems

Drug using women often have a number of health problems although these should be less severe if they are already in contact with services. Even if they have a normal body mass index (BMI) they should have their weight monitored regularly during pregnancy as a useful indicator of stability of drug use. All should be given appropriate dietary advice in the usual way.

Many drug using women have dental caries and gingival disease. Access to dental services for these women is part of comprehensive antenatal care, and attention to gum disease may even reduce the rate of preterm birth. Periodontal sepsis may also be a source of systemic infection with risk of bacterial endocarditis in women with cardiac valvular damage secondary to injecting drug use.

Women who have injected drugs often have severe limitation of vascular access due to vascular damage. While this may make venepuncture difficult it is never appropriate to allow the woman to attempt venepuncture on herself. Difficult venous access can also cause problems during labor if regional or general anesthesia is required quickly. There is also an increased risk of thromboembolic disease and women with a history of thrombosis should receive prophylaxis during pregnancy and postpartum according to guidelines (see Ch. 8). In the case of women who continue to inject into femoral vessels, there is a substantial risk of thrombotic complications. Thromboprophylaxis by anticoagulant drugs would rarely, however, be justifiable in this circumstance.

Fetal monitoring

There is no evidence of benefit from monitoring the fetus more closely than clinical circumstances would normally dictate. In addition, administered drugs may alter the fetal heart rate tracing and biophysical profile such that it is difficult to interpret using standard criteria. For example acute intoxication with sedative opiates or benzodiazepines may cause reduced fetal movements that are not necessarily indicative of fetal distress. Conversely acute maternal withdrawal from opiates will cause fetal withdrawal that may be manifest as vigorous fetal movements, not necessarily indicative of fetal well-being. Further, reduced fetal breathing will be seen on scan even with maintenance doses of methadone. Consequently if the mother is intoxicated there is no indication to intervene unless there are unequivocal signs of fetal compromise. While there is no evidence that maternal withdrawal from opiates is harmful to the fetus the same cannot be said of opiate reversal by antagonists. This can precipitate very acute fetal withdrawal and consequently severe fetal distress. In the management of maternal opiate intoxication treatment with an opiate antagonist should therefore be withheld or used as sparingly as possible.

Social management

As already discussed drug using women, even those not presently using, as well as those with a past history of drug use or women already on prescribed substitution therapy, are at risk of relapse and need referral to social and/or addiction services. However maternal drug use per se, although a potent risk factor, cannot be assumed to be associated with problems in care of the child. Rather, the aim of referral is to ensure pregnant drug using women receive appropriate support to optimize their chances of being able to provide effective parenting for their babies. If child protection issues are identified these should be addressed under standard child protection procedures. Although many drug using women have adequate parenting skills, both intoxication and the lifestyle associated with drug use can compromise parenting. Moreover, many drug using women come from dysfunctional families or have spent time being looked after by social services and thus have had little opportunity to acquire the necessary parenting skills. Drug using women should receive adequate support in providing care for their babies because socioeconomic deprivation, with or without super-imposed problem drug use can result in the birth of a sick baby whose management is very challenging to the mother.

Ongoing sharing of information is essential so regular liaison meetings should be held involving all relevant health and social services staff. A multi-disciplinary meeting held at 32 weeks' gestation and chaired by social services is recommended in both English and Scottish national guidelines. Such a meeting will allow sharing of information, identifica-tion of problems and gaps in service provision, setting of goals and planning of ongoing management. It is essential that the woman contributes to this planning process together with her partner and/or those who will provide her support.

INTRAPARTUM MANAGEMENT

Few drug using women have pregnancies that con-tinue much beyond term and most labor quickly and deliver normally. The rate of preterm labor is increased, though the majority of women deliver near term. While preterm labor is less common among women maintained on methadone it is important that such women are aware that use of heroin with methadone may precipitate labor. If delivery is imminent in an intoxicated woman, opiate reversal should be avoided if possible, even if monitoring suggests fetal compro-mise. If one succumbs to the temptation to reverse intoxication, this may precipitate fetal distress neces-sitating immediate delivery of a potentially sick baby. On the other hand, with expectant management fetal monitoring may revert to normal with avoidance of the need for delivery – hence it is best to intervene only if there is objective evidence of fetal distress. Similarly, following delivery, use of naloxone to reverse fetal sedation should be avoided if possible or undertaken with extreme caution: as its administra-tion to the sedated neonate may precipitate severe distress or shock.

There are often concerns that intrapartum pain relief will be problematic for women using opiates but in fact this is rarely the case. While epidural analgesia may seem the ideal solution it be unnecessary for drug using women who labor quickly. Alternative suggestions include the use of other analgesics or the routinely used opiate at increased doses but in general standard doses of opiate analgesia are sufficient. Pain relief in labor should therefore be given in the routine way with doses of narcotic analgesia repeated as required. If epidural analgesia using opiates is inef-fective adjusting the dose of local anesthesia may be effective. In practice problems with intrapartum anal-gesia are uncommon. Methadone is inadequate for pain relief in labor and should not be regarded as an effective substitute for usual analgesia. Equally it is important to ensure that methadone is continued during labor if due, even when opiate analgesia has been given.

POSTPARTUM MANAGEMENT

After delivery babies who are well should accompany their mothers to the postnatal ward and need not be routinely admitted to the special care nursery. Neither do mild withdrawal symptoms require admission to the special nursery provided that there is adequate care on the postnatal ward. Many babies need no spe-cific treatment for withdrawal and babies should be admitted to the special care nursery only if ill enough to warrant separation from their mother.

Breastfeeding

All babies, with the exception of those born to HIV positive women, will benefit from breastfeeding and babies born to socially disadvantaged mothers with increased rates of prematurity and low birthweight and increased risk of cot death have most to gain. As maternal cigarette smoking and problem drug use increase perinatal morbidity, babies of such women may benefit considerably from breastfeeding, with encouragement increasing numbers of women are attempting breastfeeding but continuation rates beyond 6 months are still low.

Lastly and most importantly from the mothers' point of view, breastfeeding will reduce the severity of withdrawal symptoms in babies of women using opiates and/or benzodiazepines. Many believe that feeding should be encouraged even where there is ongoing heavy drug use, for the benefit of the baby, though there is no evidence yet available. Therefore, since there is no evidence that breastfeeding in the presence of maternal drug use is harmful for the baby, drug using mothers should be encouraged to breastfeed provided their drug use is stable. The ability to successfully establish breastfeeding is acceptable proof of adequate stability. Psychosocial instability and/or high levels of use of these drugs are usually incompatible with successful establish-ment of breastfeeding.

Family planning

While many pregnancies to drug using women are unintended most are not unwanted. It is, however, important that any future pregnancy should be intended. If they are unable to care for the baby just delivering a further pregnancy should be delayed until their circumstances are appropriate; if they are able to care for the baby just delivered a further unplanned pregnancy would jeopardize their chances of continuing to care for the existing baby. It is therefore vital that these women are provided with appropriate effective contraception which should be commenced prior to postnatal discharge. Long acting progestagen contraception as an implant or intrauterine device is often most appropriate. Sterilization may sometimes seem appropriate for women who do not want any more pregnancies, especially if they are unable to care for existing children. In such circumstances however, reversible contraception preserves the option even if the choice pregnancy would never be made.

Babies of drug using mothers should remain in hospital until it is clear that the severity of any withdrawal symptoms has peaked and is on the decline. Withdrawal symptoms due to methadone have later onset and longer duration than those due to heroin but most babies, in the absence of serious health problems, will be fit for discharge within 7-10 days. While it is important to keep mother and baby together whenever possible maternal postnatal discharge should not be delayed for too long since most mothers find it hard to cope with remaining in hospital. A pre-discharge planning meeting may be appropriate and it is vital that drug using women continue to receive intensive support in the community after discharge from hospital.

CONCLUSION

The main points made in this chapter are summarized in Box 16.1. Social problems that affect pregnancy outcome should be addressed by maternity services in the same way as medical problems that affect pregnancy outcome. Consequently pregnant

---

Box 16.1 Key points in drug misuse in pregnancy

- All pregnant women should routinely have a social history taken that includes details about problem drug use.
- Problem drug use is closely associated with socio-economic deprivation so women who use drugs need multidisciplinary care, embedded in maternity services, that addresses all their problems both medical and social.
- Regular liaison meetings should be held involving health and social services with a planning meeting held at 32 weeks' gestation; maternal drug use per se is not a child protection issue and if child protection issues are identified these should be addressed separately.
- Many of the adverse effects on pregnancy outcome are indirect and due to the underlying socio-economic deprivation exacerbated by the superimposed medical and social effects of drug use.
- Drug use may cause relative but not necessarily absolute infertility. For this reason, even in the presence of amenorrhea, drug using women who do not want to become pregnant should use effective contraception.
- Antenatal opiate detoxification is acceptably safe for the fetus but management should be dictated not by theoretical considerations but by the woman's wishes and ability to cope, the aim being maintenance at the lowest dose compatible with stability.
- Drug using women should be offered screening for HIV infection according to routine practice and for HCV infection and immunity to HBV with immunization against HBV and HAV for susceptible women.
- Drug using women should receive intrapartum management according to obstetric need; analgesia should be given in the routine way with increased doses of opiates if necessary.
- Babies of drug using women should routinely go to the postnatal ward with their mothers unless their medical condition merits admission to the special care unit.
- Breastfeeding should be encouraged for all drug using women. High levels of use of drugs for which exposure of the baby would be undesirable (such as cocaine or benzodiazepines) are incompatible with successful breast feeding.
- Planning for the future should be discussed with all drug using women during their pregnancies to allow commencement of appropriate contraception before postnatal discharge.

women who have a drug and/or alcohol problem have potentially high-risk pregnancies and require specialized maternity care that is obstetrically led although much of it can be delivered in the community by midwives. They require care during pregnancy that addresses all their problems, medical and social, is delivered by a multidisciplinary service and is embedded in maternity care. Maternity care for pregnant women who use drugs should reflect their wishes but also be appropriate to their needs, acknowledging that their multiple medical and social problems may restrict the choices available to them. In the absence of reliable scientific data management of their addiction problem should not be unjustifiably directive and should be based on general principles of good practice with realistic objectives. Early identification of pregnancy, early referral to maternity services and good sharing of information will allow time to establish a positive relationship with the woman, improve the chances of providing her with the care that she needs and improve the chances of good medical and social outcomes of pregnancy. There should be greater recognition that social factors that affect pregnancy outcome necessitate provision of specialized maternity care in the same way as medical problems that affect pregnancy outcome. There is now a considerable body of evidence that if provided with appropriate care pregnant women who use drugs do attend early and regularly for maternity care. The national guidelines for England and Scotland provide information for joint health and social management of drug using families including man-agement of pregnant women who use drugs. There remains a need for increased ongoing support in the community for vulnerable families; failure to address this need will mean that long term outcomes remain compromised.

Further reading

Addis A et al 2001 Fetal effects of cocaine: an updated meta-analysis. Reproductive Toxicology 15(4): 341-369

Advisory Council on the Misuse of Drugs 2003 Hidden harm: responding to the needs of children of problem drug users. Home Office, London

British HIV Association 2001 Guidelines for the management of HIV infection in pregnant women and the prevention of mother-to-child transmission. BHIVA, London

British Medical Association 1997 The misuse of drugs. Harwood Academic Publishers, Amsterdam

Confidential Enquiry into Maternal and Child Health 2004 Why mothers die 2000-2003: The sixth report of the confidential enquiries into maternal deaths in the United Kingdom. RCOG, London

Hogg C, Chadwick T, Dale-Perera A 1997 Drug using parents – policy guidelines for inter-agency working (England and Wales). LGA Publications, London

Scottish Executive 2003 Getting our priorities right: policy and practice guidelines for working with children and families affected by problem drug use. Scottish Executive, Edinburgh

Werler M M, Sheehan J E, Mitchell A A 2003 Association of vasoconstrictive exposures with risks of gastroschisis and small intestinal atresia. Epidemiology 14:349-354

Chapter 17

Psychiatric disorders in pregnancy and the postpartum period

M. Oates

INTRODUCTION

Perinatal psychiatry is now the accepted term, both in the UK and internationally, for the study and care of women whose pregnancies and early motherhood are complicated by psychiatric disorder. The use of this term emphasizes both the frequency and importance of disorders in pregnancy as well as the more familiar postpartum disorders. It also emphasizes that not only do women become ill for the first time following childbirth but also that women with pre-existing mental illness become pregnant. It is concerned with the effects of both the illness and their treatments on the developing fetus and infant.

With few exceptions, the prevalence of psychiatric disorder during pregnancy will be much the same as among non-childbearing women of the same age. The whole range of psychiatric disorder of all types and severities can therefore complicate the management of the pregnant woman. As between 15 and 20% of all pregnant women will have a mental health problem, familiarity with these conditions is essential for the obstetrician and midwife.

It has been known since antiquity that women who have recently given birth are at a particularly elevated risk of a distinctive psychotic illness often called puerperal psychosis. This severe and life threatening condition is mercifully rare. Women are also at an increased risk of suffering from a recurrence of a pre-existing bipolar illness and of the most severe forms of depressive illness. Milder non-psychotic conditions are common place. Although there is probably not an increased risk of suffering from these conditions following childbirth, they are nonetheless distressing and frequent and contribute significantly to the workload of health professionals, particularly in primary care. To these postpartum onset conditions can be added the large number of women with pre-existing mental health problems whose conditions continue or are exacerbated following childbirth. Therefore 10 to 15% of all postpartum women will have significant mental health problems. The importance of perinatal psychiatric disorder to both maternity and psychiatric professionals also includes the issues surrounding the use of psychotropic medication in pregnancy and during breastfeeding.

The proper management of perinatal psychiatric disorder requires specialist knowledge and skills on the part of both psychiatric and maternity professionals. The particular needs of women at this time require specialist resources. In particular, if they require admission to a psychiatric unit following delivery, they need a specialist mother and baby unit. Specialist mental health teams who can work within the maternity context and provide specialist care are needed for those who are significantly ill but do not require to be in hospital.

Some serious postpartum psychiatric disorders can be anticipated. There is good evidence that women who have had a previous serious postpartum illness or a serious mental illness at an earlier time in their lives face a considerable risk of a recurrence of this condition in the days and weeks following the birth. This provides an opportunity, almost unique in psychiatry, of prediction and often preventive management. In most cases these serious illnesses are very responsive to treatment and both the short- and long-term prognosis is good. However without appropriate treatment there may be prolonged morbidity with adverse consequences, not only for the mother's but also for the infant's mental health.

Not only are perinatal psychiatric illnesses a leading cause of maternal morbidity but also of maternal mortality. The last two Confidential Enquiries into Maternal and Child Health reveal that suicide is the leading indirect cause of maternal death and overall, psychiatric disorder contributes to 25% of maternal deaths.

PSYCHIATRIC DISORDERS IN PREGNANCY

Prevalence

Psychiatric disorder in the general community is common, particularly amongst young women with children under the age of 5. In general psychiatric disorders are not associated with a reduction in fertility. Women with the whole range of psychiatric disorder will present in early pregnancy. The majority of these will be the less serious psychiatric disorders, generalized anxiety and depression, mild depressive illness as well as the less common, obsessional compulsive disorder and panic disorder. A smaller number will have bipolar illness or schizophrenia. The prevalence of psychiatric disorder at the beginning of pregnancy is therefore the same as at other times. As many as 27% of women will be taking psychotropic medication at the onset of pregnancy. It is common for these women to stop taking their medication upon the diagnosis of pregnancy. Relapses or recurrences of pre-existing non-psychotic illness are not uncommon in early pregnancy, particularly after the abrupt withdrawal of selective serotonin reuptake inhibitors (SSRI) and other antidepressants. Women who stop antipsychotic or mood stabilizer medication given for serious mental illness are also at risk of a recurrence of their condition during pregnancy.

Pregnancy is not protective of a relapse of serious mental illness particularly if medication has been stopped. Women suffer from relapses of pre-existing mental illness during pregnancy at the same rate as those who are not pregnant. However, those women who have a previous history of mental illness but have been well and stable for some time (for more than 2 years) may not be at an increased risk of a recurrence of their condition during pregnancy. These women, having been well during pregnancy and for many years previously, still face an elevated risk, at least 1:2 of becoming acutely ill following delivery:

- Women with significant mental health problems should discuss with their family physicians and psychiatrist their plans for starting a family, particularly with regard to the risks posed to their mental health and the relative risk of continuing, stopping or changing their medication before conception.
- In general, women should be advised not to stop their medication on the confirmation of pregnancy. The risk of a withdrawal syndrome or relapse of their condition is substantial and its treatment may pose a greater hazard to mother and infant than continuing the medication until an early opportunity for informed advice is taken.
- Women should be specifically asked at the early pregnancy assessment about their current and previous history of mental health problems and particular attention made to any psychotropic medication they are receiving. Those with a prior history of serious mental illness (bipolar illness, schizophrenia, serious postnatal depression, puerperal psychosis, severe OCD and panic disorder) should be seen by a specialist psychiatrist, even if they have been well for many years and a management plan put in place for their peripartum care.

Incidence

The incidence of psychiatric disorder in the first trimester of pregnancy is slightly elevated. Approximately 15% of women will develop an illness having been well for the months prior to conception. The majority of these illnesses will be relatively mild, generalized anxiety and depression and mild to moderate depressive illness. The incidence of milder illnesses declines during pregnancy. However, severe depressive illness, panic disorder and obsessional illness arising in the last trimester of pregnancy not only poses particular management problems but also may continue and deteriorate following delivery as severe postnatal depressive illness.

The incidence or new onset of serious mental illness (bipolar illness and schizophrenia) is markedly reduced during pregnancy compared to other times. Nonetheless, although relatively uncommon, these illnesses pose particular management issues for both psychiatry and obstetrics and require urgent and specialized care. These women will also be at substantial risk of a postpartum illness. (pages 301-305)

- Mental health problems are common in early pregnancy. Most are mild and will improve as the pregnancy progresses. Support and reassurance, watchful waiting and if necessary, psychological treatments will be sufficient in the majority of cases. Medication should not be the first line of treatment, particularly in the first trimester.
- The development of significant mental health problems later in pregnancy requires attention, and if serious, from a specialized psychiatrist. These illnesses are likely to continue after delivery as postnatal depression.
- Although uncommon, serious or psychotic illnesses do present in pregnancy. These should receive urgent specialized psychiatric attention.
- It is essential that mental health and maternity professionals work closely together when pregnancy is complicated by serious mental illness.

POSTNATAL PSYCHIATRIC DISORDER

In marked contrast to pregnancy, the first 90 days of the postpartum period are associated with a substantially elevated risk of becoming psychotic and of developing a serious or severe depressive illness. Women with a pre-existing serious mental illness, particularly bipolar disorder, even if they have been well for many years, are also at an elevated risk of a recurrence of their condition in this time period.

Many more women, at least 10%, will suffer from a less severe non-psychotic depressive illness often described as 'postnatal depression'. For many this will be the first time that they have ever been ill, for others it will be a recurrence of a pre-existing condition.

For some women their mental health problems may reflect difficulties in adjusting to motherhood, concerns about the baby and other difficulties in their lives. However, these may come out of the blue and not be related to adversity particularly the more serious illnesses. Postpartum illness can affect women of all ages and backgrounds (Table 17.1).

Although all types of psychiatric disorder can and do complicate the puerperium, it is the postpartum affective disorders (puerperal psychosis and severe postnatal depression) that warrant special attention because of their distinctive clinical presentation and course, their established epidemiology, and their increased incidence particularly in the first 3 months following childbirth.

Table 17.1 Incidence of postnatal psychiatric disorder

Type of disorder	Incidence (%)
Mild depression/anxiety disorder	15-30
Major depression	10
Severe depressive illness	3-5
Referral to psychiatric services	2
Admission to psychiatric unit	0.4
Puerperal psychosis	0.2

Normal emotional changes in the puerperium

During pregnancy, once the first trimester has passed, the majority of women experience a sense of well-being. Emotional changes are very variable and often individual. In contrast, after childbirth there are well described emotional and behavioral changes which are experienced by the majority of women. While essentially normal and commonplace, they may still come as an unpleasant surprise to the women themselves and be distressing and frightening. Maternity staff in hospital may be unfamiliar with these changes and consequently be either unsympathetic or, on occasion, misattribute them to an illness.

Following a normal delivery most women are happy, even ecstatic and 'high'. They feel excited, do not sleep, they have a tendency to be overactive and not get enough rest and have excessive numbers of visitors. This has been aptly described as the 'pinks'.

Almost inevitably between days 3 and 5, their emotional and behavioral state changes. This is commonly referred to as the 'blues' and affects between 50% and 80% of all new mothers. The commonest day of onset is day 5, rather than day 3. It is a state characterized by emotional lability, quickly moving from laughter to tears, heightened arousal, catastrophic thinking and exaggerated concerns, restlessness and insomnia. Acute feelings of incompetence, concerns about their feelings for the baby and the well-being of the baby are commonplace. This condition is essentially self-limiting, lasting for 48 h but may recur periodically, particularly when very tired over the next 6 to 8 weeks. This condition does not require active 'treatment' but benefits from support and reassurance and explanation. Day 5 is also the commonest day of onset of the most serious form of postnatal mental illness, puerperal psychosis. Care needs to be taken that the 'blues' is resolving as the days go by rather than escalating in both quality and severity.

Puerperal psychosis

Puerperal psychosis is by definition a psychotic illness which arises in a previously well woman within a defined time period of childbirth. The term therefore includes both those women who have a lifetime first onset psychotic illness following childbirth as well as those who have had psychotic illnesses following previous childbirths or those who have had a serious mental illness at other times but have been well in the years preceding their pregnancy. Overall, the incidence of puerperal psychosis is 2 per 1000 births and has remained relatively constant since first described in the 1850s. However, there have been some suggestions in more recent times that the incidence of postpartum onset psychosis (true puerperal psychosis) is less common than in historical times and that the incidence of postpartum recurrence of a previous history, particularly of bipolar illness has increased. Postpartum psychosis has been recognized since antiquity and across cultures. This is notable in the face of the massive changes in reproductive epidemiology, maternal and infant morbidity and mortality since these times.

Despite its rarity, woman are at substantially increased risk of becoming psychotic in the year following childbirth and massively so in the first three months following childbirth (Fig. 17.1).

Clinical features

Puerperal psychosis is an acute onset condition rapidly developing over a period of 24 to 48 h in a previously well woman. The overwhelming majority of these illnesses arise within the first 90 days following childbirth, 50% within the first week and 75% within the first 6 weeks. During the first few days of the illness, the women are very disturbed, agitated, perplexed, bewildered and very frightened. Characteristically, the symptoms are mixed and do not easily allow in the early stages for the illness to be categorized into one of the major illness categories such as schizophrenia or bipolar illness. The usual description is that of an acute undifferentiated psychosis. Their mood is usually seriously disturbed and labile, varying from profound depression to elation and irritability. They usually have a variety of delusional ideas of reference, of influence, of misidentification and paranoid delusions with suspiciousness about the motives of family and professionals. They also have frequent depressive delusions of guilt and incompetence and at other times delusions of grandiosity. In the early days, motility disturbances, confusion, disorientation and disinhibition are also very common. Puerperal psychosis typically deteriorates rapidly, the woman does not sleep and may neglect eating and drinking and other aspects of self-care. After the first few days, the illness becomes more clearly recognizable as that of a variant of bipolar illness or with a persistence of non-mood congruent delusions and hallucinations, that of schizo-affective disorder. In approximately one-third of all cases, the mood is predominantly elated (manic or schizomanic) in others, the mood is either mixed or predominantly depressive. Attention and concentration, self-care and the ordinary tasks of infant care will be seriously impaired. Whilst overt hostility to the infant is uncommon, the woman will require considerable supervision and assistance in meeting the baby's needs. The terror and delusional ideas pose a very real risk of suicide and occasional infanticide. The relative risk for suicide is between 70 and 100.

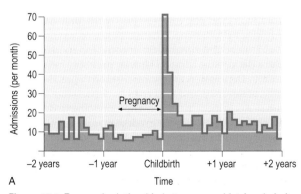

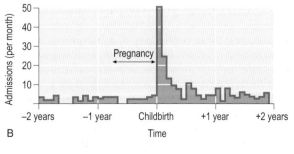

Figure 17.1 Temporal relationship between psychiatric admission and childbirth: (a) all admissions; (b) psychosis admissions.

Management

This is considered in detail on pages 301-305. The overwhelming majority of women with puerperal psychosis will need to be admitted as an emergency to a psychiatric unit. This should be to a specialized Mother and Baby Unit, the only setting in which the physical needs of mother and infant can be met and where the additional expertise is to be found.

Prognosis

Puerperal psychosis has a good short-term prognosis. With appropriate treatment, the manic states should improve within 2 weeks and the predominantly depressive states by 6 to 8 weeks. However, even before the introduction of modern psychotropic medication, puerperal psychosis was noteworthy for its propensity to fully recover within 6 months. In keeping with the probable bipolar nature of the condition, women with a predominantly manic or mixed affective psychosis may become depressed. Puerperal psychosis may relapse if the medication is not continued for many months beyond the resolution of the illness. Nonetheless, the overwhelming majority of women who suffer from puerperal psychosis can expect to fully recover and regain their premorbid level of functioning, even though they may need continuation of their medication for some time.

There is a high rate of recurrence following subsequent childbirths. This is now known to be at least 50%, perhaps higher in those with the very early onset manic conditions. The illness is likely to present in the same way and at the same time as previously.

It has long been known that women who have an episode of puerperal psychosis face a 50% risk of a serious mental illness at other times in their life. While for some women, such an illness will only be associated with subsequent childbirths, for others it may arise at other times in their life. At the time of the first episode, it is difficult to predict into which category the woman will fall. However, those women with a previous history of non-postpartum serious illness are amongst those most likely to subsequently suffer from non-postpartum as well as postpartum episodes. The older the woman is when she suffers from her life time first episode postpartum, the less likely it is that she will go on to have non-postpartum illnesses. There is evidence to suggest that even for those women who do suffer from subsequent episodes, that the frequency of the episodes is less and their overall level of functioning at long-term follow-up, better than in age-matched controls who suffered from an episode outside of the puerperium.

Risk factors

Puerperal psychosis is not as strongly associated with psychosocial risk factors as are other psychiatric conditions. It can affect women of all ages from all walks of life and from all cultures. Risk factors with a strong positive predictive value are a family history of bipolar illness, a family history of postpartum onset illness, a previous history of serious affective disorder (bipolar illness and severe unipolar depression) and a previous history of puerperal psychosis. The risk for a previous history of puerperal psychosis and bipolar illness is 1:2 and the risk for a family history of bipolar illness has been estimated at 1:3. This evidence underlines the importance of routine questioning in the early pregnancy assessment.

Classification

The coding guidelines of both ICD-10 and DSM-IV recommend that wherever possible, puerperal psychosis should be coded under other major illnesses categories but given an additional code of 099.3 mental disorders associated with childbirth. This reflects the prevailing view that puerperal psychosis is not a specific diagnostic (etiological) entity.

Postnatal depressive illness

Ten percent of all recently delivered women will suffer from a depressive illness. The studies, either prospective or cross-sectional, from which this figure is derived, are usually community studies using the Edinburgh Postnatal Depression Scale (EPDS) either as a diagnostic tool or as a screen prior to the use of other research tools. Studies using a cut-off point of 14 usually give an incidence of 10%, those using cut-off scores lower than this often reveal figures up to 15%. A cut-off score on a screening instrument is not necessarily the same thing as a clinical diagnosis of depressive illness. Nonetheless a cut-off score of 14 is said to correlate with a clinical diagnosis of major depression and the lower scores with that of major and minor depression. The incidence of women who would meet the diagnostic criteria for moderate to severe depressive illness is lower, probably between 3 and 5%. Depression following childbirth has the same range of severity and subtypes as depression at other times. According to the symptomatology, duration and severity they may be graded as mild to moderate or severe and subtypes may also be complicated by prominent anxiety and obsessional phenomena.

Postnatal depressive illness of all types and severities is therefore relatively common and represents a considerable burden of disability and distress in the recently delivered community. Although postnatal depressive illness has achieved a great deal of popular acceptance, with the exception of the most severe forms, it is in fact no more common after delivery than during pregnancy and no more common than in non-childbearing women of the same age. However, the lack of evidence of an increased risk of depressive illness following childbirth does not detract from its importance. Depressive illness of any severity occurring at a time when the expectation is of happiness and fulfillment and when major psychological and social adjustments are being made together with the often difficult task of caring for an infant, creates difficulties not found at other times in the human lifespan.

Severe depressive illness

While overall the incidence and prevalence of depressive illness in general in the year postpartum is no higher than in age-matched controls, there is evidence to suggest an increased incidence of severe depressive illness in the first 3 months. The relative risk of suffering from such an illness has been estimated at 1.7 with 3 to 5% of women suffering from a severe postnatal depressive illness.

Clinical features

Severe postnatal depressive illness has an early onset in the first few weeks following birth but unlike puerperal psychosis this tends to be gradual and not become clearly manifest until 4 to 6 weeks postpartum or later.

The core symptoms of severe postnatal depressive illness are the same as depressive illness at other times. These include the so called 'biological syndrome' now referred to as 'somatic subtype' of early morning wakening, diurnal variation of mood, slowing of mental functioning and impaired concentration and overvalued ideas of incompetence and guilt. These are often accompanied by loss of appetite and weight, loss of spontaneity and feelings of pleasure and enjoyment (anhedonia), and difficulty in coping with the tasks of everyday life. The context of new motherhood adds 'pathoplastic features', and the overvalued ideas frequently center upon the baby, mothers' feeling that they are incompetent and bad mothers with excessive worries about their own and the infant's health. These illnesses are frequently complicated by high levels of anxiety, distressing intrusive thoughts, and fears of harming the baby. Panic attacks are relatively common and may present as a psychiatric crisis. Not only do these women fear for their safety as mothers but are often concerned for their own sanity.

The distorted cognitions of a severe depressive illness, particularly the feelings of guilt and incompetence and the isolation and alienation resulting from social withdrawal may lead to suicidal ideation. Women with severe postnatal mental illness are probably at increased risk of suicide and rarely infanticide.

Management

This is considered in more detail on page 301-305. However, these conditions need to be speedily identified and treated, preferably by a specialist team. The value of early contact with those who recognize and validate the symptoms and distress, and can re-attribute the overvalued ideas of the mother and instill hope for the future cannot be underestimated. The treatment of the depressive illness is the same as the treatment of depressive illness at other times. The use of antidepressants together with good psychological care should result in an improvement of symptoms within two weeks and the resolution of the illness between 6 and 8 weeks.

Prognosis

With treatment these illnesses should fully recover. Without, spontaneous resolution may take many months and up to one-third of women can still be ill when their child is 1 year-old.

Women who have had a severe depressive (unipolar) illness face a 1:2 to 1:3 risk of a recurrence of the illness following the birth of subsequent children. They are also at elevated risk from suffering from a depressive illness at other times in their lives. However, the long-term prognosis would appear to be better than when the first episode is unrelated to pregnancy both in terms of the frequency of further episodes and in their overall functioning.

Risk factors

A variety of risk factors for postnatal depressive illness have been identified in the literature and include those associated with depressive illness at other times: lack of social support, socio-economic adversity, marital and family problems, youth and children under the age of 5. Pertinent to the maternity context can be added ambivalence about the pregnancy, high levels of anxiety during pregnancy, adverse birth experiences to name but a few. However all of these risk factors, though statistically significant are so commonplace as to have little positive predictive value. However a clustering of these risk factors might lead to those caring for the woman to be extra vigilant. Of more use are those risk factors which have a higher positive predictive value. These include a family history of severe affective disorder, a family history of severe postnatal depressive illness, developing a depressive illness in the last trimester of pregnancy and the loss of the previous infant (including stillbirth). There may also be an increased risk in those women who have conceived through IVF.

Mild/moderate depressive illness

This is the commonest of the postnatal psychiatric syndromes affecting up to 10% of all women. Although no commoner than in non-childbearing women of the same age, it can have a significant impact on a woman's adjustment to motherhood and for the care and well-being of her infant and family. This group of illnesses ranges in severity and merges with emotional distress and the common place emotional vicissitudes of early motherhood.

Clinical features
The clinical features of mild to moderate postnatal depressive illness often referred to as 'PND' are much the same as at other times. They tend to develop gradually and not become manifest until 3 months or longer after childbirth at a time when other women are successfully adjusting to motherhood. They will lack the core 'somatic subtype' of the severe depressive illness. The condition is often variable with good days and bad. The women are usually very anxious with concerns about their own abilities as a mother and the behavior and well-being of the infant. They usually feel better in company and worse on their own and tend to avoid spending time alone in the home with their infant, going out and seeking the company of others wherever possible. At the more severe end of the spectrum, they may suffer from panic attacks, intrusive unpleasant thoughts and experience variable interruption with their sleep and episodic sadness and despair. While overt hostility and aggression towards infants is uncommon, it is not uncommon for women with PND to feel irritable and to experience little joy or pleasure in their infant. They are often fearful that they might harm their infant.

Management
Early detection and treatment is essential. This is considered in more detail on pages 301-305. For the milder cases, a combination of psychological and social support and active listening from a health visitor or midwife will suffice. For others, specific psychological treatments such as cognitive behavioral psychotherapy and interpersonal psychotherapy are as, if not more effective, than antidepressants.

Prognosis
With appropriate management, postnatal depression should improve within weeks and recover by the time the infant is 6 months old. However, untreated there may be prolonged morbidity. This, particularly in the presence of continuing social adversity, has been demonstrated to have an adverse effect not only on the mother–infant relationship but also on the later social emotional and cognitive development of the child.

Risk factors
The risk factors for mild to moderate postnatal depressive illness are broadly the same as at other times. Most studies emphasize chronic social adversity, maternal youth, lack of social support, marital and family problems and more pertinent to the maternity context a previous history of mental health problems and high levels of anxiety and depression during pregnancy. However, it should be noted that postnatal depression of all severities can and does effect women from more fortunate backgrounds who are older and high achievers with much wanted pregnancies and high expectations of themselves.

ETIOLOGY OF POSTPARTUM PSYCHIATRIC DISORDER

There is a considerable overlap of the etiology and pathophysiology of postpartum psychiatric disorder with affective disorder at other times. Nonetheless, for the severe postpartum illnesses, puerperal psychosis and severe postnatal depressive illness, there are a number of features that suggest at least some specificity of the postpartum trigger and an increased vulnerability in the early postpartum period for the development of these illnesses. In general psychosocial factors combined with the increased vulnerability of the postpartum period are thought to be the main etiological factors in the milder postnatal illnesses and biological factors (genetic and neuroendocrine) in the ascendancy for the etiology of the more severe conditions.

Puerperal psychosis

The distinctive clinical features, early onset within days of delivery and the tendency to recurrence after subsequent childbirth has led some in the past to believe that puerperal psychosis was a separate clinical and diagnostic entity. However, because the majority of cases after a few days exhibit manic depressive features and respond to the treatments of manic depressive illness and because individuals with a family history of manic depressive illness are at increased risk of developing a psychotic episode in the immediate puerperal period, it is reasonable to assume that the majority of cases reflect the interaction of a manic depressive (bipolar) predisposition with the physiological and psychological effects of childbirth. This etiological theory is further supported by the finding that 50% of women who suffer from puerperal psychosis will have a further episode of bipolar illness during their lifetime. Whilst some of these women will only have episodes relating to childbirth, others will develop the illness at other times. However, it does seem that women whose lifetime first episode of psychosis arises within a month of childbirth are more likely to develop illnesses only related to childbirth.

A plausible theory is that women who develop postpartum psychoses have an estrogen a related dopamine receptor sensitivity. Variations in a serotonin transporter gene have also been associated with a subset of women with bipolar disorder that have also developed puerperal psychosis.

Postnatal depression

As at other times, the etiology of depressive illness has a complex pathophysiology and is likely to result from the interplay of genetic, neuroendocrine and psychosocial factors. In general the more severe the depressive illness the more likely it is that biological factors are in the ascendancy. It is sensible to classify these various factors as predisposing, precipitating and maintaining factors.

Predisposing factors

A previous history of depressive illness either following previous childbirth or at other times predisposes to postnatal depression, as does a family history of severe (unipolar) depressive illness indicating that the etiology of postnatal depression has at least some overlap with that of other depressive illnesses. This is further underlined by the significant proportion of women who suffer from postnatal depressive illness who go on to experience depressive illness at other times in their lives. Adverse experiences in early childhood, chronic adversity and recent life events, lack of social support, ambivalence towards the pregnancy and high levels of anxiety during pregnancy also predispose to the development of a postnatal depressive illness.

Stillbirths

Stillbirths and infant death and perhaps a traumatic experience of childbirth predispose women to developing a depressive illness after the next birth. IVF may also increase the risk of developing a postnatal depressive illness.

Precipitating factors

The obvious precipitant is childbirth itself, both as a life event and as an event that is associated with marked physical, physiological and neuroendocrine change. There has been some suggestion that adverse experience of birth may increase the risk of postnatal depression but there is no clear evidence that the mode of delivery or the site of delivery influences the prevalence of postnatal depressive illness.

Childbirth, particularly first time childbirth, is a step in the transition to motherhood. This is a time of massive psychological and social change, ceaseless activity, lack of sleep and commonly difficulties in establishing breastfeeding. It is almost impossible to tease out the contribution made by all of these to the pathogenesis of mild to moderate depressive illness. The tendency for new mothers to engage in negative self-evaluation, critically comparing themselves with the ideal of motherhood and their perception of how others are behaving may increase the vulnerability to depressive illness, particularly if there is inadequate or unsympathetic support from loved ones and health professionals.

In contrast to puerperal psychosis, which seems to be recognized throughout the world, postnatal depression may be largely a Western concept. The understanding of morbid unhappiness as an illness requiring the interventions of health professionals may not be held by those in the developing world which has implications for our own ethnic minority population.

Hormones

It is popularly believed that postnatal depression is the result of some 'hormonal disturbance'. The theory of progesterone deficiency was popularized by Dr. K. Dalton and until recently progesterone was frequently used to prevent or treat postnatal depression. There is no evidence that the progesterone levels of women who develop postnatal depressive illness are different from those of other women, nor that its use prevents or treats the illness. Indeed there is some evidence that progesterone may be 'depressogenic'. Its use can therefore not be recommended. However, there is evidence that the time of the blues is related to both the absolute and relative levels of progesterone following delivery. There is more evidence to suggest that estrogen has antidepressant effects and increases the number and sensitivity of serotonin receptors in the brain. Transdermal estrogen has been shown to be effective in the treatment of postnatal depressive illnesses, however, the lack of systematic evaluation and replication studies would not recommend its routine use.

Hypothyroidism

Depressive illness is a recognized symptom of hypothyroidism. Non-psychotic postnatal depressive illness may be associated with temporary (often subclinical) hypothyroidism that occurs in some women who develop postpartum thyroiditis in the postpartum year.

Maintaining factors

These are factors which continue to fuel the illness or prevent its recovery. Noteworthy will be inadequate or inappropriate treatment, particularly subtherapeutic doses of antidepressants or failing to continue with antidepressants for 6 months. Chronic adversity, lack of social support and significant life events may also feature as maintaining factors. However, the most commonplace maintaining factors are continuing difficulties, real or perceived, with the infant. Feeding and sleeping difficulties feature prominently. These are frequently attributed by the mother herself and sometimes by health professionals to her own mental state and a vicious cycle quickly ensues, the exhausted mother blaming herself, becoming more tense and anxious which in turn affects the infant. She vigilantly focuses on all her perceived inadequacies and compares herself unfavorably with others which may lead her to avoid company and become even more socially isolated.

Breastfeeding

Although there is no evidence that breastfeeding increases the risk of developing significant depressive illness, nor that its cessation improves depressive illness, many depressed breastfeeding mothers struggle in the early days to establish feeding and are concerned later about the quality of their breast milk and blame themselves for their infant being unsettled. All breastfeeding mothers will be up in the night and have less sleep. Continuing breastfeeding may be very important for women with depressive illness, not only because it improves their self-esteem and feeling of maternal autonomy but also because it may go some way to protect the infant, particularly boys, from the effects of the maternal illness.

Work

In general, the mental health of mothers who work is better than those who stay at home. For many, the return to work is associated with improved social contact and self-esteem. However, for others it is purely an economic necessity and they would prefer to stay at home. Whether mothers wish to return to work or feel obliged to do so, the anticipation and planning of the return to work is a frequent cause of stress and anxiety. This, combined with difficulties in finding satisfactory childcare may maintain or exacerbate a postnatal depressive illness.

MANAGEMENT

There are three components to the management of perinatal psychiatric disorders: (1) psychological treatments and social interventions; (2) pharmacological treatments; and (3) the skills, resources and services needed.

Those who are seriously mentally ill will require a combination of all three. Those with the mildest illnesses may require only psychological and social interventions which can be carried out in primary care.

Psychological treatments

All illnesses of all severities and indeed those who are not ill but experiencing commonplace episodes of distress and adjustment need good psychological care. This can only be based upon an understanding of the normal emotional and cognitive changes and common concerns of pregnancy and the puerperium. It also requires a familiarity with the symptoms and clinical features of postpartum illnesses. Good psychological care needs the professional to be able to actively listen, to validate distress, to re-attribute overvalued and negative beliefs and to instill hope. It requires the professional on the one hand not to over-medicalize and misattribute the psychopathology of everyday motherhood to an illness and at the same time to be alert to the possibility of illness.

For most women with mild depressive illness or emotional distress and difficulties adjusting, extra time given by the health visitor – 'the listening visit' – will be effective. For others, particularly those with more persistent states associated with high levels of anxiety, brief cognitive behavioral therapy treatments and brief interpersonal psychotherapy are as effective as antidepressants and may confer additional benefits in terms of improving the mother–infant relationships and satisfaction. Similar claims have been made for infant massage and other therapies that focus the mother's attention on enjoying her infant.

Social support

Lack of social support particularly when combined with adversity and life events has long been implicated in the etiology of non-psychotic depressive illness in young women. Social support not only includes practical assistance and advice and counsel but also having an emotional confidante and female friends (people who improve self-esteem). There is good evidence that organizations that are underpinned by social support theory such as Home Start and other maternal support volunteer agencies can have a beneficial effect on maternal and infant well-being and perhaps on mild postnatal depression.

Pharmacological treatment

In general psychiatric illnesses occurring during pregnancy or in the postpartum period respond to the same treatments as at other times. There are no specific treatments for perinatal psychiatric disorder. Moderate to severe depressive illnesses respond to antidepressants, psychotic illnesses to antipsychotics and mood stabilizers may be needed for those with bipolar illnesses. However, there are two particular areas which merit special attention. First, the possibility of altered pharmacokinetics of psychotropic medication in pregnancy and the immediate peripartum period and, second, the possibility of adverse consequences on the embryo and fetus during pregnancy and (via breast milk) on the developing infant.

The evidence base for the safety or adverse consequences of psychotropic medication is constantly changing both in the direction of increased concern and reassurance. Any text detailing specific advice is in danger of being quickly out of date and the reader is directed to systematic reviews and meta-analyses published by independent professional organizations or, the regularly updated information published by the National Teratology Information Service (NTIS – via Toxbase website: http://www.spib.axl.co.uk).

At least 50% of pregnancies are unplanned at the point of conception and it is known that a substantial number of women are taking psychotropic medication at that time. GPs, obstetricians and psychiatrists will therefore be asked on a frequent basis about the safety of psychotropic medication particularly antidepressants during pregnancy. No matter what the changing evidence is some general principles apply:

- The absence of evidence of harm does not equate to the evidence of safety.
- It may take 20 to 30 years after the introduction of a drug for adverse consequences to be fully realized. A good example of this is sodium valproate.
- In general there is much more evidence on older than on newer drugs although this does not necessarily mean they are safer.
- In the past most attention has been focused on the capacity of a drug to interfere with embryogenesis. The absence of any evidence linking a drug with major congenital malformations does not mean that it may not have adverse effects on the continuing development of the fetus and on the neonate.
- All psychotropic medication passes freely through the placenta. Fetal elimination of psychotropic medication will be less than that of the mother. Both the architecture and function of the fetal central nervous system continues, to develop throughout pregnancy and in infancy.
- The threshold for prescribing medication in pregnancy should be high. If there is an alternative, non-pharmacological treatment, of equal efficacy then that should be the treatment of choice.
- Serious mental illness during pregnancy requires robust treatment. Such an illness may pose a direct risk to the woman and infant through hazardous behavior including suicide or an indirect risk through the larger doses of medication that might be needed to treat an acute illness. In all cases of illness occurring during pregnancy or in a breastfeeding mother, the clinician must be able to balance the risk of not treating the mother on both mother and infant against the risk to the fetus or infant of treating the mother. The more serious the illness is, the more likely it is that the risks of not treating outweigh the risks of treating.
- The fetus and infant are no less likely to suffer from the side effects of psychotropic medication than are adults. Fetal and infant elimination of psychotropic medication may be less than adults and their central nervous system may be more sensitive to the effects of these drugs.
- Increasing blood volume, metabolism and elimination of psychotropic medication during pregnancy result in falling serum levels of antidepressants and antipsychotic and mood stabilizers in the mother (anticonvulsants and lithium). Care therefore needs to be taken when these medications are used in pregnancy to monitor maternal mental health, particularly in the last trimester of pregnancy.
- Adverse consequences of medication on the fetus and infant are dose related. If medication of

any type is used it should be used in the lowest effective dose and given in divided dosage throughout the day.

Antidepressants

Tricyclic antidepressants (imipramine, amitriptyline, dosulepin) have been in use for 40 years. There is no evidence that they are associated with major or minor congenital abnormalities or with adverse effects on the developing fetus. However, a full therapeutic dosage taken at the time of delivery is known to be associated with withdrawal effects in the neonate and with anticholinergic side effects in the newborn. Many perinatal psychiatrists therefore gently taper these antidepressants during the last few weeks of pregnancy. However this may not be possible if a woman has a profound depressive illness later in pregnancy as the reduction in the serum level of antidepressants may induce a worsening of her condition.

Selective serotonin reuptake inhibitors

Selective serotonin reuptake inhibitors (SSRIs) (for example fluoxetine, paroxetine, citalopram) have been in use for approximately 15 years and are now the antidepressants of choice in the first line treatment of depressive illness. Significant numbers of women will be taking these antidepressants at the point of conception, usually prescribed by general practitioners. Their sudden withdrawal is likely to result in a withdrawal syndrome (particularly paroxetine) and for some a relapse in the underlying condition. After years of being considered 'safe' in pregnancy, there have been recent concerns that SSRIs may be associated with an increased risk of major congenital malformation particularly ventricular septal defect and increased fetal loss. However, these findings are conflicting and have been described by the FDA as 'a weak warning signal'. Nonetheless advice has been issued against the use of paroxetine in pregnancy. There is more robust evidence that SSRIs taken late in pregnancy are associated with a neonatal withdrawal syndrome and serotonergic symptoms in the newborn.

On the basis of available evidence, it would seem sensible to advise the use of antidepressants of any type in pregnancy only when there is no effective alternative and when justified by the seriousness of the maternal illness. It is also sensible to advise women not to abruptly withdraw their medication upon the confirmation of pregnancy but rather to discuss with their physician the process of gradual withdrawal if this is indicated. Tricyclic antidepressants should be the antidepressant of choice in pregnancy.

Antipsychotics

There are two broad groups of antipsychotic medications, first, the older 'typical' antipsychotics (trifluoperazine, haloperidol, chlorpromazine) and the newer atypical antipsychotics (risperidone, olanzapine, clozapine).

The typical antipsychotics have been in use for 40 years. There is no evidence to associate the use of typical antipsychotics with major congenital malformation nor with adverse consequences on the fetus. However, theoretically they must affect the fetal brain and the use of typical antipsychotics at the point of delivery has been associated with withdrawal effects in the neonate and extra pyramidal side effects in the newborn. Withdrawal of antipsychotic medication in those suffering from enduring (chronic) bipolar illness or schizophrenia will be associated with a relapse rate in pregnancy equivalent to other times. Such a relapse will pose a considerable risk through hazardous behavior and through the inevitably higher dosage of medication required to control the illness. Therefore, these women should be advised not to withdraw their medication during pregnancy but to discuss with their physician the lowest effective dose to be taken in divided dosage throughout the pregnancy. The same principle applies to breastfeeding. Typical antipsychotics are present in breast milk. Although the amount to which the infant is exposed is likely to be very small, the added benefits of breastfeeding to the infant probably justify the continuation of breastfeeding providing that the dose required of antipsychotic is small and it is given in divided dosage. Drugs such as procyclidine that are often given to prevent extra pyramidal side effects are not recommended.

Following the recent introduction of atypical antipsychotics insufficient evidence on the use of these drugs in pregnancy and in breastfeeding exists to be assured of their safety. There has been no evidence so far that they are associated with an increased risk of major congenital malformations or fetal loss. However, there are some concerns that olanzapine may increase the risk of gestational diabetes. The use of clozapine associated with blood dyscrasias in adults, may also pose a risk to the neonate. In general therefore, the use of the newer atypical antipsychotics in pregnancy should be avoided. However, if there is evidence that these are the only effective antipsychotics for a woman with severe enduring mental illness and if previous attempts to change the atypical antipsychotic to a typical has proven deleterious then continuation of the drug may be justified. The manufacturers advise against breastfeeding while receiving atypical antipsychotics but this is reflection of lack of data rather than evidence of harm.

Mood stabilizers

Lithium carbonate is a well-established treatment for mania and a prophylactic mood stabilizing agent for those with bipolar disorder. Outside pregnancy its use involves the regular monitoring, every 3 months of serum lithium levels (which for prophylaxis should be between 0.6 and 0.8 mmol) and the annual checking of thyroid and renal function. Bipolar illness commonly has its onset in the 20s. Most young bipolar women will become pregnant. The use of lithium in the first trimester of pregnancy is associated with a substantial increase in the relative risk of developing Ebstein's anomaly. However, this is a rare condition and the absolute risk is lower than previously thought, 2 per 1000 exposed pregnancies. Lithium is also associated with an increased risk of congenital malformations including the whole range of cardiac abnormalities, an absolute risk of 8% of all exposed pregnancies. Continuing use throughout pregnancy is associated with an unquantified risk of large babies, diabetes insipidus, hypothyroidism and, following delivery, with the floppy baby syndrome. The changes in maternal hemodynamics and elimination necessitate frequent monitoring and probably an increase in the dose of lithium to maintain a steady serum level. Fetal elimination on the other hand is less than the mother's. Women with bipolar illness who have had an episode within 2 years of conception will relapse if they suddenly stop their lithium (at the same rate during pregnancy as in non-pregnant controls). After delivery, they are at substantially increased risk of relapse compared to controls. Balancing the risks of continuing maternal lithium to the fetus against the risk to both mother and fetus of stopping the lithium requires specialist skills and can only be made on an individual basis.

It is therefore critically important that all women taking lithium should discuss well in advance of conception, their medication and the risk of relapse both during pregnancy and following delivery with their psychiatrist. If the woman has been well for 2 years or longer, it may be reasonable to very slowly withdraw the lithium prior to conception. If she remains well, she should be seen frequently during pregnancy by her psychiatrist who should maintain a close liaison with both obstetrician and midwife. If, on the other hand, there is evidence of frequent relapses, and a manic episode less than 2 years before conception or previous evidence of a significant relapse following cessation of lithium, the risk of stopping the lithium

in pregnancy may be considerable. However, consideration should be given to changing the lithium to a typical antipsychotic. As in all pregnancies screening for fetal abnormalities should be offered. The mother's lithium must be monitored frequently (weekly in the last trimester of pregnancy) and attention paid to the rapid changes in maternal hemodynamics during and immediately after delivery. At this time, there may be a sudden rise in the maternal serum lithium level with a potential for lithium toxicity. The neonate will require close pediatric attention. Lithium should not be used in breastfeeding as it is present in substantial quantities in breast milk and can result in infant toxicity.

Anticonvulsants have been used as mood stabilizers for 30 years. Carbamazepine was first used in this way, sodium valproate is now increasingly the mood stabilizer of choice and recently the newer anticonvulsants such as lamotrigine and topiramate are being used A substantial number of young bipolar women will therefore be receiving this medication. Overall, anticonvulsants are associated with an increase in the baseline risk of congenital malformations particularly neural tube defects (see Ch. 14). There is no reason to believe that women receiving anticonvulsants as a mood stabilizer for bipolar illness are any less at risk. Sodium valproate at higher doses appears to be associated with a higher risk than other anticonvulsants, particularly in relation to its association with longer-term neurodevelopmental and cognitive impairments in the child. Women receiving anticonvulsant mood stabilizers should receive adequate contraception and should be advised not to become pregnant. If she has been well for some time then gradual withdrawal and supervision may be the most appropriate strategy. If not, the anticonvulsant should be substituted for another agent, such as a typical antipsychotic. If a woman accidentally becomes pregnant on sodium valproate in high dose, the dose should be reduced if possible, or the drug substituted by another. Sodium valproate should not be used in pregnancy as a mood stabilizer and probably should not be used in women of reproductive potential unless they are taking effective contraception. The advantages of breastfeeding probably outweigh the risks of taking anticonvulsant mood stabilizers during breastfeeding.

Service provision

There are a number of national recommendations for the needs of women with perinatal psychiatric disorder. The distinctive clinical features of the conditions, their propensity for sudden onset and rapid deterioration, their physical needs and the professional liaison with maternity services all require specialist skills and knowledge. The frequency of these conditions at locality level makes it difficult for general adult psychiatric services to manage the critical mass of patients required to develop and maintain their skills. The competing priorities of other psychiatric patients may make it difficult for them to give the attention and the particular rapid response required to pregnant and recently delivered women. It is also difficult for maternity services to relate to larger number of community-based teams. However, at supra-locality (regional) level the frequency of serious perinatal psychiatric disorder is sufficient to justify the joint commissioning of specialist services. Mothers who require admission to a psychiatric hospital in the early months following delivery should, unless it is positively contraindicated, be admitted to a Mother and Baby Unit. This is not only humane but also in the best interests of the infant and cost effective as it shortens inpatient stay and prevents readmission. There should be community outreach services available to every maternity service, to deal with psychiatric problems that arise after delivery but also to see women in pregnancy who are at high risk of developing a postnatal illness. The majority of women suffering from postnatal mental illness will not require to be seen by specialist psychiatric services. However, there is a need for integrated care pathways to ensure that women are effectively identified and managed in primary care and if necessary, referred on to specialist services. There is therefore a need to enhance the skills and competencies of health visitors, midwives, obstetricians and GPs to deal with the less severe illnesses themselves.

PREVENTION AND PROPHYLAXIS

Prevention

The NICE National Screening Committee and Antenatal and Postnatal Mental Health Guidelines and the SIGN Guidelines for the management of postnatal mental illness find that the risk factors for non-psychotic (mild to moderate) postnatal depressive illness do not have a sufficient positive predictive value to recommend routine screening in the antenatal period for those at risk. They also find that there is a lack of evidence to support antenatal interventions to reduce the risk of non-psychotic postnatal illness. In contrast, these bodies, together with the Children and Young Peoples and Maternity NSF and 'Why Mothers Die' all recommend that women should be screened at early pregnancy assessment for a pre-

vious or family history of serious mental illness, particularly bipolar illness because they face at least a 50% risk of recurrence of that condition following delivery.

In order to discriminate between the history of mental health problem of any type or severity, and that of a history of serious mental illness, those who undertake early pregnancy assessment will need training to refresh their knowledge of psychiatric disorder and to ask the right questions.

There is little point in screening for women at high risk of developing severe postnatal illness, if systems for the proactive peripartum management of these conditions are not in place and if resources are not available for their proper management. It is therefore recommended that all women who are at high risk of developing a severe postpartum illness by virtue of a previous history are seen by a specialist psychiatric team during the pregnancy and a written management plan placed in her records in late pregnancy and shared with the woman, her partner, her general practitioner, midwife, obstetrician and psychiatrist. The essential features of this management plan are:

- The nature of the risk, the type of illness and the time period during which the risk is at its greatest.
- The early warning signs of an illness.
- Any medication required, its dosage and day of starting
- The frequency of contact with health professionals, their names and telephone numbers
- Any provisional plans for admission in an emergency.

Prophylaxis

If the woman has a previous history of bipolar illness or puerperal psychosis, consideration should be given to starting medication on day one following delivery. For bipolar illness the use of lithium carbonate has been shown to reduce the risk of a recurrence and attenuate the illness. It is plausible that the use of antipsychotic medication may also reduce the risk of recurrence. However, lithium is not compatible with breastfeeding. Some women will not wish to take medication when they perceive there is 50% chance of them remaining well. They may also place a priority on continuing to breastfeed. On the available evidence, the best protection for a woman with a previous history of bipolar illness or mixed affective psychosis occurring either following childbirth or at other times would be to take lithium carbonate from day one, achieving a therapeutic lithium level as soon as possible. However, women with a previous history of very early onset puerperal psychosis in the first week following childbirth may be at continued risk before an effective serum lithium level is achieved. For these women, the addition of an antipsychotic will offer added protection in the early days. Breastfeeding mothers at risk of developing a bipolar or mixed affective illness may take carbamazepine or sodium valproate. However, the same problem arises with the time taken to achieve a satisfactory serum level. The evidence that antidepressants taken prophylactically may prevent the onset of a depressive psychosis is lacking. Antidepressants should be used with great caution in any woman who has a suggestion of bipolarity in her personal or family history because of the propensity of antidepressants to trigger a manic illness.

Whether or not a woman chooses to take prophylactic psychotropic medication, the most important aspect of preventive management and one that will promote early identification and the avoidance of a life threatening emergency is close surveillance and contact in the early weeks, the period of maximum risk. Specialist community perinatal psychiatric nurse together with the midwife should visit on a daily basis for the first two weeks and remain in close contact for the first six. The local Mother and Baby Unit should be notified of the woman's expected date of delivery and systems put in place for direct admission if necessary.

THE CONFIDENTIAL ENQUIRY INTO MATERNAL AND CHILD HEATH: WHY MOTHERS DIE, PSYCHIATRIC CAUSES OF MATERNAL DEATH

The last two Confidential Enquiries into Maternal and Child Health have found that in those cases reported to the Enquiry, suicide and other psychiatric causes of death are the second leading cause (indirect) of maternal death in the UK between 1997 and 2002. However, if all maternal deaths including those additionally ascertained by the Office of National Statistics Linkage Study are included, then suicide emerges as the leading cause of maternal death accounting for 15% and psychiatric conditions contribute to 25% of all maternal deaths.

The findings reveal that maternal suicide is commoner than previously thought. Overall, the maternal suicide rate appears to be equivalent to that of the general rate of suicide in the female population. Suicide in pregnancy remains relatively uncommon. The majority of suicides took place in the year follow-

ing delivery. The majority of suicides and almost all of the early suicides (first 3 months) were seriously mentally ill. Not only is the assumption of the 'protective effect of maternity' called into question but it would appear that the relative risk of suicide for seriously mentally ill women following childbirth is substantially elevated. An elevated standardized mortality ratio of 70 for women with serious mental illness in the postpartum year has previously been reported. Evidence from the Enquiries with improved case ascertainment would suggest that the SMR for serious mental illness in the 3 months postpartum is at least 100.

In contrast to other causes of maternal death, suicide was not associated with socio-economic deprivation. The majority of suicides were older, married and relatively socially advantaged. A worrying number were health professionals. This underlines the error of merging issues of maternal mental health with those of socio-economic deprivation.

A startling finding was that almost all of the suicides died violently by jumping from a height or hanging. This stands in contrast to the commonest method of suicide amongst women in general (self-poisoning) and underlines the seriousness of the illness from which the women died.

Most of those who committed suicide were seriously ill and died within 3 months of delivery. Half of these women had a previous history of having been admitted to a psychiatric hospital. In few cases had this risk been identified at booking and in even fewer had any proactive management been put into place. Had their illnesses been anticipated a substantial number of these deaths could have been avoided.

A further 10% of all maternal deaths occurred from other consequences of a psychiatric disorder. Some of these were due to accidental overdoses of illicit drugs. However, a third of these deaths occurred from physical illness. Some of these were the physical consequences of alcohol or illicit drug misuse, others from side effects of psychotropic medication. However, a worrying number of deaths, some of which took place in a psychiatric unit, were due to physical illness being missed because of the psychiatric disorder or because the physical illness had been mistakenly attributed to a psychiatric disorder. These findings underline the importance of remembering that physical illness can present as and complicate psychiatric disorder. Suicide is not the only risk associated with perinatal psychiatric disorder.

The findings of the Confidential Enquiries into Maternal and Child Health have major implications for both psychiatric and obstetric practice. If psychiatrists discussed with their patients their plans for parenthood prior to conception, if obstetricians and midwives detected those at risk of serious mental illness, if psychiatric and maternity professionals communicated freely with each other and worked together instead of within their own organizations, if specialist services were available for those women who needed them and if all had a greater understanding not only of perinatal mental illness but also of emotional changes, then not only would a substantial number of maternal deaths be avoided but also the care and outcome of other mentally ill women would be greatly improved.

Further reading

Brockington I 1996 Motherhood and mental health. Oxford University Press, Oxford

Confidential Enquiries into Maternal and Child Health 2004 Why mothers die 2000-2002. Report on confidential enquiries into maternal deaths in the United Kingdom. RCOG, London

Dean C, Kendell R E 1981 The symptomatology of puerperal illnesses. British Journal of Psychiatrists 139:128-133

Department of Health 2005 National service framework for children, young people and maternity services, maternity services standard 11. Department of Health, London

Kendal R E, Chalmers J C, Platz C 1987 Epidemiology of puerperal psychoses. British Journal of Psychiatry 150:662-673

National Screening Committee 2001 A screening for postnatal depression. Department of Health, London

Oates M 1995 Risk and childbirth in psychiatry. Advances in Psychiatric Treatment 1:146-153

Robling S A et al 2000 Long-term outcome of severe puerperal psychiatric illness: a 23 year follow-up study. Psychological Medicine 30:11263-11271

Royal College of Psychiatrists Council 2000 Perinatal maternal mental health services, report CR88. Royal College of Psychiatrists Council, London

Chapter **18**

Anesthesia and critical illness in pregnancy

J. Griffiths, R. Russell

SYNOPSIS

Risk assessment
Analgesia and anesthesia for labor and delivery
Anesthesia for Cesarean section
Cardiovascular support
Ventilatory support
Hematological support
Microbiological support
Nutritional support
Renal support

RISK ASSESSMENT

Women may develop critical illness as a direct result of pregnancy itself, a pre-existing disease may deteriorate as a result of physiological changes of pregnancy or, their illness may be purely coincidental to pregnancy. Recent editions of the Confidential Enquiries into Maternal and Child Health (CEMACH) have highlighted the importance of intensive care for these women and provide insight into those at greatest risk. Thromboembolic disease remains the leading cause of maternal mortality in the UK with severe pre-eclampsia and massive hemorrhage, which account for over 50% of intensive care unit (ICU) admissions in pregnancy, the other major causes of direct death. However, indirect causes such as cardiac and psychiatric disease now account for greater numbers of maternal deaths. Risk of mortality is greatest amongst economically and socially deprived groups, women of advanced age and those with a high body mass index (BMI).

In the developed world maternal mortality is now fortunately infrequent; consequently risk factors for critical illness amongst survivors may be missed. Morbidity data, such as those from obstetric admissions to ICU may help identify those at increased risk. It has been estimated that the need for intensive care is between 0.2-7.6 per 1000 deliveries although higher rates of up to 9 per 1000 have been reported in hospitals caring for the more socially deprived. Mortality among those admitted to ICU may be as high as 36%. However, for a variety of reasons, not all women with critical illness are admitted to ICU. Pulmonary or amniotic fluid embolism may be rapidly fatal before admission can be organized. High dependency areas, such as those for cardiac patients, may have facilities to manage those who may otherwise require ICU admission. In addition, outreach teams (see below) may review and advise on treatment outside ICU reducing the need for admission. Consequently, studies looking only at ICU admission may underestimate the true incidence of critical illness in pregnancy.

Case control studies may provide further insight into risk factors for critical illness. In the UK, severe morbidity is estimated to be associated with 12 per 1000 deliveries with a morbidity : mortality ratio of 118:1. Risk factors for morbidity are similar to those for mortality and include increasing maternal age, non-white ethnic group, pre-existing hypertension, previous postpartum hemorrhage, operative delivery, antenatal admission, multiple pregnancy and poor social circumstance. An interesting recent addition to CEMACH has been the Scottish experience of severe maternal morbidity. Here the estimated ratio of severe morbidity to maternal mortality was 49:1. Using 14 different categories such as major hemorrhage, eclampsia and pulmonary edema, management was compared with nationally accepted standards. In up to one-third of cases management was considered substandard with important lessons to be learnt.

Critical care outreach

The intensive care chapter of the most recent CEMACH report drew attention to delay in recognizing the severity of critical illness. Failure to interpret clinical signs of acute illness, mistaking them for physiological changes of pregnancy was highlighted. Maternal tachypnea, frequently observed in those whose condition was deteriorating, was often ignored or not appropriately investigated. Identification of the critically ill or deteriorating patient is the key to preventing admission or readmission to the critical care facility. As a consequence many hospitals have developed 'Critical Care Outreach Services' providing advice and help with identification and management of critically ill patients outside the ICU environment. Development of critical care outreach services was based on numerous reports indicating suboptimal management of both patients discharged from ICU and patients at risk of deterioration on hospital wards. Moreover, patients admitted to ICU from a ward area were much less likely to survive than those admitted from either accident and emergency or theatres.

Numerous physiological scoring systems have been devised to identify ward patients who are deteriorating and would benefit from critical care outreach. Examples are the Early Warning Score (EWS), Patient At Risk Score (PARS) or Modified Early Warning Score (MEWS). These are simple scoring systems that can be calculated at the patient's bedside, using routine parameters. MEWS is calculated using seven simple physiological parameters (Table 18.1). However, these scoring systems are not designed for the obstetric population whose vital signs are altered by the physiological changes of pregnancy. Of the parameters assessed, respiratory rate is one of the most important for assessing the clinical state of a patient, but is frequently not recorded. Changes in respiratory rate have been shown to be an antecedent for in-hospital cardiac arrest. Scoring systems are flexible and can be used to monitor medical as well as pre and postoperative surgical patients, and those recently discharged from ICU or attending accident and emergency. Scoring systems are designed to highlight patients at risk of deterioration ('track'), before this becomes too profound and difficult to reverse. Studies have indicated that a MEWS score of 3 or more requires urgent attention ('trigger') and should stimulate rapid assessment by a ward doctor or, if available, intensive care, outreach or emergency medical teams. If deteriorating patients are identified early, simple interventions such as oxygen or fluid therapy are often all that are required. Applied appropriately 'track and trigger' systems are able to reduce patient morbidity and mortality and prevent ICU admission. However, 'track and trigger' systems are not acting as comprehensive clinical assessment tools and are not meant to replace clinical judgment. Moreover, scores generated by such systems have no predictive value and are not an indicator for immediate ICU admission.

In some cases elective admission to ICU is planned, and in others it may follow significant deterioration in the patient's condition. Resuscitation, using the ABCDE system, should not be delayed whilst admission is arranged. Consideration of early delivery of the baby must be made as the gravid uterus may impede further resuscitative measures; left uterine displacement must be employed to avoid aortocaval compression. The airway should be protected, appropriate oxygen therapy administered, intravascular access obtained and fluid therapy instigated if the clinical situation dictates. Oxygen should be administered at

Table 18.1 Modified early warning system (MEWS)

Score	3	2	1	0	1	2	3
Respiratory rate		≤8	9-10	11-20	21-25	26-30	≥31
Pulse		≤40	41-50	51-100	101-110	111-130	≥131
Systolic BP	≤84	85-89	90-100	101-199		≥200	
GCS	≤8	9-13	14	15			
AVPU			New agitation or confusion	Alert	Voice	Pain	Unresponsive
Urine	≤10 mL/h for 2 h	≤30 mL/h for 2 h					
Temp (°C)		≤35.0	35.1-35.9	36.0-37.4	37.5-38.4	≥38.5	
SpO_2	≤87	88-91	92-94	95-100			

15 L/min via a high flow mask with reservoir bag. However, in the ward environment it is rarely possible to constantly deliver greater than 60% oxygen. Available monitoring devices should be attached and the ICU or critical care outreach team contacted as early as possible.

Physiological changes of pregnancy

Oxygen consumption increases by 60% during pregnancy predominantly to meet the metabolic needs of the developing fetus in addition to those of the mother. Minute ventilation increases throughout pregnancy primarily as a result of increasing tidal volume. By term, expiratory reserve volume decreases by 25% and in combination with a 15% reduction in residual volume, produces a 20% fall in functional residual capacity (FRC), namely the amount of gas left in the lungs at the end of normal expiration. The effect on FRC is position dependent with greater reductions occurring in the supine position and results in airway closure in 50% of term parturients. Increased oxygen demand and reduced FRC increase the risk of significant maternal oxygen desaturation during periods of apnea such as occur during induction of general anesthesia. As tracheal intubation is more difficult in the obstetric patient, adequate pre-oxygenation is imperative before anesthesia is induced.

Relative hyperventilation in pregnancy produces a respiratory alkalosis. $PaCO_2$ falls to 4.0 kPa by the end of first trimester, whilst there is only a modest increase in PaO_2 to 14 kPa. Renal compensation occurs with a fall in serum bicarbonate from 24 to 20 mmol/L, although this process is incomplete as arterial pH is at the upper limit of the normal range at around 7.44. Despite this relative alkalosis the maternal oxygen dissociation curve shifts to the right during pregnancy, probably due to elevated levels of 2,3 DPG, increasing oxygen delivery to the fetus. Excessive hyperventilation seen in labor may cause further elevation of maternal pH to values in excess of 7.50. If combined with periods of apnea, not uncommon with systemic opioids, maternal and fetal desaturation may result.

Blood volume rises by 35-40% (more in multiple pregnancy) with increases in both red cell mass and plasma volume, the latter being more significant. This physiological anemia, although aiding uteroplacental flow, may lead to difficulty with assessment of blood loss during obstetric hemorrhage as larger volumes may be lost before the onset of compensatory mechanisms. A loss of up to 25% of the mother's circulating volume may occur with little discernible change in vital signs. Inaccuracy in estimating blood loss may be further compounded by other pregnancy induced cardiovascular changes such as increased heart rate and decreased peripheral resistance. Despite increased blood volume, central venous pressure changes little in pregnancy because of increased venous capacitance.

Cardiac output increases early in the first trimester. A 30% rise in stroke volume combined with a smaller increase in heart rate result in a 50% rise in cardiac output by the end of the second trimester. Despite this, blood pressure usually falls as a result of decreased peripheral vascular resistance, reaching a nadir at mid gestation. A further rise in cardiac output occurs in labor predominantly from increased autonomic activity. Compression of the intervillous space resulting in autotransfusion increases maternal preload further elevating cardiac output. While effective regional analgesia obtunds the sympathetic response to labor pain it has little effect on pre-load. Immediately after delivery, uterine contraction expels blood from the intervillous space elevating cardiac output to levels in excess of 150% of those seen pre-pregnancy. Such increases may be of clinical significance to women with pre-existing cardiac disease. Furthermore, rapid autotransfusion may precipitate pulmonary edema in those with severe pre-eclampsia where colloid osmotic pressure is significantly reduced. Consequently, in the minutes following delivery such high-risk mothers should be closely observed, a time when many focus their attention on the newborn.

Despite obvious consequences, aortocaval compression by the gravid uterus is often overlooked. Compression of the inferior vena cava starts during the second trimester and by term it is completely occluded in up to 90% of women placed supine. This reduces stroke volume and cardiac output by up to 20%. A reduction in femoral artery pressure is also observed in advancing pregnancy signifying aortic compression. However, despite these detrimental effects of lying flat, only 60% of women become symptomatic when placed supine as they compensate by increasing systemic vascular resistance and heart rate. The former may not be possible when regional anesthesia is used. Collateral venous return by azygos and epidural veins also helps to maintain maternal cardiac output. To ensure optimal maternal and fetal cardiovascular stability, it is imperative that efforts are made to avoid placing women supine when critically ill. A simple wedge applied under right hip of the patient during Cesarean or in the ICU overcomes many of the problems of caval compression.

Platelet activity and turnover are increased in pregnancy. There is a modest decline in platelet number, but in normal pregnancy this is insufficient to produce any hemostatic problem. There is an increase in procoagulant factors, a reduction in endogenous anticoagulants and inhibition of fibrinolysis, all changes consistent with the view of pregnancy as an hypercoagulable state. Consequently, with the addition of venous stasis and vascular endothelial damage (Virchow's triad), there is an increase in risk of venous thrombosis during pregnancy and the puerperium.

During pregnancy the stomach is shifted cephalad by the gravid uterus, displacing some of the intra-abdominal portion of the esophagus into the thoracic cavity. This, combined with progesterone induced smooth muscle relaxation, reduces the efficiency of the lower esophageal sphincter. Intra-gastric pressure rises because of compression from the enlarging uterus increasing the risk of regurgitation. Should this occur, and aspiration result, the effects are determined by both volume and acidity of stomach contents. Although serum gastrin levels may rise in pregnancy, it may not be justified to conclude that gastric secretion is increased. Gastric emptying would appear to be little changed until the onset of established labor or the administration of opioids. As the risk of regurgitation is greater during pregnancy, protection of the airway is required where conscious level or airway reflexes are compromised. For induction of general anesthesia most UK anesthetists would prefer adequate starvation (6 hours for solids or semi-solids and 2 hours for clear fluids), antacid premedication and a rapid sequence induction technique using cricoid pressure from the second trimester onwards. The risk of regurgitation decreases after delivery and such precautions may not be required after 48 hours. However, in the emergency situation, or with a critically ill patient, rapid sequence induction is still advisable.

Antenatal assessment

The CEMACH reports have repeatedly highlighted the need for multi-professional care in the management of high-risk pregnancy. Anesthetists, through their experience in resuscitation and intensive care, are ideally suited to form part of this team. Although not all critical illness can be predicted, many women with significant pre-existing conditions should be reviewed by an anesthetist and/or obstetric physician during pregnancy. Many units run antenatal anesthetic assessment clinics where high-risk cases are seen. Guidelines on those who should be referred must be circulated to all professionals providing antenatal care (Table 18.2).

Antenatal anesthetic review allows adequate time for assessment, further medical review and optimization of treatment. As part of the referral process it is helpful to provide an outline of the plan regarding timing and method of delivery. Should this rely on

Table 18.2 Indications for antenatal anesthetic assessment

Cardiovascular	Congenital heart disease	Previous cardiac surgery
	Valvular heart disease	Pacemaker
	Cardiomyopathy	Pulmonary hypertension
	Ischemic heart disease	Marfan's
Respiratory	Severe asthma	Cystic fibrosis
Neurological	Severe epilepsy	Previous neurosurgery
	Myasthenia	Spina bifida
	Multiple sclerosis	
Hematology	Coagulation disorders	Thrombocytopenia
	Anticoagulant therapy	von Willebrand's disease
Musculoskeletal	Scoliosis	Achondroplasia
	Previous spinal surgery	Myotonia
	Ankylosing spondylitis	
Renal	Renal failure	Renal transplant
Endocrine	Severe obesity	Pheochromocytoma
Psychiatric	Potential difficulties with consent	
Obstetric	Severe pre-eclampsia	Placenta previa
Anesthetic	Previous GA/LA problems	Suxamethonium sensitivity
	Malignant hyperpyrexia	Needle phobia
Others	HIV	SLE
	HSV	Jehovah's Witness

the anesthetic consultation, a formal case conference with representation from all relevant parties may be considered. This facilitates decisions regarding mode of delivery, either vaginal or abdominal, whether labor is to be induced, what methods of analgesia and anesthesia are to be used, monitoring for mother and baby and which members of staff should be in attendance. Delivery of known high-risk cases in isolated maternity units is to be avoided. Once a plan is finalized it is essential that a written copy is circulated to all involved including, where appropriate, the patient.

Although antenatal anesthetic assessment identifies most high-risk cases, some women may not be seen, especially if the significance of their condition is not appreciated by those providing care during pregnancy. Furthermore, those without pre-existing problems may only present after their admission to the delivery suite. Therefore, delivery suite ward rounds with obstetricians, midwives, anesthetists and physicians, where available, should take place every day. This multi-professional approach allows a brief period for further referral, investigation and decision making. Often this may be as simple as advising regional analgesia for labor so that general anesthesia for emergency delivery may be avoided in those at increased risk.

ANALGESIA AND ANESTHESIA FOR LABOR AND DELIVERY

Pain relief in labor

The physiological response to pain in labor may be detrimental to the high-risk mother and baby. Maternal hyperventilation produces a respiratory alkalosis shifting the oxygen dissociation curve to the left. The gradient between the curves of mother and baby is therefore reduced impairing fetal oxygen delivery. Maternal catecholamine release and metabolic acidosis further compromise placental perfusion and possibly prolong labor. Many techniques have been used to relieve the pain of labor but most, with the exception of regional analgesia, have little beneficial effect on these physiological responses. Regional analgesia reduces maternal hyperventilation and endogenous catecholamine release improving metabolic condition and providing greater hemodynamic stability. Epidural solutions combining local anesthetic and opioid are most commonly used. Local anesthetics act on all nerve fibres blocking sodium channels preventing the conduction of nerve impulses. Consequently, in addition to effects on sensory pathways, motor and autonomic blockade result. Motor block is undesirable as

it reduces mobility, decreases satisfaction and may increase the number of instrumental deliveries. Autonomic block causes vasodilation producing venous pooling in the legs, reduced venous return and a fall in maternal cardiac output with hypotension. This latter effect is more marked at term when the gravid uterus further impedes venous return. Therefore no laboring woman receiving regional analgesia or anesthesia should be placed supine without adequate uterine displacement. The addition of opioids, such as fentanyl, to epidural solutions allows a reduction in local anesthetic dose minimizing motor and autonomic effects. As opioids exert their anti-nociceptive effect via specific spinal cord receptors, they have no motor or autonomic effect but may cause pruritus, nausea and vomiting. Lipid soluble opioids such as fentanyl have not been reported to cause significant maternal respiratory depression when used in appropriate doses.

Provided hypotension is avoided, regional analgesia is beneficial to the baby as placental perfusion is improved. A recent meta-analysis of fetal acidbase balance, a suitable index of the efficiency of transplacental exchange, found improved values in those babies whose mothers' had received epidural analgesia compared with those whose mothers' received systemic analgesia.

Controversy still exists regarding the effects of regional blocks on labor and delivery. Whilst epidural analgesia is frequently associated with increased intervention this does not necessarily mean that it is its cause. Regional analgesia is not a generic procedure and different protocols for management produce different outcomes. Meta-analysis of randomized studies has shown no increase in Cesarean section rates amongst women receiving epidurals although the number of vaginal instrumental deliveries may be greater depending on local practice. A small, but clinically insignificant, increase in the length of labor has also been demonstrated. To maximize the chance of spontaneous delivery low dose local anesthetic with opioid techniques should be used, whilst the appropriate use of oxytocin and delay in the second stage allowing decent of the fetal head would appear sensible. Furthermore there must be an appropriate indication for intervention, not simply performed for convenience or training. Elective instrumental delivery may, however, be appropriate for those with limited cardiac reserve where the exertions of the second stage may be detrimental.

An increasing number of women with congenital heart disease are reaching childbearing age and regional analgesia, by reducing the cardiovascular response to labor is generally very helpful provided rapid autonomic block is avoided. The diabetic patient may benefit from regional analgesia as metabolic control is more easily achieved. Furthermore, with increased risk of intervention amongst diabetic women, an effective block can be extended for operative delivery, reducing the need for emergency general anesthesia. Likewise, severe obesity may be an indication for regional analgesia. Although technically challenging, and best performed in early labor, improvements in maternal oxygenation and avoidance of general anesthesia are advantageous. Regional blocks should be recommended as the anesthetic of choice to all women scheduled for Cesarean section, and in particular to women in whom general anesthesia is thought to represent a significant risk, most notably those in whom tracheal intubation is expected to be difficult.

There are, however, a number of contraindications to regional analgesia. If a mother declines to give her consent, the reason should be sought in case her grounds for refusal are unfounded. Traumatic needle insertion in a woman with impaired coagulation may lead to an expanding vertebral canal hematoma producing ischemia and ultimately neuronal injury. Fortunately this complication is extremely uncommon (< 1 in 2-400 000) and can be treated successfully with surgical decompression. Most anesthetists are happy to perform a block when the platelet count is above 100×10^9 /L but few would proceed when the number falls below 80×10^9 /L. Between these two figures, further tests of coagulation are usually performed. Should the woman be receiving anticoagulants, the case must be discussed with a senior anesthetist. Recognized guidelines exist for those on anticoagulant therapy.

Regional blocks should not be inserted through an area of skin sepsis because of the risk of epidural abscess or meningitis. Whether blocks are contraindicated in systemic sepsis is more controversial. Many women with chorioamnionitis receive epidural analgesia without incident, although it may be prudent to give antibiotics before the block is sited. Regional blocks in the presence of hypovolemia may precipitate profound hypotension and are best avoided. Regional anesthesia is, however, now widely used for elective Cesarean section in the presence of placenta previa, although where significant bleeding has occurred or an adherent placenta is expected, general anesthesia is usually preferred. Despite the obvious benefits of regional analgesia, its use is contraindicated if staff are not available to ensure continuous monitoring. True allergy to amide local anesthetics is rare, but if proven represents another obvious contraindication. Severe neurological and cardiac disease are not by themselves absolute contraindications to regional blocks, but in certain conditions such as aortic stenosis or raised intracranial pressure, the risks may outweigh potential benefits. All cases where a possible contraindication is suspected must be referred to the anesthetist antenatally.

Epidural and combined spinal-epidural (CSE) analgesia may be used to provide effective pain relief in labor. In the latter technique an initial spinal dose lasting up to 90 min precedes epidural administration. Due to a more rapid onset, CSEs are advantageous in more advanced labor. Epidural analgesia may be maintained by either intermittent top-ups, continuous infusion or by patient-controlled bolus doses. Continuous infusion provides more uniform pain relief with greater hemodynamic stability than top-ups and may be suitable for those with cardiac disorders. Workload for midwifery staff is reduced, although that for the anesthetist may be increased, as breakthrough pain requiring supplementation is not uncommon. Patient-controlled epidural analgesia using solutions similar to that for infusion is increasing in popularity. Overall drug dosage is reduced minimizing motor block and increasing maternal satisfaction. As with infusions, the technique may be limited by the availability of suitable pumps. Unfortunately no one technique has been shown to be superior in terms of delivery outcome. If instrumental delivery is required the epidural catheter should be topped-up. For a simple lift-out delivery labor top-ups should suffice but for more complicated procedures more concentrated local anesthetic solutions are required.

All women receiving regional analgesia in labor should be continuously observed by a trained member of staff. Pulse and blood pressure should be recorded every 5 minutes after a top-up. Additional monitoring is dictated by the clinical situation and, for those with pre-existing medical problems, should have been planned before the onset of labor. Bladder care is vital and distension must be avoided otherwise postnatal atonia may result.

ANESTHESIA FOR CESAREAN SECTION

Either general or regional anesthesia (spinal, epidural or combined spinal-epidural) may be used for Cesarean section. Regional anesthesia is usually the technique of choice as it avoids the increased risk associated with general anesthesia. The decision regarding which technique to use is based on both maternal health and urgency with which the baby needs to be delivered and should be made following discussion between obstetrician and anesthetist (Table 18.3). General

Table 18.3 Classification of urgency of Cesarean section

Category	Description
1	Immediate threat to life of woman or fetus
2	Maternal or fetal compromise which is not immediately life-threatening
3	No maternal or fetal compromise but needs early delivery
4	Delivery timed to suit woman or staff

anesthesia may be preferred when immediate delivery is required (category 1) or when regional anesthesia is contraindicated or ineffective.

General anesthesia

There is no guarantee that the mother's stomach is empty and the increased risk of reflux and regurgitation in late pregnancy make aspiration more likely. This risk may be reduced with clear antacids, H2 receptor antagonists or proton pump inhibitors and restricting oral intake. While this approach is relatively straightforward for elective surgery, identifying those at greatest risk of inhibitors needing general anesthesia in labor is more challenging. Enforced starvation in labor is for many unnecessary and possibly detrimental. The risk of aspiration may be further reduced by tracheal intubation used as part of a rapid sequence induction with cricoid pressure. However, altered body habitus of term parturients and need for rapid intubation result in increased difficulty in correct placement of the tracheal tube. In the non-obstetric population, failure to intubate occurs approximately once in every 2000 cases. In obstetrics this figure increases to one in every 250 cases and failure to intubate and adequately oxygenate the mother is the most common cause of anesthetic mortality. Furthermore, laryngoscopy and tracheal intubation produce a hypertensive response in the mother. This is undesirable, especially for those with pre-eclampsia, but may be obtunded with intravenous agents such as fentanyl, magnesium or labetalol.

Maternal awareness during general anesthesia for Cesarean section has in the past been a significant problem. Fortunately, the belief that light planes of anesthesia are preferred in an attempt to avoid unnecessary depression of the newborn, is no longer widely held. Failure to achieve appropriate depth of anesthesia is in fact detrimental to both mother and baby. Maternal awareness is a harrowing experience with long lasting psychological effects while inadequate anesthesia produces a dramatic rise in catecholamine levels leading to uterine artery vasoconstriction and reduced oxygen supply to the baby. The resulting asphyxia is worse than the transient effects of placental transfer of anesthetic agents.

Volatile anesthetic agents have a tocolytic effect on the uterus. Intraoperative blood loss is greater with general anesthesia and it is prudent to infuse oxytocin once the baby is delivered until the effects of anesthesia have worn off. General anesthesia has a number of other drawbacks. The lips, teeth and tongue are vulnerable to trauma during intubation and postoperative sore throat is common. Pain relief is usually less satisfactory following general anesthesia. Systemic opioids are invariably required and resulting side effects such as nausea and vomiting more likely when compared with regional anesthesia. Mobilization may be delayed thereby increasing the risk of thromboembolism. Finally, with delivery under general anesthesia parents are unable to share the experience of childbirth.

Regional anesthesia

Spinal anesthesia is now the most popular technique for Cesarean section and is preferred to epidural anesthesia for a number of reasons. The block is usually of better quality and its onset relatively rapid, usually between 5 and 15 min. Development of narrow gauge atraumatic needles has significantly reduced the incidence of postnatal headache. However, when used as a single shot technique the duration of action of spinal anesthesia is limited to about 90 min with no facility to continue the block when surgery is prolonged. In such circumstances a combined spinal-epidural technique may be more appropriate (see below). The rapid onset of spinal when compared with epidural anesthesia creates greater hemodynamic instability, although this may be minimized by intravenous fluids, vasoconstrictors and avoidance of aortocaval compression. However, administration of generous quantities of fluids and vasoconstrictors may not be appropriate for some high-risk cases. Indeed, there has been an argument that spinal anesthesia is inappropriate for women with severe pre-eclampsia. Large fluid boluses are best avoided for fear of precipitating pulmonary edema but a number of studies have now demonstrated that in the hands of an experienced obstetric anesthetist, spinal anesthesia may be used safely. Where there are concerns regarding fluid management and cardiovascular disease, invasive monitoring of arterial and central venous pressure may be appropriate.

It is usually assumed that spinal anesthesia is better for the baby than general or epidural anesthesia. However, recently a small but statistically significant detrimental effect on neonatal acid–base balance, associated with spinal anesthesia has been demonstrated. Consequently, a beneficial effect on the health of the baby of spinal when compared with both epidural and general anesthesia cannot be assumed.

Epidural anesthesia is now most commonly used when a catheter has previously been placed to provide labor analgesia. The block may be easily extended for surgery avoiding the risks of general anesthesia. Once the decision has been made to proceed to operative delivery, the woman should be transferred to theater urgently and a larger more concentrated top-up given. A fall in maternal blood pressure may be observed, although this is usually less dramatic than that following induction of spinal anesthesia. Quality of anesthesia may not be as reliable as a spinal but the presence of an epidural catheter allows further top-ups to be given should pain develop. With larger doses of local anesthetic required for epidural anesthesia it is important to check for systemic toxicity. Visual and verbal contact must be maintained to detect early signs such as circumoral numbness. As with any anesthetic technique ECG, blood pressure and pulse oximetry should be monitored.

CSE anesthesia is preferred by some to the single shot spinal technique. The procedure usually involves passage of a spinal needle through the epidural needle before the catheter is sited, although occasionally the two are performed at separate spaces. Placement of an epidural catheter may take slightly longer but onset of anesthesia should not be significantly different from that of a spinal. CSE provides greater reliability and flexibility as the block may be extended or prolonged for complicated surgery and the catheter allows for excellent postoperative analgesia. For women with limited cardiovascular reserve, the sequential CSE, in which a small spinal dose is extended with incremental epidural top-ups is useful. In this situation high quality anesthesia from intrathecal injection is combined with the greater hemodynamic stability of the epidural, although the onset time is not as quick as with the single shot spinal.

All patients receiving either general or regional anesthesia for delivery must receive appropriate postoperative care, which may range from admission to ICU (see below) to routine recovery room care (Table 18.4). For the latter, location may vary depending on local facilities but should conform to national standards. Measurements of pulse, blood pressure, respiratory rate, temperature and oxygen saturation should be documented in addition to an assessment of analgesia. Supplemental oxygen is given as required and intravenous fluids and analgesics should be prescribed. Assessment of risk for thromboembolic

Table 18.4 Classification of patients requiring critical care services

Classification	Description
Level 0	Needs can be met through normal ward care in an acute hospital
Level 1	Patients at risk of their condition deteriorating, or those recently relocated from higher levels of care whose needs cannot be met on an acute ward without additional support from critical care team
Level 2	Patients requiring more detailed observation or intervention including support for a single failing organ system or post-operative care, and those stepping down from higher levels of care.
Level 3	Patients requiring advanced respiratory support alone or basic respiratory support together with support of at least two organ systems. This level includes all complex patients requiring support for multi-organ failure.

disease and uterine atony should be made and heparin and oxytocin prescribed as indicated. High-risk mothers or those whose clinical condition has deteriorated to an extent that level 2 or 3 support is necessary, may require more extensive organ support (Table 18.4).

CARDIOVASCULAR SUPPORT

Many patients admitted to ICU have an intravascular volume deficit or surfeit although it is often difficult to determine volume status from the complex and disordered medical record that often accompanies critically ill patients. Time spent on a careful appraisal of volume status from the fluid balance record and by assiduous clinical examination is well justified. After hemorrhage and vigorous attempts at resuscitation, many patients develop fluid overload and even pulmonary edema.

Vomiting, decreased oral intake, pyrexia, tachypnea and 'third space' losses often compound hypovolemia. Thus, administration of appropriate fluid is usually first line treatment to maintain or improve organ perfusion via an increase in stroke volume and cardiac output. The crystalloid–colloid debate is still unresolved. Systematic reviews have not demonstrated that any colloid solution is superior to any other, nor that use of colloids is associated with better outcomes than with crystalloids. As a general rule, warmed fluids should be infused rapidly until an acceptable systolic blood pressure is restored. Fluid resuscitation should be balanced with clinical condition to avoid volume overload, cardiogenic and non-cardiogenic pulmonary edema, or worsening of an existing alveolar capillary leak. Packed red cells should be given if indicated to maintain adequate blood oxygen transport capacity. Fresh frozen plasma may be the volume replacement agent of choice in a bleeding patient with a coagulopathy.

Monitoring

ECG monitoring with the CM5 lead is commonly used as it monitors anterior and lateral aspects of the left ventricle and detects over 80% of left ventricular ischemia and the majority of dysrhythmias. The CM5 lead is obtained by attaching the right arm lead to the manubrium, the left arm lead to the V5 position over the left ventricle and the indifferent lead to the left shoulder. The monitor is set to lead I. Automated non-invasive blood pressure (NIBP) devices are used when there is no direct arterial access. Most use an oscillotonometric technique and as a result the most accurate measurement is that of mean arterial pressure. As cuff width is the most important determinant of accuracy, an appropriate size must be used. Non-invasive techniques have a tendency to overestimate blood pressure when it is low and underestimate when high. Inaccurate readings may also be seen in the presence of arrhythmias. In such instances mean arterial pressure measurement should be used.

Urine output is often used as a guide to adequacy of cardiac output, although it is more a measure of renal perfusion. When perfusion is adequate urine output exceeds 0.5 mL/kg h. Urinary sodium levels can sometimes help distinguish pre-renal from intrinsic renal causes of acute renal failure. In the face of a depleted intravascular volume the urine sodium concentration is usually low (less than 20 mEq/L) while in intrinsic renal disease it is usually greater than 40 mEq/L.

Concerns regarding the safety and benefit of pulmonary artery catheters have resulted in a widespread adoption of less invasive hemodynamic monitoring techniques such as esophageal Doppler. Incorporating an ultrasound beam and Doppler shift principle, esophageal Doppler provides a minimally invasive means of real time continuous cardiac output monitoring. A small probe is inserted into the esophagus and advanced and rotated until the characteristic descending aortic trace is obtained (Fig. 18.1). Blood flow delivered to the descending aorta is then approximated

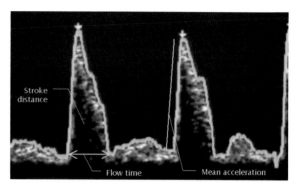

Figure 18.1 The esophageal Doppler waveform. Flow time ('the waveform base') is a reflection of left ventricular ejection and, corrected for heart rate, provides an index of preload. Mean acceleration or peak flow velocity (the 'peak of the waveform') is an indicator of myocardial contractility.

to give an estimate of cardiac output. The characteristic waveform of the esophageal Doppler gives a real time visual representation of hemodynamics. Although absolute values of cardiac output obtained by esophageal Doppler are not entirely accurate, monitoring waveform trend allows response to fluid resuscitation or inotropic therapy to be observed. Until recently insertion of the esophageal Doppler required sedation or anesthesia but recent models have been designed for use in awake patients. Transesophageal echocardiography (TEE) is becoming more widely applied on ICU as more practitioners become trained in its use. Cardiac output and end-diastolic volume can be measured and a variety of myocardial and valvular disease pathologies diagnosed.

Invasive arterial pressure is invariably measured in critically ill patients. It provides real time representation of hemodynamics and guides fluid management and inotropic therapy. It also enables repeated samples to be taken for arterial blood gas analysis. Morbidity associated with arterial cannulation is less than that associated with five or more arterial punctures. As with oscillotonometric techniques employed in NIBP measurement, mean arterial pressure is the most accurate measurement. Significant variation in the amplitude ('swing') of the arterial trace during inspiration in a mechanically ventilated patient is suggestive of volume depletion.

Central venous pressure (CVP) can be monitored using a catheter inserted via the internal jugular, subclavian or femoral vein, although the latter is less accurate in the face of raised intra-abdominal pressure. Correct placement is confirmed by easy aspiration of non-pulsatile blood through all ports of the catheter, a suitable CVP pressure trace when attached to the monitor, and for internal jugular and subcla-

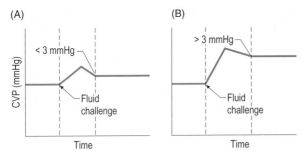

Figure 18.2 Principles of a fluid challenge. A baseline CVP measurement is obtained. A fluid challenge of 250 mL colloid is given over 10 min. If CVP rises less than 3 mmHg then a further fluid challenge may be given (A). If the CVP rises and remains >3 mmHg above baseline value in response to the fluid challenge further filling could result in pulmonary edema (B).

vian catheters, and chest X-ray to confirm that the catheter tip lies in the superior vena cava. The CVP is a surrogate marker of right ventricular filling and thus preload, and adequacy of fluid resuscitation. In the absence of significantly impaired right ventricular function or pulmonary hypertension, left ventricular filling is said to mimic right ventricular filling. An isolated value of the CVP is of less value than dynamic changes in response to fluid challenges (Fig. 18.2). Over-reliance on CVP values in the presence of pre-eclampsia may, however, be dangerous as there may be discrepancy between right- and left-sided pressures. Excessive fluid administration, in an effort to increase CVP may precipitate pulmonary edema and is inadvisable as oncotic pressure is low secondary to loss of plasma proteins and the presence of endothelial damage facilitates the passage of fluid into the lung interstitium.

Although pulmonary artery flotation catheters (PAFCs) have historically formed an important part of hemodynamic monitoring in critically ill patients, recent evidence has questioned their true benefit. Currently, there is no conclusive evidence that their use leads to improved outcomes and decreased mortality. Indeed, if used by inexperienced clinicians in the wrong group of patients, inappropriate therapies may be administered and outcome actually worsened. There may still be a role for hemodynamic monitoring using PAFCs in selected patients (e.g. complex cardiac lesions and severe pre-eclampsia) by experienced clinicians suitably trained in their use.

Mixed venous oxygen saturation ($Sv'O_2$) involves sampling pulmonary artery blood from the distal lumen of a PAFC. However, recent interest has focused on mixed 'central' venous oxygen saturation ($Scv'O_2$) obtained from sampling from the distal port of a central line. A satisfactory correlation exists between $Sv'O_2$ and $Scv'O_2$. Both values are measures of the adequacy of tissue perfusion and vary directly with cardiac output, hemoglobin and arterial saturation and inversely with metabolic rate. Normal $Sv'O_2$ is approximately 75% but is reduced when oxygen delivery falls or tissue oxygen demand increases. At levels of 30% oxygen delivery is insufficient to meet tissue oxygen demand and there is an increased potential for anaerobic metabolism and lactic acidosis. Sepsis can lead to increased values of $Sv'O_2$ reflecting a failure of the cells to utilize oxygen.

PiCCO® is a mode of hemodynamic monitoring less invasive than pulmonary artery catheterization as it utilizes information from CVP and arterial lines (normally femoral). It works by a combination of pulse contour analysis and intermittent transpulmonary thermodilution to give a continuous display of cardiac output. Data obtained using the PiCCO® correlate well with that obtained using a PAFC. It also provides information on stroke volume, systemic vascular resistance and pulse pressure variation. These latter two characteristics are similar to the traditional 'swing' on arterial tracings, and can be used to estimate circulating volume in a mechanically ventilated patient.

Inotropes

If significant hypotension or poor tissue perfusion persist despite adequate fluid resuscitation, additional pharmacological support is normally required. Vasopressors restore blood pressure and improve coronary blood flow; inotropes increase tissue oxygen delivery via an increase in cardiac output. Vasopressors must be used with extreme restraint in any patient with pre-eclampsia, however mild, unless there is a catastrophic complication leading to resistant hypotension and impaired tissue perfusion – even then they carry significant dangers.

Norepinephrine has potent alpha-adrenergic activity, with less, but significant beta-adrenergic effects. It produces significant vasoconstriction in most vascular beds and is therefore used to treat refractory hypotension. In septic patients it increases mean arterial blood pressure and systemic vascular resistance, often without altering cardiac output. Recent evidence also suggests that it increases oxygen delivery and utilization.

Epinephrine has significant alpha- and beta-adrenergic properties. Although it increases both heart rate and systemic vascular resistance, blood pressure is elevated predominantly through an increase in stroke volume. Epinephrine also increases oxygen delivery and consumption. Dysrhythmias may occur as a consequence of heightened irritability of autonomic conducting system. It also has an anti-insulin effect and can produce lactic acidosis. Given by infusion epinephrine is a useful inotrope to stabilize hemodynamics in the pre-intensive care setting, such as in the operating theatre or on the ward.

Dobutamine is a synthetic catecholamine with marked beta-1-adrenergic activity. At standard doses it produces a 25-50% increase in cardiac output. Blood pressure may rise, fall slightly or remain unchanged. At higher doses tachycardia and arrhythmias are more likely to occur. Dobutamine therapy is considered in patients with an inappropriately low cardiac output despite adequate or increased filling pressures and blood pressure. The combination of dobutamine and norepinephrine may enhance tissue perfusion in septic patients refractory to volume resuscitation. Dopamine has been used for inotropic support and oliguric renal failure. This practice was based on the belief that dopamine-induced increase in renal blood flow would improve renal function or protect the kidneys. However, recent meta-analyses have failed to demonstrate that continuous low dose dopamine prevents renal failure in critically ill adults and it is therefore no longer routinely used.

Ephedrine is a naturally occurring vasopressor amine with both direct and indirect sympathomimetic effects. It has both alpha and beta-adrenergic properties causing increased cardiac contractility and heart rate and peripheral vasoconstriction. Its hemodynamic effects are thus similar to epinephrine but it has a longer duration of action. Ephedrine has traditionally been the vasopressor of choice in obstetrics, although this has recently been challenged. Metaraminol also has direct and indirect, and alpha and beta-adrenergic properties. Its hemodynamic effects are similar to ephedrine except that overall peripheral vascular resistance is increased, producing a greater increase in mean arterial pressure. Phenylephrine has effects that mirror norepinephrine but is shorter acting. It causes peripheral vasoconstriction resulting in a rise in blood pressure, often with a reflex reduction in heart rate.

Intra-aortic balloon pumping is sometimes used in the face of frank or imminent cardiogenic shock when further medical treatment is thought likely to be ineffective.

Embolic disease

Amniotic fluid embolism is an uncommon but potentially fatal complication of childbirth accounting for an estimated 10-20% of maternal deaths. Mortality is high and is estimated at 80-90%. It is characterized by a sudden onset of cardiovascular collapse and acute hypoxia frequently followed by a systemic inflammatory reaction and DIC. The initial response of the pulmonary vasculature is intense vasoconstriction. The resultant pulmonary hypertension and hypoxia leads to right and then left heart failure. Treatment is entirely supportive with intubation, ventilation, invasive hemodynamic monitoring, correction of the inevitable profound coagulopathy and its consequences and inotropic therapy invariably required. Venous air embolism may occasionally complicate operative delivery when air in entrained into the circulation via the exposed lumen of large veins. As with amniotic fluid embolism presentation is with hypoxia, hypotension and cardiovascular collapse. Precordial auscultation may reveal a 'windmill murmur', with more definite diagnosis made by echocardiography or right ventricular Doppler studies. Treatment includes positioning in the left lateral position, ventilation with 100% oxygen, flooding the surgical site with saline and supporting the circulation with aggressive fluid loading, vasopressors and inotropes. Attempts to aspirate air through a central line placed in the right atrium are usually unsuccessful.

Venous thromboembolic disease remains the leading cause of maternal mortality in the UK. Pulmonary emboli may produce breathlessness, plueritic chest pain or sudden death. Arterial blood gases reveal hypoxemia and ECG acute right heart strain. Diagnosis is confirmed radiologically by perfusion or spiral CT scanning. Oxygen supplementation is often required in addition to anticoagulation and analgesia (see Ch. 8).

VENTILATORY SUPPORT

The aim of ventilatory support is to improve and maximize gas exchange allowing optimal oxygen delivery to the tissues and maintaining or restoring normal carbon dioxide levels in the blood. Non-invasive ventilation (NIV) using a portable ventilator may be used outside the ICU for a number of conditions causing respiratory failure (Table 18.5). NIV reduces complications associated with conventional ventilation such as the need for sedation and ventilator associated pneumonia. The most basic form of NIV is continuous positive airway pressure (CPAP) using a tight-fitting mask. Other machines are capable of providing bi-level positive airway pressure (BiPAP) that administer both positive end expiratory pressure (PEEP) and either pressure support or pressure-controlled ventilation. For many cases of hypoxemic

Table 18.5 Indications for respiratory support

Support	Indication
Non-invasive ventilation	Pulmonary edema
	Asthma
	Hypoxemic respiratory failure
	Community acquired pneumonia
	Nosocomial pneumonia
	Aspiration pneumonitis
	Trauma
	Early ARDS
	Exacerbation of COAD
	Weaning from ventilatory support
Intubation and ventilation	Respiratory arrest
	Agitation requiring sedation
	Reduced conscious level
	Hemodynamic instability
	Respiratory rate > 35
	pH < 7.30
	PaO_2 < 6 kPa
	Ineffective pulmonary toilet and secretion clearance

respiratory failure NIV is an effective alternative to conventional ventilation although 30-40% of patients ultimately require intubation. There are a variety of contraindications to NIV such as severe cardiovascular instability, impaired consciousness and an uncooperative patient. Minor complications include patient discomfort, air swallowing and nasal bridge ulceration.

Tracheal intubation and mechanical ventilation may be required should NIV be inadequate or inappropriate (Table 18.5). The goal of mechanical ventilation is to provide optimum gas exchange whilst limiting the potential for ventilator-induced lung injury. The latter may be caused by excess pressure ('barotrauma'), excess volume ('volutrauma'), repeated shear and stress injury of the opening and closing alveoli ('atelectrauma') and infection (ventilator-associated pneumonia). PEEP prevents alveolar collapse, improves oxygenation and reduces shunting and minimizing alveoli shear and stress injury and should be set at the highest level tolerated to maximize lung compliance and oxygenation. Increasing levels may, however, compromise venous return producing hemodynamic instability.

A wealth of ventilator modes exists, all with advantages and disadvantages. With poorly compliant lungs, requiring escalating levels of mechanical ventilation, pressure regulated ventilation is necessary to protect against ventilator associated lung injury.

Modern ventilation modes such as 'BiPAP' allow spontaneous ventilation during the respiratory cycle, helping to maintain diaphragmatic function. Low tidal volumes (6 mL/kg) improve outcome when compared with larger volumes (10-12 mL/kg) although it may be necessary to increase respiratory rate in order to achieve adequate minute ventilation. Increased levels of mechanical ventilation required for satisfactory gas exchange may not be tolerated causing the patient to 'fight' the ventilator. This can be rectified by increasing the level of sedation or muscle paralysis. This approach leads to decreased oxygen consumption, carbon dioxide production and ultimately the work of breathing.

High oxygen concentrations are potentially toxic to the lung if administered over long periods. Therefore, the lowest oxygen concentration required to maintain satisfactory arterial oxygen saturation should be used. The consensus view is that if possible inspired oxygen concentration should not exceed 60%. However for many patients with evolving adult respiratory distress syndrome (ARDS) this may be difficult to achieve. A variety of maneuvers have been designed to 'recruit' collapsed alveoli and improve oxygenation and reduce alveoli shear and stress injury. Inverting the normal ratio of inspiration to expiration so that expiration is much shorter than inspiration can improve oxygenation for patients who remain hypoxic. However, this strategy is often poorly tolerated and does not always result in improved gas exchange. Ventilation to dorsal regions of the lung improves when a patient is placed prone. In up to 70% of those with ARDS, prone positioning leads to more even distribution of ventilation and perfusion improving oxygenation. With escalating levels of mechanical ventilation higher arterial CO_2 levels (e.g. 60-100 mmHg) are often accepted to prevent further iatrogenic lung injury. These values are not believed to produce adverse consequences. The pH is monitored to ensure that values do not fall below 7.10.

Sedation is usually required during periods of mechanical ventilation. Nursing driven protocols managing the delivery and appropriate withdrawal of sedation have been shown to reduce the duration of mechanical ventilation, decrease length of stay on ICU, reduce the number of patients requiring tracheostomy and lead to lower levels of psychological ill-health during the recovery period.

Pulmonary edema

Under normal conditions a small amount of extracellular fluid in the lungs passes through capillary walls into the pulmonary interstitium and is removed by the lymphatic system. As with other parts of the body, Starling forces govern the net flux of fluid into the interstitial space. If more interstitial fluid accumulates than can be removed, alveolar edema eventually occurs and airways fill with fluid preventing efficient gas exchange. Pulmonary edema may develop because of alteration of Starling forces, disruption of the alveolar capillary membrane and impairment of lymphatic drainage. These mechanisms can be further classified as to whether pulmonary edema is either 'cardiogenic' (raised hydrostatic pressure) or 'non-cardiogenic' (normal hydrostatic pressure). In pregnancy complicated by pre-eclampsia, decreased oncotic pressure and capillary endothelial damage make pulmonary edema more likely especially if fluid loading, particularly with crystalloid solutions, is excessive.

Tocolytic induced pulmonary edema occurs in up to 4% of pregnant women receiving beta$_2$-adrenergic tocolytic agents to treat preterm labor especially those with multiple gestation, pre-eclampsia and sepsis. The mechanism by which pulmonary edema forms is uncertain but is probably hydrostatic in nature and is characterized by symptoms of left heart failure attributed at least partly to direct effects of beta-adrenergic stimulants on the myocardium. It is frequently associated with volume overload.

Arterial blood gas analysis demonstrates hypoxemia and normal or low CO_2. Chest X-ray features are those of the underlying condition together with those of pulmonary edema classically described as perihilar and fluffy ('bat's wing'). If pulmonary edema develops, the patient should be sat upright and high flow oxygen administered. Diuretics and opioids should be titrated carefully to avoid resultant hypovolemia with reduced placental and maternal organ perfusion. CPAP may be required and admission to high dependency or ICU is advisable. In severe cases intubation and ventilation are necessary together with vasodilators and inotropes.

Lung aspiration syndromes

Aspiration of gastric contents is more likely in the term parturient, particularly if she is exposed to general anesthesia. Intra-abdominal pressure is increased, lower esophageal sphincter tone reduced and in labor gastric emptying delayed. Severity of the condition correlates with volume, pH and particulate content of the aspirate. Large particles cause upper airway obstruction whilst small ones reach more peripheral areas causing atelectasis distal to the obstruction. Others may cause a localized pneumonitis progressing to necrotizing pneumonia, abscess

formation and empyema. Acid aspiration causes extensive lung damage starting within minutes and resulting in an acute lung injury, which may progress to adult respiratory distress syndrome. Vagally mediated bronchospasm is often evident. More severe lung injury is thought to occur with an aspirate of pH less than 2.5 and volume of greater than 25 ml. Gastric contents in previously healthy patients are free from bacterial colonization and therefore infection is not important in the early stages of acid aspiration lung injury although it may supervene. The most likely pathogens are usually anaerobic oral flora but in critically ill patients, enteric gram negative organisms dominate.

Initial management is to correct hypoxemia and instigate supportive therapy. Nebulized bronchodilators are often given if there is evidence of bronchospasm. Outpouring of protein rich fluid into the lung in severe acid aspiration may lead to relative intravascular hypovolemia. However, debate exists as to whether fluid resuscitation should be liberal or restrictive. Inotropes may be required. If there is evidence of large particulate aspiration, lobar collapse or foreign body on chest X-ray, rigid bronchoscopy is indicated. Flexible bronchoscopy should be performed in the face of semi-solid or liquid aspiration. Broad-spectrum antibiotics are used as treatment or as prophylaxis against secondary lung infection. Systemic steroids have no therapeutic role and may actually worsen outcome.

Acute lung injury and acute respiratory distress syndrome

Acute lung injury (ALI) and ARDS usually develop within 12-72 h of the precipitating event (Table 18.6). Despite recent improvements mortality remains high at about 50% for the general population and 25% in pregnancy. Less than 20% of deaths are due to refractory respiratory failure emphasizing the importance of identifying and treating the precipitating cause.

Table 18.6 Obstetric causes of ARDS

Sepsis
Aspiration
Massive hemorrhage
Pre-eclampsia
Amniotic fluid embolism
Trauma
Pneumonia

ALI and ARDS occur when inflammatory cytokines or exogenous agents injure both epi- and endothelium of the lung. These inflammatory insults may develop locally in the lung or be part of a systemic inflammatory response syndrome (SIRS). Irrespective of precipitating cause, the pathophysiological mechanisms driving the process are identical and progress through recognized phases (Table 18.7). ARDS classically affects the lung in a non-homogenous manner with CT scans taken during the initial phases showing striking asymmetry of lung involvement. Dependent posterior regions are preferentially infiltrated, consolidated or collapsed. Anterior areas are often normally or even excessively aerated during mechanical ventilation. Such heterogeneity makes effective ventilation difficult.

Although orthopnea may be present other features of congestive heart failure are rare. Arterial blood gases reveal hypoxemia that is often refractory to oxygen therapy. Initial respiratory alkalosis invariably leads to hypercapnia as dead space ventilation increases and muscle fatigue develops. As ARDS evolves the cardiovascular system is commonly affected and multi-organ failure invariably ensues. Over 50% develop renal failure. Patients with only lung involvement have 15-30% mortality. However, if three or more organs are involved this figure rises to greater than 80%. If the multi-organ failure persists beyond four days mortality is 100%.

Treatment consists of intubation with support of ventilation, oxygenation and hemodynamics. Fluid management aims to maintain intravascular volume at the lowest level consistent with adequate organ perfusion. Prone positioning invariably improves oxygenation but is not associated with improved survival. Precipitating causes should be treated to limit the evolving inflammatory cascade. A number of specific treatments have been used in ARDS although none has been shown conclusively to be of benefit. Extracorporeal membrane oxygenation (ECMO) is expensive and at present has not been associated with improved survival benefits in adult ARDS, although this is currently under investigation. Artificial surfactant, although of benefit in neonates with idiopathic respiratory distress syndrome, has proved disappointing in adults. Inhaled nitric oxide can selectively vasodilate the pulmonary vascular bed and reduce pulmonary hypertension, decrease shunting and improve gas exchange in ARDS. There are no systemic effects because nitric oxide is scavenged rapidly by hemoglobin. However, numerous large clinical trials have failed to demonstrate that improvements in oxygenation seen amongst patients treated with nitric oxide improve outcome. Inhaled prostacyclin vasodilates the pulmonary bed as effectively as nitric oxide but does not result in the same improvements in oxygenation. Corticosteroids have no role in the acute management of ARDS. High frequency oscillation ventilation provides efficient gas exchange by using very low tidal volumes and high respiratory rates. Again no survival benefit has been demonstrated in the adult population with severe ARDS.

Table 18.7 Stages of ARDS

Phases	
Initial phase	Day 3-5
	Severe oxygenation defect
	Reduced lung compliance
	Bilateral pulmonary infiltrates
	Endothelial and epithelial injury
	Leak of protein-rich edema into interstitium and air spaces
Sub-acute phase	Day 5-14
	Persistent oxygenation defect and reduced lung compliance
	Increased alveolar dead space
	Interstitial fibrosis
	Disruption of pulmonary microcirculation
Chronic	Day 14 onward
	Reduced lung compliance
	Increased dead space ventilation
	Extensive fibrosis
	Formation of bullae

HEMATOLOGICAL SUPPORT

Hemorrhage and disseminated intravascular coagulation

Major obstetric hemorrhage remains an important cause of maternal morbidity and mortality, the majority of cases resulting from uterine atony, retained products and genital tract lacerations, with amniotic fluid embolism syndrome a rare but important cause. Risk factors include a history of postpartum hemorrhage, prolonged labor and operative delivery and multiple pregnancy; there is debate as to whether grand multiparity increases risk. Initial management as with any emergency, is based on the ABCDE approach and should aim to restore circulating blood volume. Senior staff must be involved at the earliest possible stage in resuscitation and blood products need to be immediately available. Hypotension mediated endothelial injury and large volume infusion, diluting existing coagulation factors, may trigger disseminated intravascular coagulation (DIC). Renal and hepatic failure, in addition to ARDS may all result. Following initial resuscitation CVP monitoring is advisable to prevent under or over transfusion. More invasive hemodynamic monitoring (see above) may be of value if hypotension or oliguria persists despite adequate CVP or if other complications such as ARDS or sepsis develop.

DIC is characterized by inappropriate, excessive and uninhibited activation of hemostasis leading to consumption of clotting factors and platelets within the circulation. The predominant mediator driving DIC is tissue factor (thromboplastin), which activates the coagulation cascade resulting in formation of thrombin and plasmin. Thrombin formation leads to micro and macrovascular thrombosis, thrombocytopenia and microangiopathic hemolytic anemia. Circulating plasmin activates complement causing red cell and platelet lysis, increased vascular permeability, hypotension and shock. DIC also generates factor XIIa, activation of the kinin system, a reduction in antithrombin concentration and depression of protein C and S systems. Investigations are often difficult to interpret. High concentration of D-dimers are probably the most reliable, as these are formed from plasmin degradation of cross-linked fibrin and only occur when both clotting and fibrinolytic systems are activated.

Initial management is with blood products. Fresh frozen plasma contains all coagulation factors and its main inhibitors antithrombin and protein C, while cryoprecipitate is especially useful if fibrinogen is depleted. Investigation should aim to identify whether the underlying process is predominantly thrombotic or fibrinolytic in nature. Indeed, widespread macro and microvascular thrombosis and not hemorrhage have the greatest impact on morbidity and mortality. However, the use of anticoagulants in the face of DIC remains controversial and is contraindicated in a large number of patients including most parturients (with the exception of those with amniotic fluid embolus) and those with liver failure. Other therapies that may have a role in the treatment of DIC include platelet transfusions, antithrombin concentrates, inhibitors of fibrinolysis (tranexamic acid and aprotinin), recombinant factor VIIa and activated protein C. The use of these treatments requires specialist knowledge and supervision because if they are used inappropriately outcome may be worsened.

Table 18.8 Infection sepsis and SIRS

Condition	
Infection	Microbial process characterized by an inflammatory response to the presence of micro-organisms or invasion of normally sterile host tissue by these organisms.
Sepsis	Systemic response to infection, manifested by two or more of the SIRS criteria plus infection; in severe cases associated with organ dysfunction, hypoperfusion, or hypotension.
Septic shock	Sepsis-induced hypotension despite adequate fluid resuscitation, plus perfusion abnormalities, lactic acidosis, oliguria, or acute alteration in mental status. May require inotropic support
SIRS	Diagnosed by: temperature > 38°C or < 36°C; heart rate > 90 beats/min; respiratory rate > 20 breaths/min or $PaCO_2$ < 32 mmHg; WCC > 12 000 mm^{-3} or < 4000 mm^{-3}, or > 10% immature forms

MICROBIOLOGICAL SUPPORT

Tachycardia, pyrexia, elevated white cell count or CRP although strongly suggestive of infection may also be seen in pulmonary embolism or SIRS driven by a non-infective process (Table 18.8). Alternatively, a septic patient may be apyrexial or even hypothermic. Evidence of infection in an apyrexial patient include leucocytosis, tachycardia, tachypnea, hypotension and increased anion-gap acidosis. Antibiotic therapy should only follow thorough history and examination supported by relevant investigations, imaging and microbiological studies. Liaison with the local microbiology team is strongly recommended. In the absence of an established focus of infection in a deteriorating patient who may be developing multi-organ dysfunction, antibiotics should be selected to target the most likely source and cause of infection. Other important considerations when choosing an appropriate antibiotic include the patient's physiological and immune status, the presence of any indwelling lines, prior antibiotic exposure, the prevalence of and type of nosocomial infections encountered within that particular hospital environment and local sensitivities of micro-organisms commonly encountered. Invariably, broad-spectrum antibiotic cover is initially provided by beta-lactams, aminoglycosides, quinolones, vancomycin, macrolides and antifungals. Specific targeted antibiotic prescription is possible once the results of initial investigations and microbiological sensitivities are known.

Control of the source of infection is vital and should be undertaken once the patient has been stabilized. However, in some instances it may be a component of initial stabilization. For example, full resuscitation in toxic shock syndrome is not possible until the infected tampon is removed and the process arrested. Infected and ischemic tissue should be debrided, abscesses should be drained and obstruction of the urinary, biliary and gastrointestinal tracts relieved. Effective source control procedures can be expected to speed the resolution of clinical signs of severe sepsis, shorten the time to bacteriological resolution, improve wound healing, arrest the inflammatory cascade, prevent further organ dysfunction and decrease mortality.

Sepsis

Sepsis may be a life-threatening complication of pregnancy resulting from a number of infectious causes. The risk of sepsis is increased after prolonged rupture of membranes, emergency Cesarean section and with retained products of conception. Onset may be insidious but can progress to rapid deterioration. Early signs of pelvic sepsis include vomiting, diarrhea abdominal pain, tachycardia, tachypnea and pyrexia greater than 38 °C.

The pathophysiology of sepsis has been divided into five stages: the infectious insult, the preliminary systemic response, the overwhelming systemic response, compensatory anti-inflammatory reaction and immuno-modulatory failure. The SIRS observed in sepsis results in systemic vasodilation, hypotension, increased cardiac output and eventually reduced oxygen extraction by the tissues. The key pathological processes driving this process are abnormalities of endothelial function and disordered coagulation. This results in release of a variety of cytokines and tissue factors, activation of the clotting cascade and a reduction in natural inhibitors of clotting such as activated protein C. Once triggered, the downward spiral of severe sepsis is believed to be independent of the underlying infectious disease process. The combination of increased thrombosis and reduced fibrinolysis leads to disturbed microcirculatory blood flow, microcirculatory ischemia and multiple organ dysfunction and eventual multiple organ failure.

Multiple organ dysfunction syndrome

Multiple organ dysfunction syndrome (MODS) was originally described in patients with massive acute

Table 18.9 Clinical and laboratory markers of organ dysfunction

Organ system	Clinical	Laboratory
Cardiovascular	Tachycardia Hypotension Arrhythmias ↓Cardiac output	↑↓ CVP or PCWP
Endocrine	Weight loss	Hyperglycemia ↓ Albumin

Hematological	Bleeding	Thrombocytopenia
		↑ D-dimers
		Abnormal white
		  cell count
		Abnormal clotting
		  profile

Gastrointestinal	Ileus GI bleeding Acute pancreatitis Acalculous cholecystitis	↓ Intestinal pH ↑ Amylase

Hepatic	Jaundice	↑ Bilirubin
		↑ LFTs and
		  prothrombin
		  time
		↓ Albumin

Neurological	Delirium/confusion Altered consciousness	Altered EEG
Renal	Oliguria/anuria	↑ Creatinine & Urea
Respiratory	Tachypnea	$PaO_2 < 70$ mmHg $SaO_2 < 90\%$ $PaO_2/FiO_2 < 300$

Immune	Cyanosis
	Pyrexia
	Nosocomial
	  infection
		Abnormal white
		  cell count and
		  function

blood loss secondary to ruptured aortic aneurysm. It is now evident that MODS accompanies a diverse group of disorders including sepsis, trauma, pancreatitis and severe pre-eclampsia. Once initiated MODS follows a predictable clinical course irrespective of the precipitating event (Table 18.9). The first evidence of organ dysfunction is usually cardiovascular and respiratory change with the appearance of ALI or ARDS. Resulting pulmonary failure and hypoxemia are followed by hepatic and renal dysfunction and disorders of hemostatic, gastrointestinal and central nervous systems. Prognosis is related to the number of failed organ systems.

Early recognition of the septic process is vital and may be aided by the use of a 'track and trigger' system. However, many patients require ventilation to maximize oxygenation and minimize the work of breathing. Targeted and protocol driven early 'goal directed therapy' of fluid and inotropic support improves outcome from sepsis possibly by augmenting the SIRS driven by tissue hypoxia. There is little evidence to support the use of a particular inotrope in sepsis. In the face of vasodilation and reduced systemic vascular resistance that characterizes 'warm sepsis' norepinephrine is preferred. As sepsis can dampen myocardial function, dobutamine is often introduced to provide inotropy and chronotropy. Epinephrine is a useful agent when simplicity of treatment is required and is therefore often used during the initial stages of resuscitation. Circulatory shock seen in sepsis can often become resistant to treatment with the traditional catecholamine inotropes (norepinephrine and epinephrine). In this situation vasopressin or vasopressin analogues may restore adequate blood pressure and help reduce the dose of existing inotropes.

Activated protein C (APC) plays an important physiological role in the body's normal response to injury or insult. APC helps maintain the balance between coagulation and fibrinolytic pathways and helps reduce the inflammatory response through inhibition of thrombin mediated inflammatory activities and leucocyte attachment to endothelium. As levels of APC are reduced during sepsis its use may reduce mortality in sepsis.

NUTRITIONAL SUPPORT

A functioning gastrointestinal tract serves an important role in the critically ill as it allows nutrients to be absorbed, and provides important immunologic support. Stimulated gut can attenuate the stress response and protect against mucosal and gut-associated lymphoid tissue atrophy. Resultant reduction in gut permeability and enhanced immune function protect against further nosocomial infection and insult. Metabolic and nutritional demands of a critically ill patient are significant. Calorific and protein requirements are high and evidence suggests that these are best provided through the enteral route via a nasogastric or nasojejunal tube. Enteral feeding has the advantage over parenteral nutrition of representing a more physiological pattern of feeding in terms of gastric acid and gut hormone secretion. It also avoids the need for an indwelling intravascular feeding catheter. However, in critically ill patients it is not always possible to establish enteral feeding. Potential barriers include an ileus or generalized bowel hypomotility, often associated with infusion of sedatives or opiate-based analgesics. Here parenteral nutrition should be commenced and enteral feeding reinstated at the first available moment, often with the aid of prokinetic drugs. Exact caloric requirements and feeding regimens are calculated in consultation with the ICU dietitian. Much recent interest has been given to prescription of nutrients, such as glutamine, that may boost immune function. The potential benefits of this so-called 'immunonutrition' include enhanced phagocyte and lymphocyte function, improved wound healing, decreased use of antibiotics and shorter ICU stay.

Tight control of blood glucose level (4.4-6.1 mmol/L) improves survival in the critically ill. It is not clear, however, whether this beneficial effect is due to achieving near normoglycemia, or an effect of insulin itself. Potential beneficial non-glucose related effects of insulin include an anti-inflammatory action and improvement in immune function. It is well known that septic patients often display relative adrenal insufficiency and low dose hydrocortisone replacement (200-300 mg in 24 h) often reduces inotropic requirements.

RENAL SUPPORT

Acute renal failure (ARF) is uncommon in pregnancy (Table 18.10). It is characterized by a sudden and sustained fall in glomerular filtration rate associated with

Table 18.10 Etiology of acute renal failure in pregnancy

Stage	
Pre-renal	Hyperemesis
	Hemorrhage
	Cardiac failure
Renal	Acute tubular necrosis
	Pre-eclampsia/eclampsia/HELLP
	Sepsis
	Amniotic fluid embolism
	Acute fatty liver of pregnancy
	Drug induced
	Glomerulonephritis
	Pyelonephritis
Post renal	Ureteric obstruction

a loss of excretory function. This leads to accumulation of metabolic waste products and water and an increase in the serum urea and creatinine, usually with a fall in urine output. In critically ill patients ARF is often a component of multiple organ failure and its etiology is commonly multifactorial in origin. It is estimated that 10% of all patients admitted to ICU receive some form of renal replacement therapy, as ARF occurring in this setting is unlikely to resolve with conservative management.

Nephrotoxic drugs should be avoided and hemodynamic status optimized with appropriate fluid resuscitation, and when necessary inotropic support, to ensure adequate renal perfusion. Various treatments to prevent incipient renal failure including dopamine, frusemide, n-acetyl-cysteine and mannitol have not been shown to alter outcome. When oliguric renal failure develops despite optimum management, renal replacement therapy (RRT) using either arteriovenous or, more commonly, venovenous hemofiltration, is indicated. A double lumen vascular catheter is placed in a central vein, although the subclavian route is usually avoided because of the high incidence of stenosis following cannulation. Blood is drawn from the proximal lumen and pumped through an extracorporeal circuit before returning through the distal lumen of the catheter. Solutes are removed from the blood by either diffusion or convection. Diffusion is movement of solutes down a concentration gradient across a semipermeable membrane. If a pressure gradient is set up across the dialysis filter, water is pushed across the membrane carrying dissolved solutes. This process of ultrafiltration, is termed convection.

When indicated, RRT may be either continuous or intermittent. Continuous venovenous hemofiltration (CVVH) is commonly used on ICU but requires anticoagulation and has the potential for thrombocytopenia, electrolyte imbalance, hypothermia and hemodynamic instability. Blood is usually pumped through the dialysis circuit at flow rates of 100-200 mL/min and specialized replacement fluid substitutes the removed ultrafiltrate fluid. Approximately 2 L of ultrafiltrate are removed each hour. Either all or part of the ultrafiltrate is replaced depending on desired fluid balance. In contrast to hemodialysis, which excels at removing low molecular weight substances (< 500 Daltons), hemofiltration filters the blood of compounds with molecular weights as high as 30 000 Daltons. Many septic mediators (e.g. cytokines, complement) lie within this group raising the possibility that hemofiltration might benefit patients with severe sepsis. There is some evidence that high volume ultrafiltration, up to 6 L/h, may be associated with significantly lower mortality rates in septic patients.

Further reading

American College of Chest Physicians/Society of Critical Care Medicine Consensus Conference 1992 Definitions for sepsis and organ failure and guidelines for the use of innovative therapies in sepsis. Critical Care Medicine 20:864-874

Balk R A 2000 Pathogenesis and management of multiple organ dysfunction or failure in severe sepsis and septic shock. Critical Care Medicine 16: 337-352

Ball C, Kirkby M, Williams S 2003 Effect of the critical care outreach team on patient survival to discharge from hospital and readmission to critical care: non-randomised population based study. British Medical Journal 327:1014-1016

Bernard G R et al 1994 The American European Consensus Conference on ARDS: definitions, mechanisms, relevant outcomes, and clinical trial coordination. American Journal of Respiratory and Critical Care Medicine 149:818-824

Bone R C et al 1992 Definitions for sepsis and organ failure and guidelines for the use of innovative therapies in sepsis. Chest 101:1644-1655

Confidential Enquiries into Maternal and Child Health 2004 Why mothers die 2000-2002: The sixth report of the confidential enquiries into maternal death in the United Kingdom. RCOG, London

Deblieux P M, Summer W R 1996 Acute respiratory failure in pregnancy. Clinical Obstetrics and Gynecology 39(1):143-152

Department of Health 2000 Comprehensive Critical Care. A Review of Adult Critical Care Services. HMSO, London

Fernando R, Collis R 2000 Mobile epidural techniques and new drugs in labour. In: Reynolds F (ed) Regional analgesia in obstetrics. A millennium update. Springer, London, p 81-109

Greer I A 1999 Thrombosis in pregnancy: maternal and fetal issues. Lancet 353(9160):1258-1265

Hawkins J L et al 1997 Anesthesia-related deaths during obstetric delivery in the United States. Anesthesiology 86:277-284

Horlocker T T et al 2004 Regional anesthesia in the anticoagulated patient: defining the risks. Regional Anesthesia and Pain Medicine 29:S2

Johanson R et al 2003 The MOET course manual. RCOG, London

Levi M et al 1999 Disseminated intravascular coagulation. Thrombosis and Haemostasis 82: 695-705

Lucas D N et al 2000 Urgency of caesarean section: a new classification. Journal of the Royal Society of Medicine 93:346-350

Oakley C (ed) 1997 Heart Disease in Pregnancy. BMJ Publishing Group, London

Oh T E, Bersten A D, Soni N (eds) 2003 Oh's intensive care manual, 5th edn. Butterworth-Heinemann, Philadelphia, PA

Reynolds F, Seed P T 2005 Anaesthesia for caesarean section and neonatal acid-base status: a meta-analysis. Anaesthesia 60:636-653

Rivers E et al 2001 Early goal-directed therapy in the treatment of severe sepsis and septic shock. New England Journal of Medicine 345:1368-1377

Russell R, Scrutton M, Porter J 1997 Pain relief in labour. Reynolds F (ed). BMJ Publishing Group, London

The Acute Respiratory Distress Syndrome Network 2000 Ventilation with lower tidal volumes as compared with traditional tidal volumes for acute lung injury and the acute respiratory distress syndrome. New England Journal of Medicine 342:1301-1308

The Association of Anaesthetists of Great Britain and Ireland, Obstetric Anaesthetists Association 2005 Guidelines for obstetric anaesthetic services: revised edition. AAGBI, London

Van den Berghe G et al 2001 Intensive insulin therapy in critically ill patients. New England Journal of Medicine 345:1359-1367

Ware L B, Matthay M A. The acute respiratory distress syndrome. New England Journal of Medicine 342:1334-1348

Waterstone M, Bewley S, Wolfe C 2001 Incidence and predictors of severe obstetric morbidity: case-control study. British Medical Journal 322:1089-1094

Chapter 19

The neonate and maternal medical complications

P. W. Fowlie, W. McGuire

INTRODUCTION

Obstetricians, physicians and midwives caring for the woman with illness complicating pregnancy strive to balance the benefits and risks of any intervention for the mother and her fetus in order to minimize morbidity and mortality for both. Often this requires a 'trade-off' between mother and fetus. This chapter will discuss the consequences of maternal illness for the fetus and newborn infant and how to care for the neonate immediately following delivery. It will focus on the effects of preterm birth and intrauterine growth restriction, the consequences of diabetes and thyroid disease in pregnancy, the effects of maternal drug misuse in pregnancy, and the management of infants at risk of intrauterine or perinatal infection.

INTRAUTERINE GROWTH RESTRICTION AND PRETERM BIRTH

About 15 to 25% of preterm infants are delivered because of maternal or fetal complications of pregnancy. The principal causes are hypertensive disorders of pregnancy (almost always pre-eclampsia) and associated severe intrauterine fetal growth restriction. Women with diabetes, renal disease, and autoimmune disease, are also more likely to require preterm delivery because of deterioration of maternal or fetal health.

During the past 20 to 30 years changing antenatal and perinatal practice has been associated with an increase in the rate of iatrogenic preterm delivery and a fall in the incidence of still birth in the third trimester. When planning the timing and mode of delivery when maternal health is compromised or maternal disease puts the fetus at risk, it is necessary to weigh the risks to the mother and fetus of continuing the pregnancy against the risks of preterm birth and delivery. Unfortunately, there is little robust clinical evidence to suggest tools developed to assess fetal well-being (Box 19.1) are of benefit in predicting and preventing poor outcomes in high-risk pregnancies. In general, before 26 completed weeks' gestation, the

Box 19.1 Assessment of fetal growth and well-being

- Clinical assessment of growth (fundal height).
- Ultrasonography to measure head circumference and abdominal girth.
- Doppler measurement of fetoplacental blood flow velocity.
- Cardiotocography.

Box 19.2 Consequences of intrauterine growth restriction

- Fetal distress.
- Intrauterine death.
- Meconium aspiration syndrome.
- Hypothermia.
- Hypoglycemia.
- Polycythemia/hyperviscosity.
- Thrombocytopenia.

Box 19.3 Potential complications associated with preterm delivery

- Respiratory distress syndrome.
- Cardiorespiratory instability – apnea, bradycardia, desaturation, persistent patent ductus arteriosus, hypotension, persistent fetal circulation.
- Fluid imbalance.
- Metabolic disturbance – glucose homeostasis, electrolyte imbalance, jaundice.
- Intraventricular hemorrhage.
- Infection.
- Poor growth.
- Neurodevelopmental impairment.

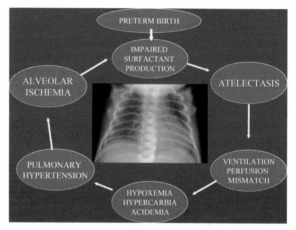

Figure 19.1 Etiology of respiratory distress.

balance of risk favors elective delivery only if the mother's health is at significant risk. Beyond 30 completed weeks' gestation, the balance often lies in favor of elective delivery if either fetal or maternal well-being is compromised. Between 26 and 30 weeks' gestation, clinical judgment is needed to determine where the balance of risk lies before deciding whether or not elective delivery is justified. The determination of such risk is site dependent. In neonatal referral units in the first world, the outcome for the infant is superior to that in units elsewhere with less developed facilities. Prolonging a pregnancy, with careful surveillance, may therefore be preferable in certain cases if advanced neonatal support for preterm babies is not available. Such decisions should be made jointly between professionals – obstetricians, physicians, neonatologists, midwives and others – and the mother and, if appropriate, her partner.

Intrauterine growth restriction due to inadequate placental support of the fetus may lead directly to a range of perinatal problems (Box 19.2). In addition, growth restricted infants delivered early because of concern about maternal or fetal health may experience the complications associated with preterm birth.

Preterm infants have to cope with additional physiological and metabolic stresses because of immaturity in the majority of organ systems. Very preterm infants (less than 32 weeks' gestation), or ill infants, often require intensive monitoring and support during this

critical period of postnatal adaptation. The more significant complications are listed in Box 19.3. Optimal care for preterm infants in the early neonatal period therefore demands attention to several key interrelated issues including respiratory and hemodynamic support, temperature control, nutritional input, and fluid and electrolyte balance.

Acute respiratory disease

Respiratory distress syndrome (RDS) of prematurity is a major cause of morbidity and mortality in preterm infants. RDS is due primarily to deficiency of pulmonary surfactant, a complex mixture of phospholipids and proteins that reduces alveolar surface tension and maintains alveolar stability (Fig. 19.1). The majority of alveolar surfactant is produced after about 30-32 weeks' gestation, so preterm infants born before then are very likely to develop RDS. Over the previous 20 to 30 years, two major advances in perinatal manage-

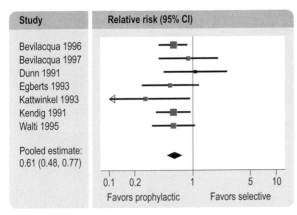

Study	Relative risk (95% CI)
Bevilacqua 1996	
Bevilacqua 1997	
Dunn 1991	
Egberts 1993	
Kattwinkel 1993	
Kendig 1991	
Walti 1995	
Pooled estimate: 0.61 (0.48, 0.77)	

0.1   0.2   1   5   10
Favors prophylactic   Favors selective

Figure 19.2 Meta-analysis of prophylactic versus selective use of surfactant to prevent mortality in preterm infants. (From Soll RF, Morley CJ 2003 Prophylactic versus selective use of surfactant in preventing morbidity and mortality in preterm infants. The Cochrane Library. 4. John Wiley & Sons Ltd, Chichester, with permission.)

ment, the use of antenatal corticosteroids and exogenous surfactant replacement, have greatly improved clinical outcomes for preterm infants with RDS.

Antenatal corticosteroid therapy (dexamethasone or betamethasone) given to women at risk of preterm delivery accelerates fetal surfactant production and lung maturation, and reduces the risk of RDS, intraventricular hemorrhage, and death by 40%. The effect of antenatal corticosteroids appears to last at least one week. Recent evidence also now suggests that repeated doses of antenatal corticosteroids in women who remain at risk of very preterm birth for more weeks after an initial course may bring short-term benefits to the neonate although long-term safety remains uncertain as animal studies have demonstrated adverse growth effects of repeated steriod doses.

Exogenous surfactant, instilled via an endotracheal tube, for the treatment or prophylaxis of RDS is associated with a 40% reduction in neonatal mortality and a 30% to 65% reduction in the risk of pneumothorax. The use of natural surfactant extracts, usually porcine or bovine, is associated with decreased mortality compared with using synthetic surfactant products. It is more effective to ensure surfactant replacement is given as soon after delivery as possible to infants at risk of developing RDS ('prophylactic therapy'), than to wait for symptoms to develop before giving treatment ('rescue therapy') (Fig. 19.2).

Chronic lung disease

The most important long-term complication of RDS is chronic lung disease of prematurity, usually defined

as a need for ventilatory support or supplemental oxygen at 36 weeks' postconceptional age. Chronic lung disease develops in about one-quarter of preterm infants who receive positive pressure ventilation for RDS. The risk is related to the degree of prematurity, severity of the initial lung disease and the duration of mechanical ventilation and oxygen administration. Despite the use of antenatal corticosteroids and surfactant replacement, the incidence of chronic lung disease has continued to rise over the past decade, possibly due to the increased survival of extremely preterm infants.

Few postnatal interventions have been shown to be effective in preventing or treating chronic lung disease. Because inflammation secondary to infection and ventilator-induced lung damage may be an important part of the disease process, corticosteroids have been used for prophylaxis and treatment of evolving or established CLD. While systemic corticosteroids administered to the newborn (dexamethasone or betamethasone) may confer short-term benefits, recent studies have raised strong concerns about long-term complications including an increased risk of cerebral palsy especially when corticosteroids are prescribed in the first few days after birth.

Hemodynamic instability

Hypotension in preterm or low birthweight infants is associated with adverse outcomes, particularly intraventricular hemorrhage and periventricular leucomalacia. Hypotension and impaired systemic perfusion may be secondary to a number of problems and management should be directed towards treating the underlying cause, for example giving volume replacement or antibiotics, as well as to specific measures to improve systemic perfusion, such as inotrope support.

In the first few days after birth, patency of the ductus arteriosus is a significant cause of hypotension and poor perfusion. Preterm infants with a patent ductus arteriosus are at increased risk of more severe and more prolonged respiratory distress syndrome, chronic lung disease, intraventricular hemorrhage, and death when compared to similar infants with closed ductus arteriosus. The patent ductus arteriosus may be closed either surgically, with transthoracic ligation, or pharmacologically, with prostaglandin synthesis inhibitors such as indomethacin of ibuprofen. There is good evidence that the prophylactic use of indomethacin in very low birthweight infants confers short-term benefits, including a reduction in the incidence of symptomatic patent ductus arteriosus, a reduced need for surgical ligation, and a

---

> ## Box 19.4 Physiological consequences of hypothermia in the neonate
>
> - Increased oxygen consumption: hypoxia.
> - Increased glucose utilization: hypoglycemia.
> - Increased energy expenditure: reduced rate of growth.
> - Reduced surfactant production: respiratory distress.
> - Vasoconstriction: poor perfusion/metabolic acidosis.
> - Delayed adjustment from fetal to newborn circulation.

reduced incidence of intraventricular hemorrhage. Despite this, the evidence does not support any neuroprotective benefit in the longer term.

Temperature control

Growth restricted and preterm infants are at risk of hypothermia because of their high surface area to volume ratio, thin non-keratinized skin, lack of insulating subcutaneous fat and thermogenic brown fat, and inability to shiver. Hypothermia is associated with a variety of adverse physiological consequences (Box 19.4).

Since the 1950s it has been established that reducing heat loss improves survival for preterm and low birthweight infants. Measures to prevent evaporative heat loss and cold stress should commence immediately following delivery. Resuscitation should always be undertaken under radiant heaters and with either immediate drying and wrapping in warmed towels or immediate placement of the newborn into a polyethylene bag. Ongoing care in incubators or under radiant heaters aims to maintain a 'neutral thermal environment', namely an ambient temperature at which oxygen consumption and energy expenditure is at the minimum to sustain vital activities.

Nutrition for growth restricted and preterm infants

Compared with term infants, preterm infants and especially those who have been growth restricted in utero, have very limited nutrient reserves at birth. Preterm infants are additionally subject to a variety of physiological and metabolic stresses that can affect their nutritional needs. Providing appropriate nutrition for growth and development is a cornerstone of their care. Early postnatal nutrition during this very critical period of brain growth may have a significant impact on clinically important outcomes, including long-term neurodevelopment.

Human breast milk is the recommended form of enteral nutrition for preterm infants. Human milk also has non-nutrient advantages for preterm infants, primarily through the delivery of immuno-protective and growth factors to the immature gut mucosa. There is evidence that preterm infants who receive human breast milk have a decreased incidence of feed intolerance and gastrointestinal disease, including necrotising enterocolitis when compared with those who receive formula milk. However, as human breast milk may not consistently provide all of the nutrient requirements of preterm infants, a variety of multi-nutrient fortifiers are available as supplements to add to human milk. If human milk is unavailable, infants may be fed any of several adapted formula milks designed to meet the nutrient requirements of preterm infants.

The most appropriate method of enteral feeding varies with the infant's gestational age and clinical condition. Well infants of gestational age greater than about 34 weeks are usually able to coordinate sucking, swallowing and breathing, and to establish breast- or bottle-feeding. In less mature infants, oral feeding may not be safe or possible because of neurological immaturity or respiratory compromise. In these infants, milk can be given through a fine feeding catheter passed via the nose or the mouth to the stomach. Very preterm infants may require a period of intravenous nutrition until enteral nutrition is fully established, or during periods when enteral nutrition is not possible because of respiratory instability, feed intolerance, serious gastrointestinal disease or other problems.

Necrotizing enterocolitis

A major concern with the introduction of enteral feeds, especially to very preterm, growth-restricted, or sick infants, is that the additional physiological strain on the immature gastrointestinal tract may predispose to the development of necrotizing enterocolitis, a syndrome of acute intestinal necrosis of unknown etiology. The incidence may be as high as 10% in very low birthweight infants with a mortality rate consistently reported as greater than 20%. Long-term morbidity may include significant neurodisability, the consequence of under-nutrition and associated infection during a very vulnerable period of growth and development. At present there is limited evidence to suggest that the way at-risk infants are fed affects the incidence of necrotizing enterocolitis. There is a need for large randomized controlled trials to determine whether strategies such as delaying the introduction of milk feeds or feeding tiny amounts of feed continuously from very early age ('trophic feeding') alter the risk of necrotizing enterocolitis.

Outcomes following preterm birth

Broadly, outcomes improve with increasing gestational age but other factors, including ethnicity and gender also influence survival and the risk of neurological handicap. The outcomes for preterm infants born after 32 weeks' gestation are similar to those of term infants. Overall, outcomes are also good for infants born at earlier gestations. The majority of infants survive without significant neurodevelopmental problems. Most serious problems associated with preterm birth (Table 19.1) occur in the 0.5% of infants who are of extremely low birthweight (< 1000 g) or are born before 28 weeks' gestation. Consequently, as the survival rate for extremely preterm infants has improved over the past decade, the overall prevalence of neurodisability following preterm birth has not fallen.

Quality of life

In the last decade, data from cohort studies have suggested that in addition to an increased risk of significant motor and sensory impairment, health-related quality of life is significantly lower in surviving extremely low birthweight children than in children born at term. However, there is also evidence that the majority of the extremely low birthweight children studied did not perceive their quality of life as being significantly different from their peers born at term.

Table 19.1 Prevalence of neuromotor and sensory findings at 18 months in extremely low birth-weight infants.

	Total (%)
Abnormal neurological examination	25
Cerebral palsy	17
Seizure disorder	5
Hydrocephalus with shunt	4
Any vision impairment	9
Hearing impairment	11

From Vohr B R et al 2000 *Pediatrics* 105:1216-1226.

INFANTS OF MOTHERS WITH MEDICAL DISEASE

Infants of diabetic mothers

It has been long recognized that maternal diabetes (both pre-gestational and gestational) can have adverse consequences for the fetus and newborn infant (Box 19.5).

Even in pregnant women with type 1 diabetes who achieve 'tight' glycemic control, maternal and perinatal complications are more common than in non-diabetic pregnancies. Whilst there is limited evidence from randomized, controlled trials that improved glycemic control in pregnant women with type 1 diabetes improves perinatal outcome, observational studies indicate that if tight control of the maternal blood glucose levels is achieved very early in (or pre-) pregnancy then the incidence of congenital abnormalities in the infant is reduced. In addition, a recent large randomized, controlled trial has provided stronger evidence that treatment of gestational diabetes reduces serious perinatal morbidity and perhaps mortality. Those caring for women with diabetes will therefore usually aim for optimum glycemic control leading up to and during pregnancy.

The management of the mature infant of the diabetic mother after birth is largely targeted towards metabolic stabilization. Because of up-regulation of insulin production in utero, the infant of the woman with diabetes may be hyperinsulinemic for the first

Box 19.5 Neonatal consequences of maternal diabetes

- Preterm birth.
- Large for gestational age/macrosomia.
- Birth injury: clavicle fracture, Erb's palsy.
- Hypoglycemia.
- Hypocalcemia.
- Hyperviscosity.
- Respiratory distress syndrome.
- Congenital anomalies (non-gestational diabetes):
  - sacral agenesis, caudal regression syndrome;
  - anencephaly, spina bifida;
  - congenital heart disease;
  - cleft lip/palate;
  - hypertrophic cardiomyopathy;
  - cataract;
  - gastrointestinal atresias;
  - hernia.

few days after birth and therefore is at risk of hypo-glycemia. Infants of diabetic mothers, particularly after glycemic control has been poor, therefore need monitoring of their blood glucose and clinical condition for the first 48 h or so after birth.

The precise definition of 'pathological hypoglycemia' is still debated but in current practice, most clinicians aim to maintain plasma glucose levels above 2 mmol/L with some centres aiming for even higher levels (> 2.6 mmol/L). If an infant is persistently hypoglycemic therapeutic options include feeding the infant on a more frequent schedule (rather than demand) or providing parenteral nutrition. These measures aim to stabilize the plasma glucose to a 'safe' level that limits the risk of neurological compromise. There are few data however, to indicate exactly what level of glycemia is 'safe' or how strong a causal association exists between neonatal hypoglycemia and adverse neurodevelopmental outcome. For this reason, clinical decisions must integrate a balance between the potential disadvantages of intervention (which may include the separation of mother and baby) and the poorly quantified neurological risks associated with hypoglycemia.

Maternal thyroid disease

Hyperthyroidism

The commonest cause of hyperthyroidism in pregnant women is Graves' disease. The hyperthyroid fetus is at increased risk of intrauterine death, preterm delivery and intra uterine growth restriction. Between 1 and 6% of babies born to mothers with Graves' disease will exhibit signs of hyperthyroidism as a result of transplacental transfer of thyroid stimulating antibody (Box 19.6). Clinical presentation of hyperthyroid symptoms in the newborn may be delayed for days and occasionally several weeks by the transplacental effects of maternal antithyroid drugs (see Ch. 5).

Management may include symptomatic treatment, for example beta-blockers to control tachycardia, as well as specific antithyroid drugs. Infants usually clear maternal thyroid stimulating antibodies within 6-12 weeks of delivery and thyroid function returns to normal. The prognosis for infants, even in those treated promptly, remains guarded however with significant mortality and increased risk of disordered growth and neurodevelopment.

Hypothyroidism

Pregnant women may be hypothyroid for a number of reasons and any of these should prompt close observation and scrutiny of the newborn infant. Thyroid agenesis or dysgenesis and inborn errors of thyroid hormone synthesis have an inherited etiology which increases the risk of similar disorder in the fetus/newborn infant. Autoimmune thyroid (Hashimoto's) disease resulting in maternal hypothyroidism also carries an inherited risk as well as the potential for transplacental transfer of antithyroid antibodies although in general these do not effect the fetal thyroid. Iodine deficiency during pregnancy and drugs used to treat maternal thyrotoxicosis (propylthiouracil and carbimazole) may also result in an under-active thyroid in the newborn. The hypothyroid newborn infant (approximately 1 : 4000 deliveries) may present with a variety of non-specific clinical features (Box 19.7). However, because of the lack of sensitivity of clinical signs, many countries now have routine screening for neonatal hypothyroidism by analysis of heel prick blood in the first days of life.

The prognosis for the hypothyroid newborn is improved with early detection and commencement of appropriate thyroid replacement therapy. Universal screening of infants for hypothyroidism within the first week after birth may not detect all cases of hypothyroidism associated with maternal autoim-

---

Box 19.6 Clinical symptoms of hyperthyroidism in the newborn infant

- Restlessness, agitation.
- Poor feeding.
- Intrauterine growth restriction.
- Poor weight gain.
- Tachycardia, tachypnea.
- Heart failure.
- Hypertension.
- Fever.
- Jaundice.
- Exophthalmos.
- Cranial synostosis.

Box 19.7 Clinical feature of hypothyroidism in the newborn infant

- Lethargy.
- Poor feeding.
- Constipation.
- Respiratory distress.
- Edema.
- Cyanosis.
- Prolonged neonatal jaundice.

mune thyroid disease. There may therefore be a role for later repeat screening through the first month or two to detect those infants who develop transient hypothyroidism because of transplacental transfer of maternal antithyroid antibody.

The mainstay of treatment is thyroxine replacement to prevent the adverse neurodevelopmental consequences of hypothyroidism. Treatment is titrated to the levels of free thyroxine, TSH and specific antibody titres in the newborn infant. In contrast to infants with disorders of thyroid development or dyshormonogenesis who will require lifelong treatment, infants of mothers with autoimmune thyroid disorders usually require treatment for up to a maximum of six months until the maternal antithyroid antibodies have naturally cleared from the infants' circulation.

Drug misuse in pregnancy

Infants of mothers who misuse illicit drugs during pregnancy are at increased risk of neonatal mortality, sudden infant death syndrome and neurodisability.

Opiates

Most infants exposed in utero to opiate either in the form of a 'street' drug such as heroin, or to a prescribed opiate analogue such as methadone develop clinical signs of withdrawal – 'neonatal abstinence syndrome'. Clinical features may develop within a few hours to days after birth (Box 19.8). The signs of neonatal withdrawal from opiate can be very nonspecific and those caring for newborn infants should be alert to the possibility even when there is no clear history of maternal ingestion.

At delivery, naloxone for hypoventilation/apnea should be avoided if there is a known history of maternal opiate misuse as an acute withdrawal syndrome may be precipitated. Scoring systems have been developed to help manage withdrawing infants. While these scores may help in defining the severity

of symptoms and assist deciding treatment strategies, they do not give a guide to ultimate prognosis. The management of neonatal opiate withdrawal aims to promote successful feeding with adequate growth in a settled infant. Active treatment of withdrawal is based on pharmacological interventions and behavioral management. Opiate replacement has been shown to limit symptoms and reduce length of stay but there is little evidence of effect on long-term outcome. Sedatives such as phenobarbitone and benzodiazepines have been used but are inferior to opiate and perhaps no better than comfort care alone. Some behavioral interventions such as waterbeds and swaddling may make infants more relaxed, as may limitation of environmental stimuli such as light, noise and handling although there is no hard evidence to support this.

Outcome for infants who experience withdrawal varies and prediction for individual babies is virtually impossible. Death in the neonatal period is extremely rare. Many studies have suggested an increased risk of adverse long-term neurodevelopmental outcome for these babies but it is difficult to account for confounding factors associated with maternal drug misuse such as poverty, low maternal education and preterm delivery. These may well be more significant than drug misuse per se in determining neurodevelopmental outcome. A similar argument attaches prime significance to confounding socio-economic factors when considering the increased risk of sudden infant death in infants of drug abusing mothers.

Cocaine

In some Western countries, the use of cocaine and its base derivative 'crack' rose markedly in the second half of the last century. Use of cocaine, like opiate, is associated with adverse pregnancy outcomes such as stillbirth, preterm birth and poor intrauterine growth. An increased risk of congenital malformations particularly of the genitourinary tract has been reported in babies exposed to cocaine in utero but no specific 'syndrome' has been described and the teratogenicity of cocaine continues to be debated. At birth, the neuroexcitatory symptoms exhibited by some babies exposed to cocaine in utero, although less commonly seen, are very similar to those seen in babies withdrawing from opiate. Such symptoms may persist for weeks or months. This group of infants is also at increased risk of adverse neurodevelopmental outcome but again the specific contribution relating to cocaine exposure is difficult to ascertain given the significant potential for confounding socio-economic factors.

Box 19.8 Clinical features associated with neonatal abstinence syndrome

- Neurological excitability/seizures.
- Gastrointestinal dysfunction and autonomic signs.
- Feeding dysfunction (incoordination, polyphagia).
- Sleep–wake cycle abnormalities.
- Vomiting.
- Dehydration.
- Poor weight gain.

Other 'illegal' social/recreational drugs

Many other pharmacological preparations are mis-used including amphetamines, marijuana, benzodiazepines, barbiturates and solvents. All have the potential to cause neonatal psychomotor behavior consistent with withdrawal with some reports suggesting symptoms may persist for up to a year. In irritable newborn infants the diagnosis should be readily considered and if confirmed, supportive measures put in place. Urine toxicology or analysis of meconium may give an indication of which substance(s) is/are involved but issues of consent and confidentiality should be considered prior to testing.

Alcohol

The effect of alcohol on the developing fetus was first described over 40 years ago but the precise relationship between alcohol and fetal outcome has still not been established. There is no clear threshold below which effects are reliably absent and this has led some to recommend complete abstinence during pregnancy. A spectrum of disorders has been described (Box 19.9).

Diagnosis in the newborn infant may not be possible at birth and the condition may not be considered until the child is much older. Management is expectant with support for mothers who may have an alcohol problem. The prognosis for the affected infant varies from mild dysmorphism only through to significantly impaired growth with microcephaly and severe neurodisability requiring support and supervision throughout childhood and adult life.

Tobacco

Smoking tobacco during and after pregnancy has adverse effects on the fetus and newborn child.

Mothers who smoke cigarettes are twice as likely to deliver before 32 weeks' gestation. There may be growth restriction in utero and there is an increased risk of respiratory tract infection, wheezy illness, sudden infant death syndrome and later behavioral disturbance. These effects result from some or all of the many toxic substances found in the combustion products of tobacco. Some of the effects are likely due to direct transfer of nicotine and its metabolite cotinine which can both be transferred across the placenta and in breast milk as well as through direct inhalation by the newborn baby (as passive smoking). In addition, women who smoke are less likely to intend to breastfeed, less likely to initiate breastfeeding, and likely to breastfeed for a shorter duration than non-smokers.

Although there are limited data to support a dose–response relationship and little evidence describing acute withdrawal symptoms, there is some evidence that antenatal smoking cessation programs can reduce the incidence of preterm birth and growth restriction. However, women from poorer socio-economic backgrounds, who are most at risk of preterm delivery, are least likely to cease smoking in pregnancy.

Neonatal sepsis and congenital infection

A number of infections some of which may present with relatively mild disease in the mother during pregnancy can have a devastating effect on the fetus (Box 19.10). This section will focus on the management of the fetus/newborn whose mother is infected with group B streptococcus, human immunodeficiency virus (HIV) or hepatitis B or C – the so-called blood-borne viruses.

Box 19.9 Fetal disorders associated with maternal intake of alcohol

- 'Fetal alcohol syndrome' – known alcohol exposure, facial dysmorphism and abnormal growth and neurodevelopment.
- 'Alcohol-related neurodevelopmental disorder' – known alcohol exposure and neurodevelopmental disorder, but no facial dysmorphism or growth disorder.
- 'Alcohol related birth defects' – known alcohol exposure in utero with an associated congenital malformation.

Box 19.10 Maternal infections that may affect the fetus/newborn infant

- Cytomegalovirus (CMV).
- Toxoplasma gondii.
- Herpes virus.
- Parvovirus.
- Rubella.
- Syphilis.
- Group B streptococcus.
- Human immunodeficiency virus.
- Hepatitis B and hepatitis C.
- Tuberculosis (TB).
- Listeria monocytogenes.
- Malaria.

Group B streptococcus

Group B streptococcus (GBS) is a commonly found commensal in the female genital tract probably originating from the gut. It may play a role in some cases of chorioamnionitis and subsequent preterm labor although the precise pathophysiology is yet to be determined. It is also the single commonest organism isolated in cases of early onset neonatal sepsis (within the first 7 days of life) with a prevalence ranging between 0.5 cases per 1000 live births to 2.0 cases per 1000 live births in different parts of the world.

When group B streptococcus is the cause of illness in the mother, e.g. urinary tract infection, it should clearly be treated. However, there is no consensus as to how best to manage asymptomatic group B streptococcus carriage. Some countries advocate universal screening of pregnant women toward the end of the third trimester with treatment of carriers with antibiotic prophylaxis during labor. In other countries screening programs targeted towards maternal and infant risk factors for GBS infection exist. Universal antibiotic prophylaxis for newborn babies has been proposed but is not practiced widely.

Evidence for most of the strategies proposed comes largely from observational studies and there is a clear need for improved epidemiological surveillance and further randomized clinical trials to assess the potential benefit (or harm) of any interventions. Robust evidence does show that antibiotic prophylaxis given to women in labor reduces the risk of early onset GBS infection but this approach does not appear to impact on the risk of late onset infection and has no effect on the overall risk of neonatal death. The potential 'benefit' of this particular intervention needs to be weighed against the possible disadvantages of such a policy including the risk of fatal anaphylaxis in women, the development of antibiotic resistant strains and the financial costs of such a program.

Regardless of any preventive strategies in place, newborn infants presenting with signs of sepsis should be treated with an antibiotic regimen that includes GBS cover until the precise causative organism is determined.

Human immunodeficiency virus

Mother-to-child transmission, either during or after pregnancy is the commonest route by which children acquire HIV infection. In developing countries, where the prevalence of HIV in pregnant women may be more than 30%, the risk of perinatal mother-to-child transmission of HIV is about 20%. Infants are at

> **Box 19.11 Effective interventions for reducing vertical transmission of HIV**
>
> - Antenatal antiretroviral therapy (ART) to reduce maternal viral load.
> - Delivery by pre-labor Cesarean section.
> - Postnatal administration of ART as post-exposure prophylaxis to the infant.
> - Avoidance of breastfeeding transmission.

further risk of acquiring infection through breastfeeding. In developed countries where antenatal and perinatal interventions are available (Box 19.11), the risk of mother-to-child transmission has been reduced to less than 2%. Current evidence indicates that the benefit of antiretroviral drugs to reduce mother to child transmission of HIV outweighs potential adverse effects of exposure of the fetus and neonate to these medications. The availability of these effective interventions therefore justifies the inclusion of universal HIV screening in routine antenatal screening programs. Screening programs must however include multidisciplinary support for women found to be infected with HIV and robust systems for screening and follow up of newborn infants. Ongoing long-term surveillance of children exposed to antiretroviral medications is needed to identify any long-term complications.

All infants born to HIV infected mothers will have anti-HIV antibody detected in plasma until up to 18 months after birth. Diagnosis (or exclusion) of HIV infection during early infancy therefore relies on serial measurement of viral RNA (or proviral DNA) by polymerase chain reaction. If these tests remain negative by 3 months after birth, parents can be reassured that HIV infection is extremely unlikely.

The prognosis for children with HIV infection in developing countries is extremely poor. Acquired immunodeficiency syndrome is now a major cause of mortality in infancy and childhood in sub-Saharan Africa. In children living in developed countries, access to health services to provide antiretroviral therapy, monitor disease progression, and prevent or treat opportunistic infection has significantly reduced morbidity and mortality.

Current consensus is that infants born to HIV-infected infants should receive the standard childhood vaccines. BCG vaccination is probably safe in the neonatal period but expert consensus advises that BCG vaccination is deferred until the infant is considered to be free of HIV infection (usually not until 3 months after birth). For children who are found to be HIV-infected, cohort studies indicate an increased risk of complications following BCG vaccination. However, as these reactions are usually mild, it may be that the risk of these complications is outweighed by the benefits of BCG vaccination in populations at high risk of tuberculosis during infancy and childhood.

Hepatitis B

More than 350 million people worldwide are chronically infected with hepatitis B virus (HBV). HBV is a major global cause of chronic liver disease, cirrhosis and hepatocellular cancer. The prevalence of HBV infection is highest in low income countries in south Asia and Africa. In these settings mother-to-child transmission is the major route of transmission. In developed countries, the overall prevalence is much lower (less than 1 in 2000) but may be higher in urban populations with higher proportions of women from Asia and Africa, or where intravenous drug misuse is more common.

In the absence of intervention, the overall risk of mother to child transmission of HBV is about 20%. However, if the mother is HBV surface antigen (HBsAg) and HBV e antigen (HBeAg) positive, the rate of transmission is around 90%. About 75% of these infants become chronically infected with HBV. The mode of delivery probably does not affect the risk of transmission.

The perinatal transmission rate of HBV can be substantially reduced to less than 10% by administration of post-exposure immunoprophylaxis to new born infants. In some countries, universal HBV vaccination is therefore offered at birth while in others a program targeted towards infants at known higher risk of acquiring HBV is preferred. In infants whose mothers are HBV positive, use of HBV vaccine alone reduces transmission by around 90%, and use of vaccine plus HBV immunoglobulin (HBIG) by around 95%. These are given in separate sites at birth or as soon as possible thereafter. It is not necessary to give HBIG to infants whose mothers had been shown to have antibodies to HBsAg.

It is necessary to follow up of infants exposed perinatally to HBV with monitoring of HBV serology and antigen status through the first year to 18 months of life in order to detect chronically infected infants. Although infected infants are not likely to develop overt clinical problems in early childhood, long-term follow-up is required to detect the onset of liver disease and to consider antiviral therapy.

Hepatitis C

The prevalence of hepatitis C (HCV) infection in pregnant women in Europe and North America ranges from about 0.2 to 3% depending on the setting and population screened. The HCV seroprevalence rate is very high in some developing countries where the practice of re-use of unsterilized injecting equipment in healthcare settings is common.

Most infants who acquire HCV infection do so in utero or in the peripartum period. Breastfeeding is not thought to be an important route of transmission. Infants who acquire HCV in utero or at birth do not develop clinically apparent liver problems in early childhood but most do develop chronic HCV infection and are likely to be at risk of longer-term problems related to chronic liver disease. There is no available vaccine for preventing HCV infection. Pharmacological treatment regimens are successful in eradicating infection in more than half of the treated individuals but these are not used in pregnancy.

The rate of mother-to-infant transmission of HCV is about 5%. Mother-to-infant transmission occurs predominantly in those women who have HCV ribonucleic acid (RNA) detected in their blood at delivery. The risk of transmission is highest in those mothers who have a high hepatitis C viral load at the time of birth. Babies of women with HCV will be antibody positive on testing for several months after birth, but this is a result of passive transfer of the antibody rather than infection. Co-infection with the HIV may also be a risk factor for transmission.

Observational studies have generally not provided evidence that the mode of delivery (Cesarean section versus vaginal delivery) affects the risk of mother-to-infant HCV transmission. Consensus statements and guidelines have concluded that elective Cesarean section does not afford the infant protection from HCV infection and that routine screening for HCV in pregnancy is not warranted. However, some other observational studies have suggested that the rate of perinatal HCV infection might be reduced if infants are delivered by Cesarean section prior to rupture of membranes.

Other viral infections

The risk to the fetus varies depending on the stage of pregnancy in which infection is acquired (Box 19.12). Diagnosis relies on recognizing an acute illness in the mother associated with seroconversion, an appropriate pattern of fetal 'disease' and/or newborn findings and the identification of either IgM directed against that virus in the infant or detection of the organism

---

Box 19.12 Possible effects of intrauterine infection on fetus/newborn

- Miscarriage or intrauterine death.
- Preterm delivery.
- Intrauterine growth restriction.
- Hematological disorder – thrombocytopenia, anemia, neutropenia.
- Congenital heart disease.
- Musculoskeletal disorder.
- Microcephaly and cerebral anomaly with neurodevelopmental morbidity.
- Congenital cataract and visual impairment.
- Sensorineural deafness.

Box 19.13 Adverse outcomes associated with the use of some anticonvulsants in pregnancy

- Neural tube defects.
- Cleft lip and palate.
- Cardiovascular abnormalities.
- Genitourinary defects.
- Limb defects.
- Developmental delay.
- Autism (putatively linked to in utero exposure to valproate).
- Neonatal bleeding.

---

in the infant's blood, cerebrospinal fluid, or urine. In general, the risk to the fetus is likely to be highest during the period of organogenesis in the first trimester, although acute maternal varicella and herpes virus infections in the days immediately before delivery carry the risk of current viremic illness in the newborn period for the baby.

Epilepsy in pregnancy

About 0.5% of pregnant women have epilepsy that may require pharmacological treatment. Unfortunately, it has long been recognized that the commonly available anticonvulsant medications (valproate, carbamazepine, phenytoin and phenobarbitone) are associated with an increased risk of teratogenicity and other adverse outcomes (Box 19.13). In most instances the absolute risk of a congenital malformation is about 5%, approximately double the rate of malformations in the general population. There is a need to balance this with the risk of adverse outcomes due to poorly controlled epilepsy.

The precise mechanism(s) whereby anticonvulsants lead to adverse outcomes seen in the child is not clearly understood. The finding that dietary supplementation with folic acid before and during pregnancy reduces the risk of congenital neural tube defect may suggest that antagonism of folic acid synthesis pathways plays a role.

The increased risk of neonatal hemorrhage in these babies may be caused by interference with vitamin K metabolism. As a result, some have recommended that vitamin K prophylaxis should be given in the third trimester to pregnant women on anticonvulsants. Regardless of maternal anticonvulsant use, neonatal vitamin K supplementation reduces the risk of serious neonatal hemorrhage and should be offered to all newborn infants.

Maternal connective tissue disease and fetal/newborn congenital heart block

More than 80% of cases of recognized complete congenital heart block are associated with maternal connective tissue disease, principally systemic lupus erythematosus (SLE) with Sjogren's syndrome, or primary Sjogren's syndrome. About 1% of pregnancies in women with SLE will present with fetal heart block although for many of the women this finding may be the first 'clinical' presentation of the disease.

Fetal heart block develops following the transplacental transfer of maternal autoantibodies (IgG Ro and IgG La) leading to the inflammatory destruction of the atrioventricular node. In addition, an immune mediated myocarditis, endocardial fibroelastosis and/ or dilated cardiomyopathy may also rarely occur. It is not clear why only a proportion of fetuses are affected when transplacental transfer of antibodies is almost universal.

Pregnancy outcome is closely related to fetal heart rate. At rates less than 50 beats/min, almost half will end in pregnancy loss. At rates greater than 60 beats/ min only 1 in 20 pregnancies end in fetal death. Treatment options in utero are extremely limited. Sympathomimetic drugs, steroids and plasmapheresis have all been associated with successful conversion to sinus rhythm but evidence of effect is restricted to small case series. Similarly, dexamethasone is used by some when partial degrees of heart block are present in an attempt to prevent progression to complete heart block. This is the subject of a current trial (2007). Fetal cardiac pacing remains an experimental intervention at present. When fetal well-being is compromised, elective delivery remains the mainstay of treatment. Here the balance between the risks associated with preterm delivery and the chances of sustaining a viable pregnancy in the presence of fetal heart failure or hydrops must be weighed.

Maternal autoimmune disorder and neonatal thrombocytopenia

In women with autoimmune disease, particularly idiopathic thrombocytopenic purpura (ITP) but also other autoimmune disease such as SLE, transplacental transfer of maternal platelet antibodies may lead to significant immune destruction of platelets in about 10% of infants at risk – neonatal autoimmune thrombocytopenia. This condition must be distinguished from alloimmune thrombocytopenia where the mother raises specific platelet antigen (PlA1) to fetal platelets in a similar manner to red cell antibodies being generated in hemolytic disease of the newborn. In alloimmune thrombocytopenia, maternal platelet count is unaffected.

It is unclear to what degree the prognosis for the newborn whose mother has ITP is related to maternal platelet count. In general, the outcome is favorable with only about 3% of infants having thrombocytopenia that causes hemostatic compromise and even fewer infants progressing to clinically important bleeding such as intraventricular hemorrhage.

Following delivery, a careful watch on the infant's clinical condition and monitoring of the platelet count is needed, as the count usually reaches its nadir around the third day of life. Bleeding is rare when platelet counts are greater than $20 \times 10^9/L$. Platelet transfusion may sustain counts at an adequate level but the effect may be short lived – a few hours. The adjunctive use of intravenous immunoglobulin or steroid may lessen the immune mediated destructive process but the precise effect of these interventions is still to be determined. As an alternative to pharmacological intervention, when the platelet count is not maintained with simple platelet transfusion, exchange transfusion may be considered in an attempt to physically remove a proportion of the active platelet antibody, which may persist for a number of weeks, from the infant circulation.

Transient neonatal myasthenia gravis

Transplacental transfer of antibodies that cause neuromuscular blockade may affect infants born to mothers with myasthenia gravis. The condition is transient lasting only days or occasionally weeks until antibody levels in the newborn fall naturally and must be distinguished from the more serious congenital forms of myotonia (as from the mother with myotonic dystrophy) which carry a grave prognosis.

Treatment of infants with transient neonatal myasthenia gravis is symptomatic: ventilatory support as required because of hypoventilation and assisted feeding, if needed, because of weakness of the oropharyngeal muscles and poorly coordinated sucking and swallowing.

Maternal malignancy

Malignancy affecting women during pregnancy is relatively rare affecting about one in a thousand pregnant women. The commoner tumors seen during pregnancy include cervical cancer, breast cancer and melanoma. Treatment options may include surgery, chemotherapy and radiotherapy all of which carry a degree of risk to the unborn child which must be balanced against maternal health risks and choice.

Surgery is relatively safe in women throughout pregnancy although risk to the fetus does rise when there are complications. Chemotherapy is associated with increased fetal loss and teratogenicity if given during the first trimester although insufficient information is available concerning effects in later pregnancy. At present, breastfeeding while receiving chemotherapy is generally contraindicated. Radiotherapy likewise carries a significant risk of fetal loss and teratogenicity especially during the first trimester. Factors such as the radiation dose, the site of the malignancy and the stage of the pregnancy will contribute to determining the overall risk to the fetus not only of death but also morbidity including microcephaly, learning difficulty and cataract.

Maternal psychiatric disease

Psychiatric disease is common and a proportion of pregnant women will exhibit some signs of psychiatric or psychological morbidity. While this may have relatively little direct effect on the unborn or newborn child, indirectly there may be risks either as a result of maternal medical treatment or because of diminished parenting capacity in the mother once the child is born. A number of psychotropic drugs are associated with an increased risk of fetal malformation and breastfeeding may be contraindicated. Women with a significant psychiatric history are at increased risk of postnatal depression which itself is associated with an increased risk of infanticide and sudden infant death (SID). The offspring of schizophrenic mothers may also be at increased risk of infanticide and SID. Determining the precise extent of risk associated with any given psychiatric condition is difficult as many cofactors such as poor social background, maternal alcohol and drug misuse are also frequently found. Regardless, the infants in these cases are extremely vulnerable and arrangements for appropriate support for the family should be made prior to delivery whenever possible.

Further reading

American Academy of Pediatrics Committee on Substance Abuse and Committee on Children With Disabilities 2000 Fetal alcohol syndrome and alcohol-related neurodevelopmental disorders. Pediatrics 106(2 Pt 1): 358-361

American Academy of Pediatrics – Committee on Drugs 1998 Neonatal drug withdrawal. Pediatrics 101(6):1079-1088

Andres R L, Day M C 2000 Perinatal complications associated with maternal tobacco use. Seminars in Neonatology 5(3):231-241

Broderick A, Jonas M M 2004 Management of hepatitis B in children. Clinics in Liver Disease 8(2):387-401

Cornblath M et al 2000 Controversies regarding definition of neonatal hypoglycemia: suggested operational thresholds. Pediatrics 105(5):1141-1145

Crowley P 1996 Prophylactic corticosteroids for preterm birth. The Cochrane Database of Systematic Reviews Issue 1.

Crowther C A et al 2006 Neonatal respiratory distress syndrome after repeat exposure to antenatal corticosteroids: a radomised controlled trial. Lancet 367(9526):1913-1919

Hawkins D et al on behalf of the BHIVA Guidelines Writing Committee 2005 Guidelines for the management of HIV infection in pregnant women and the prevention of mother-to-child transmission of HIV. HIV Medicine 6(Suppl 2):107-148

Neilson J P, Alfirevic Z 1996 Doppler ultrasound for fetal assessment in high risk pregnancies. The Cochrane Database of Systematic Reviews Issue 2.

Ogilvy-Stuart A L 2002 Neonatal thyroid disorders. Archives of Disease in Childhood. Fetal and Neonatal Edition 87(3):F165-171

Osborn D A, Jeffery H E, Cole M 2005 Opiate treatment for opiate withdrawal in newborn infants. The Cochrane Database of Systematic Reviews Issue 3.

Roberts I, Murray N A 2003 Neonatal thrombocytopenia: causes and management. Archives of Disease in Childhood. Fetal and Neonatal Edition 88(5): F359-364

Saigal S 2000 Follow-up of very low birthweight babies to adolescence. Seminars in Neonatology 5(2):107-118

Schwimmer J B, Balistreri W F 2000 Transmission, natural history, and treatment of hepatitis C virus infection in the pediatric population. Seminars in Liver Disease 20(1):37-46.

Soll R F, Blanco F 2001 Natural surfactant extract versus synthetic surfactant for neonatal respiratory distress syndrome. The Cochrane Database of Systematic Reviews Issue 2.

Soll R F, Morley C J 2003 Prophylactic versus selective use of surfactant in preventing morbidity and mortality in preterm infants. The Cochrane Database of Systematic Reviews Issue 2.

Wapner R J, Sorokin Y, Thom E A et al 2006 Single versus weekly courses of antenatal corticosteroids: evaluation of safety and efficacy. American Journal of Obstetics & Gynaecology 195(3):633-642

Chapter 20

Fetal assessment in the patient with medical complications: ultrasound and biophysical monitoring

M. M. Kennelly, S. C. Robson

SYNOPSIS

Introduction
Fetal abnormalities
Screening for fetal anomalies
Pathophysiology of fetal compromise
Monitoring the fetus in high-risk pregnancies
A pragmatic approach to antepartum surveillance

INTRODUCTION

Fetal growth and development from the earliest stage of intrauterine life can be influenced by the environment in which the conceptus develops. Maternal medical conditions can increase the risk of antepartum fetal demise with an estimated 10% of all fetal deaths being related to maternal illnesses. This risk can be posed at an early developmental stage manifesting with fetal anomalies arising from medications required or dietary deficiencies associated with the medical condition. Additionally, an adverse metabolic environment or impaired uterine/umbilical perfusion associated with the disease can jeopardize fetal well-being. Such an adverse environment can have long reaching consequences with permanent effects on structure, physiology and metabolism, resulting in the development of significant morbidity in later life. Antepartum fetal surveillance techniques aim to assess the risk of fetal death in pregnancies complicated by pre-existing maternal conditions (e.g. Type 1 diabetes mellitus), as well as those in which complications have developed (e.g. fetal growth restriction – FGR). Evidence-based observations have shown that there are different pathophysiologic processes that may place the fetus at risk and that the efficacy of the various monitoring tests depends on the underlying pathophysiologic condition. These processes include decreased uteroplacental blood flow, decreased gas exchange at the fetomaternal barrier and metabolic derangements. The clinician should recognize the nature of the fetal risk on the basis of the clinical information and then, wherever possible, apply condition-specific antenatal fetal testing, which addresses the underlying pathophysiologic processes. This chapter examines fetal screening and monitoring strategies employed in pregnancies complicated by common medical conditions.

Table 20.1 outlines medical conditions that increase perinatal morbidity and mortality according to their underlying pathophysiology. Fetal monitoring is considered mandatory in such pregnancies given the increased risk of fetal compromise. The rational approach is to use surveillance strategies based on the underlying pathophysiology. However, in some conditions (e.g. diabetes mellitus) this is poorly understood and is likely to be multifactorial. Thus, in practice, a pragmatic approach is followed using methods that are applied in other high-risk pregnancies even though the underlying pathophysiology differs.

FETAL ANOMALIES

Concerns for the fetus have centered on the possibility of malformations if drug treatment is given during organogenesis, or impaired growth or functional development if treatment is given during the second or third trimesters. Table 20.2 details an overview of drug-associated abnormalities. Reference to one of the

Table 20.1 Maternal/fetal conditions and their underlying pathophysiologic condition

Pathophysiologic process	Maternal/fetal condition
Decreased uteroplacental blood flow	Chronic hypertension
	Pre-eclampsia
	Collagen/renal/vascular disease
	Fetal growth restriction (≤34 weeks)
Decreased gas exchange	Postdates pregnancy
	Fetal growth restriction (>34 weeks)
	Sickle cell anemia
Metabolic aberrations	Fetal hyperglycemia/ gestational diabetes
	Fetal hyperinsulinemia
	Obstetric cholestasis
Fetal sepsis	Premature rupture of membranes
	Intra-amniotic infection
	Maternal fever, primary subclinical intra-amniotic infection
	Fetal infection e.g. CM, Coxsackie virus B, syphilis, toxoplasmosis
Fetal anemia	Fetomaternal hemorrhage
	Erythroblastosis fetalis
	Parvovirus B19
Fetal heart failure	Cardiac arrythmia
	Non-immune hydrops
	Placental chorioangioma
	Aneurysm of the vein of Galen
Umbilical cord accident	Umbilical cord entanglement
	Non coiled umbilical cord oligohydramnios
	Velamentous cord insertion

available online databases (e.g. http:// www.reprotox. org) will provide more comprehensive information on specific risks and timing of exposure. The agents selected refer to the most commonly accepted structural defects known to be associated with prenatal exposure. In meta-analysis of controlled observational studies, first trimester exposure to corticosteroids was not associated with a significant increase in any major malformation. However data from case-control studies show the risk of oral clefting was increased with corticosteroid exposure in early pregnancy (RR 7.1 95% CI 3.0, 16.7). No such association was found in potentially less biased prospective studies, but these have lower statistical power. Taken together these findings

suggest there is a small but genuine risk of oral clefts with corticosteroids. Specific medical disorders such as pre-gestational diabetes and epilepsy are associated with an increase in congenital anomalies. Fetuses of diabetic pregnancies are at increased risk of congenital anomalies, especially when glycemic control is poor during the periconceptional period. This risk can reach 20% and is related to the HbA1c. The specific abnormalities include cardiac and skeletal abnormalities (sacral agenesis). Non-medicated epilepsy is associated with a slightly higher risk of anomalies (4%). Both major and minor abnormalities are associated with anti-epilepric drugs (Table 20.2). One mechanism for teratogenesis is thought to be folate deficiency, especially with phenytoin and phenobarbitone. The risk of neural tube, cardiovascular and also urogenital defects is likely to be decreased by pre-conception and first trimester folic acid.

SCREENING FOR FETAL ANOMALIES

Early (11–14 weeks) ultrasound screening

Routine ultrasonography in the first trimester has proven benefits for confirming viability, gestational age assessment, nuchal translucency measurement, assignment of chorionicity in multiple pregnancies and detection of structural abnormalities. Fetal evaluation consists of a detailed examination of the skull, brain, spine, abdominal wall, extremities and visualization of stomach and bladder. More than 80% of the most common fetal malformations develop before 12 weeks' gestation; hence good visualization of the fetus should aid detection. Ultrasound at 11-14 weeks has a sensitivity of 45% for the detection of major fetal abnormalities. Several studies have evaluated the efficacy of a transvaginal scan in detecting fetal anomalies during the first and early second trimester with sensitivities ranging from 51% to 61%.

It is also possible to diminish the risk of trisomy 21 in many older mothers to below the risk of amniocentesis by finding a normal nuchal translucency (NT) measurement. Increased fetal nuchal translucency thickness between 11 to 14 weeks' gestation in the absence of aneuploidy is a common phenotypic expression of a variety of fetal malformations, dysplasias, deformations and genetic syndromes. Using the combined data of 28 studies on a total of 6153 chromosomally normal fetuses with increased NT, the prevalence of major defects was found to be 7.3%. The observed prevalence for some of the abnormalities such as anencephaly, holoprosencephaly, gastroschisis, renal abnormalities and spina bifida may not be different from that in the general population. However,

Table 20.2 Malformations associated with medications used in maternal disease

Maternal disease	Medications/teratogens	Malformation
Chronic hypertension	ACE Inhibitors, e.g. enalapril	Hypocalvaria, oligohydramnios, neonatal renal failure, FGR, pulmonary hypoplasia.
Collagen-vascular diseases Systemic lupus erythematosus Asthma	Corticosteroids, e.g. prednisolone	Possible increase risk for oral clefts
Seizure disorders	Carbamazepine	Neural tube defects, heart defects, urinary tract defects, skeletal and facial abnormalities.
	Valproic acid	Neural tube defects, cleft lip, coarctation of aorta, hypoplastic left heart, Ebstein's anomaly, fetal valproate syndrome-characteristic facies
Heart disorders e.g. prosthetic valves	Warfarin	Nasal hypoplasia, depressed nasal bridge, FGR[a], neural tube defects, scoliosis, cardiac defects, limb hypoplasia, cleft palate
Psychiatric disorders	Lithium	Cardiac abnormalities, e.g. Ebstein's anomaly

[a]FGR – Fetal growth restriction.

the prevalence of major cardiac defects, diaphragmatic hernia, exomphalos, skeletal defects and certain genetic syndromes such as congenital adrenal hyperplasia, Noonan syndrome, Smith–Lemli–Opitz syndrome and spinal muscular atrophy appear to be substantially higher than in the general population, and it is therefore likely that there is a true association between these abnormalities and increased NT. Although several studies have shown the potential of a first trimester scan in the diagnosis of fetal abnormalities, a significant number of birth defects cannot be detected or are misdiagnosed. Hence, a first trimester scan does not replace the need for a scan at 18-20 weeks.

Second trimester anomaly scan: 18–20 weeks

Routine ultrasound screening in the second trimester, when performed by experienced ultrasonographers, can detect up to 70% of major congenital anomalies. The literature provides a range of detection rates and therefore individual units should provide their own figures to inform women undergoing the '20-week' scan. Detection rates range from 25% for cardiac defects to 99% for anencephaly (Table 20.3). The antenatal detection of major congenital anomalies allows enhanced parental awareness/preparation, serial surveillance, therapeutic intervention and optimization of the time, mode and site of delivery. It also allows discussion of the option of termination of pregnancy. The use of soft markers to identify the fetus at risk of aneuploidy has been used in an erratic way. Markers

Table 20.3 Detection rates of major anomalies

Problem	Detection rate (%)
Spina bifida	90
Anencephaly	99
Hydrocephalus	60
Major congenital heart defect	25
Diaphragmatic hernia	60
Exomphalos/gastroschisis	90
Major kidney problem	85
Major limb abnormality	90
Down's syndrome	40

From RCOG (2000).

may be seen during a routine scan and when isolated are of dubious value, especially when women have already been screened for Down's syndrome (nuchal translucency or maternal serum testing). One study suggested that the use of markers increased the overall detection rate of abnormalities from 51% to 55% but increased the false positive rate from 1 in 2332 to 1 in 188. Two or more markers may be significant and should be discussed with the woman.

Fetal echocardiography

Maternal medical conditions such as diabetes mellitus and collagen vascular disease are associated with an increased risk of congenital heart disease. Pregestational diabetes is associated with numerous major cardiac anomalies including aortic coarctation, atrioventricular septal defects, tetralogy of Fallot and transposition of the great arteries. The risk of congenital heart disease has been quantified at 2% for each pregnancy on a background population risk of 7-8 per 1000 live births. Anti-epileptic drugs and lithium administration have also been linked to congenital heart defects (Table 20.2). Fetal heart scanning in the first trimester provides diagnostic information. There are two main goals in performing early fetal echocardiography as opposed to a more conventional approach at 18-20 weeks. First, to demonstrate 'normality' of situs and cardiac connections and hence to be able to reassure families at high risk of congenital heart disease as early as possible, thus minimizing anxiety. Secondly, in the event of a major abnormality being diagnosed, families have the option of interrupting the pregnancy at an earlier gestational age. There is now a growing clinical practice of first trimester cardiac scanning. The main indications are a previous family history of cardiac defects and the finding of an increased nuchal translucency thickness. Nuchal translucency of 3.5 mm is associated with a 2.5% risk while nuchal translucency of 4.5 mm has been reported to be associated with a 10% risk of cardiac defects. The issue of accuracy of first-trimester echocardiography has been addressed by Haak et al (2002) who reported 88% sensitivity and 97% specificity for the detection of heart defects by transvaginal echocardiography at 11-14 weeks in fetuses with increased nuchal translucency. In those pregnancies that terminated or demised, no major discrepancy in the diagnosis was found on pathological examination. A review by Gembruch et al (2000) showed that the transvaginal route offered greater success in demonstrating the four chambers and cross-over of the great arteries between 10-13 weeks however visualization of these structures was not always possible before 12 weeks. At 13 weeks the transabdominal approach was sufficient in over 80% of cases. In the second trimester, optimally at 20-22 weeks' gestation, complete examination of the fetal heart should be undertaken for those considered to be at high risk. A systematic approach should be followed obtaining the standard views (four chamber view, left ventricular outflow tract, right ventricular outflow tract, transverse arch view, longitudinal arch view) where maternal habitus and fetal position allow. The structures should be identified by their morphology and not by their position and hence normality can be proven rather than assumed. Screening for low-risk populations is based mainly on the four-chamber view, although some units incorporate great arteries into the assessment. Albert et al (1996) found a lower detection rate using the four chamber view alone compared to full fetal echocardiography (33% vs 92%).

Conclusion

Screening an obstetric population by means of a detailed history (past history, medications, medical condition) reveals those with an increased risk of a congenital anomaly. These women should be seen at 12-13 weeks in a fetal medicine unit (FMU).

PATHOPHYSIOLOGY OF FETAL COMPROMISE

There are a number of pathological processes implicated as possible causes of fetal compromise. These include dysmorphogenesis, fetal hypoxia, fetal acidemia and abnormalities of maternal/fetal metabolism.

Fetal hypoxia and acidemia

The proposed pathophysiology of most cases of severe FGR is that of placental disease, manifested by abnormal umbilical artery (UA) Doppler velocimetry, leading to placental respiratory failure and fetal hypoxemia. This, in turn, triggers compensatory hemodynamic changes, which include blood flow redistribution towards essential fetal organs (brain, heart and adrenal glands) at the expense of other organ systems (lungs, kidneys, bowel). There are at least two functional pathways that mediate these responses. The first pathway is a direct one, where cell function alters in the presence of diminished oxygen delivery. This effect is prominent in neurons that form the regulatory centers controlling biophysical activities. The second pathway involves the aortic arch and carotid artery chemoreceptors, which mediate the reflex redistribution of the cardiac output (Fig. 20.1). Due to their location, these chemoreceptors have a high metabolic rate and require constant perfusion with the highest oxygenated blood to remain stable. In the presence of central hypoxemia and acidemia, these receptors discharge and send afferent traffic via the vagal nerve to the cardioregulatory center. Efferent discharge from this center results in increased blood pressure, pulse rate and cardiac output in the presence of selective organ vasoconstriction. Reflex vasoconstrictive ischemia is manifest by abnormal organ function reflected in abnormal fetal biophysical parameters and liquor volume.

The compensatory phase can be recognized clinically by Doppler and ultrasound findings, including

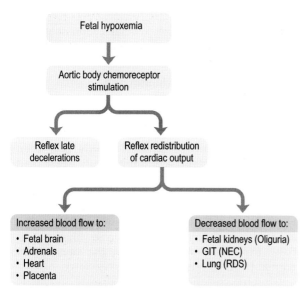

Figure 20.1 Underlying principle of hypoxia and suppression of normal function. GIT, gastrointestinal tract; NEC, necrotizing enterocolitis; RDS, respiratory distress syndrome.

decreased pulsatility index in the middle cerebral artery, decreased amniotic fluid volume and echogenicity of the bowel. The duration of the compensatory phase is variable, sometimes lasting weeks, and appears not to have deleterious short-term consequences. When these compensatory mechanisms reach their limit, myocardial dysfunction (diastolic and/or systolic) occurs. Hemodynamic decompensation is clinically recognized by abnormal venous Doppler waveforms that reflect increased pressure in the right atrium and/or dilatation of the ductus venosus and are generally associated with metabolic acidemia. Acidemia may be detected clinically by the fetal heart rate tracing as well as by the biophysical profile. Once the disease enters this decompensatory phase, the fetus is at high risk of multisystem organ failure and death. A prevalent view has been that the changes in Doppler venous waveforms occur first and are followed by fetal heart rate abnormalities and changes in the other components of the biophysical profile.

A variety of studies support the contribution of hypoxia to fetal compromise in diabetic pregnancies. Signs of fetal asphyxia before or during labor have been reported in about 20% of cases of fetal death in diabetic pregnancies. Abnormal fetal heart rate, cord blood acidosis and low Apgar scores are more commonly found in diabetic pregnancies. Fetal erythropoietin concentrations are raised in macrosomic infants of diabetic mothers and this is most likely due to relative hypoxia. Pathophysiological changes have been described in diabetic pregnancies that could result in fetal hypoxia. These include thickening of the basement membrane of the chorionic villi, which increases the diffusion distance for oxygen between the mother and the fetus and potentially lowers oxygen transfer; decreased uterine blood flow to the placental bed especially in diabetics with poor glycemic control and vascular disease; metabolic changes, especially hypergylcemia, in combination with hypoxemia, have been reported to result in lactic acidosis and fetal death in animal models. Fetal blood sampling during pregnancy and at birth in diabetic pregnancies has demonstrated significant acidemia associated with elevated lactic acid even in the absence of hypoxemia.

Fetal growth restriction (FGR)

Small for gestational age (SGA) fetuses comprise a heterogeneous group with respect to etiology, management and prognosis. In accurately dated pregnancies, approximately 80-85% of fetuses identified as being SGA are constitutionally small but healthy, 10-15% 'true' FGR cases and the remaining 5-10% of fetuses are affected by chromosomal/structural anomalies. The etiologies of FGR can be divided into fetal, placental and maternal factors. Fetal factors include karyotypic abnormalities, genetic conditions and congenital anomalies. The maternal medical conditions commonly associated with FGR are those associated with altered uteroplacental perfusion or maternal hypoxia and therefore fetal hypoxia. Medical conditions such as chronic hypertension or other vascular disease can give rise to a fetus failing to reach its growth potential. Chronic hypertension is associated with a two- to three fold increased risk of FGR. It is not clear whether a chronic reduction in uterine blood flow is a result of the vasospastic characteristics of the disorder or the result of the increased incidence of pre-eclampsia. The risk of FGR among women with diabetes is complicated by the increased risk of congenital anomalies and the type and duration of the diabetes. In general, in gestational diabetes FGR in a non-anomalous fetus is rare. This could be attributed to the elevated fetal glucose and insulin levels that are observed. In women with pre-gestational diabetes, the incidence of FGR is much greater and increases with severity and duration of the disease. This may be due to damage to the microcirculation, which is associated with diabetes. The relationship between renal disease and FGR is complex and striking with some authors quoting rates of up to 23%. Determining the etiology is complicated by the high rate of hypertension and pre-eclampsia observed among these patients. Renal transplant recipients with stable graft function in the absence of rejection or dysfunction are also at risk for prematurity and low birthweight.

Growth restriction is a frequent complication of pregnancies in women with systemic lupus erythematosus (SLE) but in many of the pregnancies hypertension and pre-eclampsia are also observed. The pathophysiology of FGR in this condition is unclear. The increase in risk for FGR, at 23%, is more than eightfold that of the general population and increases further to 65% in those with active disease. Antiphospholipid syndrome is also associated with FGR; the common mechanism for these complications appears to be intrauterine hypoxia and malnutrition due to placental thrombosis. In addition, thrombophilic disorders are associated with impaired fetal growth, which is believed to be mediated by the increased susceptibility to placental thrombosis. Normal pregnancy initiates a hypercoagulable state reflected by increased levels of several clotting factors. This precarious balance between procoagulant and anticoagulant pathways also occurs at a placental level. The low pressure and flow velocity characteristic of the placental circulation combined with the hypercoagulability of pregnancy may predispose to thrombosis. More recently the contribution of paternal and fetal thrombophilia has been recognized to be associated with placental vascular thrombosis and infarction at either side of the maternal–fetal interface. Conditions associated with maternal hypoxemia, though rare, clearly are associated with FGR. These conditions include cyanotic heart disease and severe chronic anemia as can be seen with sickle cell disease. Chronic pulmonary disease, such as severe asthma, may also be associated with impaired fetal growth.

Fetal growth restriction is independently associated with increased risk of neonatal complications, stillbirth, birth hypoxia, impaired neurodevelopment, adult type 2 diabetes and hypertension. The management should therefore focus on the identification of the fetus at risk due to placental dysfunction, and longitudinal assessment to reduce morbidity and mortality by optimal timing of delivery. Clinicians have to balance the risk of delivery too early against exposure of the fetus to hypoxemia and acidemia, which can result in damage or death. In cases of early severe FGR, aneuploidy, congenital abnormality or infection should be considered. In the absence of aneuploidy the most efficacious surveillance tool is Doppler velocimetry. There is strong evidence that pregnant women with FGR should have Doppler studies of the umbilical artery waveforms to reduce the rates of perinatal death, antenatal admissions and inductions of labour.

Altered maternal metabolism and fetal pathophysiology

An adverse intrauterine metabolic environment may adversely affect fetal well-being. In diabetes mellitus, marked oscillations of glycemic control have been postulated as a fetal risk and potentially worse than either chronic hyperglycemia or hypoglycemia. A study of glycemic variation in eight apparently well-controlled diabetic women as defined by normal HbA1c levels, whose infants were macrosomic found significant oscillations in blood glucose values, potentially explaining macrosomia in the presence of normal HbA1c levels throughout pregnancy.

Obstetric cholestasis is a liver disease specific to pregnancy. It is characterized by intrahepatic cholestasis (ICP), triggered by environmental, infectious and hormonal factors in genetically predisposed women. The diagnosis is typically based on a clinical history with a number of perturbations in aminotransferases, bilirubin and bile acids. Elevated sulfated progesterone compounds as well as impaired excretion of bile acids are found in pregnancies complicated by ICP. The disorder is associated with an increased risk of stillbirth and perinatal death. The mechanism underlying cholestasis-associated stillbirths is unknown and conventional monitoring of fetal well-being does not predict most of the cases of fetal death. Most stillbirths are not preceded by signs of chronic hypoxia, such as oligohydramnios, fetal growth restriction or by acute fetal hypoxemia as manifested by fetal heart rate changes. High levels of maternal bile acids produce abnormalities in placental transport, placental hormone production, chorionic vessel constriction and possibly fetal cardiac function, with cardiac arrhythmia a possible cause of fetal demise.

To date, no ideal method of fetal surveillance has been determined for ICP. Monitoring strategies aimed at detecting placental insufficiency cannot forecast an acute event such as an umbilical cord entanglement, or a sudden fetal cardiac decompensation or arrhythmia. Despite the limitations of antenatal fetal testing, ICP should be recognized as a condition that is associated with increased perinatal mortality and irrespective of maternal bile acid levels, intense fetal surveillance is warranted. Our unit policy is for a baseline scan when diagnosed and twice weekly computerized cardiotocography (CTG) until delivery at 37 weeks.

Screening the uteroplacental circulation/ uterine artery doppler ultrasound

Pre-eclampsia, FGR, placental abruption and some cases of fetal death during the latter half of pregnancy are believed to result from impaired placentation in early pregnancy. Impaired placentation is characterized by inadequate trophoblast invasion into the maternal spiral arteries and hence failure to develop a low-resistance uteroplacental circulation. The uteroplacental circulation can be assessed by Doppler ultrasound of the uterine arteries. Women with a previous history of a small for gestational age fetus (SGA) or pre-eclampsia/eclampsia necessitating early delivery should be referred for screening as should women at risk of FGR because of maternal disease. Studies in the past two decades have established that in pregnancies failing to establish a low resistance circulation, there is a substantial risk of complications such as pre-eclampsia, FGR and related complications. A normal waveform shows an increase in the diastolic flow and consequent fall in flow velocity indices with increasing gestation. An abnormal uterine artery waveform is usually defined as a PI > 95th centile (PI ~1.45 at 23 weeks' gestation) (Fig. 20.2). Albaiges et al (2000) reported a 40% chance of developing pre-eclampsia and 45% for delivering infants of birthweight less than the 10th percentile if the Doppler measurements are abnormal. The negative predictive value was more than 99% for adverse outcomes before 34 weeks. This suggests that uterine artery Doppler screening may be useful to determine the appropriate level of care in high-risk women. Our unit policy is to screen women with a previous history of pre-eclampsia, FGR, stillbirth or pregnancy loss (< 20 weeks) at 23 weeks using uterine artery Dopplers. Women with an abnormal waveform are offered a low dose of aspirin 75 mg daily and serial biometry, Doppler and amniotic fluid assessment at 28, 32 and 36 weeks. However if screening is normal they are considered low risk and biometry is performed at 32 weeks (Fig. 20.3).

MONITORING THE FETUS IN HIGH-RISK PREGNANCIES

Which test and how often?

The focus of monitoring in high-risk pregnancy is no longer just the prevention of fetal mortality. Fetal monitoring must account for congenital anomalies and severe morbidity as a result of growth restriction and/or the metabolic milieu of the medical condition. Thus, a broad range of potential fetal problems, in

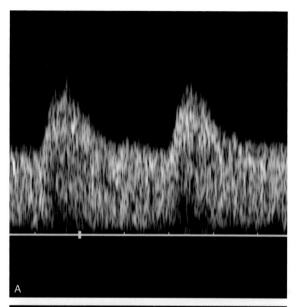

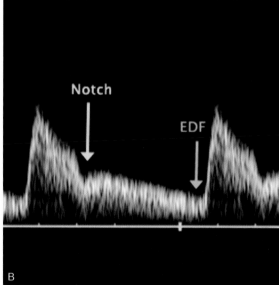

Figure 20.2 Normal flow velocity waveforms from the uterine artery at 24 weeks of gestation demonstrating (A) normal diastolic flow velocities and (B) reduced diastolic flow velocities with early diastolic notching.

addition to the maternal complications, requires individualized, serial observation with multiple testing modalities. A logical approach is as follows: definition of the population at risk, clarification of pathophysiology, application of relevant tests, and evaluation of possible neonatal impacts. The following testing modalities have been used.

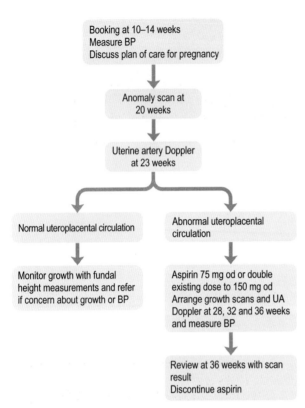

Figure 20.3 Doppler screening at 23 weeks for women at high risk of placenta-mediated disease. FGR, fetal growth restriction; BP, blood pressure.

Growth assessment: biometry

Most maternal medical disorders involve fetal growth abnormalities. Serial ultrasound biometry provides the most reliable method of assessing fetal growth. In high-risk pregnancies clinical estimates of fetal size vary greatly with sensitivities between 24% and 97%. The sensitivity of symphysial-fundal height measurement lies between 17-86% and is dependent on gestation and fetal weight with greatest accuracy between 2500 g and 4000 g. Sonographic methods provide a more accurate assessment but are still prone to error, particularly at the extremes of fetal weight. Abdominal circumference (AC) and estimated fetal weight (EFW) are the most accurate diagnostic measurements to predict SGA. In the prediction of fetuses with birth weight less than the 10th centile AC has a sensitivity of 73-95% and specificity of 51-84% whilst EFW is less sensitive at 33-89%. Abdominal circumference measured serially especially in the third trimester is probably the best indicator of a macrosomic fetus. Diabetic pregnancies should have growth assessment at 24, 28 and 32 weeks' gestation and two weekly thereafter.

Doppler ultrasound

Umbilical artery doppler (UAD)

Doppler ultrasonography non-invasively assesses vascular impedance. With advancing gestation, umbilical arterial Doppler waveforms demonstrate a progressive rise in end-diastolic velocities and a decrease in impedance indices (Fig. 20.4). End-diastolic frequencies may be detected from as early as 10 weeks and in normal pregnancies they are always present from 15 weeks. The intra- and inter-observer variations in the various indices are about 5% and 10% respectively. A number of investigators have reviewed the relationship between UAD and fetal acid – base status showing normal UAD index is inconsistent with fetal acidemia secondary to uteroplacental dysfunction. If the UAD is normal (±2 SD) one can assume the fetus is not acidemic and the CTG and biophysical profile (BPP) are normal. Doppler ultrasound studies of the umbilical artery have been evaluated by more randomized trials than any other test of fetal well-being. The Cochrane Systematic Review of Doppler ultrasound for fetal assessment in high-risk pregnancies (those complicated by hypertension or presumed impaired fetal growth) includes 11 randomized controlled trials (RCT) involving 7000 women. Compared to no Doppler, use of UAD is associated with a trend to a reduction (29%) in perinatal deaths (OR 0.71, 95% CI 0.5-1). The use of Doppler ultrasound significantly reduces the number of admissions to hospital during pregnancy (OR 0.56, 95% 0.43-0.72), rate of Cesarean section for fetal distress (OR .36, 95% 0.19-0.68) and induction of labor (OR 0.83, 95% 0.74-0.93). No benefit has been demonstrated for umbilical artery Doppler in conditions other than suspected FGR, such as post-term gestation or diabetes mellitus. In addition, it has not been shown to be of value as a screening test for detecting fetal compromise in the general obstetric population. Randomized trials comparing UA Doppler with cardiotocography also show benefits with Doppler such as less frequent antenatal monitoring and shorter inpatient stay (1.1 vs 2.5 days).

Fetal hypoxemia is associated with a diminution of umbilical artery diastolic flow and in extreme cases the flow velocities can be absent or reversed (Fig. 20.4). The adaptations of a growth-restricted fetus to hypoxemia include redistribution of the blood flow towards the brain as measured in the middle cerebral artery (MCA). The decreased resistance and increased flow in this artery is an adaptive feature of the fetus under stress and is significantly associated with an abnormal UAD. Abnormal venous Doppler indices reflect ventricular dysfunction and reflect a more advanced stage of adaptation to placental insufficiency

Normal Pulsatility Index (PI)

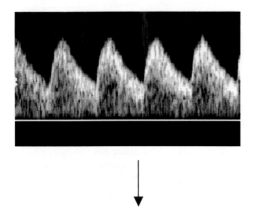

Normal PI-
Hypoxia 2%, Acidemia 0%.

Absent end diastolic flow velocities (AEDF)

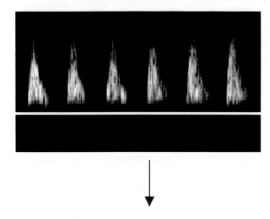

Increased PI –
Hypoxia 13-40%, Acidemia 0-20%

Reversed end diastolic flow velocities (REDF)

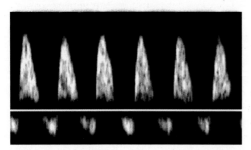

A/REDF -
Hypoxia 80-100%, Acidemia 31-88%.

Figure 20.4 Umbilical artery Doppler waveforms and relationship to fetal acid – base status.

Stage 1	Increased UA/MCA PI
	Increased UA PI
Stage 2	Absent EDF in UA
Stage 3	Reversal DV 'a' wave UV pulsations
Stage 4	Reversal MCA PI
	Tricuspid valve regurgitation

Figure 20.5 Fetal Doppler changes with progressive hypoxemia/acidemia. UA, umbilical artery; MCA, middle cerebral artery; EDF, end diastolic flow; DV, ductus venosus; UV, umbilical vein; PI, pulsatility index.

(Fig. 20.5). Hecher et al (1993) undertook a study to observe the sequence of changes in fetal monitoring modalities during FGR similar to that illustrated in Fig. 20.5. Amniotic fluid and UA pulsatility index (PI) were the first variables to become abnormal, followed by MCA and aortic Dopplers, then a decrease in short term variation of the fetal heart rate on the CTG and finally ductus venosus (DV) and inferior vena cava Dopplers. Prior to 32 weeks, the arterial Dopplers and AFI changed, on average, at least 4 weeks prior to delivery whilst the DV and CTG became abnormal 1 week before delivery.

On balance, the available evidence supports the use of Doppler in monitoring FGR. The frequency of monitoring was assessed by McCowan et al (2000); twice weekly UAD was associated with more intervention than UAD every two weeks with no improvement in perinatal outcome. Hence with a normal UAD, the frequency of follow-up can be every one to two weeks. Our current unit policy is weekly UAD. Once the UAD becomes abnormal, the consensus on management is to perform UAD twice weekly until 37 weeks and then to deliver unless evidence of compromise appears earlier. In the event of absent or reversed end diastolic flow, an alternative monitoring strategy is undertaken until 32 weeks when delivery takes place.

Middle cerebral artery (MCA) Doppler ultrasound measurement

Several investigators have observed a correlation between increased PI in the umbilical artery and decreased resistance to flow in the middle cerebral artery (Fig. 20.6). This phenomenon has been attributed to a 'brain sparing' adaptive response to fetal hypoxemia and it has been suggested that the ratio of umbilical artery PI to middle cerebral artery PI might serve as the earliest predictor of fetal compromise. The cerebral circulation, which is capable of autoregulation, vasodilates in the event of decreased perfusion

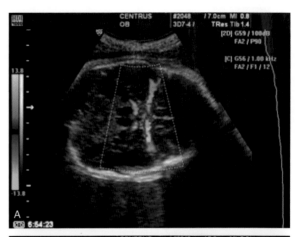

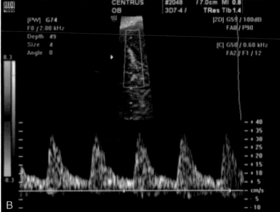

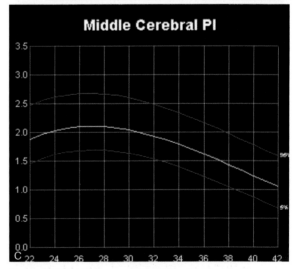

Figure 20.6 (a) Transverse view of the fetal head with color Doppler showing the circle of Willis. (b) Flow velocity waveforms from the middle cerebral artery at 32 weeks of gestation. (c) Mean (5th and 95th) centiles for pulsatility index in middle cerebral artery over gestation.

and vasoconstricts in the presence of increased perfusion pressure, giving a relatively constant blood flow despite moderate variations in perfusion pressure. The association between a FGR fetus and the brain-sparing effect is well defined, but there is less clarity on the value of MCA Doppler in predicting perinatal outcome. Several authors have reported that the reduction in MCA PI disappears in severely hypoxemic fetuses due to failure of cerebral autoregulation secondary to fetal cerebral edema and/or cardiac insufficiency. The loss of cerebral vasodilatation is a preterminal sign and demise will occur generally within 72 h. Signs of 'brain sparing' at first examination correlate with a shorter time interval to delivery. If the MCA PI is low or the ratio of UA/MCA PI is greater than 1 but UA PI is normal it may justify increasing the frequency of testing. The use of MCA Doppler is not associated with improved perinatal outcome.

Ductus venosus Doppler ultrasound measurement

Abnormal venous Doppler waveforms have been taken widely to indicate hemodynamic decompensation. An abnormal ductus venous Doppler waveform is thought to reflect increased pressure in the right atrium and/or dilatation of the ductus venosus and is usually associated with metabolic acidemia.

The ductus venosus originating from the umbilical vein can be visualized in its full length in a mid-sagittal longitudinal section of the fetal trunk (Fig. 20.7). In an oblique transverse section through the upper abdomen, its origin from the umbilical vein can be found where color Doppler indicates high velocities compared to the umbilical vein, often producing an aliasing effect. The blood flow velocity accelerates due to the narrow lumen of the ductus venosus. The ductus venosus plays a central role in the return of venous blood from the placenta. Well-oxygenated blood flows via this shunt directly towards the heart. Velocities at the inlet of the ductus venosus, immediately above the umbilical vein, are higher than at the outlet into the inferior vena cava and the sampling site should be standardized at the inlet. The typical waveform for blood flow in venous vessels consists of three phases (Fig. 20.7). The highest pressure gradient between the venous vessels and the right atrium occurs during ventricular systole (S), which results in the highest blood flow velocities towards the fetal heart during this part of the cardiac cycle. Early diastole (D), with the opening of the atrioventricular valves and passive early filling of the ventricles is associated with a second peak of forwards flow. The nadir of flow velocities coincides with atrial contrac-

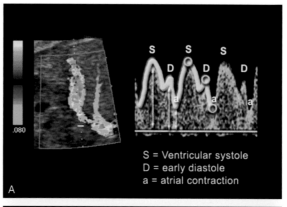

S = Ventricular systole
D = early diastole
a = atrial contraction

A

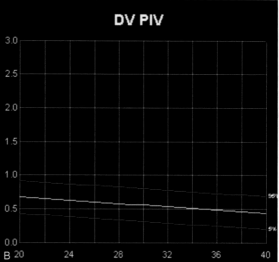

Figure 20.7 (A) Normal flow velocity waveforms of the ductus venosus visualized in a sagittal section through the fetal abdomen. The first peak indicates systole, the second early diastole and the nadir of the waveform occurs during atrial contraction. (B) PIV, which is the equivalent of pulsatility index in the ductus venosus, with gestation (mean, 5th and 95th centiles).

tion (a) during late diastole. During atrial contraction, the foramen ovale flap and the crista dividens meet, thereby preventing direct blood flow from the ductus venosus to the left atrium during the short period of closure of the foramen ovale. Increased pressure in the right atrium and/or dilatation of the ductus venosus reflects myocardial dysfunction and fetal decompensation.

Clinicians have focused on Doppler of the ductus venosus in the hope that this would allow optimal timing of delivery during the early phases of decompensation. Longitudinal studies of singleton growth restricted fetuses with abnormal umbilical artery

Doppler velocimetry have shown that venous Doppler abnormalities do not consistently precede deterioration of biophysical parameters. Hecher et al (2001) reported that among fetuses born before the 32nd week of gestation, persistent abnormalities in the fetal heart rate preceded the occurrence of an abnormal ductus venosus pulsatility index in 53% (29/55) of cases and simultaneous abnormalities were detected in 6% (3/55). Ferrazzi et al (2002) observed that more than 50% of fetuses delivered because of abnormal fetal heart rate pattern did not have venous Doppler abnormalities. Baschat et al (2001) reported that deterioration of the fetal arterial and venous systems occurred before an abnormal biophysical profile score in most cases but the interval between the two was typically only 24 h. In the remainder of cases both tests were abnormal simultaneously.

Collectively, these observations suggest that involvement of the fetal brain and heart, as detected by an abnormal fetal heart rate/biophysical profile or venous Doppler are highly variable among fetuses and do not follow a predictable pattern. Therefore, if the goal of introducing venous Doppler is to identify early entry into the decompensatory phase, these studies indicate that this can be accomplished in 50% of cases, while the data from Baschat et al (2001) suggest that the net benefit is 24 h in the majority of cases. In the absence of RCTs on the role of venous Doppler in FGR, it is clear that an abnormal venous Doppler is associated with an increase in the perinatal mortality rate in fetuses with AEDF in UA of 30-40%. Hence some authorities use this test to time delivery.

Cardiotocography (CTG)

Fetal heart rate reactivity is a reflection of the balance between the fetus's sympathetic and parasympathetic tone. It is an acquired neurologic reflex and is therefore dependent on gestational age: about 65% of healthy fetuses will have a reactive non-stress test at 28 weeks of gestation, 85% at 32 weeks of gestation and 95% at 34 weeks of gestation. Heart rate reactivity is felt to be a good indicator of normal fetal autonomic function. Fetal heart rate monitoring is the most commonly used method of evaluating fetal well-being in high-risk pregnancies overall, yet it has been poorly studied using RCTs. A Cochrane Systematic Review revealed only four published studies involving 1588 pregnancies conducted in the early 1980s, only one of which included diabetic pregnancies. In these studies, antenatal CTG appeared to have no significant effect on perinatal mortality or morbidity or on the rate of induction (41.4% vs 39.3%). Indeed, there was a trend towards an increase in perinatal deaths in the CTG

group (OR 2.85, CI 0.99-7.12). Computerized analysis (cCTG) provides a more objective assessment of heart rate variables, especially variability, however evidence is awaited that computerized analysis improves outcome. Dawes & Redman (1993) demonstrated that a low short term variability (< 3 ms) was related to metabolic acidemia (UVpH < 7.25) or intrauterine death; Guzman et al (1998) showed that in FGR the duration of reduced short term variability is significantly associated with umbilical artery pH. These results were not reproducible in low risk uncomplicated pregnancies. There have been no RCTs examining the value of CTGs in fetal assessment exclusively in diabetic pregnancies. The non-randomized studies that have been reported suggest CTG is a poorer predictor of fetal compromise than in the non-diabetic patient. False negative CTG findings are more commonly reported in diabetic than in non-diabetic pregnancies.

Biophysical profile (BPP)

The fetal BPP score is a method of determining fetal health based on a composite assessment of four dynamic fetal variables – (1) fetal breathing (FBM), (2) fetal movement (FM), (3) fetal tone (FT), (4) CTG (Table 20.4), and one long-term variable – amniotic fluid volume. The BPP was first introduced in the early 1980s and has undergone two modifications since: in 1984 the definition of oligohydramnios was liberalized from a maximum vertical pocket of ≥ 1 cm to a pocket of ≥ 2 cm, and in 1987 the CTG was recommended only when ≥ 1 of the dynamic ultrasonographic variables were abnormal. The testing method assumes that the biophysical outputs of select organ systems, be they acute or chronic, reflect the functional integrity of that system, and conversely that the absence of the select output variable be considered as evidence of dysfunction. The underlying concept is that tissue hypoxia results in suppression or loss of normal function. This loss of function affects different neural centers at different levels of hypoxia/acidemia e.g. fetal heart rate and FBM are the most sensitive to hypoxia and hence are the first to change, after which FM and then FT will be lost. Hypoxic fetuses lose these behavioral parameters in the reverse order in which they are acquired in the course of fetal development. These responses are mediated through two pathways: the direct effect of hypoxia on neuronal regulatory centers, and on aortic body chemoreceptors, which mediate changes in blood flow to various organs (Fig. 20.1).

Reports comparing the BPP score with pH in fetal blood obtained either at antepartum cordocentesis or

Table 20.4 Components of the biophysical profile

Parameter	Normal (score = 2)	Abnormal (score = 0)
CTG	≥2 accelerations of ≥ to 15 beats per minute above baseline lasting greater ≥15 s in 20 min	< qualifying accelerations during test
Amniotic fluid volume[a]	MVP ≥2 cm	MVP < 2 cm
FBM	Sustained FBM (greater than or equal to 30 seconds) in a 30 min scan	Absence of FBM or short gasps only < 30 s total
Fetal body movements	≥3 episodes of either limb or trunk movement	< 3 episodes during test
Fetal tone	Extremities in flexion at rest and ≥ equal to 1 episode of extension of extremity, hand or spine with return to flexion	Extension at rest or no return to flexion after movement

AFI = amniotic fluid index; FBM = fetal breathing movement; CTG = cardiotocography; MVP = maximum vertical pocket.
[a]Some use AFI > 5.
If ultrasound variables normal , CTG is not necessary.

at the time of elective Cesarean section, indicate a highly significant inverse relationship between BPP and pH. This study was based on 698-paired samples and the results indicated that a normal score is always associated with the absence of fetal acidemia. Prospective studies calculated a false negative rate (demise in a non-anomalous fetus within 7 days of a normal test) of 0.71-2.2 per 1000 deliveries, which, in the majority of cases, were attributed to acute causes such as fetomaternal hemorrhage. There are no prospective blinded studies to determine management according to BPP. The largest experience comes from Manitoba where the high-risk tested population had serial BPP performed with a corrected perinatal mortality rate of 1.86 compared to 7.69 in the low-risk untested population. BPP was also associated with a lower cerebral palsy rate (1.33 vs 4.74 per 1000). The Cochrane Systematic Review showed no obvious effect on pregnancy outcome. However the small number of women included in these trials (2839) and the low incidence of adverse outcome (perinatal deaths 0.8%) mean one cannot assume that the BPP is without value.

The BPP has five components, each of which scores 2 points if present (Table 20.4). A score of 8 to 10 points is considered reassuring and a reliable indicator of normal tissue oxygenation. A score of 6 points is suspicious and indicates the need for further evaluation, as there may be a probability of tissue hypoxia and central acidemia. A score of 4 points or less is ominous and indicates the need for immediate intervention. Interpretation of the biophysical profile score can be complex. For example, a fetus of 26 weeks' gestational age with preterm premature rupture of the membranes may have a score of 6 points because of oligohydramnios plus a non-reactive CTG because of gestational age, yet not be hypoxic. A low score may also reflect the fetus's behavioral state during the test, such as normal sleep or sedation from maternal use of narcotics or central nervous system depressants. Although some judgment must be made on the basis of the individual circumstances, a decreasing score has been well correlated with poor outcome and with increasing degrees of fetal acidemia.

Intervention on the basis of an abnormal biophysical profile result has been reported to yield a significant reduction in perinatal mortality, and an association exists between biophysical profile scoring and a decreased cerebral palsy rate. Dicker et al (1988) performed BPP on 98 women with insulin dependent diabetes mellitus (IDDM). Their results show a normal BPP had a good positive predictive value (≈95%) for determining an Apgar score of >7 at 1 min and 5 min. However, an abnormal BPP had a poor predictive value and sensitivity for adverse fetal outcome. Salvesan et al (1993) performed cordocentesis after BPP and fetal heart rate monitoring with computer assisted analysis, 24 h prior to delivery in 41 diabetic pregnancies at 27 to 39 weeks of gestation. The mean umbilical venous blood pH was significantly lower in diabetic pregnancies compared to normal/nondiabetic mean for gestation, and was below the 5th centile in 18 pregnancies, including all six cases of nephropathy and hypertension. There was significant association between fetal acidemia and BPP. Hence, the BPP has a high predictive value in confirming a healthy fetus in most high-risk pregnancies where the score is normal. However, it has a poor predictive value in determining fetal compromise if BPP is abnormal.

A PRAGMATIC APPROACH TO ANTEPARTUM SURVEILLANCE

A protocol for fetal monitoring cannot be applied to every possible clinical scenario, but some general principles can be followed. Each high-risk pregnancy, by virtue of its differing pathophysiology, will require an individualized approach with serial observation. The issue of when to initiate antepartum fetal surveillance and how often to perform each test is controversial. Fetal testing should not begin until interventions i.e. delivery would be undertaken. Many of the conditions listed in Table 20.1 do not jeopardize the fetus until late in pregnancy. Clearly, this should not be before 24 weeks of gestation and in most cases not before 26 weeks of gestation. If the maternal or fetal status changes, however, testing may have to be more vigilant at an earlier gestational age. Diabetic pregnancies with poor glycemic control and/or coexistent vascular disease are at risk of fetal compromise. Given the limitations of many fetal monitoring methods and the lack of randomized controlled trials, there is no agreement over the best way to monitor fetal health in diabetic pregnancies.

Our unit policy for management of the SGA/growth restricted fetus is illustrated in Fig. 20.8. This aims to delay delivery as long as possible to achieve fetal maturation while avoiding fetal acidemia. Management of the growth-restricted fetus includes a balance of the risks of intrauterine chronic hypoxia

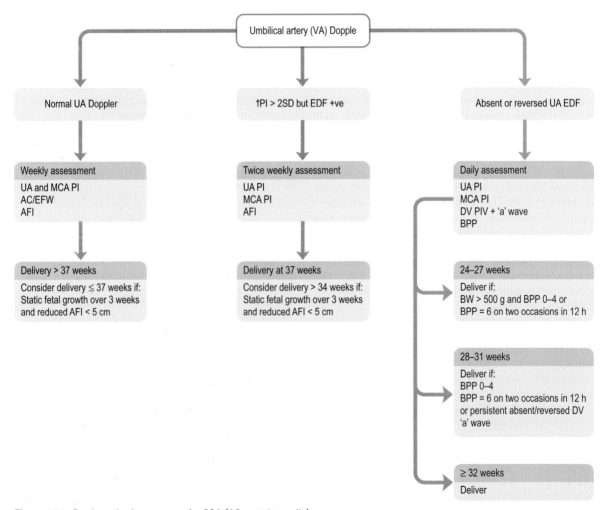

Figure 20.8 Fetal monitoring strategy for SGA (AC < 10th centile).
PI, pulsatility index; SD, standard deviation; EDF, end diastolic flow; AC/EFW, abdominal circumference/estimate fetal weight; AFI, amniotic fluid index; MCA, middle cerebral artery; DV, ductus venosus; PIV, pulsatility index DV; BPP, biophysical profile.

with the risks of prematurity. There is strong evidence that when the UA waveform is normal, the risk of mortality, cerebral hemorrhage, anemia and hypoglycemia is lower than when it is abnormal. When end-diastolic flow velocities are absent or reversed in the UA (AEDF/REDF), one study has predicted a median time interval of 7 days (range 1-26 days) until the development of an abnormal CTG. Hence AEDF in the UA mandates daily monitoring by appropriately trained staff in a unit with neonatal intensive care facilities. Depending on gestation, maternal disease and social circumstances there is a reasonable case for outpatient assessment on a daily basis with admission for delivery at 32 weeks or earlier if indicated. The optimal timing for intervention is of particular importance in the preterm FGR in whom the risk of adverse outcome due to prematurity is high. Antenatal steroids should be administered to any fetus in which delivery is anticipated before 34 weeks' gestation. The long-held belief that the stress of the intrauterine condition enhances maturation and is protective against the effects of prematurity is not supported by large population studies of FGR neonates. Management is more complicated for pregnancies between 25 to 32 weeks' gestation, where each day gained in utero may improve survival by up to 1-2%.

The only randomized controlled trial that has compared the effect of early delivery with delaying for as long as possible to increase maturity is the Growth Restriction Intervention Trial (GRIT). The GRIT Study Group (2003) showed that when delivery of fetuses with FGR presenting at a mean gestational age of 32 weeks with abnormal UAD was delayed by 4 days, there was a fivefold increase in the number of stillbirths but a twofold decrease in neonatal deaths, with no statistical difference in overall perinatal mortality. While the optimal surveillance strategy of AEDF/ REDF in the UA prior to 32 weeks has not been defined, daily assessment of BPP and ductus venosus Doppler will identify further decompensation, at which point delivery should be considered. In these situations, delivery should be by Caesarean section after the administration of steroids to reduce the incidence of respiratory distress syndrome. Over 32 weeks, the risks of complications due to prematurity are smaller than those of chronic hypoxia so AEDF in the UA alone should prompt delivery. The potential for improved clinical application of different fetal testing modalities is currently being investigated by the TRUFFLE (Trial of Umbilical and Fetal Flow in Europe) Study Group. The published protocol appeared on the Lancet website in 2003. This trial is recruiting FGR pregnancies before 32 weeks and randomizing monitoring based on one of three

investigations – computerized CTG, early DV changes, and late DV changes.

Any significant deterioration in the maternal medical status requires fetal re-evaluation, regardless of when the last assessment occurred. Although none of our current tests has ideal sensitivity and specificity, thoughtful attention to the guidelines suggested in this chapter will lead to better outcomes for pregnant patients and fetuses.

Further reading

Albaiges G, Missfelder-Lobos H, Lees C, et al 2000 One-stage screening for pregnancy for pregnancy complications by color Doppler assessment of the uterine arteries at 23 weeks' gestation. Obstetrics and Gynecology 96:559-564.

Albert T J, Landon M B, Wheller J J, et al 1996 Prenatal detection of fetal anomalies in pregnancies detected by insulin-dependent diabetes mellitus. American Journal of Obstetrics and Gynecology 174:1424-1428.

Baschat A A, Gembruch U, Harman C R 2001 The sequence of changes in Doppler & biophysical parameters as severe fetal growth restriction worsens. Ultrasound in Obstetrics and Gynecology 18:571-577.

Dawes G S, Redman C W 1993 Computerized and visual assessment of the CTG. British Journal of Obstetrics and Gynaecology 100:701-702.

Dicker D, Feldberg D, Yeshaya A, et al 1988 Fetal surveillance in insulin dependent diabetic pregnancy: predictive value of the biophysical score. American Journal of Obstetrics and Gynecology 159:800-804.

Ferrazzi E, Bozzo M, Rigano S, et al 2002 Temporal sequence of abnormal Doppler changes in the peripheral and central circulatory systems of the severely growth restricted fetus. Ultrasound in Obstetrics and Gynecology 19:140-146.

Gembruch U, Shi C, Smreck J M 2000 Biometry of the fetal heart between 10 and 17 weeks of gestation. Fetal Diagnosis and Therapy 15:20-31.

GRIT Study Group 2003 A randomised trial of timed delivery for the compromised preterm fetus: short term outcomes and Bayesian interpretation. British Journal of Obstetrics and Gynaecology 110:27-32.

Guzman E R, Vintzileos A, Egan J F, et al 1998 Antenatal prediction of fetal pH in growth restricted fetuses using computer analysis of the fetal heart rate. Journal of Maternal-Fetal Medicine 7:43-47.

Haak M, Twisk J W, Van Vught J M 2002 How successful is fetal echocardiographic examination in the first trimester of pregnancy? Ultrasound in Obstetrics and Gynecology 20:9-13.

Hecher K, Bilardo C M, Stigter R H, et al 2001 Monitoring of fetuses with intrauterine growth restriction: a longitudinal study. Ultrasound in Obstetrics and Gynecology 18:564-570.

McCowan L M, Harding J E, Stewart A W 2000 Umbilical artery Doppler studies in small for gestational age babies reflect disease severity. British Journal of Obstetrics and Gynaecology 107:916-925.

Royal College of Obstetricians and Gynaecologists 2000 Ultrasound screening for fetal abnormal: tres. RCOG, London

Salvesan D R, Freeman J, Brudenell J M, Nicolaides K H 1993 Prediction of fetal academia in pregnancies complicated by maternal diabetes by biophysical profile scoring and fetal heart rate monitoring. British Journal of Obstetrics and Gynaecology 100:227-233.

Albert T J, Landon M B, Wheller J J et al 1996 Prenatal detection of fetal anomalies in pregnancies complicated by insulin-dependent diabetes mellitus. American Journal of Obstetrics and Gynecology 174:1424-1428.

Alfirevic Z, Neilson J P 2005 Biophysical profile for fetal assessment in high-risk pregnancies. Cochrane Review. The Cochrane Library, Issue 2, Oxford.

Carvalho J S 2004 Fetal heart scanning in the first trimester. Prenatal Diagnosis 24:1060-1067.

Glantz A, Marschall, H-U, Mattsson M-A 2004 Intrahepatic cholestasis of pregnancy: relationships between bile acids and fetal complication rates. Hepatology 40:467-474.

Harding K, Evans S, Newnham J 1995 Screening for the small fetus: a study of the relative efficacies of ultrasound biometry and symphysiofundal height. Australian and New Zealand Journal of Obstetric Gynaecology 8:148-154.

Hawthorne G, Robson S, Ryall E A et al 1997 Prospective population based survey of outcome of pregnancy in diabetic women: results of the Northern Diabetic Pregnancy Audit, 1994. British Medical Journal 315:279-281.

Henrich S C, Magann E F, Brantley K L et al 2003 Detecting fetal macrosomia with abdominal circumference alone. Journal of Reproductive Medicine 48: 339-342.

Jones K L 1997 Morphogenesis and dysmorphogenesis. In: Smith DW (ed.) Recognizable Patterns of Human Malformation. Saunders, Philadelphia, p 695-705.

Kontopoulos E V, Vintzileos A M 2004 Condition-specific antepartum fetal testing. American Journal of Obstetrics and Gynecology 191:1546-1551.

Manning F A, Snijders R, Harman C R et al 1993 Fetal biophysical profile score. VI. Correlation with antepartum umbilical venous fetal pH. American Journal of Obstetric Gynecology 169:755-763.

Neilson J P 2005 Ultrasound for fetal assessment in early pregnancy. The Cochrane Library, Oxford.

Neilson J P, Alfirevic Z 2005 Doppler ultrasound for fetal assessment in high-risk pregnancies. The Cochrane Database of Systematic Reviews, Volume 1, Oxford.

Ott W J 2003 Middle cerebral artery blood flow in the fetus and central nervous complications in the neonate. Journal of Maternal-Fetal Medicine 14: 26-29.

Park-Wyllie L et al 2000 Birth defects after maternal exposure to corticosteroids: prospective cohort study and met-analysis of epidemiologic studies. Teratology 62:385-392.

Pattison N, McGowan L 2002 Cardiotocography for antepartum fetal assessment. Cochrane Review. The Cochrane Library, Issue 2, Oxford.

Pennell P B 2002 Pregnancy in the woman with epilepsy; maternal and fetal outcomes. Seminars in Neurology 22:299-308.

Royal College of Obstetricians and Gynaecologists 2002 The investigation and management of the small-for-gestational-age fetus. Guideline no. 31. RCOG, London.

Souka A P, von Kaisenberg C S, Hyett J A et al 2005 Increased nuchal translucency with normal karyotype. American Journal of Obstetrics and Gynecology 192:1005-1021.

Wong S F, Chan F Y, Cincotta R B et al 2002 Routine ultrasound screening in diabetic pregnancies. Ultrasound in Obstetrics and Gynecology 19:171-176.

Young R R 2002 Genetic toxicology: web resources. Toxicology 173:103-121.

Chapter 21

Effects of ionizing and non–ionizing radiation and electromagnetic fields in pregnancy

S. A. Lowe

INTRODUCTION

The pregnant woman is exposed constantly to a range of ionizing, non-ionizing and electromagnetic radiation in both her own environment and as a result of medical intervention. Much of the radiation that women are exposed to is incidental to the pregnancy. In some cases, additional exposure is a result of the woman's occupation, location, or her requirement for diagnostic imaging procedures. In a small number of women, therapeutic radiation may be required for treatment of cancer during pregnancy. This chapter examines the nature and magnitude of this radiation exposure and the potential effects of such radiation on the outcome of pregnancy.

DEFINITIONS IN RADIATION PHYSICS

The radiation dose of interest is the absorbed dose; the mean energy imparted per unit mass. This is expressed as gray (Gy) or milligray (mGy). One Gy is equal to 1000 mGy or 100 rad. Equal doses of different types of energizing radiation do not necessarily lead to equal detrimental effects. These differences relate to microscopic energy dissipation and are corrected for by a radiation weighting factor (w_R), which when multiplied by the dose produces a quantity expressed as the sievert (Sv). For photons and electrons, the $w_R = 1$, whilst for alpha particles the $w_R = 20$. X-rays and gamma radiation are high energy forms of electromagnetic radiation with high penetration of tissues. Medical imaging techniques including X-ray, fluoroscopy, angiography, mammography, positron emission tomography (PET), single photon emission computed tomography (SPECT), computerized tomography (CT) and most nuclear medicine procedures involve exposure to this form of radiation. In contrast, alpha and beta radiation are also high energy but less penetrating and must therefore be ingested to be used for imaging purposes. The calculation of effective dose, whole body or to specific sites, takes into account this energy dissipation.

Dose limits are generally expressed in milliSieverts (mSv). In assessing the potential effects of radiation in pregnancy, it is necessary to calculate both the maternal dose to a particular site as well as the estimated fetal absorbed dose.

Background radiation

The major radiation source for most women during pregnancy is environmental, arising from a number of sources including cosmic, gamma and radon. The magnitude of the exposure varies from 1.8 mSv per year in countries such as the UK and Australia to 7.8 mSv per year in Finland. People who work in the presence of radiation are protected by safety legislation in most countries, which limits their effective dose to 20 mSv per year, averaged over a period of five consecutive years, with a maximum of 50 mSv in any single year. The recommended dose limit for the general public is 1 mSv per year. When a pregnancy is declared by a female working in the presence of radiation, the embryo or fetus is afforded the same level of protection as the general public i.e. 1 mSv per year.

During air travel, cosmic radiation can contribute significantly to fetal absorbed dose. The intensity of cosmic radiation increases with altitude and whole body exposures of 0.001-0.003 mSv per hour on short haul routes and up to 0.005 mSv per hour on long haul flights are typical.

Accidental exposure from nuclear accidents has generally been overestimated as a source of background radiation. The Chernobyl nuclear power plant explosion in 1986 resulted in an increase in exposure to iodine isotopes and Cs-137. In the worst affected areas, whole body exposure of up to 250 mSv over 3 years was reported with the most significant dose to the thyroid. However, the general exposure beyond these areas was very low, estimated at a few mSv outside Europe, to an upper estimate of 1-2 mSv in some European countries.

Magnetic resonance imaging and non–ionizing radiation

The various forms of radio-frequency radiation including ultrasound, diathermy, microwave ovens, mobile phones and video display terminals are not sources of ionizing radiation. The potential of these energy sources to affect the fetus is probably limited to their potential to increase the fetal temperature. Magnetic resonance imaging (MRI) exposes the woman to both static and gradient magnetic fields. The machines vary in power from 0.064 to 8.0 Tesla. High field magnets produce high resolution images and faster imaging times. To date, there is no evidence of any thermal effects of MRI when used in the current manner although low field magnets are generally recommended where available. Within the suggested safety limits set by various standards committees for general and occupational exposure, sources of radio-frequency radiation have not been shown to pose a health risk to the human fetus.

ADVERSE EFFECTS OF RADIATION IN PREGNANCY

In the assessment of any adverse effects of radiation upon the fetus it is necessary to consider:

- Absorbed dose
- Timing of the exposure relative to conception
- Form of administration

X–rays and CT

In estimating the absorbed dose of radiation to the fetus, a number of techniques have been used. For plain X-rays, these include measuring the mean skin exposure and estimating absorbed dose to adjacent organs such as the ovary, or the use of wax phantoms. Dosimetry surveys even within a particular country have been found to vary by a factor of up to 30 or more for the same examination. With fluoroscopy, e.g. for embolization procedures, additional factors such as location of the beam, duration of screening, magnification and conventional versus pulsed fluoroscopy will influence dose. Digital radiography techniques may reduce fetal absorbed dose considerably. In a study of maternal pelvimetry, the use of digital radiography reduced the fetal absorbed dose by 85% (0.024 mGy versus 0.177 mGy). The fetal absorbed dose during CT scanning can be significantly reduced by reducing the number, width and spacing of the slices and by using lower dose techniques e.g. helical scanning.

In addition to the radiation technique, site and dose administered, maternal factors will influence the fetal absorbed dose. During X-rays and CT scanning the 'thickness' of the mother, which alters as pregnancy progresses, will influence the penetration of the dose and hence the fetal absorbed dose. The use of appropriate shielding will significantly reduce the fetal absorbed dose as well as the dose to adjacent maternal tissues. Table 21.1 presents approximate fetal absorbed doses for a number of common radiological procedures.

It may be seen that conventional X-ray examinations beyond the abdomen/pelvis are associated with a negligible fetal absorbed dose, which is related to right angle scatter. More direct examinations, particularly with fluoroscopy, e.g. barium enema, are associated with a more significant fetal absorbed dose. There is significantly less scatter from helical CT than standard pulmonary angiography with estimated abdomen and pelvis doses from the two procedures of 0.06-2.86 mGy and 0.2-11.5 mGy, respectively.

Nuclear medicine

In the case of nuclear medicine studies, fetal absorbed dose will represent the cumulative effect of external irradiation from the maternal tissues as well as placental transfer and fetal uptake of radiopharmaceuticals (Table 21.2). For radioisotopes that are excreted in urine, radiation from bladder contents may be a more important source. In addition, measures aimed at increasing the rate of urinary excretion may reduce the absorbed dose significantly. By using smaller administered doses and longer imaging times, the fetal absorbed dose may be further reduced. For example, in cases of suspected pulmonary embolus, the perfusion scan can be performed first and, if normal, the ventilation scan will not be needed. This will reduce the administration dose by 75%.

The special case of radioiodine requires specific mention. [131]I given for therapeutic purposes, e.g. thyroid cancer or thyrotoxicosis, crosses the placenta readily and the fetal thyroid begins to accumulate iodine from approximately the end of the first trimester. In early pregnancy, the major risk is from external gamma radiation from the maternal bladder, whilst after 12 weeks the fetal thyroid dose is much greater than the fetal whole body dose, e.g. 500-1100 mGy MBq^{-1} administered dose versus 0.06-0.08 mGy mBq^{-1}. If therapeutic doses of radioiodine are inadvertently given to a pregnant woman with thyrotoxicosis, there is a significant risk of fetal thyroid damage after 12 weeks' gestation. If pregnancy is confirmed shortly after dose administration, maternal hydration and frequent voiding should be encouraged and potassium iodide may be given as a thyroid blocking agent. The total fetal absorbed dose is still likely to be less than 100 mGy.

Investigation of suspected pulmonary embolus

The choice between ventilation perfusion scanning and helical CT pulmonary angiography for the diagnosis of pulmonary embolism in pregnancy remains controversial. The choice of test should take into account the perceived probability of pulmonary embolus, the possibility of alternate lung pathology, the clinical status of the patient and the availability of the two procedures. From the point of view of radiation risk to the fetus, neither investigation would be of concern. In a study comparing the estimated fetal

Table 21.1 Approximate fetal doses from common diagnostic procedures

	Mean (mGy)	Maximum (mGy)
Conventional X-rays		
Abdomen	1.4	4.2
Chest	<0.01	<0.01
Intravenous pyelogram	1.7	10
Lumbar spine	1.7	10
Pelvis	1.1	4
Skull	<0.01	<0.01
Thoracic spine	<0.01	<0.01
Dual X-ray absorptiometry DEXA		
Posterior anterior spine	1.7	4.9
Proximal Femur	1.0	2.7
Fluoroscopic examinations		
Barium meal	1.1	5.8
Barium enema	6.8	24
Computed tomography		
Abdomen	8.0	49
Chest	0.06	0.5
Helical chest CT	<0.01	0.13
Head	<0.005	<0.005
Lumbar spine	2.4	8.6
Pelvis	25	79

Table 21.2 Fetal whole body dose from common nuclear medicine examinations in early pregnancy and at term. Dose includes maternal and fetal-self dose contributions

		Administered activity (MBq)	Early pregnancy (mGy)	Late pregnancy (mGy)
[99m]Tc	Bone scan (phosphate)	750	4.6-4.7	1.8
[99m]Tc	Lung perfusion (MAA)	200	0.4-0.6	0.8
[99m]Tc	Lung ventilation (aerosol)	40	0.1-0.3	0.1
[99m]Tc	Thyroid scan (pertechnate)	400	3.2-4.4	3.7
[99m]Tc	Red blood cell	930	3.6-6.0	2.5
[99m]Tc	Liver colloid	300	0.5-0.6	1.1
[99m]Tc	Renal DTPA	750	5.9-9.0	3.5
[67]Ga	Abcess/tumor	190	14-18	25
[123]I	Thyroid uptake[a]	30	0.4-0.6	0.3
[131]I	Thyroid uptake[a]	0.55	0.03-0.04	0.15
[131]I	Metastases imaging[a]	40	2.0-2.9	11.0

[a]Fetal thyroid doses are much higher than fetal whole body dose.

absorbed dose from the two techniques, the mean fetal absorbed dose from helical chest CT varied with gestation between 0.003-0.02 mGy in the first trimester to 0.05-0.13 mGy in the third trimester. Increasing the pitch and reducing the dose during helical chest CT scanning reduced the fetal absorbed dose further. The radiation dose from ventilation perfusion scanning may be reduced by longer imaging times and omission of the ventilation phase if the perfusion study is normal.

It must be remembered that both CT and standard pulmonary angiography require the administration of iodine-containing contrast agents (see below) and both are associated with a significantly greater radiation dose to the maternal breast than ventilation perfusion scanning. Thoracic CT results in a radiation dose of 20-35 mGy to the breast. It has been estimated that a delivery of 10 mGy of radiation to a woman's breast before age 35 increases the risk of breast cancer by 13.6%. Helical chest CT, particularly when modified for pregnancy, is likely to deliver considerably smaller doses. In the future, magnetic resonance angiography may become the investigation of choice. (See Ch. 8.)

Radiation therapy

Data from the USA indicate that up to 4000 women per year require radiotherapy during pregnancy. This is most commonly administered as external radiation with Cobalt-60 gamma rays or X-rays. For certain cancers, radioiodine or brachytherapy with cesium-137 may be required. Estimating the potential fetal dose and providing maximal dose reduction is imperative to reduce the risk to the fetus. This may be achieved by appropriate shielding, dose fractionation and protraction of the dose. Frequently, both the patient and her doctor will try to avoid radiation therapy during pregnancy; however, the benefits of waiting until fetal viability is achieved must be balanced with the risk of disease progression. Table 21.3 gives examples of estimated dose to the fetus with radiation therapy for three different cancers.

Contrast agents

A number of X-ray and CT procedures require the administration of iodine-containing contrast agents. In radiocontrast media, the amount of inorganic iodine available to interfere with thyroid metabolism is about 0.1% of the dose administered. Non-ionic contrast agents have been shown to cross the placenta and inhibit Type II and III deiodinases, which can reduce intracellular triiodothyronine. In addition, depending on the dose of iodine, there is potential to blockade the fetal thyroid, in a manner similar to radioiodine. However, the most recent Contrast Media Safety Committee of the European Society of Urogenital Radiology guidelines conclude that there is no evidence of such a problem being of major significance in clinical practice and hence 'iodinated contrast media may be given to a pregnant patient when radiographic examination is essential.' Appropriate neonatal thyroid assessment should be performed following delivery. Only very small amounts of iodinated contrast agent are excreted into the breast milk and even less is absorbed via the oral route. Hence, there is no requirement to cease breast feeding following radiographic examinations involving the use of iodinated contrast agents.

For MRI, gadolinium is used as a tracer to enhance imaging of vascular tissue or abnormal tissue. Gadolinium is teratogenic in high doses in animal studies, but a number of studies have evaluated the administration of gadolinium contrast material during pregnancy and reported no obvious harmful effects. Administration of gadolinium contrast material in the first trimester should therefore be avoided where possible. In practice, contrast material is of limited usefulness in most obstetric applications and would more likely be required for an extra-abdominal indication such as a suspected maternal brain tumor. In such a situation, the maternal benefits would probably outweigh the potential fetal risks. The only obstetric indication for gadolinium contrast material is the evaluation of placenta accreta, usually in late pregnancy. There is no requirement to cease breastfeeding

Table 21.3 Estimated radiation dose to the fetus in several examples of radiation therapy

	Sarcoma left tibia	Glioblastoma–brain	Hodgkins disease – mantle radiation
Timing of treatment (weeks gestation)	25-30	13-19	34-40
Dose to unshielded fetus (mGy)	15	25	60
Dose to shielded fetus (mGy)	N/A	13	20

N/A – not available.

following the administration of gadolinium to the lactating woman.

RISKS OF DIAGNOSTIC RADIATION IN PREGNANCY

Experimental assessment of radiation effects has identified six specific areas of potential concern to the pregnant woman and her fetus (Table 21.4).

1. Lethality
2. Genetic damage
3. Teratogenicity
4. Growth impairment
5. Oncogenicity
6. Sterility

Radiation effects may be classified as either deterministic or stochastic. Cell killing leading to fetal death, gross malformation, developmental abnormalities or growth retardation is a *deterministic* event, i.e. there is a threshold dose below which no effect is seen and the higher the dose the greater the effect. In comparison, malignancy and hereditary abnormalities are *stochastic* effects, i.e. the absorbed dose influences the probability but not the severity of the effect.

The effects of radiation exposure in pregnancy depend on the time of exposure as well as the fetal absorbed dose. Until the placenta implants, the cells of the conceptus are hypoxic and therefore less radiosensitive. In the very early embryo, the effect of radiation is more likely to be failure to implant or undetectable death of the embryo.

Lethality

The effects of radiation upon abortion and stillbirth rates have been examined in a number of groups. There was no increase in the fetal death rate following nuclear explosions in Japan or following the nuclear accident at Chernobyl. Similarly, exposures to high levels of background radiation or to diagnostic radiation have not been associated with an increase in embryo death rates. In fact, low radiation exposure in utero (estimated 10-50 mGy) has been associated with an increased fertility rate of 10-15%. Animal studies do suggest that massive radiation exposure is associated with cell death although this has not been demonstrated in humans.

Genetic damage

The risk of developing genetic disease in future generations after irradiation with a dose of 10 mGy has been estimated between 0.012 and 0.099%. This compares with the risk of detecting chromosomal damage in a 35-year old woman of 2.26%. Although small changes in the rate of chromosomal damage are impossible to estimate, no radiation-induced transmissible gene mutations have ever been demonstrated in humans. The Japanese bomb survivors and inhabitants of areas with high background radiation have shown no significant excess of known genetic disorders.

Teratogenicity and growth impairment

There is no evidence in either humans or animals that radiation exposure in the diagnostic ranges (i.e. < 50 mGy) is associated with an increased incidence of any significant congenital malformation. In terms of the teratogenic effect of radiation, animal data provide information that may be reasonably transferable to humans. In animals, radiation at levels far in excess of those associated with diagnostic X-rays was associated with failure of implantation, abortion, growth restriction and central nervous system (CNS) effects. A number of human embryos irradiated with more than 500 mGy during the first trimester have shown evidence of CNS malformation (microcephaly), intra-

Table 21.4 Estimated threshold and median radiation dose associated with adverse effects from radiation

	Threshold	Median Dose	Gestational sensitivity (weeks)
Lethality	50-500 mGy	1000 mGy	Pre-implantation
Teratogenicity	50-250 mGy	1000 mGy	First trimester
Mental retardation	300-900 mGy	25-30 IQ pts/1000 mGy	Greatest 10-17, also 18-27
Growth impairment	250-500 mGy	N/A	All
Cancer	Probably nil	EAR* 6%/1000 mGy	All, ?greatest in first trimester
Genetic damage	N/A	1000 mGy	N/A
Sterility	N/A	1000 mGy	Throughout

*EAR = excess absolute risk.

uterine growth restriction and some skeletal anomalies. Following the massive radiation exposure of fetuses (3-17 weeks' gestation) in Hiroshima in 1945, there was an increased incidence of small head size and mental retardation, which may have been a specific response to 'fission neutron' exposure. Similar outcomes have not been reported following the accident at Chernobyl. The most recent review by the International Commission for Radiation Protection states that with regard to fetal malformation, CNS damage and death, 'a threshold of 100-200 mGy or higher' exists for all gestations. This is well in excess of the fetal absorbed doses associated with most diagnostic imaging.

Oncogenicity

A large number of epidemiological studies have been performed to assess the possible effects of prenatal radiation on the incidence of malignant disease. All are flawed by problems such as retrospective design, small study size, inadequate or inappropriate case and control selection, and variability in the determination of radiation exposure and measurement of outcome parameters. The studies in which prenatal radiation exposure has been associated with an increased incidence of malignancy have found a relative risk ratio (RR) for all cancers of between 1.5 and 2.4. However, a number of other studies have failed to establish any statistically significant association between prenatal exposure to radiation and childhood malignancy. At least part of the increased risk associated with irradiation could be accounted for by the fact that mothers with a higher incidence of illness during pregnancy (a susceptibility that might be associated with an increased risk of tumor in their offspring) had a greater incidence of exposure to diagnostic radiation. Taking into account this factor, the RR for cancer mortality in their children was reduced from 1.9 to 1.4. In their most recent review, Wakeford and Little (2002) concluded 'the reality of the statistical association between childhood cancer and antenatal X-ray exposure is not doubted but its explanation remains contentious.'

The largest study in this area remains the case-control study of Stewart et al now known as the Oxford Survey of Childhood Cancer (OSCC). Radiation exposure data both in utero and in childhood were obtained by patient recall although subsequent assessment of the medical records demonstrated the relative accuracy of this method. From this study, the relative risk for leukemia prior to the age of 10 was 1.92 [95% Confidence Interval 1.12, 3.28] for women

having abdominal radiation and 1.19 [0.63, 2.16] for non-abdominal X-ray examinations. For all malignant disease the corresponding relative risks were 2.28 [1.31, 3.97] and 1.15 [0.68, 1.94]. In 1962, MacMahon et al reported similar findings in their case control study performed in the USA using chart review to determine the radiation exposure in utero.

Most of the studies in which a significant risk of oncogenicity was found failed to establish an association between the dose of radiation and the oncogenic effects. The exception was again the OSCC which interpolated a linear relationship between dose of radiation and excess risk of malignancy. At a dose of 'one film', the estimated excess risk was approximately 0.3 (0.1, 0.6), rising to 1.0 (0.5, 3.0) with a dose of five films, an excess relative risk of 0.194 per film. The very crude measurement of dose based on numbers of films and the very large confidence intervals of these results must cast some doubt on their assumptions. In a large study by MacMahon, no significant association between radiation dose and cancer mortality was detected. However, there is some circumstantial evidence that improvement in radiographic techniques and reductions in radiation doses since the 1950s have been associated with a decreasing incidence of cancer deaths amongst children. However, these data do not indicate whether this association is causal. Against the proposition are the results from Hiroshima, the lack of specificity of the malignancies experienced and the data from a number of case control and twin studies.

The children exposed in utero in Hiroshima and Nagasaki have not experienced any corresponding excess incidence of cancer. The average dose received by these 1253 children was just over 300 mGy and two cases of childhood cancer (not leukemia) were observed versus none in the control group. This equates to an Excess Absolute Risk (EAR) coefficient of 0.7% [-0.12, 2.6] compared with the same measure derived from the OSCC data of 8.04% [4.42, 11.99]. More recently, following the nuclear accident at Chernobyl in 1986, there has been no detectable increase in childhood malignancy according to the International Advisory Committee set up to assess the radiological consequences of this disaster.

Dividing cells are more sensitive to injury from radiation than other cells and therefore it might be postulated that the rapidly growing fetus might be particularly susceptible to radiation, particularly in the first trimester. In general, the highest radiation exposures were in women in early pregnancy, before confirmation of the pregnancy. Although the studies of both MacMahon and Stewart suggest an increased risk at these times, the small numbers involved do not allow a statistically significant risk ratio to be determined. Court Brown also noted that amongst the offspring of the 750 pregnant women identified as having been irradiated in the first trimester, there were no cases of leukemia with an average follow-up period of 6 years.

The increase in total malignancy associated with radiation is in contrast to the effects of postnatal radiation in which there has been a specific association with leukemia. The excess risk per Gy is also much greater for in utero exposure, predominantly third trimester, than for childhood exposure. In the studies by Stewart and MacMahon, there was no excess risk of leukemia (compared to other malignancies) although in another study such an increased risk was found. Diamond et al concluded that the relative risk of leukemia amongst white children was increased in fetuses exposed to radiation compared with non-exposed controls. This statement was based on an incidence of 10 cases of leukemia amongst approximately 30 000 children; 6 cases in the exposed group and 4 in the control group. There was no excess of leukemia deaths amongst black children in the same study. They postulated that this may reflect either differences in the selection of subjects amongst the white group or possibly some difference in the susceptibility to radiation damage amongst white and black fetuses. Kaplan found a significantly increased risk of leukemia when radiation exposed children were compared with their non-exposed siblings but not when compared with a control group derived from their playmates. Harvey et al reported the converse in a study of twins in which the relative risk ratio of solid cancers was greater than that for leukemia. Hopton identified two important diagnostic subgroups with a significantly high incidence of in utero radiation exposure: children dying of leukemia aged less than 2 years (RR 4.96 [95% confidence intervals 1.39, 17.7]) and cases of the rare tumor, histiocytosis X (RR 6.2 [1.89, 19.99]). This was not confirmed in the studies by Bithell or MacMahon. Stewart also noted an exceptional risk of teratoma in children of 12 women exposed to greater than '7 films'.

Most cohort studies have failed to detect an association between radiation exposure in utero and malignancy. More recently, two European case-control studies with database ascertainment of cancer cases and comprising a total of 3289 case-control pairs have failed to demonstrate any association between recalled radiation exposure in pregnancy and risk of childhood malignancy. This compares with 15 276 case-control pairs in the most recent OSCC.

Diagnostic imaging in pregnancy

For practical purposes, no specific counseling is required for women undergoing diagnostic imaging with a predicted fetal absorbed dose of less than 10 mGy. This includes all X-ray and CT scanning not involving the abdomen. For direct exposures or nuclear scanning with a potential exposure > 10 mGy, the women should be counseled on a risk/benefit basis. The specific risk appears to be childhood malignancy, but, as described above, for each 10 mGy exposure, theoretical projections suggest a maximum risk of 1 additional cancer death per 1700 exposures. This must be balanced against the benefit of the imaging or treatment in terms of management of the maternal condition. Typical examples include ureteric obstruction requiring an intravenous pyelogram (IVP) or contrast CT, trauma to the abdomen or malignancy.

In general, the clinician ordering the imaging should be responsible for counseling the patient and obtaining informed consent in consultation with the radiologist or nuclear physician. There are no diagnostic imaging procedures that can be considered a risk factor for genetic damage, malformation or neurodevelopmental effects based on current knowledge. It is particularly important to liaise with the radiologist or nuclear physician to ensure the most appropriate imaging is performed to obtain maximal information with minimal fetal absorbed dose. If possible, diagnostic imaging should be delayed until after delivery if the information is not likely to alter immediate management.

CONCLUSION

In summary, although there are some inconsistencies in these studies, they suggest that diagnostic imaging of the abdomen/pelvis (but not other sites) with fetal exposure is associated with a small but recognizable increased risk of malignancy, which is probably dose related. The National Radiological Protection Board has adopted an excess absolute risk (EAR) coefficient for cancer incidence under 15 years of age following low dose irradiation in utero of 0.006% per mGy compared with a risk of 0.0018% per mGy for a dose received just after birth. This assumes there is no threshold dose below which the risk is not increased. However, in absolute terms, for an individual, this represents an additional 1 excess cancer death per 1700 children exposed in utero to a 10 mGy dose. The risk is equal in the second and third trimesters but may be greater in the first trimester than later in pregnancy.

A summary is given in Box 21.1.

Box 21.1 Precautions and management of radiation exposure

- Minimize all radiation exposure to mother and fetus by selecting the most appropriate imaging modality for the clinical situation.
- Inform the radiologist and radiographer that the patient is pregnant so they may make appropriate provision.
- Obtain accurate estimates of the fetal absorbed dose.
- If the estimated fetal absorbed dose is <10 mGy, no specific counseling is required.
- If direct pelvic or abdominal radiation is considered necessary during pregnancy, the patient should be counseled regarding the benefits and risks of the procedure stressing the very low incidence of complications and the importance of the information to be derived.
- The evidence regarding the value of delaying radiation exposure until after the first trimester is not well substantiated but on theoretical grounds, if such delay will not alter the management, it should be considered.
- Avoid contrast media in pregnancy if possible.
- Ultrasound and MRI remain the safest alternative to ionizing radiation.

Further reading

Brent R L 1999 Utilisation of developmental basic science principles in the evaluation of reproductive risks from pre- and post-conception environmental radiation exposure. Teratology 59:182-204.

Cook JV, Kyrion J 2005 Radiation from CT and Perfusion scanning in pregnancy. British Medical Journal 331

Fry F A 1991 International Chernobyl project. Radiological Protection Bulletin 124:12-18.

Harjulehto T, Aro T, Rita H et al 1989 The accident at Chernobyl and the outcome of pregnancy in Finland. British Medical Journal 298:995-997.

Lowe S A 2004 Diagnostic radiography in pregnancy: risks and reality. Australian and New Zealand Journal of Obstetrics and Gynaecology 44(3):191-196.

Stovall M, Blackwell C R, Cundiff J et al 1995 Fetal dose from radiotherapy with photon beams: report of AAPM Radiation Therapy Committee Task Group No. 36. Medical Physics 22(1):63-82.

Valentin J 2000 Pregnancy and medical radiation. Annals of the ICRP 30(1):1-43.

Valentin J 2002 Biological effects after prenatal irradiation (embryo and fetus). ICRP Publication 90 Approved by the Commission in October 2002. Annals of the ICRP 33(1-2):1-206.

Wakeford R, Little M P 2002 Childhood cancer after low-level intrauterine exposure to radiation. Journal of Radiological Protection 22:A123-A127.

Webb J A W, Thomsen H S, Morcos S K 2005 The use of iodinated and gadolinium contrast media during pregnancy and lactation. European Radiology 15:1234-1240.

Chapter 22

Laboratory values in normal pregnancy

M. Ramsay

SYNOPSIS

Introduction
Hematological values
Inflammatory markers and immunological tests
Biochemical values

INTRODUCTION

Major changes in maternal physiological and metabolic processes occur in pregnancy, as a response to orchestrated hormonal changes. As a result, laboratory measurements can be profoundly different in pregnancy and may further change as gestation advances. An accurate knowledge of normal laboratory values during pregnancy and the puerperium is essential to allow correct diagnosis of new disease states and to follow the course of a chronic disease, recognizing where changing values are 'normal' as opposed to indicating deterioration of health.

Information about laboratory values in pregnancy has been derived from either longitudinal studies of a cohort of healthy women studied at intervals during pregnancy and the puerperium, or from cross-sectional studies where single samples are taken from women across the spread of gestation. Longitudinal studies are ideally suited to understanding changes in laboratory values as gestation advances; cross-sectional studies are better at defining the extremes of normal ranges in a healthy population. It is important also to appreciate that different laboratories may use different assays or analysis techniques, so their quoted 'adult normal ranges' may differ. Thus, an important principle is to know whether the pregnancy normal ranges are equivalent to, higher or lower than standard adult ranges.

HEMATOLOGICAL VALUES

Full blood count

Hemoglobin values decrease in the first trimester of pregnancy, whether or not iron and folate supplements have been given. Typical mean values of 12 g dL^{-1} are found. Late pregnancy values are influenced by hematinic supplementation; one study found mean (±SD) hemoglobin values at 36 weeks of 11.07 (±0.84) g dL^{-1} in women who did not have supplements and 12.66 (±0.81) g dL^{-1} in those who had received supplements from the start of the second trimester.

Total white cell count is increased in pregnancy, with particularly high values in the late third trimester and early puerperium. Typical ranges are 6-16 and 9-25 × 10^9 L^{-1}, respectively. The main increase is in neutrophil count, with lymphocytes, monocytes, eosinophils and basophils remaining within typical adult ranges throughout gestation. Immature granulocytes are often found in peripheral blood smears during pregnancy. Even by 6-8 weeks following delivery, white cell counts remain elevated.

Platelet count has been shown to decrease through the third trimester of healthy pregnancies and this is attributed to excessive destruction of platelets. In a study of 6770 women in late pregnancy, the 50th and 2.5th centile counts were 213 and 116 × 10^9 L^{-1}, respectively. The younger platelets have larger mean volumes. Platelet count increases following delivery, reaching peak values 6-14 days postpartum; these changes are particularly marked in women who have had pre-eclampsia.

Hematinics

Iron stores, as judged by serum ferritin, become depleted during pregnancy, even in women given iron supplements. In the late third trimester, one study found mean values of 13 mg L^{-1} in women not receiving iron supplements and 41 mg L^{-1} in those who were. Ferritin levels return to normal by 8 weeks following delivery.

Serum folate levels decrease as gestation advances, but remain within adult normal ranges. Red cell folate levels depend on diet and folate supplements, but generally are a little higher during than outside pregnancy. Red cell folate is lower in women who smoke. By 6 weeks post partum, red cell folate levels are close to normal adult ranges, but serum folate levels can remain low for up to 6 months, especially in lactating women.

Plasma homocysteine values are significantly lower throughout pregnancy and further suppressed in women taking folate supplements. One study found the 5th and 95th centiles during pregnancy to be approximately 5 and 20 micromol L^{-1}, compared to 7 and 38 micromol L^{-1} at 6 weeks postpartum.

Vitamin B_{12} levels are approximately 100 pmol L^{-1} lower in pregnancy than in the non-pregnant state. Levels are back to normal by 6 weeks postpartum. There is no evidence that low vitamin B_{12} found in pregnancy is a deficiency state, since women with normal ferritin but low B_{12} levels have normal hemoglobin and red cell counts.

Coagulation tests

Major changes occur during pregnancy in several coagulation factors, naturally occurring anticoagulants and fibrinolytic factors. Pregnancy is a hypercoagulable state, evidenced firstly by relatively shorter clotting times, compared to control plasma, for the intrinsic, extrinsic and common pathways in a standard coagulation screen. Specific clotting factors are increased (VII, VIII, X and fibrinogen) due to increased production in the liver. Typical fibrinogen levels in the third trimester are 3-6 g L^{-1}. The natural anticoagulant protein S is found at progressively lower levels during pregnancy. Accurate diagnosis of protein S deficiency usually requires repeat estimation 6-12 weeks postpartum. Protein C levels do not change significantly during pregnancy. Antithrombin levels are low during labor and pre-eclampsia, but return to normal by 1 week postpartum. Fibrinolytic activity is suppressed during pregnancy. Fibrin degradation products and D-dimers are elevated in late normal pregnancy. In one study looking at D-dimers, in a laboratory whose reference range in non-pregnant women was < 0.5 mg L^{-1}, 34 out of 35 healthy women had D-dimer levels of ≥ 0.5 mg L^{-1} at term. This indicates that clot formation and destruction is an active process in pregnancy and limits the usefulness of these tests in the diagnosis of venous thromboembolism.

INFLAMMATORY MARKERS AND IMMUNOLOGICAL TESTS

Erythrocyte sedimentation rate (ESR) is high in pregnancy, due to elevated plasma fibrinogen and other globulins. It may exceed 30 mm in the first hour and thus has limited usefulness as a marker of inflammation. C-reactive protein levels have been shown to remain unchanged during healthy pregnancies, so elevated values are useful in the diagnosis of inflammatory states. However, C-reactive protein levels may be transiently elevated in the few hours following delivery. Complement factors C3 and C4 are significantly elevated in the third trimesters of pregnancy. There are no longitudinal studies of C3 degradation products; cross-sectional studies have found either normal or elevated values during pregnancy. Circulating immune complexes are low in pregnancy.

BIOCHEMICAL VALUES

Renal function

Changes in renal function are found in pregnancy, as a consequence of the increase in renal blood flow and glomerular filtration, which are approximately 50% above non-pregnant values by the end of the first trimester. The most marked changes are in 24-h creatinine clearance, which increases from a typical range of 80-100 mL min^{-1} in non-pregnant women to values of 130-150 mL min^{-1} in the late second trimester. Longitudinal studies have shown there is a normal slight decline in creatinine clearance measurements in the late third trimester. Plasma urea and creatinine levels are lower during pregnancy; typical upper ranges of normal are approximately 3.5 mmol L^{-1} for urea and 70 µmol L^{-1} for creatinine in the third trimester. Serum osmolality is found to be approximately 280 m/s mol kg^{-1} even early in the first trimester, compared with typical non-pregnant values of 290 m/s mol kg^{-1}. Serum sodium, potassium and chloride values do not change significantly during pregnancy, but bicarbonate and phosphate values decrease.

Glycosuria is common in healthy women during pregnancy and does not relate to elevated plasma glucose levels. Total urinary protein and albumin excretion are increased after 20 weeks gestation, with generally accepted upper limits of normal as 300 mg and 20 mg per 24 h, respectively. Protein : creatinine ratio (PCR) measurements on spot urine tests have been shown to correlate well with total protein estimates in 24-h urine samples. A threshold of 30 mg protein per mmol creatinine is strongly predictive of ≥ 300 mg 24 h^{-1} proteinuria. The 95% reference range for urinary albumin : creatinine (ACR) ratio on an early morning urine in healthy pregnancy is 1-2 mg albumin per mmol creatinine, with a small rise towards term. With automated PCR and ACR desktop assays available, it is now possible to diagnose significant proteinuria more rapidly and precisely. Aminoaciduria has also been reported to increase during pregnancy.

Liver enzymes and function

Large cross-sectional studies of liver enzymes in healthy pregnancies have demonstrated lower normal ranges for gamma glutamyl transferase (GGT), aspartate transaminase (AST) and alanine transaminase (ALT) than in the general adult population. Typically, the upper limit of the pregnancy range for GGT, AST and ALT is approximately 80% of that found outside pregnancy. After delivery, especially after Cesarean section, these liver enzymes are elevated for a few days at most. Alkaline phosphatase levels are often doubled in pregnancy, due to production of placental isoenzymes. Bilirubin levels remain within normal adult reference ranges throughout pregnancy and the puerperium.

Total serum protein and albumin concentrations are decreased in pregnancy, leading to a decrease in colloid osmotic pressure. There are no significant changes in serum immunoglobulin levels during pregnancy.

Serum copper levels are increased in pregnancy and serum zinc decreased, as compared to nonpregnant values.

Commercial assays for bile acids measure total levels of the four main bile acids (cholic, deoxycholic, chenodeoxycholic and lithocholic acids) and their taurine and glycine conjugates. Studies of individual bile acids show that chenodeoxycholic acid levels almost double during pregnancy, but the other bile acids have stable levels. The upper limit of the adult normal range is quoted as 5 micromol L^{-1}, but a pragmatic 'abnormal' limit is set as > 13 micromol L^{-1} during pregnancy. This level has been identified as differentiating women with obstetric cholestasis from those without the condition although other hepatic disorders also may provoke an increase in serum levels of bile acids.

Fasting plasma triglyceride levels increase approximately threefold during pregnancy and plasma cholesterol levels double. These changes happen gradually during gestation, reaching maximal values at term. Lipid levels decrease soon after delivery, but are still higher at 6 weeks postpartum than in the normal nonpregnant state. Lipid levels are not affected by lactation.

Carbohydrate metabolism

Fasting plasma glucose levels are lower in pregnancy. These changes are apparent by the end of the first trimester and there is continued decline in most women through the second and third trimesters, with typical mean values of ≤ 4 mmol L^{-1}. In response to a known glucose load, the rise in plasma glucose measured at 1, 2 or 3 hours is exaggerated as pregnancy advances. The diagnosis of gestational diabetes requires demonstration of an abnormal glucose tolerance test (GTT). There is no international agreement about the upper limits of normal for the GTT in pregnancy (see Ch. 5 Gestational diabetes) and each practitioner should be familiar with national accepted normal limits. Serum fructosamine and glycosylated hemoglobin are generally found to be lower in the second and third trimesters than in the nonpregnant state; however, the precise normal ranges depend on individual laboratories.

Thyroid function

Serum total thyroxine (T$_4$), tri-iodothyronine (T$_3$) and thyroid binding globulin are elevated during pregnancy. However, the free levels of T$_4$ and T$_3$ are decreased and lie within the lower part of the normal adult reference ranges throughout pregnancy. Thyroid stimulating hormone (TSH) levels may be low towards the end of the first trimester, but thereafter levels increase, remaining within the normal adult reference ranges.

Adrenal function

Studies of glucocorticoid function in pregnancy are confusing, due to the assortment of different tests available, instability of substances being measured and circadian rhythms. All measures of cortisol (total, bound and free levels) are elevated in pregnancy. Normal diurnal patterns are maintained, with highest values at 08:00 h, lowest values at midnight. The cortisol response to an adrenocorticotrophic hormone (ACTH) challenge is unchanged in pregnancy. Cortisol levels suppress in a normal fashion following the administration of oral dexamethasone.

Plasma epinephrine and norepinephrine levels show very little change during pregnancy from non-pregnant values. There are diurnal changes with lowest levels of these catecholamines at night. No specific studies of urinary vanillylmandelic acid (VMA) or urinary catecholamines have been reported during pregnancy, but they are likely to be within the normal adult range and should be used to interrogate the possibility of pheochromocytoma.

Prolactin

There is a wide normal range for prolactin values in late pregnancy. The 10th and 90th centiles in one study were 55-180 microgram L^{-1} in the late third trimester, reflecting a 10- to 20-fold increase during pregnancy. Prolactin levels have a diurnal pattern, with highest values at night. Prolactin levels decrease markedly during labor, but there is a rapid rise in levels in the two hours following delivery, except in women who have elective Cesarean deliveries. Prolactin levels remain elevated in women who breast feed, but otherwise return to normal values by 3 weeks postpartum.

Calcium metabolism

Ionized calcium levels remain constant during pregnancy, although total calcium decreases, in line with lower serum albumin. Parathyroid hormone levels are low in pregnancy and reach their lowest values in the middle trimester (< 10 ng L^{-1}). Typical values measured 6 weeks after delivery are approximately 25 ng L^{-1}. Calcitonin levels do not change during pregnancy. Levels of 1,25-dihydroxyvitamin D rise during gestation and are significantly higher than during the puerperium. Typical values are 70 ng L^{-1} in early pregnancy, 100-150 ng L^{-1} in second and third trimesters, <60 ng L^{-1} in the puerperium.

Box 22.1 Key points

- Recognize that the physiological changes of pregnancy cause changes in common laboratory values.
- Interpret laboratory values from known pregnancy-derived ranges, not just from adult normal ranges.
- Remember that values can change with advancing gestation, during labor or in the puerperium; some values are affected by mode of delivery or lactation status.
- If in doubt, look up pregnancy-specific reference graphs or tables.

Further reading

Aune B, Gjesdal K, Oian P 1999 Late onset postpartum thrombocytosis in preeclampsia. Acta Obstetricia et Gynecologica Scandinavia 78:866-870.

Biswas S, Rodeck C H 1976 Plasma prolactin levels during pregnancy. British Journal of Obstetrics and Gynaecology 83:683-687.

Boehlen F, Hohfeld P, Extermann et al 2000 Platelet count at term pregnancy: a reappraisal of the threshold. Obstetrics and Gynecology 95:29-33.

Cikot R J L M, Steegers-Theunissen R P M, Thomas C M G et al 2001 Longitudinal vitamin and homocysteine levels in normal pregnancy. British Journal of Nutrition 85:49-58.

Davison J M, Dunlop W 1980 Renal haemodynamics and tubular function in normal human pregnancy. Kidney International 18:152-161.

Edelstam G, Lowbeer C, Kral G et al 2001 New reference ranges for routine blood samples and human neutrophilic lipocalin during third trimester pregnancy. Scandinavian Journal of Clinical Laboratory Investigation 61:583-592.

Fenton V, Cavill I, Fisher J 1977 Iron stores in pregnancy. British Journal of Haematology 37:45-149.

Forest J-C, Garrido-Russo M, Lemay A et al 1983 Reference values for the oral glucose tolerance test at each trimester of pregnancy. American Journal of Clinical Pathology 80:828-831.

Girling J C, Dow E, Smith J H 1997 Liver function tests in pre-eclampsia: importance of comparison with a reference range derived for normal pregnancy. British Journal of Obstetrics and Gynaecology 104: 246-250.

Maybury H, Waugh J 2004 Proteinuria in pregnancy – just what is significant? Fetal and Maternal Medicine Review 16:71-95.

Pitkin R M, Reynolds W A, Williams G A et al 1979 Calcium metabolism in normal pregnancy: a longitudinal study. American Journal of Obstetrics and Gynecology 133:781-787.

Ramsay M M, James D K, Steer P J et al 2000 Normal values in pregnancy, 2nd edn. Saunders, London, p 16-55.

Robertson E G, Cheyne G A 1972 Plasma biochemistry in relation to the oedema of pregnancy. Journal of Obstetrics and Gynaecology of the British Commonwealth 79:769-776.

Seki K, Makimura N, Mitsui C et al 1991 Calcium-regulating hormones and osteocalcin levels during pregnancy: a longitudinal study. American Journal of Obstetrics and Gynecology 164: 1248-1252.

Stirling Y, Woolf L, North W R S et al 1984 Haemostasis in normal pregnancy. Thrombosis and Haemostasis (Stuttgart) 52:176-182.

Taylor D J, Lind T 1979 Red cell mass during and after normal pregnancy. British Journal of Obstetrics and Gynaecology 86:364-370.

Index